PHYTOPATHOGENIC PROKARYOTES

Volume 2

Contributors

Anne J. Anderson
J. W. Brewer
T. A. Chen
E. L. Civerolo
David L. Coplin
Albert H. Ellingboe
D. W. Fulbright
D. J. Hagedorn
M. D. Harrison
M. J. Holliday
A. L. Jones
Clarence I. Kado
N. T. Keen
Zoltan Klement
George H. Lacy
J. V. Leary
C. H. Liao
Paul F. Lurquin
John L. McIntyre
Donald J. Merlo
Mark S. Mount
Suresh S. Patil
M. C. M. Pérombelon
David A. Rosenberger
Alfred W. Saettler
John P. Sleesman
James R. Venette
Anne K. Vidaver
J. M. Wells

SB731
.P55
v.2

PHYTOPATHOGENIC PROKARYOTES

Edited by

Mark S. Mount
Department of Pathology
University of Massachusetts
Amherst, Massachusetts

George H. Lacy
Department of Plant Pathology and Physiology
Virginia Polytechnic Institute and State University
Blacksburg, Virginia

Volume 2

1982

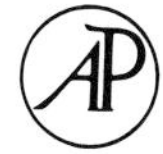

ACADEMIC PRESS

A Subsidiary of Harcourt Brace Jovanovich, Publishers

New York London
Paris San Diego San Francisco São Paulo Sydney Tokyo Toronto

COPYRIGHT © 1982, BY ACADEMIC PRESS, INC.
ALL RIGHTS RESERVED.
NO PART OF THIS PUBLICATION MAY BE REPRODUCED OR TRANSMITTED IN ANY FORM OR BY ANY MEANS, ELECTRONIC OR MECHANICAL, INCLUDING PHOTOCOPY, RECORDING, OR ANY INFORMATION STORAGE AND RETRIEVAL SYSTEM, WITHOUT PERMISSION IN WRITING FROM THE PUBLISHER.

ACADEMIC PRESS, INC.
111 Fifth Avenue, New York, New York 10003

United Kingdom Edition published by
ACADEMIC PRESS, INC. (LONDON) LTD.
24/28 Oval Road, London NW1 7DX

Library of Congress Cataloging in Publication Data
Main entry under title:

Phytopathogenic prokaryotes.

Includes bibliographical references and index.
1. Micro-organisms, Phytopathogenic. 2. Plant diseases. 3. Micro-organisms, Phytopathogenic--Control. 4. Bacteria, Phytopathogenic. 5. Bacterial diseases of plants. 6. Bacteria, Phytopathogenic--Control. I. Mount, Mark S. II. Lacy, George H. [DNLM: 1. Plants--Microbiology. 2. Plant diseases. 3. Prokaryotic cells. 4. Cells. QW 60 P578]
SB731.P55 1982 632'.32 82-13954
ISBN 0-12-509002-1 (v.2)

PRINTED IN THE UNITED STATES OF AMERICA

82 83 84 85 9 8 7 6 5 4 3 2 1

The Editors
Dedicate This Volume to
Their Wives,
Patricia Mount and Ruth Lacy
for
Their Patience, Understanding, and Support

Contents

Contributors

Numbers in parentheses indicate the pages on which the authors' contributions begin.

Anne J. Anderson (119), Department of Biology, Utah State University, Logan, Utah 84322

J. W. Brewer (31), Department of Zoology and Entomology, Colorado State University, Fort Collins, Colorado 80523

T. A. Chen (417), Department of Plant Pathology, Rutgers University, New Brunswick, New Jersey 08930

E. L. Civerolo (343), Fruit Laboratory, Horticultural Science Institute, USDA-ARS, Beltsville, Maryland 20705

David L. Coplin (255), Department of Plant Pathology, Ohio Agricultural Research and Development Center, Wooster, Ohio 44619

Albert H. Ellingboe (103), International Plant Research Institute, San Carlos, California 94070

D. W. Fulbright (229), Department of Botany and Plant Pathology, Michigan State University, East Lansing, Michigan 48824

D. J. Hagedorn (361), Department of Plant Pathology, University of Wisconsin, Madison, Wisconsin 53706

M. D. Harrison (31), Department of Botany and Plant Pathology, Colorado State University, Fort Collins, Colorado 80523

M. J. Holliday (179), Biochemical Department, E. I. DuPont de Nemours, Wilmington, Delaware 19898

A. L. Jones (399), Department of Botany and Plant Pathology, Michigan State University, East Lansing, Michigan 48824

Clarence I. Kado (303), Davis Crown Gall Research Group, Department of Plant Pathology, University of California, Davis, California 95616

N. T. Keen (179), Department of Plant Pathology, University of California, Riverside, California 92521

Zoltan Klement (149), Research Institute for Plant Protection, Budapest, Hungary

George H. Lacy (221), Department of Plant Pathology and Physiology, Virginia Polytechnic Institute and State University, Blacksburg, Virginia 24061

J. V. Leary (229), Department of Plant Pathology, University of California, Riverside, California 92521

C. H. Liao (417), Department of Plant Pathology, Rutgers University, New Brunswick, New Jersey 08930

Paul F. Lurquin (303), Program in Genetics and Cell Biology, Washington State University, Pullman, Washington 99164

John L. McIntyre (137), Syracuse Research Laboratory, Allied Chemicals, Solvay, New York, 13209

Donald J. Merlo (281), AgriGenetics Research Park, Madison, Wisconsin 53716

Mark S. Mount (329), Department of Plant Pathology, University of Massachusetts, Amherst, Massachusetts 01003

Suresh S. Patil (221), Department of Plant Pathology, University of Hawaii, Honolulu, Hawaii 96822

M. C. M. Pérombelon (55), Scottish Crop Research Institute, Invergowerie, Dundee DD2 5DA, Scotland

David A. Rosenberger (71), New York State Agricultural Experiment Station, Hudson Valley Laboratory, Highland, New York 12528

Alfred W. Saettler (329), ARS-USDA, Department of Botany and Plant Pathology, Michigan State University, East Lansing, Michigan 48824

John P. Sleesman (447), Mobay Chemical Corporation, Agricultural Chemicals Division, Howe, Indiana 46746

James R. Venette (3), Department of Plant Pathology, North Dakota State University, Fargo, North Dakota 58105

Anne K. Vidaver (387), Department of Plant Pathology, University of Nebraska, Lincoln, Nebraska 68583

J. M. Wells (417), USDA, Post Harvest Pathology, Department of Plant Pathology, Rutgers University, New Brunswick, New Jersey 08930

Preface

This is the second volume of "Phytopathogenic Prokaryotes" a treatise intended to increase our understanding of these organisms. This two-volume work is a source of information for those interested in current research dealing with interactions among prokaryotes and their hosts. We anticipate that the information, opinions, and speculation contained herein will stimulate new thought and research in this important area of phytopathology.

In the first volume we included chapters on the basic nature of phytopathogenic prokaryotes, how they are classified, how they penetrate into and become established in plants, present hypotheses for the development of pathogenesis and relationships with vectors, interactions of prokaryotes and their hosts in the phylloplane and the rhizosphere, and the mechanisms for pathogenesis.

In this second volume we continue to develop additional concepts of host–pathogen coevolution. Part I concentrates on the movement of pathogens from one host to another. The concepts presented are essential for understanding the epidemiology, and, therefore, the control of diseases caused by prokaryotes. Parts II and III elaborate on the dynamic nature of host–parasite interactions. First, we consider methods by which hosts may evolve to minimize damage caused by their pathogens. Second, we present the mechanisms for rapid genetic change available to the pathogen to counteract host defenses. The ultimate goal of phytopathology is to control plant–prokaryote interactions for the benefit of mankind. The fourth part therefore emphasizes control of diseases caused by prokaryotes. Manipulation of plant–prokaryote interactions to break the disease cycle or minimize losses is discussed in regard to cultural practices, host breeding, biological control, and chemical control. Together both volumes establish new perspectives and stimulate new ideas for the realization of this goal.

In the last part, important aspects of technology needed to study phytopathogenic prokaryotes are included. The culture of fastidious prokaryotic plant pathogens is discussed and preservation techniques are reviewed.

Again, the Editors thank all the contributors to this Treatise for their enthusiasm and scholarship.

Mark S. Mount
George H. Lacy

Miles C. Horton, Sr. Research Center
Salt Pond Mountain
Giles County, Virginia

Contents of Volume 1

Part **I**

Epidemiology and Dispersal

This first section of the treatise deals with how phytopathogenic prokaryotes find their hosts. Controls for diseases caused by these pathogens often depend on limiting their access to plants. Therefore, the chapters included here are important for understanding the biology of plant-associated prokaryotes as well as minimizing economic losses from the diseases they cause. In Chapter 1, J. R. Venette reviews dispersal of bacterial plant pathogens with some emphasis on pseudomonads and xanthomonads causing leaf spots and blights. M. D. Harrison and J. W. Brewer discuss the field dispersal of soft rot bacteria in Chapter 2. The effects of the environment, bacterial populations, and host impairment are related to the distribution of soft rot bacteria, their contamination of host plants, latency, and disease development by M. C. M. Pérombelon in Chapter 3. How fastidious walled and wall-less prokaryotes are transmitted by insects is reviewed by D. A. Rosenberger in Chapter 4.

Chapter **1**

How Bacteria Find Their Hosts

JAMES R. VENETTE

Phytopathogenic Prokaryotes, Vol. 2

Copyright © 1982 by Academic Press, Inc.
All rights of reproduction in any form reserved.
ISBN 0-12-509002-1

I. INTRODUCTION

A. Mechanisms of Transport

This chapter deals with the mechanisms by which bacteria are transmitted from one plant to another. Plant pathogenic bacteria are simple organisms which usually lack spores or other elaborate survival structures and do not have mechanisms for launching themselves into the air as do many fungi. Yet the bacteria are remarkably well adapted to passive transmission by wind-splashed rain, seeds, insects, vegetatively propagated stock, irrigation water, cultural implements, and other agents.

The transmission process is often complex. A review of the Commonwealth Mycological Institute Descriptions of Phytopathogenic Bacteria indicates that of 59 bacteria, 5 have a single mode of transmission and 13 are spread in 5 or more ways.

Cox (1966) has pointed out that dissemination methods are not equally efficient, and that attention to one or two of the primary methods may result in satisfactory disease control. In some instances, variants of a pathogen became better adapted to a mode of transmission once thought minor and thereby escape control (Buddenhagen and Elsasser, 1962).

The dispersal mechanisms are highly dependent on environmental conditions. For example, wind-driven rainsplash may be important in dissemination of leaf blight pathogens in regions of high rainfall and unimportant as a means of disseminating bacteria among plants grown with furrow irrigation in an arid region (Rotem and Palti, 1969; Menzies, 1967). If sprinkler irrigation is used in the arid region, watersplash dissemination may once again become an important agent of dispersal (LeBaron *et al.*, 1976; Schnathorst, 1966).

Many bacteria produce an extracellular capsule or slime which may protect the bacteria from harmful environmental stresses. *En masse*, bacteria and their capsules form a matrix, commonly called ooze or exudate. The matrix readily disassociate in water. Dried exudate may be dispersed as flakes or strands. Moist exudate adheres to passing vectors.

B. Bacteria

This discussion centers on the readily cultured bacteria as presented by Schaad (1980). These bacteria are members of the genera *Xanthomonas, Pseudomonas, Erwinia, Corynebacterium,* and *Agrobacterium.* Other bacteria such as species of *Bacillus, Clostridium,* and *Streptomyces* have been described as pathogens, and some strains of the mutualistic symbionts, *Rhizobium,* could be classified as pathogenic. Dispersal of fastidious vascular tissue-limited bacteria is presented in other chapters.

C. Finding Their Hosts

Plant pathogenic bacteria usually find their hosts by accidental encounter. Actions of phoretic agents dictate successful transmission. However, the process is not random. The specific crops cultivated limit the number of plant species which grow in an area. Therefore, tools for cultivating and insects attracted to that plant species may spread pathogenic inocula in several fields cropped to the same host. If, for instance, contaminated irrigation water is reused, it is likely that it would be reapplied to another field containing the same crop species.

The term "find," meaning seeking the suspect, might also be appropriate for some plant pathogenic bacteria. Many species are mobile and their mobility may assist the bacteria in moving through the soil (Wallace, 1978). Motile bacteria are chemotactically responsive and the chemotaxis may assist the bacteria in locating infection courts (Mulrean and Schroth, 1979; Raymundo and Ries, 1980). While ordinarily motile bacteria cause more infections than nonmotile mutants, motility does not appear to be mandatory for successful host invasion (Napoli and Alberscheim, 1980; Panopoulos and Schroth, 1974). Bacteria from aqueous suspension may adhere to leaf surfaces (Leben and Whitmoyer, 1979; Haas and Rotem, 1976). It is generally accepted that plant pathogenic bacteria do not move more than a few centimeters under their own power.

D. What Is a Host?

Agrios (1978) has defined host as a plant that is invaded by a parasite and from which the parasite obtains its nutrients. Roberts and Boothroyd (1972) have defined host as a living organism from which a parasite derives its sustenance. Bateman (1978) affirms the nutrient-based relationship which designates host–parasite interactions. Unfortunately, most definitions do not adequately reflect the relative nature of the interaction. Relativity is imposed by plant nutrition, age, tissues or organs affected, temperature, and a variety of other factors that limit the compatible association.

Determination of host is generally based on development of symptoms on inoculated plants. Often this is the result of placing a large number of bacterial cells (via wounds, leaf intromission, etc.) in an appropriate infection court. If the plant and pathogen are compatible, characteristic symptoms are manifested and the plant is called a host for that parasitic bacterial species.

Less clear are host–parasite relationships in which visible symptoms are not produced. Some bacterial pathogens survive within apparently healthy tissues as latent endophytes (Hayward, 1974). Certainly the plant is a host, but because these bacteria do not rapidly reproduce and generate symptoms, we may conjecture that the host is not susceptible to disease under those particular conditions. Why such controlled survival is perpetuated is not known.

From an ecological standpoint, an invasive bacterium meets not only the host, but also the dynamic complement of associated microflora and microfauna. Every microorganism present may interact with the pathogen. In complex environments like the soil, probably all of the various symbiotic interactions described by Starr (1975) occur. Also, each of the interactions is mediated by the physical environment surrounding the host plant. In this context, the plant acts as a habitat, and bacteria that successfully establish themselves on or in a plant fill a unique ecological niche. If the ecological principle that no two similar species occupy the same ecological niche (Gause, 1934) applies to bacteria, then we may assume that different bacteria isolated from on or in plant tissue occupy different niches. If niches are filled, introduction of other bacteria may not be possible. However, increasing the numbers of introduced bacteria, such as in tests to establish minimum infection doses, may sufficiently modify the microbial balance to allow the bacterium to become established.

If we consider a host as a plant which provides a habitat supportive of a plant pathogenic bacterial population and recognize that the degree of support may vary from none (e.g., latent infection) to nearly total (e.g., obvious disease symptoms), we avoid the complication of describing survival of pathogens on "nonhost" plants.

II. HOW PLANTS ARE FREED FROM BACTERIA

Both natural and artificial processes disassociate pathogens from their hosts. Bacteria vary in the intimacy of association they maintain with their hosts. Some bacteria such as *Corynebacterium michiganense* pv. *sepedonicum* (Spieckermann & Kotthoff) Dye & Kemp and *Xanthomonas campestris* pv. *phaseoli* (Smith) Dye maintain close association through vegetative and seed-borne transmission. Other bacteria, such as *Ag-*

robacterium tumefaciens (Smith & Townsend) Conn, maintain a more loose association and progeny from infected plants must infect from exogenous sources. Understanding the processes by which plants are freed from their bacterial pathogens is important if we are to apportion relative values to recontamination mechanisms. For example, aerosol transport of bacterial pathogens may be less important in initiating epiphytotics if the pathogen is readily carried in and disseminated from infected seed.

A. Natural

Since genes for resistance to various plant pathogens have been described and used in control programs, we must assume that natural selection operates to free hosts from, at least, some components of the pathogen population. This would constitute a genetic method for freeing some plants from some pathogenic bacteria.

Cultivation of plants in regions where the pathogen cannot readily spread should eventually result in plants and seed free from bacterial contamination. For example, bean (*Phaseolus vulgaris* L.) seed has been grown in arid regions using furrow irrigation to promote plant growth and minimize bacterial spread via watersplash. This program has reduced the amount of seed-borne contamination and has allowed profitable crop production when this seed is used in higher rainfall areas (Butcher *et al.*, 1967; Grogan and Kimble, 1967; Guthrie *et al.*, 1975). Claims that bean seeds were blight-free (Butcher *et al.*, 1969; Guthrie *et al.*, 1975), however, were based on methods not sufficiently sensitive to detect low numbers of bacteria.

Fermentation of tomato (*Lycopersicon esculentum* Mill.) fruits during the seed extraction process eliminates *C. m.* pv. *michiganense* (Smith) Jensen and *Pseudomonas solanacearum* (Smith) Smith (Chester, 1942). Apparently, the fermentation products, acetic and lactic acid, are lethal to the bacteria. Blood (1937) suggested that a soak in acetic acid helped eliminate bacteria.

Selection of vegetative cuttings from noninfected potato (*Solanum tuberosum* L.) plants has effectively eliminated *Erwinia carotovora* subsp. *atroseptica* (van Hall) Dye from plants which serve as source material in potato certification programs (Pérombelon and Kelman, 1980). Shepard and Claflin (1975) point out that meristem culture should similarly be an effective technique to eliminate *Erwinia* and *Corynebacterium* pathogens. However, Rattink and Vruggink (1979) claim that meristem or tissue culture cannot eliminate *X. c.* pv. *begoniae* (Takimoto) Dye from begonia (*Begonia* spp.).

Some plant pathogens do not complete their disease cycles in association with their host plant, nor as saprophytic soil inhabitants. Thus, each new generation of plants must be reinfested. For example, *Erwinia tracheiphila* (Smith) Bergey *et al.*, which causes bacterial wilt of cucurbits, is not seed-borne and thus each new generation of plants is freed from the disease until the spotted cucumber beetle (*Diabrotica undecimpunctata* Oliva.) or the striped cucumber beetle (*D. vittata* Fabr.) reinoculates the plants. If the beetles are not allowed to feed on the cucurbits, then the host has escaped from its pathogen.

B. Chemical and Physical Treatments

Chemical and physical treatments of seeds and vegetative plant parts have been used in attempts to eliminate bacteria. Formaldehyde was used to disinfect tobacco (*Nicotiana tabacum* L.) seed contaminated with *Pseudomonas syringae* pv. *tabaci* (Wolf & Foster) Young *et al.* (Bradbury, 1967), cereal grains infected with pseudomonad and xanthomonad pathogens (Garrard, 1951), and potatoes infected with blackleg pathogens (Morse, 1911). Peroxide has been used to eliminate *X. c.* pv. *citri* (Hasse) Dye from citrus seed (Limber and Frink, 1953).

Ark and Alcorn (1956), Leben and Keitt (1954), Dekker (1963), Sharvelle (1979), Thirumalachar (1979), and others have reviewed the use of antibiotics as disinfectants. Reports that streptomycin formulations could cure infected plants or significantly reduce bacterial contamination are frequent (Hildreth, 1969; Humaydan *et al.*, 1980; Keyworth and Howell, 1961; Stoddard, 1957; Taylor, 1973; Thirumalachar, 1979; Thomas, 1959, etc.). However, these reports should be viewed with caution because techniques sufficiently sensitive to detect low populations of bacteria were often not available. In many cases the reports on effectiveness of an antibiotic have engendered little commercial application. The unavailability of effective bactericides has caused concern among phytobacteriologists who have called for a national cooperative effort toward their development (see Jones, this volume, Chapter 19).

Heat treatments have been recommended for control of *X. c.* pv. *oryzae* (Ishiyama) Dye on rice (*Oryzae sativa* L.) (Sinha and Nene, 1967), and *X. campestris* pv. *incanae* (Kendrick & Baker) Dye on stock (Garrard, 1951). Hot water seed treatment has been used to control *X. c.* pv. *campestris* (Pammel) Dowson on crucifer seed (Clayton, 1925; Walker, 1924) and recent recommendations combine heat and chemical treatment (Schaad *et al.*, 1980). While heat may provide practical control, it does not completely eliminate the pathogen (Srinivasan *et al.*, 1973), nor is it equally effective on all lines of crucifer seed (Clayton,

1925). Ralph (1977) failed to eliminate bacteria from infected bean seeds and trash using aerated steam at 55 and 60°C and suggested that thermal resistance may be widespread among bacterial plant pathogens.

Crosse (1971) has reviewed the use of chemicals as seed treatments. Until recently mercury compounds were the most frequently recommended. Other materials were copper, quaternary ammonium compounds, sodium hypochlorite, malachite green, phenacridane chloride, acids, and antibiotics. Seed treatments are most effective against surface-borne contaminants, and in many cases provided practical control. Seldom are bacteria completely eliminated from all treated seeds. Similarly, bacteria are not easily eliminated from vegetative planting material.

C. Movement of Variant Strains

In many cases the problem is not that the bacteria are disassociated from their hosts, but rather a variant strain of a bacterial pathogen becomes distributed among a population of hosts. If the success of bacterial pathogens is based on the numbers of individuals which can be generated in a short time (Agrios, 1978), it is the variability of the individuals within that population which ensures that success. Species of plant pathogens have been recognized as variable in their ability to multiply in their host (Halluka *et al.*, 1978), colony size and aggressiveness (Kidby *et al.*, 1977; Rao and Devadath, 1978), color of colonies (Okimoto and Furuta, 1977), serological response (DeBoer *et al.*, 1979), virulence (Reddy and Kauffman, 1978; Sands *et al.*, 1978; Schuster *et al.*, 1975; Thakur *et al.*, 1978), ability to attack different plant parts (Hill *et al.*, 1972; Mew, 1978; Vallardes-Sanchez *et al.*, 1979), temperature sensitivity (Chamberlain, 1952; Skirvin *et al.*, 1978), phage sensitivity (Mathew and Patel, 1979; Persley and Crosse, 1978), bacteriocin, plasmid, and pectolytic diversity (Gonzalez and Vidavor, 1979), symptom expression (Barakat, 1979; Chamberlain, 1952; Cunfer *et al.*, 1979), as well as recognized differences in biochemical requirements and physiological responses.

Stable characteristics are used to categorize variant strains at the subspecific level. For example, *Erwinia carotovora* (Jones) Bergey *et al.* strains which do not grow at 37°C, form reducing sugars from sucrose, and utilize α-methyl glucoside are called subsp. *atroseptica*. Similarly, variants of *X. c.* pv. *phaseoli* which produce a soluble dark pigment on nutrient agar are called *X. c.* pv. *phaseoli* var. *fuscans* (Burkholder) Starr & Burkholder. Whether or not these characteristics have adaptive value in nature remains unknown.

Adaptive variation is better recognized when cultivars of a crop are differentially attacked by variants of a pathogen. Generally these variants are designated races although other epithets such as "pathogen group" (Horino, 1978), varieties, pathovars, and *forma specialis* have been used. Horino (1978) categorizes *X. c.* pv. *oryzae* into five pathogen groups based on reactions to four rice differentials. At last report 17 races of *X. c.* pv. *malvacearum* (Smith) Dye had been characterized (Brinkerhoff, 1970). Crosse *et al.* (1966) described seven races of *P. s.* pv. *glycinea* (Coerper) Young *et al.* and Thomas and Leary (1980) recently added an eighth. *Pseudomonas syringae* pv. *phaseolicola* (Burkholder) Dye is separated into two races based on reaction on red Mexican kidney bean (Walker and Patel, 1964). Buddenhagen *et al.* (1962) separated *P. solanacearum* into three races based primarily on host range. Variants of *P. solanacearum* perhaps best exemplify movement of adaptive variants into the host population. Buddenhagen (1965) described how a variant designated SFR, which caused copious ooze on banana *Musa paradisiaca* subsp. (L.) Kuntze inflorescenses, was readily transported by insects (Buddenhagen and Elsasser, 1962) and was rapidly transported over a wide geographic area. Native strains from wild *Heliconia* spp. that were designated "D" strains were poorly transmitted and were not aggressive on slow growing bananas. Culturing bananas near *Heliconia* spp. allowed selection of a variant strain "B" which spread among bananas via root connections.

Selective pressure exerted by cultural practices may also influence pathogen spread. Variants of *Erwinia amylovora* (Burrill) Winslow *et al.* resistant to streptomycin became widely dispersed in orchards on the west coast of the United States where minimal doses of the antibiotic had previously effected control (Schroth *et al.*, 1974).

Variation and selection lead to the development of gamodemes which are localized populations sharing a common gene pool and filling an ecological niche (Briggs and Walters, 1969). This phenomenon causes some question about the value of designating races.

III. BACTERIA IN THE GROWING MILIEU

A. Soil

Buddenhagen (1965) described soil-borne bacteria as transient visitors, resident visitors, and residents. Transient visitors have no population increase and rapid population decline in soil. Populations of resident visitors, such as soft rotting *Erwinias,* decline gradually, or they increase depending on hosts. Residents such as soft-rotting pseudomonads and *Bacillus* spp. maintain their populations in the soil. Schuster and Coyne (1974) claimed most foliar bacterial pathogens survive in soil as transient visitors. A great number of bacterial pathogens would be so classified including *X. c.* pv. *malvacearum* (Brinkerhoff and Fink, 1964), *X. c.* pv. *phaseoli* (Sabet and Ishag, 1969), *X. c.* pv. *vesicatoria* (Doidge) Dye (Peterson, 1963), *E. stewartii* (Smith) Dye (Ivanoff, 1933; Pepper, 1967), *Corynebacterium nebraskense* (Schuster *et al.*) Vidaver & Mandel (Schuster *et al.*, 1973), *P. syringae* pv. *syringae* van Hall (Hoitink *et al.*, 1968), *P. s.* pv. *glycinea* (Graham, 1953), *X. c.* pv. *phaseoli* var. *sojense* (Hedges) Starr & Burkholder (Fett, 1979), and *X. c.* pv. *oryzae* (Hsieh and Buddenhagen, 1975).

Most foliar pathogens do not survive well if they are dissociated from plant tissues. For example, *X. c.* pv. *campestris* survives less than 2 weeks in soil in late summer (Schaad and White, 1974) with a half life of 4 days; *E. rubrifaciens* Wilson *et al.* from dripping walnut (*Jugland regia* L.) trees survived no more than 4 months in semitropical winter soil (Schaad and Wilson, 1970), and *X. c.* pv. *translucens* (Jones *et al.*) Dye did not survive long in nonsterile soil (Boosalis, 1952).

Because the pathogen does not survive long periods in soil does not automatically dismiss this phase as being unimportant in epidemiology of the pathogens. It is possible that rain-splashed, bacteria-laden soil particles may disseminate the pathogen (Manns, 1909) or may dry on foliage and offer protection to the pathogens.

Menzies (1963) pointed out that organic plant debris tends to favor survival of soil pathogens with saprophytic activity. For example, *X. c.* pv. *malvacearum* was recovered from 6-, 7-, and 17-year-old dried cotton (*Gossypium hirsutum* L.) plants (Ark, 1958; Schnathorst, 1964, 1969).

In the field, such long-term survival may not be possible. In fact, most researchers are more interested in the ability of the pathogen to survive from one growing period to the next and serve as primary inoculum. Contaminated plant debris serves as an overwintering mechanism for many pathogens and survival is increased if these debris remain on the surface rather than being buried deep in the soil. Generally, the bacterial populations decline rapidly as the organic residue decomposes, and deep burial provides the moisture, temperature, and other conditions which hasten decomposition. *Xanthomonas campestris* pv. *malvacearum* survived 40–107 days until the supporting cotton debris was thoroughly decomposed (Brinkerhoff and Fink, 1964). Decomposition of the cotton took twice as long at winter temperatures than it did at greenhouse temperatures. In India, *X. c.* pv. *malvacearum* survived 6 months on the soil surface and only 3 months when the cotton debris was buried 15 cm (Verma *et al.*, 1978). Bacterial pathogens of beans overwinter better on the soil surface than buried 20 cm (Schuster 1967, 1970; Schuster *et al.*, 1965). In the dry season, in the Sudan, *X. c.* pv. *phaseoli* survives in dried debris (Sabet and Ishag, 1969). Natti (1967), Schuster (1967), and Schuster *et al.* (1965) showed that *P. s.* pv. *phaseolicola* overwintered in the soil. In Brazil, the soybean *Glycine max.* (L.) Merr. pathogen, *P. s.* pv. *glycinea*, was not recovered from buried debris 91 days later. Similarly, *X. c.* pv. *phaseoli* var. *sojensis* was not recovered from buried debris but did survive in low numbers for 7 months in debris on the soil surface (Fett, 1979). In the United States, all three bacterial pathogens of soybean overwinter in infected debris (Graham, 1953; Kennedy, 1965, 1969). *Corynebacterium michiganense* cv. *michiganense* survived 36 weeks at −20°C in infected leaves in sterile and nonsterile soil, but only about 3 weeks at 5–35°C (Basu, 1970). *Pseudomonas solanacearum*, survived 7 weeks in decomposing debris in soil (Erinle, 1978).

B. Irrigation Water

Irrigation water provides not only the medium for bacterial transmission, but also provides the moisture important to establishing infections. Sprinkler irrigation is more effective in spreading bacterial pathogens than surface irrigation. Bacterial pathogens of beans, *X. c.* pv. *phaseoli* and *P. s.* pv. *phaseolicola*, are effectively spread by sprinkler irrigation (Menzies, 1954). The duration of sprinkling does not affect severity of halo blight of bean caused by *P. s.* pv. *phaseolicola* but sprinkled plants had more infections than furrow irrigated plants (LeBaron *et al.*, 1976). *X. c.* pv. *vesicatoria* spread rapidly and was more severe on sprinkler-irrigated, compared to furrow-irrigated, tomatoes (Volcani, 1969). In California, bacterial blight of cotton was associated with the use of overhead sprinkler irrigation (Schnathorst *et al.*, 1960), and in Arizona, *X. c.* pv. *malvacearum* was spread by both surface and sprinkler irrigation. Flood irrigation moved the pathogen downhill and laterally from an infected area to the end of an experimental plot, a distance of 7.6 m (King and Brinkerhoff, 1949).

In some irrigation systems, runoff water is passed through successive fields before it is returned to a drainage. Thus bacterial pathogens may be easily spread from field to field. In other irrigation systems, runoff water is collected in a sump or basin then reapplied to the field. Bacterial pathogens have been detected in the water in these sumps and a control procedure based on addition of chlorine to the irrigation water has been developed (Steadman, 1979).

Flooding, intentional or accidental, may disseminate pathogenic bacteria. For example, *Erwinia chrysanthemi* Burkholder *et al.* which causes bacterial foot rot of rice is spread in paddy water (Goto, 1979). Also *X. c.* pv. *ampelina* Panagopoulos was spread to roots of grapevine (*Vitis vinifera* L.) when plants were flooded to control frost damage (Ride *et al.*, 1978). Flooding can reduce survival of *P. solanacearum* in the soil (Erinle, 1978). Flooding also kills *X. c.* pv. *malvacearum* in dried plant debris (Andrews, 1937).

IV. DISSEMINATION BY VEGETATIVELY PROPAGATED PLANT PARTS

A review of the Commonwealth Mycological Descriptions of Bacterial Diseases indicates that over 40% of the listed pathogens are transmitted on vegetatively propagated plant material. Among the most notable examples are the citrus canker pathogen, *X. c.* pv. *citri* (Hasse) Dye, *A. tumefaciens* the rotting pathogens, *E. chrysanthemi* and *X. c.* pv. *pelargoni* (Brown) Dye; and the pathogens of potatoes, *Erwinia carotovora* subsp. *carotovora*, (Jones) Bergey *et al.*, *E. c.* subsp. *atroseptica*, and *C. michiganense* cv. *sepedonicum*. Dissemination of the soft-rotting pathogens in seed stock of potato has also been recently reviewed (Perombelon and Kelman, 1980).

Bacteria surviving in vegetative materials are easily transported and serve effectively as primary inoculum. Since the bacteria are well adapted to concomitant survival with the host, the need for finding a host is minimal. Dispersal of bacteria to other plants often occurs during cultural manipulation (cutting, planting, pruning, grafting, etc.). Diseases caused by these pathogens are among the most difficult to control.

V. DISSEMINATION IN SEED

It could be argued that the bacteria never leave their host if they are transmitted in or on the seed; therefore, they have little need to find hosts. Schuster and Coyne (1974), Noble *et al.* (1958), and Kennedy (1979) have reviewed seed-borne transmission.

Kiraly *et al.* (1970) summarized types of seed contamination as those with bacteria adhering to the seed coat, those with bacteria lodged among the seed hairs, and those in which the bacteria are beneath the seed coat or in deeper seed tissues. Understanding the nature of seed contamination is important if treatments are to eliminate the pathogens.

Noble (1957) pointed out that seed lots may carry contaminants which are not closely associated with individual seeds. Rye grass (*Lolium* sp.) may be contaminated with galls of *Anguina agrostis* Steinbuck and these galls may carry pathogenic corynebacteria. In association with active nematodes, these corynebacteria may incite disease, but without the nematodes, the bacteria are innocuous (Sabet, 1954).

Not all seed is contaminated from the parent plants. For example, cotton seed became contaminated after processing in a delinter that had previously treated seed infested with *X. c.* pv. *malvacearum* (Schnathorst, 1964). Also bean seed may become contaminated by dust in the harvesting and conditioning process (Grogan and Kimble, 1967). A high percentage (32%) of cotton seed became infested after seed was soaked in water to hasten germination (Schnathorst *et al.*, 1960).

VI. INSECT TRANSMISSION

Early studies on bacterial diseases of plants showed that honeybees and perhaps other insects were able to transport *E. amylovora*, the fire blight pathogen, to apparently healthy blossoms of apple (*Malus sylvestris* Mill.). Since that time, a large volume of literature and several reviews have elucidated many relationships between bacteria and their insect vectors. This literature has been recently and critically reviewed (Harrison *et al.*, 1980; Harrison and Brewer, this volume, Chapter 2; Purcell, Vol. 1, Chapter 6). These reviewers point out that insects also assist in bacterial survival, dissemination, and penetration into host tissues.

Dissemination apparently ranges from intimate associations to accidental contamination. Intimate associations would include transmission of bacteria with a limited host range by insects restricted to a small group of plants. Examples would include transmission of *E. stewartii* by the corn flea beetle (*Chaetocnema pulicaria* Melsh.) and *E. tracheiphila* spread by the striped and spotted cucumber beetles.

Carter's (1962) suggestion that *E. tracheiphila* is totally dependent on the activities of cucumber beetles for survival, dissemination, and inoculation would make this a very intimate example of the associations. Harrison *et al.* (1980) claim that the literature does not support such a contention, and that the main function of the beetles is in transmission of the pathogen. No other means of transmission are known; thus, the intimate association for transmission is apparently still valid.

The corn flea beetle is not the sole agent for transmission of *E. stewartii*, but it is the primary vector. Disease control procedures based on successful overwintering of infested adult beetles have been developed. The bacterium can survive more than a month in the digestive tract of active beetles but there is not conclusive evidence that the bacterium can overwinter there. There is no evidence to suggest that the bacterium enhances the reproduction or survival of the beetle.

The apple maggot (*Rhagoletis pomonella* Walsh) carries *P. melophthora* (nomenspecies *sensu* Allen & Riker) as an external and internal contaminant. The insect larvae cannot develop normally in the absence of apple tissue rotted by the bacterium. The bacteria are apparently introduced as contaminants on the surface of the eggs through oviposition wounds.

Similarly, *P. s.* pv. *savastanoi* (Smith) Young *et al.* which incites olive (*Olea europaea* L.) knot may be carried in the digestive tract throughout the life of the olive fruit fly [*Dacus oleae* (Gmelin)]. The pathogen is transmitted in internally contaminated eggs deposited in the olive during oviposition. Harrison *et al.* (1980) questioned whether the bacterium forms a significant part of the intestinal microflora, but agree that in some cases, the bacterium is transmitted to olive via internally contaminated eggs. Apparently the bacterium makes host nutrients available to the developing larvae.

Mutualistic symbiotic relationships have developed between strains of *E. carotovora* (Jones) Bergey *et al.* and several insects: the black onionfly (*Tritoxa flexa* Wiedemann), the onion maggot (*Hylemya antiqua* Meigen), and the iris borer (*Macronoctua onusta* Grote). Larval stages of the black onionfly and onion maggot do not fully develop in the absence of bacterial infection which provides nutrients otherwise unavailable to the insect. Both insects deposit externally contaminated eggs and larval feeding provides wounds for bacterial entry. The onion maggot maintains the soft rot pathogen overwinter in the puparia. The iris borer maintains *E. carotovora,* causal agent of soft rot of iris (*Iris* spp.), in the digestive tract and uses bacterially macerated host tissue as a food base. The bacterium can be deposited in fecal pellets. The importance of the bacterium in insect development has not been investigated. Insects are probably not important in secondary spread of the disease. The seed corn maggot (*Hylemya platura* Meigen) transmits *E. carotovora* soft rot and blackleg of potatoes via externally contaminated eggs deposited at oviposition. The bacteria are normal inhabitants of the insect gut, and provide modified host materials for the insect. The bacteria may overwinter in the pupae but the importance of the bacteria to larval development may be minor.

Often bacteria are transmitted on insects which are contaminated during their foraging, or nectar/pollen collecting activities. Generally no long-term insect–bacterial associations are established. Many bacterial diseases are thus casually or accidently transmitted. The most studied example is that of fire blight of apple, pear (*Pyrus communis* L.), and related species. Bees and other insects are contaminated during visits to infected blossoms and spread the pathogen to healthy blossoms. Insects may spread the pathogen to leaf and shoot surfaces and thereby establish epiphytic populations. Insects visit oozing cankers which harbor the overwintering bacteria and transport the bacteria to blossoms or leaf surfaces.

Nematodes may also carry pathogenic bacteria. Saprozoic nematodes passed viable pathogens through the intestine and were judged to be significant in disseminating the bacteria (Jensen, 1967; Chantanao and Jensen, 1969). Plant pathogenic nematodes can carry pathogenic bacteria as surface contaminants (Pitcher, 1963; Pitcher and Cross, 1958). Birds (Anonymous, 1979), earthworms (Perombelon and Lowe, 1970), mites (Smith *et al.*, 1912), and a variety of other fauna have also been associated with transmission.

VII. TRANSMISSION VIA COLLATERAL HOSTS

Weeds, volunteer crop plants, and other cropped plants have all been implicated in the maintenance and dispersal of plant pathogenic bacteria. *Solanum cineaeum* (R. Br.) and *S. nigrum* L. (black nightshade) supported *P. solanacearum* biotype II (Graham and Lloyd, 1978). *Corynebacterium michiganse* pv. *tritici* (Hutchinson) Dye & Kemp and an associated nematode *Anguina tritici* (Steinbuck) Filip. caused tundu (yellow spike disease) on *Lolium tumulentum* L., *Polypogon monspeliensis* (L.) Desf., and *Phalaris minor* Retz. (Dahiya and Bhatti, 1980). Red vine, *Brunnichia cirrhosa* Gaertn., and *Dolichos biflorus* L. (Patel *et al.*, 1949) served as hosts of *X. c.* pv. *phaseoli* var. *sojense* (Jones, 1961). *Solanum muricatum* and *S. mammosum* are perennial weeds susceptible to *C. michiganense* (Ark and Thompson, 1960) and in California, perennial nightshade (*S. elaeagnifolium* Cav.) served as an overwintering host for the pathogen (Baines, 1947). All *Brassica* species and *Boerhaavia erecta* L., *Matthiola incana* (L.) R. Br., *Raphanus sativus* L., *Lepidium sativum* L., and *Capsella bursa pastoris* (L.) Medic can serve as hosts of *X. c.* pv. *campestris* (Young, 1969).

If a pathogen can incite disease in weeds or other cultivated crops, it is often said to have a wide host range. *Pseudomonas solanacearum* (Kelman, 1953), *E. carotovora* (Perombelon and Kelman, 1980), *P. s.* pv. *tabaci* (Wolf & Foster) Young *et al.* (Bradbury, 1967), *E. rhapontici* (Millard) Burkholder (Sellwood and Lelliott, 1978), *A. tumefaciens* (DeCleene and DeLey, 1976), and *P. s.* pv. *syringae* are among the bacteria with the widest host ranges. Recent changes in the taxonomic positions of many bacteria has modified our species concept and many bacteria originally designated species are now pathovars or subspecies in a more inclusive species (Dye *et al.*, 1980). It may be argued that we have artificially increased the host ranges of some of the bacterial pathogens. The action was necessary in view of the increasing body of knowledge on bacterial genetics and techniques for identification. Perhaps early workers reported even wider host ranges for bacteria than actually exist. One reason for this is the hypersensitive reaction (HR) which was not recognized until the mid 1960s (Klement *et al.*, 1964). The HR reaction induced by incompatible bacteria in a nonhost plant may have been classified as a pathogenic response (Kiraly *et al.*, 1970).

Many plants support an epiphytic microbial population which may include plant pathogenic bacteria (Leben, 1965). For example, hairy vetch (*Vicia villosa* Roth.) supported *P. s.* pv. *syringae* pathogenic to beans (Ercolani *et al.*, 1974), and both grasses and broadleaf plants supported pseudomonads pathogenic to wild cherry (*Prunus* sp.) (Lattore and Jones, 1979). *Xanthomonas campestris* pv. *phaseoli* grew epiphytically on leaves of crop and weed species for up to 21 days. The pathogen was able to spread among beans and weeds such as lambquarters (*Chenopodium album* L.) and pigweed (*Amaranthus retroflexus* L.) within 12 days after field inoculation (Cafati and Saettler, 1980).

Epiphytic populations appear to be highly variable with respect to total number of pathogens, relative proportion of pathogens to other organisms, age and resistance of the host plant, and presence of toxicants applied to the leaf. Substances toxic to the host plant may also change the relative numbers of epiphytic bacteria (Fry and Ramsay, 1977).

In general, epiphytes are now recognized as both sources of inoculum and as a transitory stage prior to induction of pathogenesis. They may serve to maintain the pathogen in the absence of the primary host. It appears that selection pressure may modify the pathogens which survive on "nonhosts." For example, *C. m.* pv. *michiganense* isolated from perennial nightshade (*Solanum douglasii*) was able to attack both nightshade and tomato while an isolate from tomato was pathogenic on tomato but not on nightshade (Baines, 1947). A strain of *X. c.* pv. *translucens* (Jones *et al.*) Dye f. sp. *undulosa sensu* (Smith *et al.*) Hagborg which infected *Bromus commutatus* Schrad and *Bromus tectorum* L. and overwintered on these weed species was not extremely virulent on wheat (*Triticum aestivum* L.) or barley (*Hordeum vulgare* L.). Therefore, the strain was not considered important in epidemiology of the grain pathogen (Boosalis, 1955).

A number of soil-invading bacteria have been shown to survive on the roots of "nonhost" species. There appears to be some selection for survival within the rhizosphere and some pathogens may be retained preferentially (Diachun and Valleau, 1946). Unless the weed roots are transported (by rogueing to remove weeds), rhizosphere survival may have little epidemiological significance. If one considers rhizosphere survival as an adaptive modification which has prolonged the soil phase of some invasive bacteria, the soil phase becomes more important. For the role of rhizosphere survival on weeds see the chapter by M. Stanghellini (Vol. 1, Chapter 10).

VIII. AIRBORNE DISPERSAL

A. Pollen and Fungal Spores

The fact that bacteria can colonize buds and flowers makes transport via pollen probable. In 1944, Ark isolated *X. c.* pv. *juglandis* (Pierce) Dye from the pollen produced by walnut. Later, Miller and Bollen (1946) discounted the importance of contaminated pollen grains in dispersal and attributed most of the spread to rainsplash. Ercolani (1962) demonstrated that pollen transmission of *X. c.* pv. *juglandis* does occur. Ivanhoff (1933) suggested that *E. stewartii* was also pollen-borne.

Because pathogenic fungi and bacteria often are closely associated on plant surfaces, contamination of fungal propagules by the bacteria seems highly probable. Many fungi have developed mechanisms to aid in airborne dispersal, and any bacterium which contaminated the fungal spores could share in the fungal adaptation for air dispersal. While the scenario is plausable, reports supporting it are few. Yarwood (1969) assayed 200 uredospores from bean leaves concurrently infected with rust *Uromoyces phaseoli* Pers. (Wint.) and *P. s.* pv. *phaseolicola* inducing halo blight. He was unable to detect bacteria on the uredospores and concluded that the rust fungus does not function as a vector for bacteria. We do know, however, that spores of plant pathogenic fungi do support an epiphytic microflora. French *et al.* (1964) isolated *Bacillus* spp. and *P. fluorescens* Migula from wheat stem rust (*Puccinia graminis* f. sp. *tritici* Eriks. & E. Henn.) spores, and Doherty and Preece (1978) obtained from uredospores of *Puccinia porri* (Sow) Wint. a strain of *Bacillus cereus* Frankland & Frankland which was antagonistic to the development of leek (*Allium porrum* L.) rust. Pon *et al.* (1954) have demonstrated that *E. uredovora* (Pon *et al.*) Dye, a pathogen on uredia of cereal rusts, was spread on contaminated uredospores.

B. Rainsplash

Faulwetter (1917a) related rainfall and wind direction to spread of *X. c.* pv. *malvacearum,* causal agent of angular leafspot, from inoculated plants to a relatively disease free field of cotton. Later, in a classic set of experiments, Faulwetter (1917b) studied the mechanisms of splash dispersal. By dripping water drops of various sizes onto surfaces covered with marker solutions and observing the resulting splash droplets, he determined that (1) single drops onto a dry surface do not cause splashing, (2) the distance of splash in still air varies as the size of the drop varies although not in direct proportion, (3) in still air, larger droplets traveled farther than the smaller droplets, and (4) in moving air (16 km/hr) smaller droplets traveled 6 m further than larger ones. Rainsplash is one type of airborne inoculum. Gregory *et al.* (1959) have shown that impact of water drops can generate thousands of splash droplets; most of these contain inoculum propagules.

Rainsplash can transport bacteria from the soil surface to upper portions of a plant. Manns (1909) found *P. avenae* Manns, the bacterium causing bladeblight of oats (*Avena sativa* L.), could be moved from the soil to leaves by spattering rains.

Rainsplash can also disperse bacteria from plants on which the bacteria are residing as epiphytes. *P. syringae* pv. *syringae,* which causes brownspot of beans, can be spread to the natural host by rainsplash from hairy vetch, a common weed, where the bacterium exists as an epiphyte (Ercolani *et al.,* 1974).

Windblown rain has been shown to be effective in spread of a number of bacterial diseases including fire blight of pear and apple (Bauske, 1967; Beer, 1979; Stevens *et al.,* 1918), bacterial blight of walnut caused by *X. c.* pv. *juglandis* (Miller *et al.,* 1945), filbert (*Corylus* spp.) blight caused by *X. c.* pv. *corylina* (Miller *et al.*) Starr & Burkholder (Miller, 1936), bacterial canker of tomato (*C. m.* pv. *michiganense*) (Cass Smith and Goos, 1946; Cox, 1966), halo blight of bean (Butcher *et al.,* 1967; Walker and Patel, 1964; Wilson, 1947), bacterial spot of pepper (*Capsicum frutescens* L.) caused by *X. c.* pv. *vesicatoria* (Weber, 1932), bacterial blight of soybean (Daft and Leben, 1972), bacterial canker and blossom blight of stone-fruits caused by *P. s.* pv. *morsprunorum* (Wormald) Young *et al.* or by *P. s.* pv. *syringae* (Crosse, 1966), and black rot of cauliflower (*Brassica oleracea* var. *botrytis* L.) caused by *X. c.* pv. *campestris* (Clayton, 1929).

C. Dew or Fog Drip

Several investigators have implicated dew drip in spread of bacterial pathogens from one portion of the plant to healthy tissues on another portion. Rolfs (1915), in discussing dispersal of angular leafspot of cotton, states that wet weather is important in spread of the pathogen but even in dry weather, evening dews will furnish enough water for spread. Spread is enhanced by movement of leaves in wind which brings healthy leaves in contact with bacteria-laden diseased leaves.

Faulwetter (1917b) claimed that dew drip may be quite important in splash dispersal. In experiments, he showed drops from leaves falling 30 cm onto a thin film of water caused splash droplets which spread 50–80 cm from the source. Dunegan (1932) indicated that dew may effectively disperse the bacterium causing bacterial spot of peach [*Prunus persica* (L.) Batsch].

D. Sprinkler Irrigation Splash

Sprinkler irrigation can be important in spread of some bacterial diseases. Almost all comments about rainsplash apply to sprinkler irrigation spread, except that drops from sprinklers can be larger than natural raindrops. The force from larger drops increases the distance that splash droplets travel (Faulwetter, 1917b).

In dry climates where rain or dew seldom occurs, sprinkler irrigation can be the primary method of dispersal. For example in Israel, bacterial spot of tomato became a serious problem in the 1960s after sprinkler irrigation became the primary method of providing water to tomato plants (Volcani, 1969). In the San Joaquin valley of California, angular leaf spot of cotton appeared only sporadically until about 1951. When sprinklers came into wide use in growing cotton, the disease became prevalent and virtually every occurrence of the disease was associated with overhead irrigation (Schnathorst *et al.*, 1960).

When sprinklers are used in more moist climates, the results can be devastating. In 1963, an epidemic of bacterial blight of peas (*Pisum sativum* L.) caused by *P. s.* pv. *pisi* (Sackett) Young *et al.* occurred on about 506 ha of peas under sprinkler irrigation in Wisconsin (Hagedorn and Wade, 1964). Although other factors such as infected seed, high winds and rain were implicated in the epidemic, the use of the sprinklers were considered important in spread of the disease.

E. Airborne Debris

Phytobacteria might become airborne as infected leaves or plant debris. There is little doubt that bacteria can live in plant tissues, overwinter there, and possibly be blown about to serve as inoculum. For example, Rolfs (1935) reported that a single whirlwind scattered dry cotton leaves infected with *X. c.* pv. *malvacearum* over an area of 40 ha in 20 min.

F. Airborne Dust

In 1942, Brown published one of the few reports on dust dispersal of a phytobacterium. From observations on over 486 ha of cotton in Arizona, he determined that *X. c.* pv. *malvacearum* was spread by a dust storm from a field of infected cotton which lay upwind of apparently disease-free fields. Due to the pattern of resulting disease, lack of rainfall, and lack of disease in a comparable set of control fields, he concluded that dust must have been the method of dissemination. Unfortunately, no samples of air or dust were taken to verify his conclusions. Lloyd (1969) found *Streptomyces* attached to airborne dust particles and showed that wind or agricultural implements increased the concentration of the streptomycete propagules in the air. Clafin *et al.* (1973) showed that windblown soil containing bacteria-infested debris caused infection of alfalfa (*Medicago sativa* L.) and bean. Vakili (1967) and Sackett (1916) indicated that dust abrasion increased likelihood of plant infection.

G. Aerial Strands

Many phytobacterial diseases are characterized by bacterial ooze or slime. In the case of fire blight of fruit trees the exudate can be extruded in the form of long aerial strand up to 100 mm long and 6–300 μm in diameter (Eden-Green and Billing, 1972). Temperature and humidity were not the only factors governing exudate or strand production (Paulin and Lachuad, 1978). Similar strands can be formed by *P. s.* pv. *mori* on mulberry (*Morus alba* L.) (Smith, 1920), *P. s.* pv. *pisi* on pea (Skoric, 1927), and *Pseudomonas* and *Xanthomonas* pathogens on beans (Venette, unpublished). The epidemiological significance of these strands is unknown (Beer, 1979), but Eden-Green and Billing (1972) speculate that these may break apart into fine fragments which could be carried by dry wind to host plants.

H. Aerosols

Smith (1911) theorized that since dust or dry wind-borne bacteria require half a day or more to rehydrate, they are probably not the primary inocula for inducing disease. Rather, fresh hydrated cells which come from the interior of infected leaves, would be the primary inoculum. Crosse (1957) agreed and said that since bacteria lack adaptive structures for launching cells into the air and are not able to penetrate the dry protective surfaces of plants, it is improbable that wind dissemination is comparable to that of fungal spores for the spread of disease. However, Gorlenko (1965) felt that phytobacteria can be dispersed in dry air, but offered no data or references to support his claim. Gregory (1959) suggested that small water droplets containing bacteria might evaporate quickly, thus leaving the particle truly airborne. Venette and Kennedy (1975) detected airborne *P. s.* pv. *glycinea* bacteria from a field of infected soybeans during rainstorms and sprinkler irrigation. Predominant particle size was within the size range 2.1–3.3 μm, and an average of 151 bacteria per cubic meter of air was detected during rainstorms. Lindemann *et al.* (1978) showed that bacterial aerosols are produced by wind blowing over dry foliage. They concluded that bacteria from vegetation were a major source of airborne contamination. Fast wind gusts (Shaw *et al.*, 1978) are probably of sufficient velocity to liberate surface-borne bacteria. Electrostatic forces may assist in liberation (Fish, 1972).

Southey and Harper (1971) found in laboratory tests that *E. amylovora* survived for 3 hr as airborne particles suspended in air with relative humidities between 40 and 90%. When bacteria, adhering to microthreads, were exposed to open air, the viability decreased more rapidly than in laboratory tests, but significant numbers of bacteria remained alive for 2 hr. Graham *et al.* (1979) showed *E. c.* subsp. *atroseptica* could survive on microthreads exposed to open air and that airborne spread, especially during cool, humid weather was possible. Similarly, tests on *Rhizobium meliloti* Dangeard (Won and Ross, 1969) showed the bacterium survived as airborne particles for test periods of 5 hr and that survival was maximal at high relative humidities and minimal at low relative humidity. Venette (1975, 1979) observed that *P. s.* pv. *glycinea*, *P. s.* pv. *phaseolicola*, and *X. c.* pv. *phaseoli* survived as airborne particles better in humid air. Survival for nearly 3 hr indicated long distance transmission is possible. Graham and Harrison (1975) determined that water drops impacting stems of potatoes infected with *E. c.* subsp. *atroseptica* generated airborne bacterial particles which could be detected 60–90 min after generation. Similar studies were later quantitated (Graham *et al.*, 1977). Venette (1975) demonstrated that the number of airborne *P. s.* pv. *glycinea* was related to the number of water drops which impacted wet leaves.

Xanthomonas campestris pv. *malvacearum*, pseudomonads, and other bacteria were trapped from the field aerosol in India (Wadje and Deshpande, 1978). These bacterial populations were greatest during the two wet seasons and the few plant pathogens that were detected occurred only during these periods. Pathogenic bacteria may be made airborne via pulverization of potato vines (Perombelon *et al.*, 1979) or thrashing operations (Venette, unpublished) or when wind erosion makes contaminated soil airborne (Delany and Zenchelsky, 1976; Zenchelsky *et al.*, 1975).

From aerosols, airborne particles may be deposited directly (Klepper and Craig, 1975; Wedding *et al.*, 1975). Airborne *P. s.* pv. *glycinea* bacteria deposited directly onto soybean leaves caused infections and established epiphytic populations (Surico *et al.*, 1981). Leaf structure and surface waxes may affect deposition (Forster, 1977). Washout by precipitation may cause bacteria to be deposited. Venette (1975) has shown that water drops passed through airborne *P. s.* pv. *glycinea* effectively collect the bacteria.

IX. ACTIVITIES OF MAN

A. Worldwide

The activities of man are certainly important in the international dissemination of bacterial diseases. Rapoport *et al.* (1976) claimed that oceans, mountain ranges, and rivers have ceased to be great geographical barriers and, instead, have been transformed into routes of dispersal for the interchange of species. Man has opened new roads and people, animals, plants, and agricultural products with all their respective parasites are being distributed more widely.

Examples of worldwide distribution are many: *X. c.* pv. *citri* on fruit and citrus stocks from Japan was introduced into the United States (Stakman and Harrar, 1957). *Erwinia amylovora* was introduced into Japan, New Zealand, and Europe (Schroth *et al.*, 1974; Stakman and Harrar, 1957), and *C. m.* pv. *michiganense* was introduced into England from a country where the disease was widely distributed (Moore, 1957).

Pathogens are often introduced into new areas when new crops are introduced. *Pseudomonas syringae* pv. *glycinea* was probably introduced into the United States and Russia with the introduction of soybean culture from the Orient (Kennedy and Tachibana, 1973) and bean pathogens were introduced on seed in the Columbia River basin of Washington when noncultivated desert land was brought into crop production (Menzies, 1952).

B. Cultural

Cultural techniques also favor distribution of some plant pathogenic bacteria. *Corynebacterium michiganense* pv. *sepedonicum* is spread to noninfected potato seed on cutting knives contaminated from infected tubers. The bacterium also survives on machinery, clothing, bags, and in storage areas (Nelson, 1978). *Pseudomonas solanacearum* (Moko disease of banana) and *X. axonoperis* Starr & Garces (Gummosis of grasses) are spread by machetes used in harvesting (Kelman, 1953; Castano *et al.*, 1964). Cabbage (*Brassica oleraceae* var. *capitata* L.) black rot, caused by *X. c.* pv. *campestris* (Strandberg, 1973), is spread by cultivation equipment and bacterial blight of beans is spread by the wheels of center pivot irrigation systems (Bissonnett, personal communication). Sackett (1916) suggested a spiketooth harrow spread *P. s.* pv. *pisi* among pea plants and farm equipment may spread *P. alboprecipitans* Rosen in corn (*Zea mays.* L.) (Gitaitis, 1978). See Civerolo (this volume, Chapter 16) for a discussion of the use of cultural practices for disease control.

X. CONCLUSIONS

This report emphasizes that the mechanisms by which bacteria find their hosts are diverse. While several modes of dissemination for bacterial plant pathogens might be recognized, the relative importance of each of the mechanisms is seldom designated. Because we currently lack efficient chemical control agents and have difficulty developing and maintaining crop plants resistant to bacterial disease, we must make careful appraisal of the relative importance of various methods of dispersal. Following such studies, we may more strategically employ available control practices to minimize losses from the bacterial diseases. Saettler and Mount (this volume, Chapter 15) discuss strategies for manipulating plant–prokaryote interactions for disease control.

References

Addy, S. K., and Dhal, N. K. (1978). *Indian Phytopathol.* **31,** 64–69.
Agrios, G. N. (1978). "Plant Pathology," 2nd ed. Academic Press, New York.
Andrews, F. W. (1937). *Emp. J. Exp. Agric.* **5,** 204–218.
Andrews, J. H., and Kenerley, C. M. (1979). *Can. J. Microbiol.* **25,** 1331–1344.
Anon. (1979). *Rep. EPPO Colloq. Fire Blight, Wageningen, 1977, EPPO Bull.* **9,** 3–5.
Ark, P. A. (1944). *Phytopathology* **34,** 330–334.
Ark, P. A. (1958). *Plant Dis. Rep.* **42,** 1293.
Ark, P. A., and Alcorn, S. M. (1956). *Plant Dis. Rep.* **40,** 85–92.
Ark, P. A., and Thompson, J. P. (1960). *Plant Dis. Rep.* **44,** 98–99.
Baines, R. C. (1947). *Phytopathology* **37,** 359.
Barakat, F. M. (1979). *Proc. Egypt. Phytopathol. Congr., 3rd* pp. 299–310.
Bashan, Y., Okon, Y., and Henis, Y. (1978). *Phytoparasitica* **6,** 135–143.
Basu, P. K. (1970). *Phytopathology* **60,** 825–827.
Bateman, D. F. (1978). *In* "Plant Disease" (J. G. Horsfall and E. B. Cowling, eds.), Vol. III, pp. 53–83. Academic Press, New York.
Bauske, R. J. (1967). *Proc. Am. Soc. Hortic. Sci.* **91,** 795–801.
Bazin, M. J. (1978). *Ann. Appl. Biol.* **89,** 159–162.
Beer, S. V. (1979). *Rep. EPPO Colloq. Fire Blight, Wageningen, 1977 EPPO Bull.* **9,** 13–25.
Blood, H. L. (1937). *Science* **86,** 199–200.
Boosalis, M. G. 1955. *Plant Dis. Rep.* **39,** 751–754.
Bradbury, J. F. (1967). Commonwealth Mycological Institute Descriptions of Pathogenic Fungi and Bacteria. No. 129. Kew, Surrey, England.
Briggs, D., and Waters, S. M. (1969). "Plant Variation and Evolution." McGraw-Hill, New York.
Brinkerhoff, L. A. (1970). *Annu. Rev. Phytopathol.* **8,** 85–110.
Brinkerhoff, L. A., and Fink, G. B. (1964). *Phytopathology* **54,** 1198–1201.
Brown, J. G. (1942). *Phytopathology* **32,** 81–90.
Brown, J. G., and Heep, D. M. (1946). *Sci. Civ.* **2696,** 208.
Buddenhagen, I. W. (1961). *Trop. Agric.* (*Trinidad*) **38,** 107–121.
Buddenhagen, I. W. (1965). *In* "Ecology of Soil-Borne Plant Pathogens" (K. F. Baker and W. C. Snyder, eds.), pp. 269–284. Univ. of California Press, Berkeley.
Buddenhagen, I. W., and Elsasser, T. A. (1962). *Nature* (*London*) **194,** 164–165.
Buddenhagen, I. W., Sequeira, L., and Kelman, A. (1962). *Phytopathology* **52,** 726.
Butcher, C. L., Dean, L. L., and Laferriere, L. (1967). *Plant Dis. Rep.* **51,** 310–311.
Butcher, C. L., Dean, L. L., and Guthrie, J. W. (1969). *Plant Dis. Rep.* **53,** 894–896.
Cafati, C. R., and Saetteler, A. W. (1980). *Plant Dis.* **64,** 194–196.
Carter, W. (1962). "Insects in Relation to Plant Disease." Wiley (Interscience), New York.
Cass Smith, W. P., and Goos, O. M. (1946). *J. Dep. Agric. West Aust.* **23,** 147–156.
Castano, J. J., Thurston, H. D., and Crowder, L. V. (1964). *Agric. Trop.* **20,** 379–387.
Chamberlain, D. W. (1952). *Phytopathology* **42,** 299–300.
Chantanao, A., and Jensen, H. J. (1969). *J. Nematol.* **1,** 216–218.
Chester, K. S. (1942). "The Nature and Prevention of Plant Diseases." Blakiston, Philadelphia, Pennsylvania.
Claflin, L. E., Stuteville, D. L., and Armbrust, D. V. (1973). *Phytopathology* **63,** 1417–1419.
Clayton, E. E. (1925). *Phytopathology* **15,** 49.
Clayton, E. E. (1929). *N.Y. Agric. Exp. Sta. Bull.* **576.**
Cox, R. S. (1966). *Plant Dis. Rep.* **50,** 699–700.
Coyne, D. P., and Schuster, M. L. (1979). *Annu. Rep. Bean Improv. Coop.* **22,** 21–22.

Crosse, J. E. (1955a). *Rep. East Malling Res. Sta.* pp. 121–125.
Crosse, J. E. (1955b). *J. Hortic. Sci.* **30**, 131–142.
Crosse, J. E. (1957). *In* "Biological Aspects of the Transmission of Disease" (C. Horton-Smith, ed.), pp. 7–12. Oliver & Boyd, Edinburgh.
Crosse, J. E. (1966). *Annu. Rev. Phytopathol.* **4**, 291–310.
Crosse, J. E. (1971). *Proc. Br. Insectic. Fungic. Conf., 6th* pp. 694–705.
Crosse, J. E., Kennedy, B. W., Lambert, J. W., and Cooper, R. L. (1966). *Plant Dis. Rep.* **50**, 557–560.
Cunfer, B. M., Schaad, N. W., and Morey, D. D. (1979). *Ga. Agric. Res.* **20**, 14–16.
Daft, G. C., and Leben, C. (1972). *Phytopathology* **62**, 57–62.
Dahiya, R. S., and Bhatti, D. S. (1980). *Haryana Agric. Univ. J. Res.* **102**, 257.
Davis, R. D. (1976). *Soil Biol. Biochem.* **8**, 429–433.
De Boer, S. H., Copeman, R. J., and Vruggink, H. (1979). *Phytopathology* **69**, 316–319.
DeCleene, M., and DeLey, J. (1976). *Bot. Rev.* **42**, 389–466.
Dekker, J. (1963). *Annu. Rev. Microbiol.* **17**, 243–262.
Delany, A. C., and Zenchelsky, S. (1976). *Soil Sci.* **121**, 146–155.
Diachun, S., and Valleau, W. D. (1946). *Phytopathology* **36**, 277–280.
Doherty, M. A., and Preece, T. F. (1978). *Proc. Int. Conf. Plant Pathog. Bact., 4th, Angers* p. 977 (Abstr.).
Dunegan, J. C. (1932). *U.S. Dept. Agric. Tech. Bull.* **273**, 53 pp.
Dye, D. W., Bradbury, J. F., Goto, M., Hayward, A. C., Lelliot, R. A., and Schroth, M. N. (1980). *Rev. Plant Pathol.* **59**, 153–168.
Eden-Green, S. J., and Billing, E. (1972). *Plant Pathol.* **21**, 121–123.
Ercolani, G. L. (1962). *Phytopathol. Mediterr.* **2**, 1–10 (from *Rev. Appl. Mycol.* **42**, 223).
Ercolani, G. L., Hagedorn, D. J., Kelman, A., and Rand, R. E. (1974). *Phytopathology* **64**, 1330–1339.
Erinle, I. D. (1978). *Proc. Int. Conf. Plant Pathog. Bact., 4th, Angers* p. 884.
Faulwetter, R. C. (1917a). *J. Agric. Res.* **8**, 457–475.
Faulwetter, R. C. (1917b). *J. Agric. Res.* **10**, 639–648.
Fett, W. F. (1979). *Plant Dis. Rep.* **63**, 79–83.
Fish, B. K. (1972). *Science* **175**, 1239–1240.
Forster, G. F. (1977). *Trans. Br. Mycol. Soc.* **68**, 245–250.
French, R. C., Novotny, J. F., and Searles, R. B. (1964). *Phytopathology* **54**, 970–973.
Fry, J. C., and Ramsay, A. J. (1977). *Limnol. Oceanogr.* **22**, 556–562.
Garrard, E. H. (1951). *Ont. Dep. Agric. Bull.* 478.
Gause, G. F. (1934). "The Struggle for Existence." Williams & Williams, Baltimore, Maryland.
Gitaitis, R. D., Stall, R. E., and Strandberg, J. O. (1978). *Phytopathology* **68**, 227–231.
Gonzalez, C. F., and Vidauer, A. K. (1979). *J. Gen. Microbiol.* **110**, 161–170.
Gorlenko, M. V. (1965). "Bacterial Diseases of Plants." Israel Program for Scientific Translations, Jerusalem.
Goto, M. (1979). *Plant Dis. Rep.* **63**, 100.
Graham, D. C., and Harrison, M. D. (1975). *Phytopathology* **65**, 739–731.
Graham, D. C., Quinn, C. E., and Bradley, L. F. (1977). *J. Appl. Bacteriol.* **43**, 413–424.
Graham, D. C., Quinn, C. E., Sells, I. A., and Harrison, M. D. (1979). *J. Appl. Bacteriol.* **46**, 367–376.
Graham, J. B., and Istock, C. A. (1979). *Science* **204**, 637–638.
Graham, J. H. (1953). *Phytopathology* **43**, 189–192.
Graham, J. H., and Lloyd, A. B. (1978). *J. Aust. Inst. Agric. Sci.* **44**, 124–126.
Gregory, P. H., Githrie, E. J., and Bunce, M. E. (1959). *J. Gen. Microbiol.* **20**, 328–354.

Grogan, R. G., and Kimble, K. A. (1967). *Phytopathology* **57,** 28–31.

Guthrie, J. W., Dean, L. L., Butcher, C. L., Fenwick, H. S., and Finley, A. M. (1975). *Univ. Idaho Agric. Exp. Sta. Bull.* 550.

Haas, J. H., and Rotem, J. (1976). *Phytopathology* **66,** 992–997.

Hagedorn, D. J., and Wade, E. K. (1964). *Plant Dis. Rep.* **48,** 318–320.

Halluka, M., Schuster, M. L., Weihing, J. L., and Coyne, D. P. (1978). *Fitopatol. Brasil.* **3,** 13–26.

Harrison, M. D., Brewer, J. W., and Merrill, L. D. (1980). *In* "Vectors of Plant Pathogens" (K. F. Harris and K. Maramorosch, eds.), pp. 201–292. Academic Press, New York.

Hayward. A. C. (1974). *Annu. Rev. Phytopathol.* **12,** 87–97.

Hildreth, R. C. (1960). *Proc. Int. Congr. Crop Protect., 4th, Hamburg, 1957* **2,** 1587–1589.

Hill, K., Coyne, D. P., and Schuster, M. L. (1972). *J. Am. Soc. Hortic. Sci.* **97,** 494–498.

Hoitink, H. A. J., Hagedorn, D. J., and McCoy, E. (1968). *Can. J. Microbiol.* **14,** 437–441.

Horino, O. (1978). *Ann. Phytopathol. Soc. Jpn.* **44,** 297–304.

Hsieh, S. P. Y., and Buddenhagen, I. W. (1975). *Phytopathology* **65,** 513–519.

Humaydan, H. S., Harman, G. E., Nedrow, B. L., and DiNitto, L. V. (1980). *Phytopathology* 70, 127–131.

Ivanhoff, S. S. (1933). *J. Agric. Res.* **47,** 749–770.

Jensen, H. J. (1967). *Plant Dis. Rep.* **51,** 98–102.

Jones, J. P. (1961). *Phytopathology* **51,** 206.

Kelman, A. (1953). *North Carol. Agric. Exp. Sta. Tech. Bull.* 99.

Kennedy, B. W. (1965). *Phytopathology* **55,** 415–417.

Kennedy, B. W. (1969). *Phytopathology* **59,** 1618–1619.

Kennedy, B. W. (1979). *In* "Seed Pathology Problems in Progress" (J. T. Yorinori, J. B. Sinclair, Y. R. Mehta, and S. K. Mohan, eds.), pp. 155–160. Parana, Brazil.

Kennedy, B. W., and Tachibana, H. (1973). *In* "Soybeans: Improvement, Production and Uses." Agronomy Series #16, Am. Soc. Agronomy, Madison, Wisconsin.

Keyworth, W. G., and Howell, S. J. (1961). *Ann. Appl. Biol.* **49,** 173–194.

Kidby, D., Sandford, P., Herman, A., and Cadmus, M. (1977). *Appl. Environ. Microbiol.* **33,** 840–845.

King, C. J., and Brinkerhoff, L. A. (1949). *Phytopathology* **39,** 88–90.

Kiraly, Z., Klement, Z., Solymosy, F., and Voros, J. (1970). "Methods in Plant Pathology." Akademiai Kiado, Budapest.

Klement, Z., Farkas, G. L., and Lovrekovich, L. (1964). *Phytopathology* **54,** 474–477.

Klepper, B., and Craig, D. K. (1975). *J. Environ. Qual.* **4,** 495–499.

Latorre, B. A., and Jones, A. L. (1979). *Phytopathology* **69,** 1122–1125.

Leben, C. (1965). *Annu. Rev. Phytopathology* **3,** 209–230.

Leben, C., and Keitt, G. W. (1954). *Agric. Food Chem.* **2,** 234–239.

Leben, C., and Whitmoyer, R. E. (1979). *Can. J. Microbiol.* **25,** 896–901.

LeBaron, M., McMaster, G., and Guthrie, J. (1976). *Univ. Idaho Curr. Info. Ser.* 359.

Limber, D. P., and Frink, P. R. (1953). *In* "Plant Diseases, The Yearbook of Agriculture," pp. 159–161. U.S. Dept. of Agriculture, Washington, D.C.

Lindemann, J. *et al.* (1978). *Bull. Am. Meteorol. Soc.* **59,** 1516.

Lloyd, A. B. (1969). *J. Gen. Microbiol.* **57,** 35–40.

Manns, T. F. (1909). *Ohio Agric. Exp. Sta. Bull.* 210.

Mathew, J., and Patel, P. N. (1979). *Phytopathol. Z.* **94,** 3–7.

Menzies, J. D. (1952). *Plant Dis. Rep.* **36,** 44–47.

Menzies, J. D. (1954). *Phytopathology* **44,** 553.

Menzies, J. D. (1959). *Phytopathology* **49,** 648–652.

Menzies, J. D. (1963). *Bot. Rev.* **29,** 79–122.

Menzies, J. D. (1967). *In* "Irrigation of Agricultural Lands" (R. M. Hagan, H. B. Haise, and T. W. Edminster, eds.), pp. 1058–1064. Am. Soc. Agron. Irrigation Series 11, Madison, Wisconsin.

Mew, T. W. (1978). *Proc. Int. Conf. Plant Pathog. Bact., 4th, Angers* pp. 371–374.

Miller, P. W. (1936). *Oreg. Agric. Ext. Bull.* 486.

Miller, P. W., and Bollen, W. B. (1946). *Oreg. Agric. Exp. Sta. Tech. Bull.* 9.

Miller, P. W., Schuster, C. E., and Stephenson, R. E. (1945). *Oreg. Agric. Exp. Sta. Bull.* 435.

Mizukami, T., and Wakimoto, S. (1969). *Annu. Rev. Phytopathol.* **7**, 51–72.

Moore, W. C. (1957). *In* "Biological Aspects of the Transmission of Disease" (C. Horton-Smith, ed), pp. 135–139. Oliver & Boyd, Edinburgh.

Morse, W. J. (1911). *Maine Agric. Exp. Sta. Bull.* **194**, 201–228.

Mulrean, E. N., and Schroth, M. N. (1979). *Phytopathology* **69**, 1039.

Napoli, C., and Albersheim, P. (1980). *J. Bacteriol.* **141**, 979–980.

Natti, J. J. (1967). *Phytopathology* **57**, 343.

Nelson, G. A. (1978). *Am. Potato J.* **55**, 449–452.

Noble, M. (1957). *In* "Biological Aspects in the Transmission of Disease" (C. Horton-Smith, ed.), pp. 81–85. Oliver & Boyd, Edinburgh.

Noble, M., deTempe, J., and Neergaard, P. (1958). "An Annotated List of Seed-borne Diseases." Commonwealth Mycological Inst., Kew.

Okimoto, Y., and Furuta, T. (1977). *Bull. Fac. Agric. Tamagawa Univ.* **17**, 19–25.

Panopoulos, N. J., and Schroth, M. N. (1974). *Phytopathology* **64**, 1389–1397.

Patel, M. K., Kulkarni, R. S., and Dhande, G. W. (1949). *Curr. Sci. (India)* **18**, 83–84.

Patel, P. N., Trivedi, B. M., Rekhi, S. S., Town, P. A., and Rao, Y. P. (1970). *Plant Protect. Bull. FAO* **18**, 136–141.

Paulin, J. P., and Lachaud, G. (1978). *Acta Hortic.* **86**, 31–38.

Pepper, E. H. (1967). *Am. Phytopathol. Soc. Monogr.* **4**.

Perombelon, M. C. M., and Kelman, A. (1980). *Annu. Rev. Phytopathol.* **18**, 361–387.

Perombelon, M. C. M., and Lowe, R. (1970). *Rep. Scott. Hortic. Inst.* **1969**, 31–32.

Perombelon, M. C. M., Fox, R. A., and Lowe, R. (1979). *Phytopathol. Z.* **94**, 249–260.

Perombelon, M. C. M., Lowe, R., Quinn, C. E., and Sells, A. (1980). *Potato Res.* **23**, 413–425.

Persley, G. J., and Crosse, J. E. (1978). *Ann. Appl. Biol.* **89**, 219–222.

Peterson, G. H. (1963). *Phytopathology* **53**, 765–767.

Pitcher, R. S. (1963). *Phytopathology* **53**, 35–39.

Pitcher, R. S., and Cross, J. E. (1958). *Nematologica* **3**, 244–256.

Pon, D. S., Townsend, C. E., Wessman, G. E., Schmitt, C. G., and Kingsolver, C. H. (1954). *Phytopathology* **44**, 707–710.

Ralph, W. (1977). *Seed Sci. Technol.* **5**, 559–565.

Rao, C. S., and Devadath, S. (1977). *Indian Phytopathol.* **30**, 233–236.

Rapoport, E. H., Ezcurra, E., and Drausal, B. (1976). *J. Biogeogr.* **3**, 365–372.

Rattink, H., and Vruggink, H. (1979). *Med. Fac. Landbouww Rijksuniv. Gent.* **44**, 439–443.

Raymundo, A. K., and Ries, S. M. (1980). *Phytopathology* **70**, 1066–1069.

Reddy, A. P. K., and Kauffman, H. E. (1977). *Indian Phytopathol.* **30**, 106–111.

Ride, M., Ride, S., and Novoa, D. (1978). *Proc. Int. Conf. Plant Pathog. Bact., 4th, Angers,* pp. 969–971.

Roberts, D. A., and Boothroyd, C. W. (1972). "Fundamentals of Plant Pathology." Freeman, San Francisco, California.

Robinson, J. B., Salonius, P. O., and Chase, F. E. (1965). *Can. J. Microbiol.* **11**, 746–748.

Rolfs, F. M. (1915). *South Carol. Agric. Exp. Sta. Bull.* 184.

Rolfs, F. M. (1935). *Phytopathology* **25**, 971.

Rotem, J., and Palti, J. (1969). *Annu. Rev. Phytopathol.* **7,** 267–288.
Sabet, K. A. (1954). *Ann. Appl. Biol.* **41,** 606–611.
Sabet, K. A., and Ishaq, F. (1969). *Ann. Appl. Biol.* **64,** 65–74.
Sackett, W. G. (1916). *Color. Agric. Exp. Sta. Bull.* 218.
Sands, D. C., Warren, G., Myers, D. F., and Scharen, A. L. (1978). *Proc. Int. Conf. Plant Pathog. Bact., 4th, Angers* pp. 39–45.
Schaad, N. W. (1980). *In* "Laboratory Guide for Identification of Plant Pathogenic Bacteria" (N. W. Schaad, ed.), pp. 1–10. Am. Phytopathol. Soc., St. Paul, Minnesota.
Schaad, N. W., and White, W. C. (1974). *Phytopathology* **64,** 1518–1520.
Schaad, N. W., and Wilson, E. E. (1970). *Phytopathology* **60,** 557–558.
Schaad, N. W., Gabrielson, R. L., and Mulanax, M. W. (1980). *Appl. Environ. Microbiol.* **39,** 803–807.
Schnathorst, W. C. (1964). *Phytopathology* **54,** 1009–1011.
Schnathorst, W. C. (1966). *Plant Dis. Rep.* **50,** 168–171.
Schnathorst, W. C. (1969). *Phytopathology* **59,** 707.
Schnathorst, W. C., Halisky, P. M., and Martin, R. P. (1960). *Plant Dis. Rep.* **44,** 603–608.
Schroth, M. N., Thomson, S. V., Hildebrand, D. C., and Moller, W. J. (1974). *Annu. Rev. Phytopathol.* **12,** 389–412.
Schuster, M. L. (1967). *Phytopathology* **57,** 830.
Schuster, M. L. (1970). *Bean Improve. Coop.* **13,** 68–70.
Schuster, M. L., Hoff, B., and Compton, W. A. (1975). *Plant Dis. Rep.* **59,** 101–105.
Schuster, M. L., and Coyne, D. P. (1974). *Annu. Rev. Phytopathol.* **12,** 199–221.
Schuster, M. L., Coyne, D. P., and Kerr, E. D. (1965). *Phytopathology* **55,** 1075.
Schuster, M. L., Hoff, B., Mandel, M., and Lazar, I. (1973). *Proc. Annu. Corn Sorghum Res. Conf., Chicago* **27,** 176–191.
Sellwood, J. E., and Lelliott, R. A. (1978). *Plant Pathol.* **27,** 120–124.
Sharvelle, E. G. (1979). "Plant Disease Control." AVI Publ., Westport, Connecticut.
Shaw *et al.* (1978). *Bull. Am. Meterol. Soc.* **59,** 1517.
Shepard, J. F., and Claflin, L. E. (1975). *Annu. Rev. Phytopathol.* **13,** 271–273.
Sinha, S. K. and Nene, Y. L. (1967). *Plant Dis. Rep.* **51,** 882–883.
Skirvin, R. M., Otterbacher, A. G., and Ries, S. M. (1978). *HortScience* **13,** 444.
Skoric, V. (1927). *Phytopathology* **17,** 611–627.
Smith, E. F. (1911). "Bacteria in Relation to Plant Diseases," Vol. 2. Carnegie Inst. Wash. Publ. No. 27.
Smith, E. F. (1920). "An Introduction to Bacterial Diseases of Plants." Sanders, Philadelphia, Pennsylvania.
Smith, R. E., Smith, C. O., and Ramsey, H. J. (1912). *Calif. Agric. Exp. Sta. Bull.* **231,** 119–398.
Southey, R. F. W., and Harper, G. J. (1971). *J. Appl. Bacteriol.* **34,** 547–556.
Srinivasan, M. C., Neergaard, P., and Mathur, S. B. (1973). *Seed Sci. Technol.* **1,** 853–859.
Stakman, E. C., and Harrar, J. G. (1957). "Principles of Plant Pathology." Ronald, New York.
Starr, M. P. (1975). *In* "Symbiosis" (D. H. Jennings and D. L. Lee, eds.), pp. 1–20. Cambridge Univ. Press, London and New York.
Steadman, J. R. (1979). Tech. Res. Project B-032-NEB. Neb. Water Resources Ctr.
Sterne, R. E., McCarver, T. H., and Courtney, M. L. (1979). *Ark. Farm Res.* **28,** 9.
Stevens, F. L., Ruth, W. A., and Spooner, C. S. (1918). *Science* **48,** 449.
Stoddard, E. M. (1957). *Plant Dis. Rep.* **41,** 536.
Strandberg, J. (1973). *Phytopathology* **63,** 998–1001.
Surico, G., Kennedy, B. W., and Ercolani, G. L. (1981). *Phytopathology* **71,** 532–536.

Tachibana, H., and Shih, M. (1966). *Phytopathology* **56,** 903.
Taylor, J. D. (1973). *Annu. Rep., 23rd, 1972, Natl. Veg. Res. Sta., Wellesbourne, Warwick.*
Thakur, R. P., Kumar, S., Patel, P. N., and Verma, J. P. (1978). *Indian Phytopathol.* **31,** 52–56.
Thirumalachar, M. J. (1979). *In* "Seed Pathology—Problems and Progress" (J. L. Yorinori, J. B. Sinclair, Y. R. Mehta, and S. K. Mohan, eds.), pp. 208–220. Inst. Agric. Parana, Brazil.
Thomas, C. A. (1959). *Phytopathology* **49,** 461–463.
Thomas, M. D., and Leary, J. V. (1980). *Phytopathology* **70,** 310–312.
Vakili, N. G. (1967). *Phytopathology* **57,** 1099–1103.
Valladares-Sanchez, N. E., Coyne, D. P., and Schuster, M. L. (1979). *J. Am. Soc. Hortic. Sci.* **104,** 648–654.
Venette, J. R. (1975). Ph.D. thesis, University of Minnesota, St. Paul.
Venette, J. R. (1979). *Bean Improve. Coop. Natl. Dry Bean Council Res. Conf.* **23,** 80–81.
Venette, J. R., and Kennedy, B. W. (1975). *Phytopathology* **65,** 737–738.
Verma, J. P., Nayak, M. L., and Singh, R. P. (1977). *Indian Phytopathol.* **30,** 361–365.
Volcani, Z. (1969). *Plant Dis. Rep.* **53,** 459–461.
Wadje, S. S., and Deshpande, K. S. (1977). *Indian Phytopathol.* **30,** 506–508.
Wakimoto, S. (1955). *Agric. Hortic.* **30,** 1501.
Walker, J. C. (1924). *U.S. Dep. Agric. Circ.* 311.
Walker, J. C., and Patel, P. N. (1964). *Phytopathology* **54,** 952–954.
Wallace, H. R. (1978). *In* "Plant Disease. An Advanced Treatise" (J. G. Horsfall, and E. B. Cowling, eds.), Vol. 2, pp. 181–202. Academic Press, New York.
Weber, G. T. (1932). *Univ. Fla. Agric. Ext. Sta. Bull.* 244.
Wedding, J. B., Carlson, R. W., Stukel, J. J., and Bazzaz, F. A. (1975). *Environ. Sci. Tech.* **9,** 151–153.
Wilson, R. D. (1947). *Agric. Gaz. New South Wales* **58,** 15–20.
Wimalajeewa, D. L. S. (1980). *Aust. J. Exp. Agric. Anim. Husband.* **20,** 102–104.
Won, W. D., and Ross, H. (1969). *Appl. Microbiol.* **18,** 555–557.
Yarwood, C. E. (1969). *Phytopathology* **59,** 1302–1305.
Young, J. M. (1969). *Plant Dis. Rep.* **53,** 820–821.
Zaumeyer, W. J., and Thomas, H. R. (1957). *U.S. Dep. Agric. Tech. Bull.* 868.
Zenchelsky, S. T., Delany, A. C., and Pickett, R. A., II. (1975). Rutgers Univ. and National Center Atmos. Res. pp. 129–132.

Chapter **2**

Field Dispersal of Soft Rot Bacteria

M. D. HARRISON *and* **J. W. BREWER**

I. INTRODUCTION

Soft rot bacteria break down plant structures by enzymatically macerating parenchymatous tissues. Bacteria in several genera over a wide geographic area produce soft rot symptoms and cause serious

Phytopathogenic Prokaryotes, Vol. 2

Copyright © 1982 by Academic Press, Inc.
All rights of reproduction in any form reserved.

ISBN 0-12-509002-1

losses of food and other plant products. Recent estimations suggest that such losses may reach $50–$100 million annually on a world wide basis (Pérombelon and Kelman, 1980).

The dispersal of inoculum is of fundamental importance in the biology of soft rot bacteria, as with any plant disease. Research on the dispersal of bacteria, especially *Erwinia* spp., has been stimulated by the relatively recent evidence that these bacteria are not common inhabitants of soil, at least in temperate areas (DeBoer *et al.*, 1979; Graham and Harper, 1967; Lazar and Bucur, 1964; Logan, 1968; Naumann, 1976).

Production of *Erwinia*-free potato (*Solanum tuberosum* L.) seed stocks by stem cutting methods and the subsequent discovery that these clean stocks become recontaminated rapidly from unknown sources during propagation (Graham, 1976; Graham and Hardie, 1971; Pérombelon, 1976; Sampson, 1977) led to extensive investigations of *Erwinia* inoculum sources and means of dispersal. Several previously unknown or poorly understood means of dispersal have been studied, and an understanding of these mechanisms has helped to explain the contamination of clean stocks in the absence of soil-borne and tuber-borne inoculum. Unfortunately, no other soft rot bacteria have been studied as intensively as *Erwinia*. For other soft rot bacteria including *Clostridium*, *Pseudomonas*, and *Bacillus* the soil is also considered to be the main source of inoculum much as it was for *Erwinia* for many years.

II. DISPERSAL BY INSECTS

A. Importance

The importance of insects as dispersal agents for bacteria has become increasingly apparent in recent years (Harrison *et al.*, 1980). Previously it was believed that dispersal by insects was of importance only in those cases where (1) specialized relationships existed between the vector and the pathogen or, (2) where many insect species could act as vectors of a specific bacterium. For example, cucurbit wilt caused by *Erwinia tracheiphila* (Smith) Bergey *et al.* would not be an important pathogen without the close biological relationship between the bacterium and its beetle vectors *Acalymma vittata* (Fabricius) and *Diabrotica undecimpunctata howardi* Barber (Harrison *et al.*, 1980). Conversely, the fact that the fire blight bacterium *Erwinia amylovora* (Burrill) Winslow *et al.* is incidentally spread by 100 or more insect species contributes significantly to its importance as a pathogen (Harrison *et al.*, 1980).

It is now clear that a wide variety of insects can act as general vectors of bacteria, especially soft rot forms, mainly through incidental associations between the two types of organisms. For example, Kloepper *et al.*, (1979) demonstrated that contamination of insects with soft rot bacteria occurs commonly in areas where these diseases are found. These workers reported that 10 genera of 9 families of Diptera collected in the San Luis Valley region of Colorado were contaminated with either *Erwinia carotovora* subsp. *atroseptica* (van Hall) Dye (*Eca*) or *E. carotovora* subsp. *carotovora* (Jones) Bergey *et al.* (*Ecc*). The incidence of contaminated insects, collected from a variety of habitats, was highest in early spring, but decreased as the season progressed, probably as a result of declining inoculum abundance. Chiu *et al.* (1958) also reported that contaminated insects were abundant in Chinese cabbage (*Brassica oleracea* var. *capitata* L.) fields with 30–76% of five common insect species carrying *Ecc*. We expect that bacterial contamination on insects is probably common in nature, as suggested by the work of Gilbert (1980) who reported that fruit flies (*Drosophila* sp.) and some Hymenoptera were frequent carriers of bacteria in a forest situation.

It seems that virtually any insect group that commonly visits rotting vegetable material and healthy plants may act as vectors of soft rot bacteria. Of course, insects that are normally associated with specific crops are likely to be more important vectors than general insect visitors, particularly in crops where soft rot bacteria cause serious economic losses. It is now clear, however, that the great abundance of the nonspecific insect visitors makes them extremely important in the dispersal of soft rot bacteria.

B. Vector–Pathogen Relationships

As noted, most relationships between insects and soft rot bacteria are nonobligate and often largely incidental. In some cases insects are not even differentially attracted to soft rotted versus healthy plant material (Brewer *et al.*, 1980) but any insects that do visit an inoculum source become contaminated and are potential vectors. In only a few cases are there close biological relationships between insects and soft rot bacteria that are highly beneficial to one or both of the organisms involved. These close associations, however, result in increased success of both organisms and thus frequently cause serious economic losses. One example of such a close relationship is the association between the onion maggot *Hylemya antiqua* (Meigen) and soft rot of onions (*Allium cepa* L.) caused by *E. carotovora* (Jones) Bergey *et al.* The work of Friend *et al.*

(1959) suggests that these insects require bacteria to break down onion tissue for adequate nutrition since they did not survive on sterile onion tissue. The bacteria are transmitted to healthy plants via the eggs and larvae of *H. antiqua* and may also overwinter within the puparium.

In general, however, the associations between insects and bacteria have little value to the insects but aid dispersal and survival of the bacteria. Such aid may arise from one or more combinations of the following ways outlined by Harrison *et al.* (1980).

1. Insects may aid the survival of the bacterium. For example, *E. carotovora*, the causal agent of several soft rot diseases of vegetables including onion, lettuce (*Lactuca sativa* L.), celery (*Apium graveolens* var. *dulce* DC), and potato, as well as iris (*Iris* spp.), may survive within its insect vectors (Leach, 1940). More recently, we (Brewer *et al.*, 1981) reported that both *Ecc* and *Eca* survive internally in two insect vectors, *Drosophila melanogaster* Meigen and *D. busckii* Coquillet for 48 to 72 hr. These organisms survive only 2 hr or less in unprotected situations (Graham *et al.*, 1979). Insect protection may be especially valuable during adverse periods since these bacteria, like almost all other plant pathogens, do not possess a resistant stage (spores).
2. Insects may disseminate either the primary or secondary inoculum from diseased to healthy plants. *Drosophila melanogaster* and other Diptera have been shown to be effective vectors of *Ecc* and *Eca* to wounded, healthy potato plants in the laboratory and the field (Kloepper *et al.*, 1979, 1981; Molina *et al.*, 1974). Other examples of this association are discussed by Harrison *et al.* (1980).
3. Insects may provide wounds necessary for the entry of soft rot bacteria into healthy hosts. This relationship involves the wounding of the healthy plant by the insect, followed by invasion of bacteria from another source, or by those bacteria already on the plant. An example is the association between bacterial soft rot of iris caused by *E. carotovora* and transmitted by larvae of the iris borer moth *Macronoctua onusta* Grote. Apparently injuries caused by these larvae are necessary for entrance of the bacterium (Thanos, 1948) and control of the disease depends on effective insect control (Howard and Leach, 1962, 1963). Thanos (1948) suggested that the insect and bacteria were intimately associated, but it now seems probable that the larvae act mainly as a wounding agent, allowing entry of bacteria already present on the plant surface or in the soil debris (Harrison *et al.*, 1980).
4. Insects may help bacteria circumvent unfavorable environmental conditions. An example is heart rot of celery caused by *E. carotovora*, and transmitted by two species of Diptera, *Scaptomyza graminum* (Fal-

len) and *Elachiptera costata* (Lowe). During normal moist periods the insects deposit their eggs and the bacteria on the outer leaves of the plant where both survive well. During dry weather the insects consistently deposit their eggs, and the bacteria, on the inner leaves of the celery plant where both are better protected from drying, irradiation, and heat (Leach, 1927). The result is that the bacteria survive well during the dry adverse weather when they would not do so during such times on the outer leaves.

5. Insects may provide substrates for the growth of bacterial pathogens. This is reportedly the case in the coffee industry where a saprophytic species of *Xanthomonas* sometimes grows on substrates provided by fruit fly larvae on coffee (*Coffea arabica* L.) berries causing an objectionable odor in the product (Stolp, 1960).

C. Inoculum Sources

Much past research on insect dispersal of soft rot bacteria was based upon the premise that the soil was a primary source of inoculum (Leach, 1930). There are still unresolved questions about the nature of the soil–bacteria relationships of the *Erwinia* group, as discussed more completely later in this chapter. It now appears that in most areas, soil is not a general inoculum source for insect vectors of these bacteria except in cases where susceptible crops are grown continuously without rotation (Mew *et al.*, 1976). Soil may, however, be a major inoculum source for other soft rot bacteria including *Clostridium, Pseudomonas, Bacillus,* and others but little research has been conducted on insect transmission of these groups (Harrison *et al.*, 1980).

A major inoculum source for the soft rot bacteria of cultivated crops is probably cull piles, refuse dumps, and other areas where waste vegetable matter is discarded. Kloepper *et al.* (1979) surveyed the insect fauna from various habitats in the San Luis Valley region of Colorado for the presence of two varieties of *E. carotovora*. *Erwinia*-contaminated insects were collected from a variety of areas including settling ponds near potato warehouses, potato cull piles on growers' farms, municipal dumps, and growing crops of lettuce and potatoes. The predominant sources of *Erwinia* contamination, however, were the potato cull piles found in the vicinity of potato fields. These cull piles are probably also overwintering and/or breeding sites for several insect groups.

Harrison *et al.* (1977) found that 3–5% of the insects collected from potato cull piles in Scotland were contaminated with either *Ecc* or *Eca*. The same bacterial serotypes found on injured plants in an *Erwinia*-free potato crop in Scotland were isolated from insects collected from a nearby vegetable dump (Graham *et al.*, 1976).

Another potential inoculum source is the healthy plant itself. *Erwinia* cells may persist on potato foliage for considerable periods of time, and even increase in numbers in the presence of sufficient moisture (Harrison, 1980; Pérombelon, 1979a). These researchers working in Scotland (Pérombelon) and Colorado (Harrison) under greatly differing environmental conditions demonstrated that bacteria could be detected for weeks under some conditions. Insects seem to be attracted by any moisture, especially plant wounds exuding fluid (Graham *et al.*, 1976). Thus, the survival and/or reproduction of *Erwinia* cells on moist foliage could represent an important inoculum source that would be extremely attractive to potential insect vectors in those areas. Increasingly common overhead irrigation in many areas of the arid western United States increases the probability that these epiphytic bacteria are an important inoculum source.

Plant debris is another source of inoculum and one that probably accounts for the presence and survival of *Erwinia* in the soil. It has been estimated that up to 100,000 potato tubers/ha may remain in the field after harvest, many of which are likely to be infected with soft rot bacteria (Pérombelon, 1975). These scattered sources of inoculum may be utilized by insects for breeding sites in much the same way as cull piles.

Soft rot bacteria may also survive in association with volunteer plants of the infected crop and unless these plants are destroyed the bacteria they harbor will also survive. Studies have shown that diseased plants act as reservoirs of infection so that adjacent healthy plants become infected more often than those more distant (Pérombelon, 1973).

It seems clear from the foregoing considerations that much of the bacterial inoculum which is available for contaminating insect vectors could be avoided by better husbandry. At least inoculum levels and the incidence of insect transmission could be greatly reduced by more thorough sanitation, and better cultural and harvesting practices.

D. Distance

The distance over which insects transport soft rot bacteria probably varies considerably depending upon characteristics of the vector and the environmental conditions at the time dispersal occurs. Soil-inhabiting vectors like the seed corn maggot *Hylemya platura* (Meigen), that may transmit potato blackleg to potato seed pieces, probably are not involved in spread of the bacteria over substantial distances since the larvae do not travel far. Likewise, larvae of the iris borer *Macronoctua onusta* Grote that transmit soft rot of iris appear to be mainly involved in primary rather than secondary dissemination of the inoculum since Howard and Leach (1963) noted that borer larvae do not move readily from plant to plant.

In contrast, fruit flies, *Drosophila* spp., which are effective vectors of potato blackleg bacteria (Kloepper *et al.*, 1979, 1981; Molina *et al.*, 1974) are known to move considerable distances within a short period of time. For example, Yerington and Warner (1961) reported that *D. melanogaster* could travel up to 7 km upwind within 24 hr. Phillips and Kelman (1978) used a unique serotype of *Ecc* to test dissemination of blackleg bacteria by insects in Wisconsin. They inoculated potato tubers with this serotype and later demonstrated that it was present on insects, and on potato foliage and tubers in the field up to 26 m from the inoculum source. Kloepper *et al.* (1981) have reported data which strongly suggest that insects emerging from a potato cull pile can transmit potato blackleg bacteria to artificially injured potato plants as far as 183 m from the inoculum source (the maximum distance in the test). Brewer *et al.* (1981) demonstrated that the same bacterial strain could survive 48–72 hr inside the known vectors *Drosophila melanogaster* and *D. busckii* and for 24–48 hr on the exterior of these insects. These workers suggested that it would be possible for the blackleg bacteria to be transmitted up to 21 km from the inoculum source. Of course, much greater distances would be possible with the aid of the wind. Thus, potato blackleg could be theoretically spread from a few inoculum sources throughout a wide area by these insects in a very short time given the proper environmental conditions.

Among the large variety of insect species visiting decaying vegetable matter are some potential vectors which are more powerful fliers than *Drosophila* and consequently would probably disperse bacteria over even greater distances. No data are available on dispersal distances of various vectors of soft rot bacteria. However, distance of travel of insects is not associated necessarily with their flight capabilities since strong winds can increase the range of weak fliers considerably. For example, aphids seem to use their wings primarily to escape the quiet boundary layer of air next to plant and soil surfaces and then are transported long distances by the wind currents and it is possible that dipterous insects, the most common vectors of *Erwinia*, could do likewise.

It now seems probable that insects carry soft rot bacteria much further than has been considered possible in the past. What is certain is that soft rot bacteria survive for relatively long periods in association with at least some of the vectors, that these insects can move considerable distances, and many insects actively seek plant wounds. Together, these factors create an effective dispersal mechanism for soft rot bacteria.

E. Extent and Significance

The general opinion about the importance of insect dispersal of soft rot bacteria, especially *Erwinia,* has changed very greatly since the discovery that these bacteria are not commonly soil-borne. Much of the recent research on insect transmission of this group of bacteria has been concerned with *Erwinia* spp., especially those that cause potato blackleg (Harrison *et al.,* 1980). One reason for the intensive work in this area is that major efforts have been, and are still being, made to produce and maintain *Erwinia*-free potato seed stock. Thus any potential sources of recontamination are of major concern. The frequent occurrence of *Erwinia* contamination of aerial portions of potato plants in supposedly *Erwinia*-free fields (Graham, 1976; Graham and Hardie, 1971; Pérombelon, 1976; Sampson, 1977) suggests that insects carry these bacteria from some inoculum source to the seed stock. As discussed later in this chapter, some potato tubers may carry *Erwinia* infection without visible symptoms and large scale planting of such "disease-free" material could seriously damage the industry. Consequently, even low levels of insect dispersal of *Erwinia* in certain seed-producing areas could have serious consequences. Unfortunately, it appears from recent research that such dispersal is common (Graham *et al.,* 1976; Harrison *et al.,* 1977; Kloepper *et al.,* 1979) and can occur over relatively long distances (Kloepper *et al.,* 1981).

The fact that many of the insect species involved have been commonly observed at moist plant wounds suggests that the vectors are efficient in locating such wounds. This behavioral pattern is important since many insects that occur in crop situations do not cause plant wounds and might not normally be considered potential vectors. Such insects, however, may be very effective vectors if plants have been wounded (Kloepper *et al.,* 1981), and many crops subject to attack by soft rot bacteria are also very susceptible to injury by hail or high winds, and perhaps more importantly, by machinery during normal cultural operations. Insect visitation of moist wounds is very common in the arid western United States but it appears that even in humid areas insects also frequently visit such wounds. In Wisconsin, for example, heavy outbreaks of blackleg bacteria in the aerial portions of potato plants have occurred following hail damage. These outbreaks were associated with the presence of various species of *Diptera* carrying soft rot erwinias (A. Kelman and K. Chapman, unpublished).

The potential damage of insect–bacterial associations is emphasized by our data (Brewer *et al.*, 1981) which suggest that under the proper environmental conditions *Drosophila* spp. could distribute *Erwinia* throughout the potato seed producing region of Colorado from a few inoculum sources in a matter of weeks.

It seems very likely that insects are important dispersal agents for soft rot bacteria in most if not all potato growing regions of the world. Insects are probably most important in the initial reintroduction of *Erwinia* into *Erwinia*-free crops. The likelihood of gross recontamination of crops by insects seems slight but after introduction the bacteria could multiply and then be spread rapidly during harvesting and handling operations. Although relatively little information is available at present on insects as vectors of soft rot bacteria in other crops, they are probably responsible for substantial levels of bacterial transmission to above ground plant structures.

The incidence of successful disease transmission could be greatly reduced through minor changes in cultural and sanitation practices. As one example, the elimination of vegetable cull piles would reduce the number of insects available as potential vectors, since these areas are major breeding sites, and at the same time would eliminate a major inoculum source of the soft rot bacteria. Such measures would be impractical if the soil were a major source of inoculum as was once believed; since it is not, efforts should be made to promote these and other control procedures among growers.

III. DISPERSAL IN AEROSOLS

A. Occurrence

Dispersal of bacterial plant pathogens by rainsplash and windblown rain has been recognized for many years but the importance of their dispersal in aerosols has only been recognized since 1973 (Graham and Harrison, 1975; Pérombelon and Lowe, 1973; Venette and Kennedy, 1975). The recognition that bacteria can be airborne as aerosols over a significant distance has introduced a new dimension to soft rot epidemiology. Currently only four species of phytopathogenic bacteria, *E. carotovora* (Quinn *et al.*, 1980; Pérombelon *et al.*, 1979), *Pseudomonas syringae* pv. *glycinea* (Coerper) Young *et al.* (Venette and Kennedy, 1975), *Xanthomonas campestris* pv. *phaseoli* (Erw. Smith) Dye (Venette, 1979), and *Pseudomonas syringae* pv. *phaseolicola* (Burkholder) Young *et al.* (Venette, 1979) have been shown to be dispersed in aerosols. Undoubtedly other species will be added to the list as this dispersal mechanism is investigated more fully.

Among the soft rot bacteria, aerosol dispersal has been investigated only for *Erwinia*. Studies with *Ecc* and *Eca* have been quite intensive and the phenomenon is reasonably well understood for these organisms. *Erwinia* aerosols are commonly present in the atmosphere, especially in cool, moist environments, and they are very probably responsible for at least some recontamination of *Erwinia*-free potato seed crops (Graham, 1976; Graham and Harrison, 1975; Graham *et al.*, 1979; Harrison, 1980; Pérombelon, 1979a,b; Pérombelon *et al.*, 1979).

B. Generation

Two mechanisms are known by which *Erwinia* aerosols are produced: (1) the impact of water drops (raindrops or drops from overhead sprinklers) on infected plant material (Graham and Harrison, 1975; Quinn *et al.*, 1980; Harrison, 1980), and (2) the mechanical pulverization (beating) of potato stems and leaves prior to harvesting (Pérombelon, 1979a, Pérombelon *et al.*, 1979).

Extensive sampling of air in the field in Scotland and the United States has shown that *Erwinia* aerosols are commonly generated by these mechanisms. In Colorado (Harrison, unpublished; Harrison, 1980) air samples collected down wind from potato crops during the operation of overhead sprinklers during four growing seasons have shown both *Ecc* and *Eca* are present in the air even in a dry climate. The bacteria are present most often during the night and morning hours when the weather is cool and humid and they appear most commonly after August 10. Similar but more extensive sampling in Scotland by Quinn *et al.* (1980) from August 1977 to October 1979 showed *Ecc* and *Eca* occur regularly in the air, often in relatively high numbers, during and immediately after rainfall from July until the end of the year. No viable cells were ever collected during dry periods. These studies support the view that the impact of water drops on infected tissue is a major generator of *Erwinia* aerosols. The amount of aerosol in the air is related to the intensity of rainfall and *Erwinia* populations in the air decline rapidly when rainfall ceases (Quinn *et al.*, 1980). Pérombelon (1977) and Pérombelon *et al.* (1979) likewise showed that *Erwinia* aerosols could regularly be detected downwind from potato crops being mechanically pulverized.

In all cases, regardless of the mechanism by which *Erwinia* aerosols are generated, *Ecc* has been collected more commonly than *Eca* from the air in the field. The reasons for the predominance of *Ecc* are not clear except that *Ecc* seems to survive better than *Eca* under poor conditions (see below).

C. Survival, Dispersal, and Deposition

The generation of aerosols has little epidemiological significance unless the cells remain viable sufficiently long to be dispersed a significant distance and deposited on susceptible crops. Considerable effort has therefore been made to determine the ability of *Erwinia* cells to survive in aerosols under different environmental conditions. When survival was studied by Graham *et al.* (1979) and Pérombelon and associates (1979) using "captive aerosol" techniques in which cells are deposited on spiders' webbing and exposed to the environment, it was found that the aerosolized cells survived much better than previously thought. Up to 50% of the aerosolized *Erwinia* population can survive for 5–10 min under temperature and moisture conditions which are common in the field in many parts of the world (18°C and 65% RH). Under more favorable conditions (12–12.5°C and 86–90% RH with rain falling) approximately 10% of the population remained viable for 1 hr and numbers of viable cells were still present after 2 hr. The bacteria survive poorly during warm dry periods and *Ecc* survives better than *Eca* in less favorable environments. Thus viable cells are present in the air for sufficient time to be dispersed considerable distances by light to moderate winds. In fact, Graham *et al.* (1977) and Pérombelon *et al.* (1979) concluded that viable cells could be easily carried for several hundred meters by the wind.

Detailed laboratory studies using simulated raindrops and pulverized material in the specialized chamber described by Graham and Harrison (1975) have shown that 10^8 *Erwinia* cells/ha could be generated by either mechanism from a crop containing only 2% visibly infected plants (Graham *et al.*, 1977; Pérombelon *et al.*, 1979).

The atmospheric diffusion and deposition models of Gregory (1945, 1961, 1973), Pasquill (1961), and Chamberlain (1953) show that when this number of cells is present in the air, a significant number of cells could be deposited on potato foliage as far as 100–1000 m downwind from the source (Graham *et al.*, 1977; Pérombelon *et al.*, 1979). Pérombelon *et al.* (1979) calculated that $\sim 10^2$ cells/m^2 would be deposited on potato foliage 100 m downwind from a source of 10^8 bacterial cells, and many fewer cells ($\sim$1–5/m^2 at 1000 m and $\sim$0.1 cells/m^2 at 10,000 m) would be deposited at greater distances. Thus, it appears that an effective dispersal distance of *at least* 100 m is probable and distances much greater than this are possible depending on the prevailing atmospheric conditions.

Field experience has shown that viable *Erwinia* cells can be detected in the air as much as 183 m downwind from overhead sprinklers in Colorado (Harrison, 1980) and at least 800 m away from known *Erwinia* sources (potato crops) in Scotland (C. E. Quinn, personal communication). In fact, large numbers of viable *Erwinia* cells have been captured from the air during times of the year or in locations in Scotland when no potato crops could be found in the vicinity of the sampling site (Quinn *et al.* 1980).

In summation, it appears from the considerable accumulated data that *Erwinia carotovora* can be dispersed substantial distances in aerosols, especially in cool, moist climates and also in warmer, drier climates during times of the day favorable for cell survival.

D. Extent and Significance

All attempts to monitor the presence of airborne viable *Erwinia* cells in the vicinity of sources of bacteria (primarily potato crops) have met with surprising success regardless of the precise sampling location. Since bacteria can be regularly found in the air in wet (Quinn *et al.*, 1980) as well as dry climates (Harrison, 1980), aerosol dispersal may have considerable significance in soft rot epidemiology. This coupled with the facts that significant numbers of cells can be present at least 100 m (and probably further) downwind from their source and that known *Erwinia* serotypes released upwind from *Erwinia*-free crops (or present in surrounding crops) have subsequently been isolated from the tubers harvested from the clean crop provide compelling evidence for the significance of this means of dispersal (Graham *et al.*, 1979; Lapwood, 1976; Quinn *et al.*, 1980).

Aerosol dispersal creates severe problems for achieving isolation of healthy from diseased crops to prevent contamination during propagation. In few major potato-producing areas is it possible to provide at least 100 m isolation from other potato fields.

Important questions regarding the significance of aerosol dispersal of soft rot erwinias have been raised in two major areas. First, since relatively few viable cells may be introduced per unit area into fields located moderate distances downwind from the bacterial source, there may not be enough cells to establish infection. Second, the chance for cells being deposited on injured tissues is small and the survival of cells deposited on uninjured tissues may be too short to result in a threat to a crop. *Erwinia* cells deposited on potato stems and leaves in the field persist for considerable periods of time and even increase in numbers during wet periods (Harrison, 1980; Pérombelon, 1979a). Viable cells could be detected for at least 7 weeks after deposition in relatively cool and moist Scotland and for at least 10–15 days under warm and dry conditions in Colorado. This suggests that a few cells deposited from aerosols could survive and perhaps increase in numbers in the interim and pose a significant threat when infection courts become available due to injury, tuber harvesting, etc. Furthermore, it has been shown that marked strains of *Erwinia* applied to the surface of potato plants in the field in September can be detected in tubers harvested from the crop in October (Pérombelon, 1979a).

Thus current evidence indicates that *Erwinia* can be carried considerable distances in aerosols, deposited on potato foliage in sufficient numbers to survive and reach the developing tubers by being washed off the foliage and into the soil where they penetrate lenticels or wounds. This means of contamination is probably very significant for reintroducing the pathogen to *Erwinia*-free crops. Once this has been accomplished, spread within the field may occur rapidly depending on various factors such as atmospheric conditions, the activity of insects, and the use of agricultural implements.

The role of aerosols as a means of dispersing other soft rot bacteria has not been investigated but we expect this means of spread to be significant.

IV. DISPERSAL THROUGH SOIL

A. Occurrence

As in the case of aerosol dispersal, little is known about the dispersal of soft rot bacteria through soil except for the genus *Erwinia,* apart from the fact that these organisms all have a soil phase and some like pectolytic *Pseudomonas* spp., *Bacillus* spp., and *Clostridium* spp. can commonly be isolated from the soil.

The relationship of *E. carotovora* to soil and its dispersal through this medium has attracted considerable attention for many years. Whereas the issue of the soil-borne nature (or lack thereof) of *Erwinia* is not yet resolved, the bulk of the recent evidence indicates that in most temperate regions where 2 to 5 or more year rotations with nonsusceptible crops are practiced, *Erwinia* is not a soil inhabitant. Rather it is a transient invader which survives in detectable numbers for relatively short periods of time (Burr and Schroth, 1977; De Boer *et al.* 1979; Graham,

1958; Lazar and Bucur, 1964; Logan, 1968; Pérombelon and Lowe, 1970; Voronkovich, 1960). With few exceptions *Erwinia* can be isolated from field soils only during the season following the production of a susceptible crop such as potatoes (De Boer *et al.*, 1979) and then only occasionally. In circumstances where susceptible crops are grown continuously in certain fields *Erwinia* appears to be present more or less constantly (Mew *et al.*, 1976).

Erwinia are introduced into the soil when contaminated seed tubers are planted. Bacterial decay of the mother tubers releases large numbers of cells into the soil. The bacteria are then dispersed through the soil and contaminate progeny tubers on the same plant and those adjacent to it, extending the degree of contamination in a crop (Pérombelon, 1974). Spread may occur for some distance from a rotting tuber along potato rows (Lapwood 1976); bacteria have been isolated at least 1–3 m from their source (Graham and Harper, 1967; Pérombelon and Lowe, 1971). Graham and Harper (1967) have suggested that they may be dispersed considerably longer distances under certain conditions.

B. Means of Dispersal

1. Water Movement

Although *Erwinia* cells, for which the bulk of the data regarding movement in the soil has been developed, are motile, this probably plays no significant role in their dispersal in the soil. The only likely means by which viable cells could be moved quickly for a meter or more and contaminate large percentages of progeny tubers is with the soil water (Graham and Harper, 1967; Harris and Lapwood, 1977; Pérombelon, 1976; Pérombelon *et al.*, 1976). Since *Erwinia* cells are apparently located superficially on soil particles (Kikumoto and Sakamoto, 1969) they are probably easily removed by water moving through the soil and thus redistributed. Water suspensions of cells move readily with the water passing upward in a dry soil column, but do not move in a saturated column (Pérombelon, 1973) thus emphasizing the need for moving water to disperse the cells widely. Pérombelon (1973, 1976) showed clearly that *Erwinia* move downward in the soil as they are leached from rotting tubers during rainy periods, then are redistributed into the upper levels of the soil (and uniformly in the hill) as the surface of the soil dries and water is redistributed by evapotranspiration forces.

Distribution of *Erwinia* cells within the potato hills during dry periods was discontinuous but they were generally in the vicinity of the rotting mother tubers demonstrating the importance of water in the distribution of bacteria. This same movement of water through the soil probably results in the movement of cells along rows for considerable distances but the precise distances that *Erwinia* and cells of other soft rot bacteria can be dispersed in this way is not known. The studies performed to date (Graham and Harper, 1967; Harris and Lapwood, 1977; Lapwood, 1976; Pérombelon and Lowe, 1971) have all been done in areas where rainfall is the sole source of moisture. No definitive studies have been done in areas where irrigation (especially surface or row irrigation) is common to determine how far viable cells of soft rot bacteria can be dispersed when large volumes of water are applied regularly in this way.

2. *Dispersal by Soil Organisms*

Movement of bacterial cells through the soil by water is obviously the most important mechanism by which dispersal for significant distances occurs. There are, however, other possible means by which soil dispersal can occur which may be significant in soft epidemiology. Soil fauna including earthworms (Pérombelon and Lowe, 1970) and nematodes (Chantanao and Jensen, 1969; Thorne, 1961) may be contaminated with soft rot bacteria, especially *Erwinia*. The bacteria can, at least in some cases, pass through the intestinal tracts of nematodes in a viable condition and be deposited in the soil with feces (Chantanao and Jensen, 1969). Although these animals do not move long distances in the soil they could perhaps be responsible for introducing soft rot bacteria into "clean" areas of fields where they could be more widely dispersed by soil water or other means. They could also be responsible for dispersing bacteria across field rows more effectively than water (Lapwood, 1976). This mechanism could result in the introduction of bacteria into *Erwinia*-free crops planted adjacent to contaminated crops or soils when adequate separation is not provided.

C. Extent and Significance

The movement of soft rot bacteria (especially *Erwinia* spp.) through the soil is an extremely important phenomenon which must occur in all parts of the world where crops are grown. When environmental conditions favor survival of *Erwinia* cells in soil (cool, moist conditions) movement of the bacterium through the soil, especially by water, can result in 100% contamination of developing daughter tubers. The soil provides a medium through which dispersal from plant to plant can readily occur. Thus, if a few individual plants become infected from distant sources via aerosols or insects, etc., contamination of adjacent plants via the soil bridge is practically unavoidable if conditions favor bacterial survival and movement.

V. DISPERSAL BY CULTURAL PRACTICES

A. Occurrence

Like most bacterial pathogens, spread of soft rot bacteria occurs during seed handling, planting, cultivation, irrigation, and harvesting operations. Little is known about the importance of cultural operations in the spread of soft rots caused by other bacteria. Therefore, discussion will be restricted to this genus. Several common field operations have been implicated in *Erwinia* transmission.

B. Mechanisms

1. Dispersal on Machinery

Seed potato tubers are subject to extensive mechanical manipulation during the planting, harvesting, sorting, and storing operations. Considerable information has been accumulated showing that *Erwinia* bacteria are commonly dispersed during these operations. The potato tuber is the major source of *Erwinia* inoculum (Graham and Hardie, 1971; Pérombelon, 1974), thus machines used for handling seed potatoes are commonly contaminated with the organism and contribute to the spread from contaminated seed sources to *Erwinia*-free ones. Potato seed cutters used commonly in North America are especially important means of dispersing the bacteria since they not only serve as sources of inoculum but also deposit it directly onto wounded tuber surfaces. In Colorado (M. D. Harrison, unpublished data), all seed cutters sampled were extensively contaminated with *Erwinia* cells as were high percentages of the seed potatoes cut by these machines. Similarly, other potato handling or cultivating equipment including graders and elevators (Graham and Hardie, 1971), harvesting equipment (Graham and Harper, 1967; Maas Geesteranus, 1972), tractor and sprayer wheels (Graham and Hardie, 1971; Naumann, 1976), and probably also planting equipment, especially that used to handle cut seed pieces, are contaminated with *Erwinia* and contribute to contamination of potato crops. All of these mechanical operations not only provide inoculum sources via surface contamination, but also create wounds on tubers facilitating entry and establishment of the pathogen.

Even though *Erwinia* apparently does not survive for long periods on contaminated harvesting and field preparation machinery (Ficke *et al.*, 1973a) it certainly survives for sufficient time (up to 2 weeks) to be a significant factor in the spread of the organism. *Erwinia* may survive for longer periods of time on machinery stored in protected locations where the bacteria are not exposed to sunlight and other adverse environmental conditions especially if the cells are protected by soil and machine parts. Graham and Quinn (unpublished data) showed that graders remained contaminated for up to 100 days after use when housed in a dark shed. Further investigations should be made into this aspect of *Erwinia* epidemiology.

2. *Dispersal on Plant Parts and Seeds*

The extensive movement of seeds and vegetatively propagated plant material from country to country or from farm to farm represents a major means by which soft rot bacteria are dispersed over considerable distances. The association of soft rot bacteria with true seed is not common. Sands *et al.* (1976) reported that *Ecc* cells could be isolated from tobacco (*Nicotiana tabacum* L.) seed stored up to 5 months, but there are no additional data which suggest that seed contamination is common.

The regular association of soft rot bacteria with vegetative plant parts used for propagation has undoubtedly resulted in widespread dispersal around the world. This association is best understood for *Erwinia* spp. associated with potato tubers. It is well known that large percentages of seed potatoes can harbor *Erwinia* cells for long periods without developing soft rot symptoms (De Boer and Kelman, 1978; Ficke *et al.*, 1973b; Graham and Hardie, 1971; Pérombelon, 1972). When such seed stocks are shipped from location to location, the bacteria are introduced into new areas. Such latent infections are difficult to detect and usually pass unnoticed until problems develop in the growing crop.

3. *Dispersal by Irrigation Water*

In regions where crops are irrigated, the potential for dispersal of soft rot bacteria is great. As mentioned earlier water provides an ideal long-range dispersal medium since during transport bacterial cells are not exposed to unfavorable conditions such as desiccation and irradiation.

When diseased tissue is exposed to moving water, bacterial cells are released into the water. The extent to which this happens in the case of bacterial soft rots in the field is generally unknown. Studies in Japan (Goto, 1979) have shown that *Erwinia chrysanthemi* Burkeholder *et al.* infection in rice (*Oryza sativa* L.) is readily and quickly spread from a few infected plants in a field plot to a high percentage of the healthy population via irrigation. This phenomenon probably also occurs in the case of other soft rot diseases in irrigated crops but no definite data are available.

The recent discovery that *Erwinia* (especially *Ecc*) can be regularly isolated from a large percentage of lakes, streams, reservoirs, and ditches in arable areas as well as in remote locations where susceptible crops are not grown, in Scotland and the United States (M. C. M. Pérombelon, personal communication; Graham *et al.*, unpublished data; McCarter-Zorner, 1980; McCarter-Zorner *et al.*, 1983) adds a new dimension to soft rot epidemiology. This suggests that when water from such contaminated sources is used to irrigate susceptible crops, bacteria are being applied also. These organisms could be available to cause disease when appropriate infection courts were available if they become established in the rhizospheres of appropriate plants. Research on this source of inoculum is in progress and the full significance of irrigation water as a source of inoculum and means of dispersal will not be known until it is completed.

C. Extent and Significance

Dispersal of soft rot bacteria by contaminated machinery and equipment and with contaminated vegetative propagation material is widespread and important. Although these means of dispersal are widely recognized, it has proved to be difficult to eliminate them and dispersal continues to be a serious problem. Complicated equipment required for large sale production of potatoes and other vegetables has proved impossible to disinfect completely. Even high pressure washing followed by the application of disinfectants failed to totally eliminate *Erwinia* (M. D. Harrison and G. D. Franc, unpublished data). No doubt this will continue to be a means of contaminating *Erwinia*-free stocks and spreading the bacteria rapidly within and among seed stocks until better machinery designs to facilitate more effective cleaning and disinfecting or more effective chemical disinfectants, or both, are available. Contaminated vegetative planting materials pose an especially difficult problem for growers since bacterial infections in such materials are often latent and detectable only by special and time-consuming laboratory procedures. Until clean stocks are much more widely available or until rapid, accurate, practical diagnostic procedures are developed to detect contaminated planting stocks, contaminated planting materials will continue to be a significant source of organisms and an efficient means of dispersing bacteria for long distances.

The potential significance of the presence of soft rot erwinias in streams and reservoirs which serve as sources of irrigation water cannot yet be fully appreciated. The final analysis of this inoculum source and dispersal means must await the results of current research. The widespread use of irrigation, however, for production of soft rot susceptible crops provides some indication of its possible consequences. Serious outbreaks of bacterial stalk rot of corn (*Zea mays* L.) in North Carolina and Wisconsin occurred only in crops irrigated by overhead sprinklers using water pumped from farm ponds and streams, suggesting that water dispersal of soft rotting organisms may be very important (Hoppe and Kelman, 1969; Kelman *et al.*, 1957). Water was not proved to be the source of the pathogen in these cases, since it is possible that overhead irrigation merely acted as a predisposing agent to bacterial infection. Whether or not soft rot organisms are present in water pumped from deep or shallow wells is vitally important and needs to be answered in the immediate future.

VI. OTHER MEANS OF DISPERSAL

The only other means of dispersal of soft rot bacteria in the field besides those discussed above is the possible dispersal of *Erwinia* by birds. Feare *et al.* (1974) and Graham and Hardie (1971) suggested that rooks (*Corvur frugillegus* L.) may be responsible for some dispersal of *Erwinia* in the field. This means of dispersal may be one way by which the bacteria can be introduced into *Erwinia*-free seed stocks. These birds feed on rotting seed and developing tubers around mid-summer when other sources of food become scarce. There is observational evidence which indicates that the birds attack *Erwinia*-infected plots preferentially (D. C. Graham, personal communication). Since they also feed on healthy developing tubers it is probable that they do introduce bacteria into *Erwinia*-free stocks and establish infection foci for bacterial spread. The full extent and significance of this means of dispersal are unknown.

VII. SUMMARY

Soft rot bacteria, in particular *Erwinia*, are dispersed in the field by a variety of mechanisms. A large number of insects, particularly Diptera, have been shown to be important vectors of these bacteria, although in general the association between insects and bacteria is an incidental one. Insects spread soft rot bacteria within individual fields but they are probably most important in the initial introduction of the pathogens into disease-free areas. The fact that insects breed and/or overwinter in cull piles which also act as inoculum sources greatly increases the probability of such insects being important disease vectors.

Viable cells of these bacteria are also dispersed in aerosols in both moist and dry climates. Current research on potato soft rots indicates that bacterial cells can be carried considerable distances and still establish infection in healthy plants. Aerosol dispersal has thus become a significant factor in the epidemiology of soft rot in potatoes and probably in other crops as well.

Soil dispersal of bacterial soft rot pathogens is thought to occur mainly by the action of water movement and to some extent by soil invertebrates. The evidence suggests that bacterial cells are moved by soil water and this is probably the most important means of dispersal for significant distances through the soil. Water movement seems to account for bacterial dispersal in potato hills and probably is the mechanism involved in transport of pathogens for considerable distances along rows. Soil fauna, including earthworms and nematodes, are known to be contaminated with viable cells of soft rotting bacteria and may be responsible for some movement through the soil, especially across rows where water movement is thought to be less effective.

One of the most important means of dispersing soft rot bacteria is through cultural practices. These bacteria are spread during seed handling, planting, cultivation, irrigation, and harvesting operations. In one instance, 100% of the potato seed cutting machinery examined was contaminated with soft rot bacteria. Dispersal by such machines and other cultural practices increases the difficulty of controlling their spread.

Additional research is needed on all of the mechanisms of bacterial dispersal discussed above. It is especially important, however, to determine the role of airborne aerosols in the spread of these pathogens. This is most important, perhaps, in areas where irrigation is commonly practiced since application methods and water quantities could possibly be modified to reduce aerosol formation. The role of insects as vectors of these pathogens also needs further study, especially as disease spread is related to natural and man-caused plant injuries. The role of water movement, particularly irrigation water, in dispersal of bacterial pathogens also needs further research. Lastly, research on, and development of crop handling machinery that does not contribute to the spread of disease, or which can be efficiently disinfected, is desperately needed.

Acknowledgments

We gratefully acknowledge the careful reviews and constructive suggestions of Ms. Laura Merrill, the University of California, Berkeley, Ms. Mary Hathaway, Harvard University, Ms. Mary Walmsley, Drs. W. Don Fronk, Joseph Hill, and Gary McIntyre, Colorado State University, and Dr. D. C. Graham and Mr. C. E. Quinn, Department of Agriculture and Fisheries for Scotland, Edinburgh. We also wish to express our sincere appreciation to Ms. Jane Wilkins and Ms. Nancy Flaming for careful editing and typing of this manuscript.

References

Brewer, J. W., Harrison, M. D., and Winston, J. A. (1980). *Am. Potato J.* **57,** 219–224.

Brewer, J. W., Harrison, M. D., and Winston, J. A. (1981). *Am. Potato J.* **58,** 339–349.

Burr, T. J., and Schroth, M. N. (1977). *Phytopathology* **76,** 1382–1387.

Chamberlain, A. C. (1953). *Atom. Energy Res. Estab. Rep.* AERE/HP/R 1261, pp. 1–28. London, HMSO.

Chantano, A., and Jensen, J. H. (1969). *J. Nematol.* **1,** 216–218.

Chiu, W. F., Yuen, C. S., and Wu, C. A. (1958). *Acta Phytopathol. Sin.* **4,** 8–15 (In Chinese; original not seen. Cited from Pérombelon, M., and Kelman, A. (1980). *Annu. Rev. Phytopathol.* **18,** 361–387.)

De Boer, S. H., and Kelman, A. (1978). *Potato Res.* **21,** 65–80.

De Boer, S. H., Allan, E., and Kelman, A. (1979). *Am. Potato J.* **56,** 243–252.

Feare, C. J., Dennet, G. M., and Patterson, I. J. (1974). *J. Appl. Ecol.* **11,** 867–914.

Ficke, W., Skadow, K., Muller, H. H., Naumann, K., and Zielke, R. (1973a). *Arch. Phytopathol. Pflanzenschutz* **9,** 371–381. [Abstract in *Rev. Plant Pathol.* **53** (4101), 1974.]

Ficke, W., Naumann, K., Skadow, K., Muller, H. J., and Zielke, R. (1973b). *Arch. Phytopathol. Pflanzenschutz* **9,** 281–293. [Abstract in *Rev. Plant Pathol.* **53** (3597), 1974.]

Friend, W. G., Salkeld, E. H., and Stevenson, I. L. (1959). *Ann. N.Y. Acad. Sci.* **77,** 384–393.

Gilbert, D. C. (1980). *Oecologia* **46,** 135–137.

Goto, M. (1979). *Plant Dis. Rep.* **63,** 100–103.

Graham, D. C. (1958). *Nature (London)* **181,** 61.

Graham, D. C. (1976). *EPPO Bull.* **6**(4), 243–245.

Graham, D. C., and Hardie, J. L. (1971). *Proc. Br. Insectic. Fungic. Conf., 6th* **1,** 219–224.

Graham, D. C., and Harper, P. C. (1967). *Scott. Agric.* **46,** 68–74.

Graham, D. C., and Harrison, M. D. (1975). *Phytopathology* **65,** 739–741.

Graham, D. C., Quinn, C. E., and Harrison, M. D. (1976). *Potato Res.* **19,** 3–20.

Graham, D. C., Quinn, C. E., and Bradley, L. F. (1977). *J. Appl. Bacteriol.* **43,** 413–424.

Graham, D. C., Quinn, C. E., Sells, I. A., and Harrison, M. D. (1979). *J. Appl. Bacteriol.* **46,** 367–376.

Gregory, P. H. (1945). *Trans. Br. Mycol. Soc.* **28,** 26–72.

Gregory, P. H. (1961). "The Microbiology of the Atmosphere." Hill, London.

Gregory, P. H. (1973). "The Microbiology of the Atmosphere," 2nd ed. Hill, London.

Harris, R. I., and Lapwood, D. H. (1977). *Potato Res.* **20,** 285–294.

Harrison, M. D. (1980). *Ann. N.Y. Acad. Sci.* **353,** 94–104.

Harrison, M. D., Quinn, C. E., Sells, I. A., and Graham, D. C. (1977). *Potato Res.* **20,** 37–52.

Harrison, M. D., Brewer, J. W., and Merrill, L. (1980). *In* "Vectors of Plant Pathogens" (K. F. Harris and K. Maramorosch, eds.). Academic Press, New York.

Hoppe, P. E., and Kelman, A. (1969). *Plant Dis. Rep.* **53,** 66–70.
Howard, C. M., and Leach, J. G. (1962). Phytopathology **52,** 1219 (Abstr.).
Howard, C. M., and Leach, J. G. (1963). *Phytopathology* **53,** 1190–1193.
Kelman, A., Person, L. H., and Hebert, T. T. (1957). *Plant Dis. Rep.* **41,** 798–802.
Kikumoto, T., and Sakamoto, M. (1969). *Ann. Phytopathol. Soc. Jpn.* **35,** 29–35.
Kloepper, J. W., Harrison, M. D., and Brewer, J. W. (1979). *Am. Potato J.* **56,** 351–361.
Kloepper, J. W., Brewer, J. W., and Harrison, M. D. (1981). *Am. Potato J.* **58,** 165–175.
Lapwood, D. H. (1976). *Bull. OEPP* **6,** 237–239.
Lazar, I., and Bucur, E. L. (1964). *Eur. Potato J.* **7,** 102–111.
Leach, J. G. (1927). *Phytopathology* **17,** 663–667.
Leach, J. G. (1930). *Phytopathology* **20,** 215–228.
Leach, J. G. (1940). "Insect Transmission of Plant Diseases." McGraw-Hill, New York.
Logan, C. (1968). *Rec. Agric. Res. Minist. Agric. North Ireland* **17,** 115–121.
McCarter-Zorner, N. J. (1980). M.Sc. thesis, Colorado State University.
McCarter-Zorner, N. J., Franc, G. D., Harrison, M. D., Quinn, C. E., Sells, J. A., and Graham, D. C. (1983). In preparation.
Maas Geesteranus, H. P. (1972). *Bedrijfsontwikkeling* **3,** 941–945.
Mew, T. W., Ho, W. C., and Chu, L. (1976). *Phytopathology* **66,** 1325–1327.
Molina, J. J., Harrison, M. D., and Brewer, J. W. (1974). *Am. Potato J.* **51,** 245–250.
Naumann, K. (1976). *Tagungsber. Akad. Landwirtschaftswiss DDR* **140,** 139–148.
Pasquill, F. (1961). *Met. Mag.* **90,** 33–49.
Pérombelon, M. C. M. (1972). *Ann. Appl. Biol.* **71,** 111–117.
Pérombelon, M. C. M. (1973). Ph.D. thesis, Dundee University, Dundee, Scotland.
Pérombelon, M. C. M. (1974). *Potato Res.* **17,** 187–199.
Pérombelon, M. C. M. (1975). *Potato Res.* **18,** 205–219.
Pérombelon, M. C. M. (1976). *Phytopathol. Z.* **85,** 97–116.
Pérombelon, M. C. M. (1977). *Proc. Symp. Probl. Pest Dis. Control Br., Invergowrie, Dundee,* pp. 39–40.
Pérombelon, M. C. M. (1979a). *Proc. Int. Conf. Plant Pathol. Bacteriol., 4th, Angers,* pp. 563–565.
Pérombelon, M. C. M. (1979b). *Proc. Int. Conf. Plant Pathog. Bact., 4th, Angers,* pp. 749–752.
Pérombelon, M. C. M., and Kelman, A. (1980). *Annu. Rev. Phytopathol.* **18,** 361–387.
Pérombelon, M. C. M., and Lowe, R. (1970). *Rep. Scott. Hortic. Res. Inst. 1969,* pp. 31–32.
Pérombelon, M. C. M., and Lowe, R. (1971). *Rep. Scott. Hortic. Res. Inst. 1970,* pp. 50–51.
Pérombelon, M. C. M., and Lowe, R. (1973). *Rep. Scott. Hortic. Res. Inst. 1972,* pp. 52–53.
Pérombelon, M. C. M., Lowe, R., and Ballantine, E. M. (1976). *Potato Res.* **19,** 335–347.
Pérombelon, M. C. M., Fox, R. A., and Lowe, R. (1979). *Phytopathol. Z.* **94,** 249–260.
Phillips, J. A., and Kelman, A. (1978). *Am. Potato J.* **55,** 389 (Abstr.).
Quinn, C. E., Sells, I. A., and Graham, D. C. (1980). *J. App. Bacteriol.* **49,** 175–181.
Sampson, P. J. (1977). *Am. Potato J.* **54,** 1–9.
Sands, D. C., McIntyre, J. L., and Taylor, G. (1976). *Proc. Am. Phytopathol. Soc.* **3,** 270 (Abstr.).
Stolp, H. (1960). *Phytopathol. Z.* **39,** 1–15.
Thanos, A. (1948). M.Sc. thesis, West Virginia University, Morgantown.
Thorne, G. (1961). "Principles of Nematology." McGraw-Hill, New York.

Venette, J. R. (1979). *Proc. Conf. Bean Improve. Coop. Natl. Dry Bean Council* pp. 80–81.
Venette, J. R., and Kennedy, B. W. (1975). *Phytopathology* **65**, 737–738.
Voronkovich, I. V. (1960). *Bull. Soc. Nat. Moscow (Biol.)* **65**, 95 (In Russian) (Abstract in *Rev. Appl. Mycol.* **40**, 202, 1961).
Yerington, A. O., and Warner, R. W. (1961). *J. Econ. Entomol.* **54**, 425–428.

Chapter **3**

The Impaired Host and Soft Rot Bacteria

M. C. M. PÉROMBELON

I. INTRODUCTION

Soft rot bacteria have many hosts with a worldwide distribution. They are economically important because of the crop loss they can cause both in the field and after harvest in transit and in storage. They mainly damage parenchymatous tissue which they rot by macerating agents (pectic enzymes) and the nature of the symptoms often depends on the organ attacked. On some crops, the symptom is not primarily a rot but a general stunting and wilting caused by attacks on below-ground parts of the plant. Wilting may also be caused by direct attack on the stems but it is not clear whether stunting and wilting are caused by the action of pectic enzymes alone and/or by toxins produced by the bacteria. Undoubtedly the action of pectic enzymes is the dominant cause of symptom expression and the soft rot syndrome.

An ability to produce pectic enzymes *in vitro* does not imply that an organism will be found to rot plant tissues. Indeed, although many

Phytopathogenic Prokaryotes, Vol. 2

Copyright © 1982 by Academic Press, Inc.
All rights of reproduction in any form reserved.
ISBN 0-12-509002-1

bacteria and fungi can produce these enzymes *in vitro*, only a few species have been associated with field symptoms or the decay of plant products in store. Among these few species, those of *Erwinia* are the most common and often behave as true plant pathogens able to cause systemic infection and vascular disorders. Nevertheless, Pérombelon and Kelman (1980) consider that they are mostly opportunist pathogens able to initiate disease only when there is a coincidence of a particular set of conditions. They require a combination of a favorable environment, a minimum number of bacterial cells in the infection court, and some impairment of the host's resistance mechanisms (Pérombelon and Kelman, 1980).

This theme of coincidence of environment, bacterial numbers, and host impairment will be discussed in relation to the distribution of soft rot bacteria, contamination of host plants, and factors affecting symptom development.

II. THE SOFT ROT BACTERIA

Among the species of pectolytic bacteria associated with crop loss are *Erwinia* spp., *Bacillus subtilis* (Ehernberg) Cohn, *B. megaterium* de Bary, *B. polymyxa* (Prazmowski) Mace, *Pseudomonas marginalis* (Brown) Stevens, *P. viridiflava* (Burkholder, Dowson), and pectolytic species of other pseudomonads and of the genera *Corynebacterium*, *Clostridium*, and *Flavobacterium* (Dowson, 1944; Jackson and Henry, 1946; Lelliott, 1974; Lund and Nicholls, 1970; Obi, 1981; Pérombelon, 1972a, 1979b; Rudd-Jones and Dowson, 1950; Sampson and Hayward, 1971; Tsuchiya *et al.*, 1980). Of those named, only species of *Erwinia* and *Clostridium* are economically important in temperate areas. In warmer climates species of the other genera may play an important role [e.g., *Bacillus* spp., whose pathogenicity is often greater at high temperatures (Dowson, 1943; Jackson and Henry, 1946)].

Clostridium is a genus of generally Gram-positive spore-forming strict anaerobes. The taxonomy of the soft rotting forms is still largely unresolved but there are probably several species which may be placed into three broad groups on the basis of colony pigmentation and their spore morphology (Lund, 1979). Little is known of their biology but they are present in most soils and their pathogenicity may be affected by temperature. Although long associated with and investigated in relation to the commercial retting of flax (*Linum usitatissimum* L.) (Prévot *et al.*, 1967), only recently have they been clearly implicated as a cause of rot in stored potato (*Solanum tuberosum* L.) tubers (Lund and Wyatt, 1972; Pérombelon *et al.*, 1979b). They have also been implicated as a probable cause of a crop field symptom—cavity spot in carrots (*Daucus carota* L.) (Perry, 1981; Perry and Harrison, 1979).

The species of *Erwinia* are Gram-negative, non-spore-forming facultative anaerobes. The species most extensively studied belong to the carotovora group (Lelliott, 1974). They include *E. carotovora* subsp. *carotovora* (Jones) Bergey *et al.* (*Ecc*), *E. carotovora* subsp. *atroseptica* (van Hall) Dye (*Eca*), and *E. chrysanthemi* Burkholder *et al.* (*Echr*). The taxonomy of the species named has been examined (Dickey, 1979; Dye, 1969; Graham, 1972) and their ecology reviewed (Pérombelon and Kelman, 1980). Characteristically, they produce large quantities of pectic enzymes and although they are closely related biochemically and serologically, they nevertheless differ in temperature optima and requirements. Strains of *Ecc*, but not of *Eca* will grow at 37°C and, whereas most strains of the former are inhibited at 39°C, those of *Echr* grow relatively well at >39°C. These temperature characteristics are reflected in their host range as affected by geographical distribution. Thus, *Eca* is usually associated with the potato which, until recently, has traditionally been a cool climate crop. In contrast, *Echr* is a recognized pathogen of a wide range of tropical and subtropical crops including maize (*Zea mays* L.), pineapple [*Ananas comosus* (L.) Merr.], and rice (*Oryza sativa* L.), as well as those grown as greenhouse crops in temperate regions. The host range and geographical distribution of *Ecc* is wider and it has been associated with a range of symptoms on many plant species in both the temperate and tropical zones.

III. CROP CONTAMINATION

Information on the extent of and the route by which host plants are contaminated by soft rot bacteria is limited. Most of the published information is on potatoes and, in turn, on species of *Erwinia*. Their ecology and epidemiology has recently been reviewed in detail by Pérombelon and Kelman (1980) and only a summary is presented here.

It is convenient to consider potato crop contamination as a system of two separate but interlocking cycles for *Ecc* and *Eca*, very little being known about *Echr*. First there is a cycle that can occur within a single plant although in field crops progeny tubers of adjacent plants may also be contaminated. The seed or mother tuber is, in terms of bacterial numbers, the main source of the bacteria that contaminate progeny tubers. Moreover, whereas stem lesions, at least in temperate climates, are caused only by *Eca,* mother tubers are rotted by both *Eca* and *Ecc.* When the contaminated mother tuber rots, as it usually does, it liberates bacteria into the soil to contaminate adjacent progeny tubers. Stem lesions, though they may be important, are much rarer than rotted mother tubers because they nearly always arise as a result of, but by no means necessarily, as a sequel to rotting of the mother tuber. Indirect evidence (Pérombelon, 1976) suggests that high levels of soil water encourage both mother tuber decay and movement of the bacteria to daughter tubers, affecting both their liability to and the level of their contamination. These contamination levels do not progressively increase during the growing season, but they tend to fluctuate, often falling to quite low levels during dry periods and increasing again after heavy rain (Pérombelon, 1976). This last observation not only reinforces the concept of the soil as the most important route (cf. contamination via the stolons) but also indicates that at least in the early stages, contamination is limited to the tuber surface which morphologically includes the lenticels. The numbers of cells of *E. carotovora* per lenticel rarely exceeds 10^2 even in heavily contaminated crops and, usually, only a few cells are present (Burr and Schroth, 1977; Pérombelon, 1973). Nevertheless, although essentially superficial, the bacteria in lenticels can survive in apparently undiminished numbers during winter storage (Pérombelon, 1973). The route from stem lesions to the tuber surface and lenticels must also be affected by rainfall, initially, when bacterial cells are washed from lesions into the soil.

The second external cycle is considered as that not associated with an individual plant but one that may involve adjacent plants, potato plants distant in a field, or other sources at any distance. Farm machinery, both in the field and in stores, storage containers, and crop detritus in or about stores have all been implicated as factors aiding dispersal or contamination. Infection is usually a sequel to direct contact either with tubers in store, or in the field to the tuber and the growing plant. The plant may also be contaminated by airborne bacteria either passively vectored on insects or deposited from aerosols. The numbers of bacterial cells per unit area derived from these sources clearly will vary greatly but it is usually very low (Pérombelon *et al.,* 1979a). However, absolute numerical levels are of little importance if the bacteria can multiply *in situ.* The importance of the phylloplane as a site for landing, multiplication, and then dispersal into the soil by rain wash has been demonstrated (Pérombelon, 1981a). Other known sources, whose relative importance has yet to be assessed, are ponds, lakes, streams and rivers—surface water generally when used for irrigation or as a source of rain-generated aerosols—and the rhizospheres of other crop plants and weeds (Pérombelon, 1981b).

The soil harbors a large range of bacteria able to rot plant tissue and, either directly or indirectly after rhizosphere multiplication, it may be an important reservoir of these ubiquitous bacteria for many plant species. Not surprisingly, it is common to find that plants are contaminated by more than one species. Thus in potatoes, pectolytic *Pseudomonas* spp. and *Clostridium* spp. may readily be detected or become self-evident. In Scotland (Pérombelon *et al.*, 1980) and in Germany (Nauman *et al.*, 1978) both *Ecc* and *Eca* occur in similar proportions in potato seed stocks. Nauman *et al.* (1978) found that the combined totals of *Pseudomonas* spp., *Bacillus* spp., and *Clostridium* spp. comprised only 11% of his isolates of pectolytic bacteria from tubers in Germany. Pérombelon *et al.* (1979b) and Campos *et al.* (1981) in Wisconsin found that erwinias were commonly present in a high proportion of the tuber samples from which clostridia were isolated.

IV. LATENCY

Apparently healthy plants may harbor a wide range of bacteria. It is generally accepted that lacking the ability of fungi to directly penetrate plant tissue, bacteria gain access through natural openings (e.g., stomata) or via natural wounds (e.g., wind damage, breakage in root systems, etc). Some of these bacteria may have little pathogenic potential but they will have an *in situ* advantage as potential competitive saprophytes at the onset of plant or tissue senescence. Among others there may be some having the potential to induce decay and these include species of the genera *Erwinia, Pseudomonas,* and *Bacillus* (De Boer and Copeman, 1974; Hollis, 1951; Meneley and Stanghellini, 1972, 1974; Sturdy and Cole, 1974). Cells both of *Rhizobium* spp. (other than in nodules) and of *Erwinia* spp. have been detected within plant cells (Davey and Cocking, 1972; Meneley and Stanghellini, 1975) and Jones and Paton (1973) have also suggested that *Erwinia* spp. may be present in plant cells as L forms.

In growing potato crops, in addition to those already present in tuber lenticels, bacteria may gain entry via fresh wounds in the protective epidermis above ground when plants are damaged by, for example, farm implements, birds, and insects—any or all of which may also act as vectors. At and soon after harvest, bacteria from the soil or at the tuber surface may be impacted into inner tissue, by-passing the protective periderm, when tubers are mechanically damaged. A survey in the United Kingdom (Potato Marketing Board, 1974) showed that nearly a quarter of all harvested potatoes had suffered some damage by the time they went into storage.

The numbers of bacterial cells found in potential infection courts following any of the above routes are usually small and there may be several reasons, alone or in combination, why they do not induce decay. First, they may be cut off from potentially susceptible tissue by the normal process of wound barrier formation. Second, they may be killed either by metabolic products from the host or by the presence of antagonists impacted into the wound with them. Third, even if they remain viable, some additional physical or physiological damage to the host may be required to release nutrients and impair tissue resistance, thus enabling them to multiply *in situ*. It appears that only when their numbers have reached some critical level in combination with other favorable factors, not fully understood, will a progressive lesion develop.

The transition from a latent (or quiescent) to an active stage is undoubtedly affected by local O_2 concentration. At low levels, the bacteria can grow as facultative anaerobes, but several oxygen-dependent and temperature-moderated mechanisms are involved in resistance to them. These include the oxidation of phenolic compounds to antibacterial quinones, the production of antibacterial phytoalexins, as well as suberization and wound periderm formation (Lund, 1979).

Although anaerobic conditions, or very low O_2 concentrations, may eventually cause cell death in many plant tissues, some leakage of cell contents is induced before the cells or tissue have reached a state leading irreversibly to death. Nutrients are more obviously released by wounding when tubers are punctured to enhance their decay as in the procedure advocated by De Boer and Kelman (1978). The numbers of bacterial cells within lenticels can be raised to levels far higher than those encountered in nature by the now widely used technique of vacuum infiltration. Potato tubers are placed in bacterial suspensions, of varying concentrations, subjected to vacuum which is then abruptly released. Despite the high numbers which can thereby be infiltrated into lenticels, rotting does not necessarily ensue. In contrast, hypodermic injection (which necessarily wounds tissue and thereby releases nutrients) of high concentrations of bacteria can lead to rotting (De Boer and Kelman, 1978).

The transition from the latent to the active state followed by rotting in a potato tuber is evidently affected by a number of factors which may interact both quantitatively and qualitatively in nature. No single experimental system could test the hypotheses that must necessarily be adduced in attempts to explain the natural phenomena, but the brief and simple points made above do provide persuasive indirect evidence for at least some of the factors involved.

V. DISEASE DEVELOPMENT

A. Pathogenicity and Temperature Interactions

The development of a disease (i.e., pathogenesis) cannot adequately be studied without defining its associated symptoms. It is important to state at the outset of this section that temperature affects not only the distribution and host range of *Ecc, Eca,* and *Echr,* but their symptoms also. The type of blackleg symptom caused by *Eca* is typically a black wet rot of the stem base which often extends to the upper part under moist conditions. However, the symptoms caused by *Ecc* and *Echr* are variable; often the stem has a brown translucent appearance especially at intermediate temperatures, but at higher temperatures as found in the lowland tropical zone in Peru the symptoms are similar to those caused by *Eca* (E. R. French and L. de Lindo, personal communication). To avoid confusion it may be advisable to substitute for blackleg the term bacterial stem rot to describe symptoms caused by all soft rot erwinias.

Temperature is the main factor affecting the relative virulence of soft rot bacteria and its level may determine which organism predominates in a lesion. When assessed by the effective median dose (ED_{50}) for induction of decay in potato tubers, *Ecc, Eca,* and pectolytic clostridia were equally virulent at 22°C, but there were marked differences at 16°C, *Eca* being the most, *Ecc* the intermediate, and clostridia the least virulent (Pérombelon *et al.*, 1979b). When potatoes were inoculated by simultaneously injecting *Eca* and clostridia in a 1 : 1 ratio, in the rotted tubers *Eca* became dominant at 16°C whereas the clostridia were dominant at 20°C. When naturally contaminated tubers developed extensive lesions during incubation at 16°C, *Ecc* predominated and clostridia were fewer although both population numbers were high, but following incubation at 22°C both populations were greatly reduced. The decrease has been attributed to the accumulation of toxic gases, organic acids, and higher alcohols which are probable by-products of the rapid growth of clostridia at 22°C (Prévot *et al.*, 1967). When *Ecc* and *Eca* were jointly inoculated into tubers and incubated, *Eca* predominated at low temperatures (ca. 16°C) and *Ecc* at high temperatures (ca. 26°C) (Pérombelon and Ghanekar, 1978; Pérombelon *et al.*, 1979b). Only at ca. 22°C do both bacteria grow *in planta* at equal rates (Pérombelon, 1979) and from the foregoing it is evident that the wrong choice of incubation temperature may lead to erroneous or misleading results in diagnostic or experimental work when associating causes and effects.

The differential effects of temperature on the relative virulence of *Ecc* and *Eca* may have at least two explanations. First, the absolute growth rate of *Eca in vitro* is always lower than that of *Ecc* including the rates at the temperature (ca. 28°C) that is the optimum for both (Wells, 1974). Second, the level of production of one of the pectic enzymes, endopolygalacturonic transeliminase (PGTE), by *Eca* is greater at 15 than at 30°C, whereas that of *Ecc* is equally high at both temperatures (Pérombelon and Ghanekar, 1979).

Chatterjee and Starr (1977) have demonstrated the importance of PGTE in pathogenicity because mutant strains of *Echr* that have lost both their virulence and the ability to produce large quantities of PGTE had their virulence restored by chromosomal transfer of loci for PGTE production from wild-type virulent strains.

Graham and Dowson (1960) obtained isolates of *Eca, Ecc,* and *Echr* from different hosts and countries. When they inoculated potato stems, all three erwinias induced stem rots at 25°C or higher but at temperatures below 19°C typical symptoms developed only with *Eca.* In parallel with the results obtained with tubers, Pérombelon and Lowe (1979) found that when they coinoculated *Ecc* and *Eca* into potato stems, *Eca* predominated at 15°C and *Ecc* at 30°C, although the differential effect was not as great as they had obtained in tubers.

In Scotland, as in most cool temperate areas, *Ecc* and *Eca* are present in most seed stocks but only *Eca* is commonly isolated as a cause of stem rots (Pérombelon, 1973). Under somewhat warmer conditions in Oregon, stem rot is mostly caused by *Eca* early in the growing season (June) whereas later (July–August) *Ecc* becomes dominant (Powelson, 1980). In Colorado, Molina and Harrison (1980) recovered *Ecc* more often than *Eca* from stem lesions in crops planted either late, when soil temperature was high, or in crops planted in the warmer parts of the state while at sites with intermediate soil temperatures both bacteria were recovered with equal frequency. In hot desert or semidesert regions, as in parts of Arizona or Southwest Australia where soil temperature is often higher than 35°C, *Ecc* predominates (Cother, 1980; Stanghellini and Menely, 1975). Stem rot in Southwest Australia (Cother, 1980) and Japan (Tanii and Baba, 1971) may also be caused by *Echr.*

B. Infection of the Growing Plant

Most plants are superficially contaminated with but rarely infected by soft rot bacteria. In temperate climates, symptom development following infection by soft rot bacteria is associated with erwinias and only unusually with species of other genera. Symptom expression often seems capricious and little is known qualitatively or quantitatively about factors affecting its development. The eventual outcome of infection and subsequent disease development may be gross maceration and rotting of affected parts but the initial symptoms may be diverse and remote from the site of primary infection. In potatoes, for example, the first symptoms of infection at the base of the stem just above or below ground may be no more than a yellowing and/or curling of the leaves or a slight wilting, nonspecific symptoms similar to those of drought that occur, however, when soil moisture is adequate. Under wet conditions affected stems rot; otherwise they may simply wither, dry, and die. In temperate regions, these, or more severe symptoms on potatoes are usually caused by *Eca* and, just as it is rare to find other bacteria causing such symptoms, so it is unusual for *Eca* to be found on other hosts, although it can infect crops such as carrots and calabrese (*Brassica oleracea* ssp. *italica* Plenk) (Pérombelon and Lowe, 1971), tomato (*Lycopersicon esculentum* Mill.) (Barzic *et al.,* 1976), sunflower (*Helianthus annusis* L.) (Fucikovsky *et al.,* 1978), and celery (*Apium graveolens* L.) (M. Lemattre, personal communication). Strains of erwinias isolated from a given host are often more virulent when reinoculated to that host than those obtained from other species (Lacy *et al.,* 1979; McIntyre *et al.,* 1978) but true host specificity either does not occur or has not yet been proved. The common association of one strain with a particular host, as with *Eca* noted above, is of ecological and environmental rather than pathological origin. It is not surprising that attempts to define pathovars on the basis of host susceptibility or resistance ranges by artificial inoculation have failed. Not only is there a lack of specificity per se but, in consequence, and as Dickey (1981) has shown for *Echr,* a given host may yield isolates that could have been derived from different hosts.

Disease of the aerial parts of plants may be initiated at sites where the bacteria enter through wounds caused by insects and other agents [e.g., as in cassava (*Manihot esculenta* Crantz), maize, and sunflower]. Alternatively, the bacteria may move upward from roots or storage organs or their presence in those roots or storage organs alone may induce symptoms in the upper part of the plant. Regardless of the mode of entry, soft rot erwinias can be described as vascular pathogens because on the one hand they may cause wilt symptoms typical of many true vascular pathogens such as *Verticillium* spp., *Fusarium* spp., or *Pseudomonas solanecearum* (Smith) Smith, and on the other they can spread systemically via the vascular system before symptoms develop. Histopathological studies on potato (Artschwager, 1920), carnation (*Dianthus caryophyllus* L.) (Wolf and Nelson, 1969), and *Chrysanthemum* sp. (Pennypacker *et al.,* 1981a) showed that the bacteria move out of xylem vessels to infect adjoining parenchymatous tissue. Hellmers and Dowson (1953) found that spreading lesions failed to develop when soft rot erwinias were inoculated into the interfascicular regions of stems of potato, tomato, and tobacco (*Nicotiana tobacum* L.), but they caused extensive lesions when inoculated directly into the vascular bundles. As with wilt fungi, symptoms following vascular infection could result from the production of gum-like material and tyloses in the xylem elements with consequent restriction of water flow (Pennypacker *et al.*, 1981b). The suggestion by Lazar *et al.* (1970) that symptoms might be caused by endotoxins produced by soft rot erwinias merits further investigation. Pennypacker *et al.* (1971a,b) examined the histopathology of infection by *Ecc* and *Echr* of wilt-susceptible and -resistant cultivars of *Chrysanthemum*. Systemic infection by both erwinias in a susceptible cultivar was followed by bacterial multiplication in the xylem elements and the development of symptoms typical of bacterial blight. In contrast, in a resistant cultivar symptoms were caused only by *Echr* which alone increased in numbers, the spread and multiplication of *Ecc* being restricted by more intensive host reactions—hypertrophy, hyperplasia, and the production of chromophilic cells around infected vascular bundles with the formation of suberin.

In contrast to the nature of pathogenesis in *Chrysanthemum*, stem rot of potato is invariably associated with decay of the parent or seed tuber. Stem rot is not a necessary sequel to tuber rot, but it is clear that conditions in the soil are important for symptom initiation. Factors which favor rotting of mother tubers, and thus favor the growth of erwinias, are likely to be conducive to symptom expression in stems. Moreover, rotting of the seed tubers and multiplication of erwinias are more likely to be rapid if the initial numbers of the bacteria are high rather than low (Aleck and Harrison, 1978; Pérombelon and Lowe, 1978). Stem rot may still develop if the initial inoculum is low provided environmental conditions favor seed tuber decay, for example, during wet periods or wet seasons when the soil becomes waterlogged and the mother tuber is subject, in part, to very low O_2 concentrations or even anaerobiosis. Pérombelon and Lowe (1979) have shown that in Scotland stem rot symptoms tend to appear during the first half of the growing season during and soon after periods when the soil water deficit has been low or near zero for periods of 10–14 days. Locally, within a tuber, anaerobiosis may permit growth of pectolytic clostridia which may inhibit the erwinias (Pérombelon *et al.*, 1979). It might be supposed that only periods of low O_2 that are inimical to tuber tissue resistance favor the initiation of rots, but the return of aerobic conditions when clostridia are inhibited permits rapid growth of erwinias. Thus alternating periods of heavy rain and dryness may enhance stem rot incidence and, indeed, alternating moisture regimes have been associated with high numbers of erwinias under experimental conditions in the laboratory (Pérombelon, 1972b). The hypothesis is in agreement with the common observation that "black leg" incidence is greater in freely drained sandy soils than in clay or loamy soils especially in areas or seasons when there are frequent heavy showers (Van den Boom, 1967).

In hot regions, there is a dual effect in potato crops due to high temperature affecting both tuber rotting in the soil and symptom expression in the stem. Some consequences indicated in the following passage are common knowledge, but the semiquantitative relationships suggested, while possible or even probable, have yet to be studied and confirmed. Blanking, caused by preemergence rotting of the mother tuber, and the incidence of stem rot may both be high in the same crop and are invariably higher than in temperate regions. High temperatures early in the growing season may cause severe losses due to blanking but, because most mother tubers liable to rot have already done so, the subsequent incidence of stem rot may be comparatively low. If, however, initial temperatures are moderate there may be much less blanking, but the potential for tuber rot is then expressed later in the season by consequential severe levels of stem rot (Aleck and Harrison, 1978). High levels of stem rot later in the season, associated with somewhat later decay of the mother tuber, have also been associated in hot regions with high levels of contamination of progeny seed tubers. Very late development of stem rots may be associated with the transition from latent to active infection in potato stems, concomitant with the onset of senescence. Similarly, symptoms of blight caused by *Echr* in *Saintpaulia ionantha* Wendl. in glasshouse grown crops also tend to occur at the end of the growing season (Lemattre and Narcy, 1972).

C. Infection and Decay of Storage Organs

Naturally contaminated progeny tubers rarely rot in the soil. Experimentally in the laboratory, such tubers cannot be induced to rot under anaerobic conditions with or without an increase in CO_2 levels and even under conditions of high humidity—providing temperature fluctuations do not cause dew formation leading to water films on the surface. Bacteria on the surface of tubers (including the lenticels, see above) are unlikely to gain access to the inner tissues of tubers in soils if they are relatively well aerated and not water logged nor will they under normal storage conditions.

With prolonged exposure to high humidity due, for example, to poor storage conditions or in wet soils, lenticels tend to proliferate (Pérombelon and Lowe, 1975) and concomitant increases in CO_2 concentrations further promote lenticel enlargement (Howard *et al.*, 1968). The water economy of tubers is such that they are usually in a condition of internal water stress (Epstein and Grant, 1973; Gander and Tanner, 1976), and they may readily absorb water at a rate dependent on the extent of stress as moderated by the degree of suberization of the periderm. The effects of water stress and lenticel enlargement are readily illustrated and may be seen when nonturgid tubers [water loss from, say, sprouting or silver scurf—*Helminthosporium solani* (Durr & Mont)] are planted in moist soil when they quickly become fully turgid. Susceptibility of tuber tissue to decay is greater when its water status is high than when it is low (Fernando and Stevenson, 1952; Kelman *et al.*, 1978; Pérombelon and Lowe, 1975). A similar relationship was found in Chinese cabbage (*Brassica* sp.) (Tanaka and Kikumoto, 1976). How decay is affected by tissue water status is not known; however, it is relevant to note that pectic enzyme activity of *Echr* was found to be directly related to the water potential of potato tissue (Alberghina *et al.*, 1973) and that plant cells at incipient plasmolysis are not readily killed by pectic enzymes (Tribe, 1955).

As the water status of a tuber increases, cortical cells below the lenticels swell, stretch the phelloderm, and then rupture the suberized layer (Pérombelon and Lowe, 1975). If a film of a free water is present the motile bacteria may move into the tuber. A continuous film of water will, moreover, have other effects. If it covers much of the tuber surface, respiration will cause rapid internal depletion of O_2 (within 2.5 hr at 22°C, see Burton and Wiggington, 1970) and the resultant progress toward anaerobiosis induces more changes. The intercellular spaces normally do not contain free water because tuber tissue is under water stress, but with O_2 depletion, cell membranes lose their integrity. Solutes and water then leak into the intercellular spaces (Pérombelon and Lowe, 1975; Stiles, 1927), allowing the bacteria to become motile and providing them with nutrients. Oxygen-dependent resistance mechanisms will fail and both aerobic and facultative anaerobic bacteria will grow and the pectolytic forms will start to macerate adjoining tissue.

Decreasing O_2 concentration leads to an exponential increase in the amount of decay (De Boer and Kelman, 1978) and it thus seems likely that tuber resistance is proportional to O_2 levels favoring growth of soft rot erwinias because they grow better *in vitro* under aerobic than anaerobic conditions, although Wells (1974) found that both *Ecc* and *Eca* fail to grow in liquid cultures at any concentration of O_2 in the absence of CO_2. However, CO_2, a growth factor for many bacteria, is unlikely to be limiting *in vivo* because it is produced by plant tissue and by other bacteria in incipient lesions.

Studies of dose–response relationships indicate that under moist, anaerobic conditions $<10^2$ cells per microsite is sufficient to start a lesion in potato tubers (De Boer and Kelman, 1978; Pérombelon, 1972c; Pérombelon *et al.*, 1979). Indeed, extrapolation suggests that a single viable bacterial cell may do so. In contrast, under aerobic conditions the number needed may be as high as 10^6–10^7 at temperatures $<30°C$ (De Boer and Kelman, 1978; Zielke, 1976). Temperatures above 30°C—whatever their other effects—enhance tuber susceptibility and the numbers of bacteria needed are then less than at lower temperatures (Sellam *et al.*, 1980). Higher temperatures of ca. 60°C cause further stress and the accompanying liability to decay has been associated with increases of membrane permeability (Nielsen, 1946; Nielsen and Todd, 1946). In contrast, low storage temperatures cause an increase in both total sugar content and the proportion of reducing sugars and, although absolute levels may be affected by cultivar and storage time, a positive correlation between reducing sugar content and susceptibility to soft rot caused by *Eca* has been reported by Otazu and Secor (1981). In general, potato tubers in store tend to become more resistant to decay with time and De Boer and Kelman (1978) have suggested that this may be associated with water loss but no increase in water deficit (measured by psychometry) was detected in two cultivars during 3 months of storage from February to April although their resistance increased markedly (Pérombelon, unpublished).

Acknowledgment

I am grateful to R. H. Fox for helpful discussions during the preparation of this chapter.

References

Alberghina, A., Mazzucchi, U., and Pupillo, P. (1973). *Phytopathol. Z.* **78**, 204–213.
Aleck, J. R., and Harrison, M. D. (1978). *Am. Potato J.* **55**, 479–494.
Artschwager, E. R. (1920). *J. Agric. Res.* **20**, 325–330.
Barzic, M. R., Samson, R., and Trigalet, A. (1976). *Ann. Phytopathol.* **8**, 237–240.
Burr, T. J., and Schroth, M. N. (1977). *Phytopathology* **67**, 1382–1387.
Burton, W. G., and Wigginton, M. J. (1970). *Potato Res.* **13**, 180–186.
Campos, E., Maher, E. A., and Kelman, A. (1981). *Phytopathology* **71**, 207 (Abstr.).
Chatterjee, A. K., and Starr, M. P. (1977). *J. Bacteriol.* **132**, 862–869.
Cother, E. J. (1980). *Potato Res.* **23**, 75–84.
Davey, M. R., and Cocking, E. C. (1972). *Nature (London)* **239**, 455–456.
De Boer, S. H., and Copeman, R. J. (1974). *Can. J. Plant Sci.* **54**, 115–122.
De Boer, S. H., and Kelman, A. (1978). *Potato Res.* **21**, 65–80.
Dickey, R. S. (1979). *Phytopathology* **69**, 277–284.
Dickey, R. S. (1981). *Phytopathology* **71**, 23–29.

Dowson, W. J. (1943). *Nature (London)* **152,** 331.
Dowson, W. J. (1944). *Nature (London)* **154,** 557.
Dye, D. W. (1969). *N.Z. J. Sci.* **12,** 81–97.
Epstein, E., and Grant, W. J. (1973). *Agron. J.* **65,** 400–404.
Fernando, M., and Stevenson, G. (1952). *Ann. Bot.* **16,** 103–114.
Fucikovsky, L., Rodriguez, M., and Cartin, L. (1978). *Proc. Int. Conf. Plant Pathog. Bact., 4th, Angers* **11,** 603–606.
Gander, P. W., and Tanner, C. B. (1976). *Am. Potato J.* **53,** 1–14.
Graham, D. C. (1972). *Proc. Int. Conf. Plant Pathog. Bact., 3rd, Wageningen, 1971* pp. 273–279.
Graham, D. C., and Dowson, W. J. (1960). *Ann. Appl. Biol.* **48,** 51–57.
Hellmers, E., and Dowson, W. J. (1953). *Acta Agric. Scand.* **111,** 103–112.
Hollis, J. P. (1951). *Phytopathology* **41,** 350–366.
Howard, F. D., Flocker, W. J., and Yamaguchi, M. (1968). *Phytopathology* **45,** 438 (Abstr.).
Jackson, A. W., and Henry, B. S. (1946). *Can. J. Res. Sect. C* **24,** 39–46.
Jones, S. M., and Paton, A. M. (1973). *J. Appl. Bacteriol.* **36,** 729–737.
Kelman, A., Baughn, J. W., and Maher, E. A. (1978). *Phytopathol. News* **12,** 178 (Abstr.)
Lacy, G. M., Hirano, S. S., Victoria, J. I., Kelman, A., and Upper, C. D. (1979). *Phytopathology* **69,** 757–763.
Lazar, I., Savulescu, A., Popovici, I., and Grou, E. (1970). *Int. Symp. Slovak Acad. Sci., 1966.*
Lelliott, R. A. (1974). *In* "Bergey's Manual of Determinative Bacteriology" (R. E. Buchanan and S. E. Gibbons, eds.), 8th ed., pp. 332–339. Williams & Wilkins, Baltimore, Maryland.
Lemattre, M., and Narcy, J. P. (1972). *Extract Procès-Verbal Feb. 16, Acad. Agric. Franc.* pp. 227–231.
Lund, B. M. (1979). *Soc. Appl. Bacteriol. Tech. Ser.* **12,** 14–49.
Lund, B. M., and Nicholls, J. C. (1970). *Potato Res.* **13,** 210–214.
Lund, B. M., and Wyatt, G. M. (1972). *Potato Res.* **15,** 174–179.
McIntyre, J. L., Sands, D. C., and Taylor, G. S. (1978). *Phytopathology* **68,** 435–440.
Meneley, J. C., and Stanghellini, M. E. (1972). *Phytopathology* **62,** 779 (Abstr.).
Meneley, J. C., and Stanghellini, M. E. (1974). *J. Food Sci.* **39,** 1267–1268.
Meneley, J. C., and Stanghellini, M. E. (1975). *Phytopathology* **65,** 670–673.
Molina, J. J., and Harrison, M. D. (1980). *Am. Potato J.* **57,** 351–363.
Naumann, K., Zielke, R., and Peter, K. (1978). *Arch. Phytopathol. Pflanzenschutz* **14,** 151–161.
Nielsen, L. W. (1946). *Am. Potato J.* **23,** 41–57.
Nielsen, L. W., and Todd, F. A. (1946). *Am. Potato J.* **23,** 73–87.
Obi, S. K. C. (1981). *Appl. Environ. Microbiol.* **41,** 563–567.
Otazu, V., and Secor, G. A. (1981). *Phytopathology* **71,** 290–295.
Pennypacker, B. W., Dickey, R. S., and Nelson, P. E. (1981a). *Phytopathology* **71,** 138–140.
Pennypacker, B. W., Smith, C. M., Dickey, R. S., and Nelson, P. E. (1981b). *Phytopathology* **71,** 141–148.
Pérombelon, M. C. M. (1972a). *Ann. Appl. Biol.* **71,** 111–117.
Pérombelon, M. C. M. (1972b). *Plant Dis. Rep.* **56,** 552–554.
Pérombelon, M. C. M. (1973). *Ann. Appl. Biol.* **74,** 59–65.
Pérombelon, M. C. M. (1979). *Potato Res.* **22,** 63–68.
Pérombelon, M. C. M. (1981a). *In* "Microbial Ecology of the Phylloplane" (J. P. Blakeman, ed.), pp. 411–431. Academic Press, New York.
Pérombelon, M. C. M. (1981b). *Triennial Conf. EAPR, 8th, Munich,* pp. 90–91 (Abstr.).

Pérombelon, M. C. M., and Ghanekar, A. (1978). *Rep. Scott. Hortic. Inst. 1977* p. 76.
Pérombelon, M. C. M., and Ghanekar, A. (1979). *Rep. Scott. Hortic. Inst. 1978* p. 31.
Pérombelon, M. C. M., and Kelman, A. (1980). *Annu. Rev. Phytopathol.* **18,** 361–387.
Pérombelon, M. C. M., and Lowe, R. (1971). *Rep. Scott. Hortic. Inst. 1970* pp. 32–33.
Pérombelon, M. C. M., and Lowe, R. (1975). *Potato Res.* **18,** 64–82.
Pérombelon, M. C. M., and Lowe, R. (1978). *Rep. Scott. Hortic. Inst. 1977* pp. 84–85.
Pérombelon, M. C. M., and Lowe, R. (1979). *Rep. Scott. Hortic. Inst. 1978* pp. 86–87.
Pérombelon, M. C. M., Fox, R. A., and Lowe, R. (1979a). *Phytopathol. Z.* **94,** 249–260.
Pérombelon, M. C. M., Gullings-Handley, J., and Kelman, A. (1979b). *Phytopathology* **69,** 167–173.
Pérombelon, M. C. M., Lowe, R., Quinn, C. E., and Sells, A. (1980). *Potato Res.* **23,** 413–425.
Perry, D. A., and Harrison, J. G. (1979). *Ann. Appl. Biol.* **93,** 101–108.
Perry, D. A. (1981). *Ann. Appl. Biol.* (in press).
Potato Marketing Board (1974). Report on a National Damage Survey, 1973, London.
Powelson, M. L. (1980). *Am. Potato J.* **57,** 301–306.
Prévot, A. R., Turpin, A., and Kaiser, P. (1967). *In* "Les Bactéries Anaerobies," pp. 878–949. Dunod, Paris.
Rudd-Jones, D., and Dowson, W. J. (1950). *Ann. Appl. Biol.* **37,** 563–569.
Sampson, P. J., and Hayward, A. C. (1971). *Aust. J. Biol. Sci.* **24,** 917–923.
Sellam, M. A., Rushdi, M. H., and Abd-El-Aal, S. A. (1980). *Anz. Schaedlingskd. Pflanz. Umweltschutz* **53,** 185–189.
Stiles, W. (1927). *Protoplasma* **2,** 577–601.
Sturdy, M. L., and Cole, A. L. J. (1976). *Ann. Bot.* **19,** 351–368.
Tanaka, T., and Kikumoto, T. (1976). *Bull. Inst. Agric. Res. Tohoku Univ.* **27,** 89–101.
Tanii, A., and Baba, T. (1971). *Hokkaido Prefect. Agric. Exp. Sta. Bull.* **24,** 1–10.
Tribe, H. T. (1955). *Ann. Appl. Biol.* **19,** 351–368.
Tsuchiya, Y., Ohata, K., and Shirata, A. (1980). *Bull. Natl. Inst. Agric. Sci.* **34,** 51–73.
Van den Boom, T. (1967). *Phytopathol. Z.* **58,** 239–276.
Wells, J. M. (1974). *Phytopathology* **64,** 1012–1015.
Wolf, R. T., and Nelson, P. E. (1969). *Phytopathology* **59,** 1802–1808.
Zielke, R. (1976). *Arch. Phytopathol. Pflanzenschutz (Berlin)* **12,** 27–41.

Chapter **4**

Fastidious Prokaryotes: Epidemiology of the Hidden Pathogens

DAVID A. ROSENBERGER

Copyright © 1982 by Academic Press, Inc.
All rights of reproduction in any form reserved.
ISBN 0-12-509002-1

I. INTRODUCTION

A. Definitions

The fastidious prokaryotes are minute organisms which for many years remained hidden in their plant and insect hosts because they could not be grown on simple culture media preparations. The plant pathogenic fastidious prokaryotes include spiroplasmas, mycoplasma-like organisms (MLOs), the fastidious bacteria commonly called rickettsialike bacteria (RLB), and the small coryneform bacteria associated with ratoon-stunting disease of sugarcane. The taxonomic position of MLOs is still unclear since the term is used primarily for those plant disease agents which have not yet been cultured or characterized. To date, all of the MLOs isolated from plants and insects have proven to be spiroplasmas rather than true mycoplasmas. However, the term "mycoplasma" is now commonly used to refer to all members of the *Mollicutes* (Maramorosch, 1981). Spiroplasmas and true mycoplasmas are both in the class *Mollicutes,* but spiroplasmas have a larger genome than mycoplasmas, and most but not all spiroplasmas occur in helical forms (Maramorosch, 1981; Townsend *et al.,* 1977). Spiroplasmas and MLOs have no cell wall and require sterols for growth. In plants, spiroplasmas and MLOs are usually found in the phloem tissue although some spiroplasmas have been found in flower nectar (Davis, 1978) and recent evidence suggests some MLOs may move through parenchyma cells (Ulrychova and Petru, 1980).

Some of the fastidious bacteria were originally called rickettsialike organisms because their size and morphology as observed in electron micrographs suggested they might be rickettsia (Goheen *et al.,* 1973; Hopkins and Mollenhauer, 1973). The subsequent culture and partial characterization of the RLB causing Pierce's disease of grapevines indicates these bacteria are not true rickettsia (Davis *et al.,* 1978), but their taxonomic position has not yet been determined. The RLB have been divided into three groups, however, based on the plant tissue they invade. Hopkins (1977) has listed diseases caused by xylem-limited RLB, phloem-limited RLB, and non-tissue-restricted RLB.

B. Objectives

In this chapter we shall investigate the factors involved in dissemination of RLB and mycoplasmas (spiroplasmas and MLOs). Although mycoplasmas and RLB are in different taxonomic classes, many similarities exist in the epidemiologies of diseases caused by these organisms.

Both mycoplasmas and RLB depend almost entirely on homopteran vectors for dissemination, both are relatively temperature sensitive, and, with the exception of the non-tissue-restricted RLB and the flower nectar spiroplasmas, both invade plants exclusively through vascular tissues.

Most of the subsequent discussion will involve epidemiological aspects of leafhopper vectored diseases. In fact, this chapter could have been titled "Epidemiology of Leafhopper-Vectored Fastidious Prokaryotes" because most of the known vectors of mycoplasmas and RLB are leafhoppers. Relatively little work has been done on non-leafhopper vectors of fastidious prokaryotes. Mycoplasmas are transmitted primarily by phloem-feeding leafhoppers from the subfamily Deltocephalinae. The known leafhopper vectors of phloem-limited RLB fall in the subfamily Agalliinae and the xylem-limited RLB are transmitted primarily by leafhoppers from the subfamily Cicadellinae (Nielson, 1979). Classes of non-leafhopper vectors of fastidious prokaryotes include the psyllids which vector the MLO causing pear decline (Jensen *et al.*, 1964) and the phloem-limited RLB causing citrus greening (Martinez and Wallace, 1967; Olson and Rogers, 1969). Cercopid froghoppers can vector the RLB causing Pierce's disease and the MLO causing peach yellows (Purcell, 1979a; Severin, 1950a). There have also been reports of fulgorids, piesmids, and aphids vectoring MLOs and/or RLBs (Harris, 1979). In addition to dissemination by insect vectors, some of the fastidious prokaryotes have been disseminated through man's use of contaminated nursery stock and plant-propagating materials.

Rather than reviewing all of the diseases caused by fastidious prokaryotes and listing all of the known vectors, we shall use representative pathogen-vector disease systems to illustrate the problems, basic principles, and complex interrelationships encountered in epidemiological studies of fastidious prokaryotes. For the benefit of readers unfamiliar with diseases caused by fastidious prokaryotes, we shall start with brief historical reviews of aster yellows, X-disease, Pierce's disease, and phony peach disease. Most of the examples in our subsequent discussion will be drawn from these four pathogen-vector disease systems. Readers interested in more complete lists of mycoplasma and RLB vectors are referred to recent reviews by Harris (1979) and Chiykowski (1981).

C. Terminology

Familiarity with some terms unique to insect-vector research is important for understanding research reports dealing with insect vectors.

The term "acquisition" is used to refer to the process whereby a vector acquires a pathogen from a diseased plant. The acquisition access period is the time the insect is allowed to feed on diseased plants. The inoculation access period is the time insects are allowed to feed on healthy test plants (or indicator plants) which will later be observed for disease development.

Circulative transmission and noncirculative transmission are terms used to describe two mechanisms of insect transmission. Circulative transmission occurs when the insect ingests the pathogen and the pathogen then invades the cells of the insect host. Mycoplasmas and some viruses are known to multiply within their insect vectors and they are considered propagative circulative pathogens. Usually the circulative pathogen reaches the hemolymph of its insect vector after invading the gut wall. The pathogen then circulates throughout the insect, invades numerous other body tissues, and is finally injected into healthy plants in normal excretions from infected salivary glands. In circulative transmission, the insect vectors become infective (able to transmit the pathogen) only after the pathogen has invaded the salivary glands, but they remain infective for long periods, often for as long as they live. The period between acquisition and the time insects become infective is called the incubation period. For mycoplasmas, the incubation period within the insect vector ranges from 8 to 30 or more days depending on the mycoplasma and vector species involved.

Noncirculative transmission is a more mechanical process wherein the pathogen does not invade the insect host but is transferred from plant to plant on the stylet or other mouthparts of the vector. No incubation period is required for noncirculative transmission and the insect vectors usually lose infectivity relatively quickly after leaving an infected host plant. Because of the short retention of the pathogen by the vector, noncirculative transmission is also known as nonpersistent or semipersistent transmission.

Plant-infecting mycoplasmas are circulative within their insect vectors whereas many viruses are noncirculative. The RLB causing Pierce's disease of grapes is noncirculative but multiplies within the foregut of its insect vectors (Purcell *et al.*, 1979). Although the mechanisms of transmission have not been determined for other fastidious bacteria, the mechanism described for Pierce's disease bacterium may apply to other xylem-limited RLB as well. Phloem-limited RLB have short incubation periods, long retention in their insect vectors, and are the only fastidious prokaryotes known to be transmitted transovarially (through the eggs) from one generation of leafhoppers to the next (Hopkins, 1977).

II. OVERVIEWS OF FOUR DISEASES

A. Aster Yellows

Aster yellows affects more than 175 species of plants and commonly causes commercial losses in lettuce (*Lactuca sativa* L.), celery (*Apium graveolens* var. *dulce* DC), carrots (*Daucus carota* var. *sativa* DC), and potatoes (*Solanum tuberosum* L.) (Chiykowski and Chapman, 1965). Aster yellows was first reported by Smith (1902) shortly after it appeared in plantings of China asters [*Callistephus chinensis* (L.) Nees]. The aster yellows disease found in California in 1925 was initially assumed to be identical to the east coast strain, but Severin (1929) showed that the western pathogen could be transmitted to *Zinnia elegans* Jacq. and celery whereas the eastern strain had not been found in those plants. The western strain, subsequently known as California aster yellows or celery-infecting aster yellows, spread to eastern United States by 1952 (Magie *et al.*, 1953). The two strains of aster yellows were carefully compared by Kunkel (1955) who showed that the eastern strain could infect zinnia and celery if young seedlings were exposed to infective leafhoppers. Kunkel concluded that the eastern and western strains of aster yellows were very similar although in most host plants the western strain caused more severe stunting and production of axillary rosettes whereas plants infected with the eastern strain developed an abundance of long, spindly, axillary shoots.

Insect transmission of aster yellows was first reported by Kunkel (1926) who showed that the pathogen was vectored by the aster leafhopper, *Macrosteles fascifrons* (Stal), following a 10-day incubation period within the insect. This appears to be the first report of insect transmission of a fastidious prokaryote, although Kunkel (1926) considered it a virus transmission similar to leafhopper transmissions previously reported for curly top virus of sugar beets, rice mozaic virus, and potato leafroll virus. Other leafhopper vectors reported for aster yellows in North America include *Colladonus montanus* (Van Duzee), *C. geminatus* (Van Duzee) (Severin, 1934), *Texananus lathropi* (Baker), *T. latipex* DeLong, *T. oregonus* (Ball), *T. pergradus* DeLong, *T. spatulatus* (Van Duzee), *Paraphlepsius apertinus* (Osborn & Lathrop) (Severin, 1945), *Gyponana angulata* (Spangberg) (Severin, 1946), *Acinopterus angulatus* Lawson (Severin, 1947a), *Scaphytopius irroratus* (Van Duzee), *S. acutus delongi* Young, *Chlorotettix similis* De Long, *Fieberiella florii* (Stal), *Euscelidius variegatus* (Kirschbaum) (Severin, 1947b), *Idiodonus heidmanni* (Ball), *C. flavocapitatus* (Van Duzee), *C. holmesi* Bliven, *C. intricatus* (Ball), *C. kir-*

kaldyi (Ball), *C. rupinatus* (Ball) (Severin, 1948), *Excultanus incurvatus* (Osborn & Lathrop) (Severin, 1950), *S. acutus* (Say) (Chiykowski, 1962), *Endria inimica* (Say) (Chiykowski, 1963), *Elymana sulphurella* Zetterstedt (Chiykowski and Sinha, 1969), and *Aprodes bicinta* (Schrank) (Chiykowski, 1977). Some of the vectors have been taxonomically reclassified since they were first reported and the taxa listed above are from a recent listing by Nielson (1979).

The first MLOs observed in plants were aster yellows mycoplasma (Doi *et al.*, 1967). Recently a spiroplasma identical to *Spiroplasma citri*, the organism which caused citrus stubborn (Saglio *et al.*, 1971) was isolated from plants with aster yellows symptoms (Maramorosch, 1979; Purcell *et al.*, 1981a). At first these isolations were taken as evidence that aster yellows is caused by a spiroplasma, but later evidence suggested that aster yellows-diseased plants from which spiroplasma were recovered were dually infected with the aster yellows MLO and with *Spiroplasma citri* (Smith *et al.*, 1981). There is as yet no solid evidence that the aster yellows MLO is a spiroplasma. The aster yellows agent has not been successfully maintained in pure culture for more than a few days (Smith *et al.*, 1981).

B. X-Disease of Stone Fruits

X-Disease was first noted in a Connecticut peach [*Prunus persica* (L.) Batsch] orchard (Stoddard, 1947), but the disease spread rapidly through most of the peach-growing areas of New York, Ontario, Michigan, Ohio, and Illinois. A similar disease, first called cherry buckskin and later known as western X-disease, was found in California infecting sweet cherry (*Prunus avium* L.) in 1928 (Rawlins and Horne, 1931) and in peach in 1932 (Thomas *et al.*, 1940). Western X-disease gradually spread through much of the stone fruit areas of California, Oregon, Washington, Idaho, Colorado, Utah, and Texas. Numerous strains have been reported for both X-disease (Gilmer *et al.*, 1954) and western X-disease (Rawlins and Thomas, 1941). The peach yellow leaf roll disease reported from California is probably the most severe strain of X-disease (Jensen *et al.*, 1964; Nyland and Schlocker, 1951; Purcell *et al.*, 1981b). Several researchers have suggested X-disease and western X are caused by the same or closely related organisms (Gilmer and Blodgett, 1976; Richards and Cochran, 1957). For purposes of clarity in this discussion, the term "X-disease" will be used to embrace all of the various strains of the disease in both the eastern and western United States and we shall refer to the specific strains as eastern X-disease and western X-disease.

X-Disease has been found infecting peach, nectarine [*P. persica* var. *nectarina* (Ait.) Maxim.], Japanese plum (*P. salicina* Lindl.), sweet and tart cherries (*P. cerasus* L.), and the common and western chokecherries, *Prunus virginiana* L. and *P. demissa* (Nutt.) Walp. (Gilmer and Blodgett, 1976). Symptoms on peach include yellowing of leaves and development of red, water-soaked spots on leaves followed by leaf tattering and early defoliation. Cherries on mahaleb (*P. mahaleb* L.) rootstock wilt suddenly and die in mid-summer after contracting the disease whereas cherries on mazzard (*P. avium*) rootstock decline more slowly but produce small fruit which fail to ripen on infected limbs. Symptoms in the wild chokecherry hosts include the development of fall coloration during mid-summer and shortened internodes on growing terminal shoots.

X-Disease, like other diseases caused by fastidious prokaryotes, was assumed to be a virus disease until mycoplasma were observed in phloem cells of diseased plants (Granett and Gilmer, 1971; MacBeath *et al.*, 1972) and infectious leafhoppers (Nasu *et al.*, 1970). Recently several researchers have reported success in culturing a spiroplasma from plants infected with X-disease (Purcell *et al.*, 1981a), but some of the cultured isolates were not pathogenic. It now appears likely that the spiroplasma may have been recovered X-diseased plants dually infected with the X-disease MLO and with *Spiroplasma citri*. Dual infections by *S. citri* and an MLO have been documented in periwinkle and weeds (Calavan and Oldfield, 1979).

Vectors of the western X-disease mycoplasma include *Colladonus geminatus* (Van Duzee) (Wolfe *et al.*, 1951b), *C. montanus* (Van Duzee), *Scaphytopius acutus* (Say), *Fieberiella florii* (Stal), *Graphocephala confluens* (Uhler) (Anthon and Wolfe, 1951; Wolfe and Anthon, 1953), *Euscelidius variegatus* (Kirschbaum) (Jensen, 1957), *Osbornellus borealis* De Long & Mohr (Jensen, 1969), *S: nitridus* (De Long), and *Acinopterus angulatus* (Lawson) (Purcell, 1979b). Because *G. confluens* is a xylem-feeding leafhopper, some experts have suggested the single report of transmission by this species needs further confirmation (Frazier, 1965). Vector species identified for the eastern X-disease mycoplasma are *C. clitellarius* (Say), *S. acutus, F. florii, Paraphlepsius irroratus* (Say), *Norvelina seminuda* (Say) (Gilmer *et al.*, 1966), *Orientus ishidae* (Matsumara), and several unidentified species of *Scaphoideus* (Rosenberger and Jones, 1978).

C. Pierce's Disease of Grapes

Pierce's disease was first observed in 1884 in vineyards near Anaheim, California (Pierce, 1892). The disease spread rapidly through most of the vineyard areas of southern California causing the death of many acres of vines in the 1880s and 1890s (Hewitt, 1958). By 1921 Pierce's disease had reached the northern California grape (*Vitis* spp.) areas, but it spread more slowly in northern California vineyards (Hewitt, 1970). Pierce's disease has destroyed more than 31,000 ha of grapes in California, and the disease is so endemic in the Gulf Coast States that it is a major limiting factor in grape culture in that area (Hewitt, 1958, 1970).

Symptoms of Pierce's disease vary with grape variety and climatic conditions. Symptoms often include delayed growth in spring, mottling, dwarfing and burning of leaves, wilting of fruit, and uneven cane maturity (Hewitt, 1970). The disease kills vines of *Vitis lambrusca* L. and *V. vinifera* L. and thus causes economic damage to most commercial grape varieties. Under field conditions, however, differences exist in varietal susceptibility (Purcell, 1974).

Hewitt (1939) suggested a virus was the causal organism for Pierce's disease and later investigations showed the pathogen was xylem-limited (Hewitt *et al.*, 1942; Houston *et al.*, 1947). Pierce's disease was thus attributed to a xylem-limited virus until RLB were observed in the xylem of infected plants (Goheen *et al.*, 1973; Hopkins and Mollenhauer, 1973). The bacterium causing Pierce's disease has been isolated from infected grapevines and from almond trees (*Prunus amygdalus* Batsch) where it causes almond leaf scorch (Davis *et al.*, 1978, 1980). Other hosts for Pierce's disease bacteria are alfalfa (*Medicago sativa* L.) where it causes alfalfa dwarf (Goheen *et al.*, 1973), citrus (*Citrus sinensis* Isbeck) (Hopkins *et al.*, 1978), and the numerous weed hosts identified by Freitag (1951), Raju *et al.* (1980), and Adlerz and Hopkins (1981). The Pierce's disease bacterium is serologically related to the xylem-limited bacterium causing phony peach disease (Davis *et al.*, 1979), plum (*Prunus* spp.) leaf scald, young tree decline of citrus (Raju *et al.*, 1981), and leaf scorch of elm (*Ulmus* spp.), sycamore (*Platanus* spp.), and oak (*Quercus* spp.) (Hearon *et al.*, 1980).

Pierce's disease is vectored by at least 26 different species of xylem-feeding leafhoppers and froghoppers (Hewitt, 1970), but the most important vector species in California are the sharpshooter leafhoppers *Carneocephala fulgida* Nottingham, *Draeculacephala minerva* Ball, and *Graphocephala atrapunctata* (Signoret) (Hewitt *et al.*, 1942; Purcell, 1975). Vector species present in Florida are *Carneocephala flaviceps* (Riley), *Draeculacephala portola* Ball, *Homalodisca coagulata* (Say), *H. lacerta* (Fowler), and *Oncometopia orbona* (Fabricius) (Kaloostian *et al.*, 1962; Stoner, 1953). *O. nigricans* is probably the most important vector in Florida due to its wide host range and high populations in grape (Adlerz and Hopkins, 1979). Freitag and Frazier (1954) showed infective sharpshooter leafhoppers may be captured throughout the year in southern California, but Adlerz and Hopkins (1979) found the transmission period in Florida was limited to several weeks during spring and early summer.

D. Phony Peach Disease

Phony peach disease was first observed in Georgia around 1890 (Hutchins, 1933). The disease gradually spread west as far as Texas and north to central Illinois, Kentucky, and North Carolina. By 1935 local patterns of disease spread had been established: the disease spread rapidly in infected orchards in the Coastal plains from South Carolina to Texas but more slowly in the Piedmont areas and upper Mississippi and lower Ohio River Valleys (Turner and Pollard, 1959b).

Peach trees affected by phony peach disease show shortened internodes, greater-than-usual lateral branching, and darker-than-normal foliage color. Infected trees develop flowers and leaves earlier than healthy trees and retain leaves longer in the fall. Fruit on infected trees are smaller, ripen earlier, and are more highly colored than fruit on healthy trees.

In addition to peach trees, apricots (*Prunus armeniaca* L.), almonds, and many species of wild plums are hosts for the phony peach bacterium (Hutchins, 1933). Infections in the wild plum *Prunus angustifolia* Marsh. and some other plums produce no symptoms. Wells *et al.* (1980) found an organism similar to the phony peach bacterium in Johnson grass [*Sorghum halpense* (L.) Pers.] and suggested that perennial weeds may also harbor phony peach disease. More recently, Timmer *et al.* (1981) isolated from ragweed (*Ambrosia* spp.) a bacterium serologically similar to the phony-peach bacterium and showed that the ragweed bacterium is transmitted by two of the phony peach vectors.

An extensive search for the vectors of phony peach showed that the sharpshooter leafhoppers *Homalodisca coagulata* (Say), *Oncometopia orbona* (Fabricius), *Cuerna costalis* (Fabricius), *Graphocephala versuta* (Say) (Turner, 1949), *H. insolita* (Walker), *Draeculacephala portola* Ball, and *Oncometopia nigricans* (Walker) (Nielson, 1979; Turner and Pollard, 1955) can all transmit the phony peach bacterium. The life histories of the five most important vectors were described by Turner and Pollard (1959a).

Rickettsialike bacteria were observed in the xylem of peach trees with phony peach disease in 1973 (Hopkins *et al.*, 1973), but the causal organism could not be isolated on the JD3 medium used for culture of Pierce's disease bacterium although the two bacteria are closely related serologically (Davis *et al.*, 1980). The phony peach bacterium has since been isolated on several other artificial media (Davis *et al.*, 1981; Wells *et al.*, 1981).

III. FASTIDIOUS PROKARYOTES IN THEIR PLANT HOSTS

A. Prokaryote Movement

The systemic nature of diseases caused by fastidious prokaryotes attests to the invasive ability of these organisms, but the processes involved in the invasion of plants by fastidious prokaryotes following insect inoculation are one of the least studied aspects of fastidious prokaryote epidemiology. The spread of the pathogens within plants is as important as spread between plants because within-plant movement affects the length of the incubation period in the plant, the availability of inoculum to vector insects feeding on portions of recently inoculated plants distal to the inoculation site, and possibly the ability of pathogens to survive winter in their plant hosts. Because of the paucity of research reports dealing directly with the fastidious prokaryote movement in plants, much of the following discussion is based on field observations and hypotheses which help to explain those observations.

After they are injected into plant phloem or xylem by insect vectors, most of the fastidious prokaryotes invade their plant hosts by multiplying and spreading through the host–plant vascular tissue. The mechanism by which mycoplasma and RLB move through vascular tissue and/or resist being moved within plants has not been determined. During the era when all fastidious prokaryotes were assumed to be viruses, the pathogens were assumed to move as inanimate suspended particles in the vascular stream. Even after the discovery of mycoplasma and RLB, there was little reason to think the pathogens played an active role in their own dispersal throughout plant vascular systems. However, the discovery of the helical morphology and motility of spiroplasmas raises the possibility that with spiroplasmas at least, the pathogen's motility may contribute to its invasion of inoculated plants.

The rate of pathogen movement within plants has not been accurately determined for any of the fastidious prokaryotes, but the rate probably varies with the pathogen, the host plant species, the amount of inoculum introduced, and perhaps with the time of year inoculation occurs. Differences in the rate of pathogen movement within different host plant species may explain some of the differences in X-disease symptom development in infected peach and chokecherry. X-Disease symptoms often appear on only one limb or one scaffold of a peach tree during the first year of infection indicating a slow invasion rate. However, partially infected chokecherry bushes are relatively uncommon, suggesting that the pathogen moves through chokecherry more quickly than through peach. Stoddard (1947) suggested the X-disease pathogen overwinters only in the roots of infected peach trees and is translocated from the roots to the top of the tree each spring because he could transmit X-disease with root patches but not with buds collected from X-diseased peach trees in winter. However, Rosenberger and Jones (1977b) showed X-disease mycoplasmas persist in a low percentage of peach buds even during the coldest part of winter and questioned the earlier theory that the mycoplasma are rapidly translocated throughout the tree crown each spring.

The movement of fastidious prokaryotes in plant vascular systems could conceivably be inhibited by physical obstructions and/or physiological resistance mechanisms within plants. Mycoplasma infecting plant phloem must move from one phloem cell to the next via the sieve plate pores. Electron micrographs have shown mycoplasma traversing the sieve plate pores (MacBeath *et al.*, 1972; Maramorosch *et al.*, 1970) and suggest the phloem sieve plate may provide a physical barrier which slows the flow of mycoplasma through plants. McCoy (1979) showed that the accumulation of mycoplasma in and around sieve-plate pores is an artifact produced by the turgor pressure surge which occurs when sieve tubes are injured. He indicated functioning sieve plate pores are usually large enough to allow mycoplasmas to pass through them. The relationship between the size of the sieve plate pores and the size of the infecting mycoplasmas could nevertheless affect the rate at which mycoplasmas pass from cell to cell. The normal buildup of callose around older sieve plate pores (Esau and Cheadle, 1959) might also inhibit mycoplasma movement during certain times of year. Conceivably, a plant with sieve plate pores too small to allow easy passage of mycoplasma (if any such plants exist) might show some degree of field resistance to the disease because the pathogen would be unable to invade beyond the point of inoculation. Because none of the necessary histological studies have been done, we can only wonder if small sieve plate pores are found in the several cultivars of peach, apricot, plum, and cherry which Gilmer and Blodgett (1976) list as immune to infection by the X-disease mycoplasma.

Physiological responses of plants to invasion by vascular pathogens have been reviewed by Beckman (1964). He proposed that vascular occlusion is a common plant defense against vascular pathogens. Later Hampson and Sinclair (1973) and Banko and Helton (1974) showed that xylem plugging in peach occurs in advance of xylem invasion by *Cytospora* fungi and helps to slow the fungal invasion. An abundance of gums and tyloses have been observed in the xylem of grape and alfalfa infected with Pierce's disease bacteria and in peach trees with symptoms of phony peach disease (Esau, 1948; Houston *et al.*, 1947). Whether the xylem plugging in RLB-infected plants is a host defensive mechanism which occurs in advance of the pathogen invasion or whether the xylem plugging results from vessel damage caused directly by the RLB pathogen has not been determined. In more recent work with grapevines infected with Pierce's disease bacteria, Mollenhauer and Hopkins (1976) reported that gums and tyloses were more abundant in xylem vessels of leaf petioles from Muscadine grapes than in similar tissue from the more susceptible bunch grapes. Although the latter report provides some indirect evidence that vessel occlusion is involved in reducing the movement of RLB in grapes, much more work is needed to clarify the existence and effectiveness of plant defense mechanisms active against the fastidious prokaryotes.

A rapid rate of pathogen invasion in inoculated plants may be either an advantage or a disadvantage for pathogen survival depending on other aspects of the pathogen's epidemiology. A slow rate of pathogen invasion produces a slow increase in surface area of diseased foliage and initially reduces the chances for vectors to find and feed on diseased foliage. Thus, a slow rate of plant invasion by the pathogen should decrease the proportion of vectors which become infective in a given area and should decrease the rate of disease spread in the field. However, a rapidly invaded plant may survive for only a relatively short period of time compared to plants in which invasion occurs more slowly. A pathogen such as the aster yellows mycoplasma which often kills its host plants within several months requires more frequent vector transfers than a pathogen such as the X-disease mycoplasma which commonly survives in the same host plant for 3 to 5 years.

Slow plant invasion following inoculations late in the growing season may limit the pathogen's ability to survive within the plant. In deciduous host plants, fastidious prokaryotes inoculated into leaves late in the season will fail to cause systemic infections if they have not moved beyond the leaves prior to leaf-fall in autumn. Purcell (1975, 1981) showed that vines inoculated with Pierce's disease late in the season often fail to develop disease. He suggested late-season inoculations failed to cause disease because the succulent portion of the vine usually inoculated late in the season is often removed during winter pruning. Failure of the pathogen to invade a significant portion of the host plant may also increase the chances that the pathogen will not survive cold winter temperatures.

B. Effects of Temperature on Prokaryote Survival

Very little effort has been devoted to determining how environmental factors affect the survival and growth rate of fastidious prokaryotes within their plant hosts. Probably the assumed viral etiology of diseases caused by fastidious prokaryotes caused researchers to overlook the possibility that temperature might directly affect the functioning of these pathogens within their plant hosts. Perhaps researchers assumed pathogens within host tissues are protected from the extreme temperature fluctuations experienced by pathogens found on a plant surface. The fallacy of this assumption is amply illustrated by noting the 34°C fluctuation in temperature recorded in bark of peach trees during a single 6-hr period during winter (Martsolf *et al.*, 1975). As we shall see, failure to consider the temperature-sensitive nature of fastidious prokaryotes in inoculated plants has caused considerable confusion in the interpretation of research results.

Although researchers have tended to overlook the effects of ambient temperatures on prokaryote survival in plants, the heat-labile nature of the pathogens causing yellows diseases was noted in 1936. Kunkel (1936) showed that the pathogens causing several peach diseases now attributable to mycoplasmas are inactivated in budwood if the wood is immersed in water at 50°C for 3–4 min. Other researchers reported the X-disease pathogen could be inactivated with 6–7 min of treatment in water at 50°C (Hildebrand, 1953) and by 16 min in water at 48°C (Stoddard, 1947). The effects of cold temperature on pathogen survival was not seriously considered as an epidemiological factor until Hopkins (1976) and Purcell (1977) proposed that cold winter temperatures may limit the northern spread of Pierce's disease.

In California's Napa Valley, Pierce's disease is more prevalent in the vicinity of shaded riverbank vegetation and the incidence of diseased grapevines declines rapidly with distance from the river (Purcell, 1974). Purcell (1975) later showed that the early season (April–May) distribution of the major vector, *Hordinia circellata,* was closely correlated with the incidence of diseased vines. Purcell (1975) also found the natural infectivity and distribution of *H. circellata* within vineyards increased during the growing season, but the disease distribution patterns suggested the absence of secondary disease spread. The lack of secondary spread despite the presence of infective vectors was attributed to seasonal changes in the susceptibility of host plants and/or the failure of late season infections to persist through the dormant season. Later reports (Purcell, 1977, 1980, 1981) verified that grapevines infected with Pierce's disease could be freed of disease by exposure to cold winter temperatures. These reports also showed that late season inoculations result in weak infections which often fail to survive winter conditions.

Factors contributing to the failure of late season infections to persist through winter have not been evaluated. It is not known if plant defense mechanisms or other conditions in the vascular tissues actually cause a reduction in the rate of plant invasion late in the season, or if the slower rate of pathogen invasion can be attributed to cooler temperatures reducing the pathogen growth rate. In either case, one may assume that following late-season inoculations the pathogen often fails to reach the roots or larger woody parts of a tree where winter temperatures are moderated by the soil or by the larger mass of woody tissues. Trunks and branches absorb and hold more heat from solar radiation than smaller twigs and canes. Infections limited to small twigs or vine extremities would be exposed to unmoderated winter temperatures.

C. Plant Invasion and Vector Transmission: Two Separate Steps

The failure of epidemiologists to recognize that vector transmission of the pathogen and plant invasion by the pathogen are two separate processes may cause significant misinterpretation of leafhopper transmission data. Peach trees inoculated with phony peach bacteria or X-disease mycoplasma and grapes inoculated with Pierce's disease bacteria often fail to develop symptoms until the year after inoculation. With these diseases, failure of the pathogen to survive the first winter (prior to symptom development) in its host plant cannot be easily distinguished from failure of leafhopper vectors to transmit the pathogen.

In the initial search for phony peach vectors, much of the work was done near Chattanooga in an area free of phony peach disease (Turner and Pollard, 1959b). However, during 5 years of extensive testing, no successful transmissions were recorded although the same vectors which had been tested in Chattanooga later transmitted the phony peach bacteria at other locations. The failure of Turner and Pollard to find vectors in the Chattanooga location may well have resulted from failure of inoculum to survive the winter in infected plants, and that factor may also explain why the Chattanooga area was free of phony peach (Purcell, 1979a).

Failure to separate vector transmission from the plant invasion process may also cause an overestimation of the potential for disease spread if experimentally inoculated plants are not maintained under normal environmental conditions during the plant incubation period. Thus, the report by Rosenberger and Jones (1978) showing that leafhoppers transmit X-disease to indicator plants in the field in September should not be interpreted to mean September inoculations are important in the field spread of X-disease in Michigan. Indicator plants used in their study were not exposed to normal winter conditions following inoculation. The indicator plants were given only a minimal dormancy period in a cooler at 2°C and plants were then forced in a greenhouse and observed for symptom development. The short dormancy period and mild temperature probably favored survival of late-season infections which could not have survived more severe winter conditions. A more reliable estimate of the *effective* inoculation period for X-disease in peaches might be Stoddard's (1947) estimate based on observations of disease spread following chokecherry removal. He suggested most peach trees developing symptoms were inoculated between mid-June and mid-July. The actual cut-off date for inoculations which survive winter conditions probably varies with the pathogen, the host plant species, the part of the plant inoculated, and the severity of the winter conditions.

D. Prokaryote Titer

No method has been developed for determining the titer of fastidious prokaryotes in diseased plants, but the number of infectious prokaryote units per plant cell and/or the proportion of infected plant cells in an infected plant may directly affect both the ability of insect vectors to acquire the pathogen while feeding and the probabilities for the pathogen's overwinter survival in the plant host. The absence of an established method for determining pathogen titer within plants has precluded any direct studies on the relationship of pathogen titer and vector transmission. However, combining electron microscope observations with vector transmission studies can provide some indirect, non-quantitative evidence about how pathogen titer in various host plants may affect acquisition of the X-disease mycoplasma by vectors.

Shortly after X-disease became a commercial problem in eastern peach orchards, Hildebrand and Palmiter (1942) noted that the disease did not appear to spread from diseased to healthy peach trees but it did spread rapidly into peach orchards from surrounding chokecherries. Rosenberger and Jones (1977a) noted severe X-disease in one peach orchard adjacent to an old cherry orchard in Michigan, and Jones (1981) later reported X-disease can also spread from infected cherry orchards to peaches. Prior to the discovery of plant mycoplasmas, no one could explain why leafhoppers failed to acquire eastern X-disease from infected peach trees.

Electron microscope studies of the X-disease mycoplasma showed striking differences in the apparent titer of the pathogen in different host plants. Jones *et al.* (1974) noted that mycoplasma were relatively easy to find in phloem cells of X-diseased chokecherry and sour cherry and in peach infected with little peach disease, but mycoplasma were relatively uncommon in thin sections from X-diseased peach trees. These differences in the abundance of mycoplasma as observed with the electron microscope suggest the mycoplasma titer is higher in chokecherry and sour cherry than in peach. Thus, one reason peach to peach spread of X-disease may be rare in eastern United States may be that vectors feeding on diseased trees will rarely encounter mycoplasma in the phloem. Vectors feeding on infected tart cherry or chokecherry are much more likely to encounter mycoplasma. If the failure of leafhoppers to acquire X-disease mycoplasma from peach in eastern United States is caused by low pathogen titer in peach, then vectors would still be expected to acquire the mycoplasma from peach on the rare occasions when they encounter mycoplasma in the phloem. Such low probability encounters could explain some of the cases of slow X-disease spread in eastern peach orchards where no alternate host plants could be found (Lukens *et al.*, 1971; Rosenberger and Jones, 1977a). An extremely low transmission frequency from X-diseased peach would almost preclude detecting peach to peach spread with small numbers of caged leafhoppers.

There is virtually no experimental evidence to explain how prokaryote titer affects overwinter survival of the prokaryote in infected plants. We can only suggest a probable pattern for seasonal rise and fall of prokaryote populations in infected plants. Fastidious bacteria and mycoplasma have no known resting stage or protective structures to carry them through periods of adverse temperature. Multiplication of these pathogens is assumed to decrease as temperatures decline, and the pathogen populations within plants decline when natural mortality exceeds the rate of multiplication. Adlerz and Hopkins (1979) have shown that the availability of Pierce's disease bacterium declines in late summer, and Rosenberger and Jones (1977b) showed by bud inoculation of indicator plants that the X-disease mycoplasma was present in more buds in summer than during other times of year. Possibly factors other than temperature contribute to decline of pathogen titer in late summer. Hopkins (1981) noted bacterial populations in grape declined even before temperatures dropped in autumn.

Two mechanisms might be at work in temperature-dependent declines of prokaryote populations within plants. The decline in pathogen titer during winter may be a gradual process of population depletion during extended periods of temperature too low to allow pathogen growth, or pathogen populations may collapse rapidly following temperature stresses which directly contribute to pathogen mortality. The latter mechanism would explain the "curing" effect of heat treatments on yellows infected plants, but as yet there is no firm evidence that a short cold period will cause a high rate of pathogen mortality. In fact, Purcell (1980) found a poor correlation between daily minimum temperature and the percentage of exposed grapevines recovering from Pierce's disease.

Correlating gradual declines in plant pathogen titers with temperature would be difficult without some prior information on the pathogen's growth response to temperature when grown in pure culture. With their relatively short generation times, fastidious bacteria and mycoplasma may benefit from daily periods of warm temperature even when nights are cold. Thus, survival of the pathogen during winter may be correlated less closely with average daily temperatures than with the number of hours during which temperatures within the host tissue are above the minimum temperature required for pathogen growth.

E. Noncrop Host Plants

Noncrop hosts or "alternate hosts" of fastidious prokaryotes often function as inoculum sources for insect vectors which later inoculate crop plants. Noncrop hosts have also served as "bridges" between crop areas and as overwintering inoculum reservoirs. To understand how disease spreads through commercial crops the epidemiologist must be able to identify other host plants which may contribute to an epidemic.

One of the more striking examples of an alternate host contributing to disease spread in a commercial crop is the role of wild chokecherry in the spread of eastern X-disease of peach. As noted earlier, peach to peach spread of X-disease is not important in eastern United States. Hildebrand and Palmiter (1942) reported no X-disease infections were found more than 63 m away from diseased chokecherries and Stoddard (1947) noted a row by row decrease in X-disease in nursery stock as the distance from X-diseased chokecherries increased. The association between chokecherries and X-diseased peach trees led to the standard recommendation of removing all chokecherries within 160 m of peach orchards (Parker *et al.*, 1963). More recently, recommendations have included separating new peach plantings from older plantings of sweet and tart cherry because cultivated cherry orchards can also provide X-disease inoculum for peach orchards (Jones, 1981).

In addition to its function as an X-disease inoculum reservoir, chokecherry has also functioned as a host bridge for the X-disease mycoplasma between commercial stone fruit plantings. Wild chokecherry is the only known, commonly occurring wild host for X-disease in northeastern North America and the abundance of wild chokecherry throughout this area apparently enabled X-disease to spread from Connecticut to Michigan in less than 10 years (Stoddard, 1947; Cation, 1941). Although the western chokecherry is less important as an inoculum source for within-orchard spread of X-disease in western United States, Richards and Cochran (1957) noted that the western chokecherry contributed to spread between orchards.

A high incidence of Pierce's disease in grapes in California has been associated with alternate host plants along river banks (Purcell, 1975) and irrigated pastures (Hewitt *et al.*, 1942). Pierce's disease has also been more severe where vineyards adjoined alfalfa fields showing symptoms of alfalfa dwarf, a disease caused by the Pierce's disease bacterium (Hewitt *et al.*, 1946). Alfalfa dwarf is more severe in weedy alfalfa fields where weeds also act as hosts for the causal bacterium (Purcell, 1979a). In all of the above instances, the importance of the alternate hosts for the bacterium is increased by the fact that these alternate hosts also provide preferred habitat for the insect vectors of Pierce's disease.

Aster yellows is a commercial problem primarily in annual crops. Perennial weed hosts are therefore important sources of overwintering inoculum. Wallis (1960) and Hagel and Landis (1967) listed more than 70 biennial and perennial host plants for aster yellows. Fall planted barley (*Hordeum vulgare* L.) and wheat (*Triticum aestivum* L.) may also serve as overwintering hosts for aster yellows (Banttari, 1965; Chiykowski, 1963).

The presence of alternate hosts can seriously compromise the value of removing diseased plants from commercial plantings. Winkler *et al.* (1949) found that removing grapevines infected with Pierce's disease did not reduce disease spread and Frietag (1951) and Purcell (1974) showed this failure was related to the presence of weed hosts around the fields. In an attempt to limit the spread of phony peach disease, infected peach trees were marked and removed from orchards in southeastern United States. Because wild plum is also a host for phony peach (Hutchins and Rue, 1949), wild plum and other wild *Prunus* were also removed from areas surrounding orchards. Roguing diseased trees and wild *Prunus* was not conclusively proven to be effective (KenKnight, 1961), and disease incidence has increased periodically despite roguing efforts (Hopkins, 1977). Wells *et al.* (1980) reported finding an RLB in Johnson grass which was antigenically similar to the phony peach RLB. Timmer *et al.* (1981) found a similar RLB in ragweed. If the RLB in Johnson grass or ragweed proves capable of causing phony disease in peach, the presence of these weed hosts may explain the limited effectiveness of earlier roguing efforts, especially since Turner and Pollard (1955) reported that one of the phony disease vectors, *H. insolita,* feeds and breeds on Johnson grass.

IV. FASTIDIOUS PROKARYOTES IN THEIR VECTOR HOSTS

A. Transmission of Mycoplasmas

How mycoplasmas invade their insect vectors has been examined in more detail than their invasion of plant hosts. Kunkel (1926) began the investigation of mycoplasma–vector relationships by testing the effect of the aster yellows pathogen on vector longevity. Although he reported that infective aster leafhoppers lived just as long as noninfective leafhoppers, Littau and Maramorosch (1956, 1960) later showed aster yellows is pathogenic to its insect vectors. Jensen (1959, 1962, 1971) found that the western X-disease pathogen reduced both the lifespan and reproductive potential of *C. montanus.* The mean lifespan for infected leafhoppers was reduced from 55 to 38 days and 30% of infective females were sterile. Fecundity was severely reduced in another 30% of the females.

The cytopathological effects of the X-disease mycoplasma on its vector *C. montanus* were examined in a series of reports by Whitcomb *et al.* (1967, 1968a,b,c). Cytopathological symptoms were found in the salivary, neural, adipose, and alimentary tracts of infective vectors. Whitcomb *et al.* (1967) found lesions in neural tissue but never in salivary tissues of noninfective leafhoppers which had been injected with mycoplasma (see next paragraph for an explanation of leafhopper injection). Whitcomb *et al.* (1968a) also showed that the gut wall is affected only in leafhoppers which acquire X-disease by feeding, not in leafhoppers injected with mycoplasma. Taken all together, the cytopathological evidence shows mycoplasmas invade the gut wall after being ingested by leafhoppers. The mycoplasmas then circulate through the hemolymph, infect other body tissues including the salivary glands, and are then excreted into plants with normal excretions during feeding. The length of an incubation period for a pathogen in its insect vector apparently is determined by the amount of time required for the pathogen to move through the gut wall and into the salivary glands.

In vector transmission experiments, leafhopper acquisition of mycoplasma from diseased plants is a time-consuming and often inefficient process: only a small proportion of the vectors feeding on a diseased plant may become infective and many vectors may die before completion of the incubation period. To circumvent these difficulties, many investigators have used a technique pioneered by Storey (1933) and further refined by Black (1940) in which the pathogen is injected into the hemolymph of leafhopper vectors. With this procedure, a large number of infective vectors are ground in a buffer solution, the solution is clarified by centrifugation, and 0.002 to 0.2 μl of the clarified solution are injected into anesthetized leafhoppers through a fine, pulled-glass needle inserted into the abdomen between the third and fourth sternites. Using this technique, as many as 1000 insects per hour can be injected (Markham and Townsend, 1979), the precise time that the mycoplasma enters the leafhopper is known, and the incubation period is shortened. Nearly 100% of the injected vectors will be infective compared to less than 50% for many vectors given acquisition access periods on diseased plants. The use of microinjection to inoculate vectors has been reviewed by Markham and Townsend (1979).

Although the injection of leafhoppers allows mycoplasma to invade the vectors without traversing the gut wall, Sinha and Chiykowski (1967) have shown that *Agallia constricta* Van Duzee, a leafhopper which fails to acquire aster yellows from infected plants, will also fail to transmit aster yellows following injection with the pathogen. Townsend and Markham (1976) showed the spiroplasmas causing corn (*Zea mays* L.) stunt and citrus stubborn could survive and multiply when injected into nonvector insects, and although salivary glands of the nonvector insect became infected, they transmitted the spiroplasma to very few plants. Thus, neither the gut wall nor the salivary glands can be considered as simple barriers which by themselves prevent nonvector leafhoppers from acquiring and transmitting mycoplasma. Rather, the ability of a vector to transmit a specific mycoplasma appears to depend on many factors including both vector feeding habits and susceptibility of specific vector tissues to invasion by the mycoplasma.

B. Transmission of Xylem-Limited RLB

The transmission mechanism for xylem-limited RLB is much simpler than the mechanism involved in transmission of mycoplasmas, but it differs from all previously described leafhopper transmission mechanisms and was not finally explained until 1979. Severin (1949) and Purcell (1976) working with Pierce's disease noted that the adult sharpshooter vectors had incubation periods as short as 2 hr and then remained infective for long periods, often until they died. The retention of the virus by the vectors suggested circulative transmission, but the incubation period appeared too short to fit the circulative transmission pattern. After insects injected with Pierce's disease failed to become infective and insects failed to retain the virus during molts, Purcell and Finlay (1979) concluded circulative transmission was not involved.

The mechanism of transmission was finally clarified when Purcell *et al.* (1979) found Pierce's disease bacteria adhering to the wall of the esophagus in infective leafhoppers. Bacteria ingested with xylem sap apparently survive and multiply in the foregut of insect vectors and are egested into xylem again during normal feeding processes. The location of the bacteria within the vectors also explained the loss of infectivity following vector molts because the linings of the foregut and esophagus are lost during molting.

Although this transmission mechanism has been proved only for Pierce's disease, other xylem-limited RLB may be transmitted by the same mechanism since they also have short incubation periods and long pathogen retention by their vectors.

V. HOW VECTOR BIOLOGY AFFECTS DISEASE SPREAD

A. Vector Host Preference

The importance of vector host preference is illustrated by Kunkel's (1926) observation that marigolds are susceptible to aster yellows but are seldom infected in the field because the aster yellows leafhopper does not normally feed on marigolds. The patterns of disease incidence within a commercial planting may reflect the distribution of preferred vector host plants and/or good vector habitat. Thus, Pierce's disease was more prevalent in areas of Napa Valley vineyards bordering the Napa River because vectors readily colonized many of the weed hosts common to the riverbottom (Purcell, 1974). Rosenberger and Jones (1977a) noted X-disease was more severe in low areas of some peach orchards and suggested the lush grass in these low spots may have attracted more vectors to the area.

Habitat and/or host preferences limit the economic importance of many insect vector species. Although 26 species of insects are known to transmit the Pierce's disease bacterium, only three species are commonly found in California vineyards (Hewitt, 1970), and the incidence of these species depends on the ecology of the area surrounding the orchard. *Draeculacephala minerva* and *Carneocephala fulgida* are the most important vectors in the central valley of California where vineyards are close to irrigated pastures and alfalfa, but the dendrophilous *Graphocephala atropunctata* is the major vector in the Napa Valley and coastal areas where vineyards border wooded areas (Hewitt *et al.*, 1942; Purcell, 1975). The other 23 vectors of Pierce's disease may be important in disseminating Pierce's disease among noncrop host plants, but because of their habitat and host preference they are comparatively less important in California vineyards. Similarly, the *Scaphoideus* vectors of X-disease prefer woodland habitat and may have contributed significantly to the spread of X-disease in chokecherry, but they are far less common in peach orchards than other vectors and are unlikely to contribute to the spread of X-disease in orchards (Rosenberger and Jones, 1978; Taboada *et al.*, 1975).

Vector host preferences may also affect a vector's ability to survive in sprayed croplands. *Scaphytopius acutus* and *Paraphlepsius irroratus*, the major vectors of X-disease in eastern North America (Gilmer *et al.*, 1966; Rosenberger and Jones, 1978), breed and feed primarily on grasses (De Long, 1948; Osborn, 1912). Because they appear to feed on trees only occasionally, these vectors may survive orchard insecticides more readily than vectors which feed primarily on trees (Rosenberger and Jones, 1978).

Vector preferences could conceivably increase the probability of vectors feeding on diseased plants instead of adjacent healthy plants. Sticky traps used in leafhopper surveys are commonly painted yellow because that color is effective in attracting leafhoppers (Taboada *et al.*, 1975). Many of the mycoplasma diseases cause yellowing of fôliage which could increase the attractiveness of diseased plants to leafhoppers.

B. Vector Movement and Dispersal

Vector movement from one feeding site to another is an obvious requisite for dissemination of fastidious prokaryotes. Vector movement often appears unpredictable but occasionally falls into patterns which can be attributed to seasonal changes in the vector's host plant preferences, to wind patterns, or to ecological disturbances. The importance of long distance leafhopper migration was demonstrated when Carter (1930) and Dorst and Davis (1937) showed that in western United States the beet leafhopper *Circulifer tenellus* (Baker), the vector of beet curly top virus, annually migrates from arid hill country across several hundred miles of desert to the irrigated beet fields. Long distance migration of *C. tenellus* may have contributed to epidemics of brittleroot of horseradish, a disease caused by *Spiroplasma citri* (Fletcher *et al.*, 1981). Brittleroot has been a problem in southern Illinois primarily during seasons when *C. tenellus* populations are high.

Long distance migration of the aster leafhopper from the Ozark area of Missouri to Wisconsin was documented by Drake and Chapman (1965) and Chiykowski and Chapman (1965). The migration of the aster leafhopper is stimulated by the ripening of small grain host plants in Missouri. The leafhoppers are carried northward on wind currents in spring storms and arrive in Minnesota and Wisconsin before leafhoppers hatching from eggs in those areas have become adults. Some of the migrating aster leafhoppers acquire aster yellows mycoplasma during or prior to their migration and are therefore infective upon arrival in Wisconsin (Drake and Chapman, 1965). The early arrival of infective leafhoppers in Wisconsin increased early season spread of aster yellows in commercial crops. McClure (1980) suggested that X-disease vectors in Connecticut move from hedgerow plants to orchards during summer, possibly because vegetation in hedgerows stops growing earlier.

A vector's ability to fly long distances may also affect its economic importance as a vector. *Paraphlepsius irroratus,* the major X-disease vector in Michigan, is a strong flier. It was captured more than 9 miles from land in the Delaware Bay (Stearns and MacCreary, 1938) and is known to occur in virtual swarms (Steyskal, 1945). The flying ability of this vector may be one reason X-disease spreads more rapidly in Michigan than in New York where *P. irroratus* is less common (Rosenberger and Jones, 1978).

VI. FUTURE FOR EPIDEMIOLOGICAL RESEARCH

A. Handicaps in Epidemiological Research

One of the major problems in research with fastidious prokaryotes has been and continues to be our inability to grow these hidden pathogens on simple culture media. The fact that no bacterium or other organism could be isolated from diseased plants led to the commonly accepted idea that diseases caused by mycoplasmas and fastidious bacteria were viral in nature. Much of our knowledge of insect vectors of fastidious prokaryotes stems from research performed prior to 1967 when all of these pathogens were considered viruses. The discovery of mycoplasmas and RLB neither negated nor diminished the value of earlier vector research, but earlier researchers would undoubtedly have profitted from knowing the true identity of the pathogens with which they were working. Knowing minimum temperatures for pathogen growth and survival in culture might have stimulated studies on pathogen survival in plants and might have contributed to an earlier recognition that winter temperatures may affect pathogen survival.

Although nearly 15 years have passed since MLOs were first described in plants by Doi *et al.* (1967), relatively few of the fastidious prokaryotes have been grown in pure culture and characterized. In some cases where successful isolations of mycoplasma or RLB have been reported, the organism initially isolated has proven to be a contaminant (Purcell *et al.*, 1977) or only a few of the isolates recovered from diseased plants have been proven pathogenic (Purcell *et al.*, 1981a). A culture medium suitable for isolation of one organism may prove unsatisfactory for culture of a similar organism as is the case with the RLBs causing Pierce's disease and phony peach (Davis *et al.*, 1980). Because of the difficulty in acquiring and maintaining cultures of fastidious prokaryotes, most vector researchers must still work with cultures which are maintained by frequent transfers from diseased to healthy host plants and the relationships between organisms causing different diseases cannot be determined in a definite manner.

A second problem encountered in researching the epidemiology of fastidious prokaryotes is the need for interdisciplinary cooperation. Expertise in plant pathology, entomology, microbiology, and ecology is often needed in the course of a single study. The epidemiologist must be able to recognize and describe the disease symptoms in various host plants. He should be familiar enough with insect taxonomy to be able to recognize common vector species, and knowledge of insect ecology is important for understanding vector distribution in the field. The epidemiologist should have the expertise and facilities for maintaining insect colonies and he may need to identify and catalog the weed hosts of both the vectors and the pathogen. If he wishes to isolate the causal organism or make serological comparisons among various organisms, the epidemiologist will need the skills of a microbiologist. Electron microscopy may be useful for observing the pathogen. Because few scientists have the expertise and the facilities needed for work in all of the epidemiology-related areas mentioned above, the epidemiologist must often depend on cooperators from other disciplines.

A third problem encountered in epidemiological research is the long-term nature of many studies. The pace of investigations may be slowed by lengthy incubation periods in the vector and/or in the host plant. For example, the X-disease mycoplasma has an incubation period of 23–40 or more days in its insect vectors and 3 weeks in celery. Thus, an experiment testing transmission with a suspected vector species will require a total of about 2 months before any results are available if celery is used as the acquisition host plant and the test plant. If peach trees or other woody indicator plants are used, results may not be evident until the season following inoculation. Some vector species have only one generation per year and survive poorly in captivity. In such cases the epidemiologist may have only 2 or 3 weeks per year during which he can capture suspected vectors in the field and test their ability to transmit the pathogens involved. Determining vector populations in the field also requires multiyear data because population patterns vary greatly from one season to the next (Rosenberger and Jones, 1978).

Despite the difficulties encountered in researching the epidemiology of diseases caused by fastidious prokaryotes, such research is needed both to explain field observations of disease incidence and to provide insight for selecting control measures. The epidemiologist must use his interdisciplinary expertise to put together all the pieces in the puzzle. Only as the various pieces fall into place can we fully understand how the vectors, the pathogens, and the host plants interact together to cause disease in the field.

B. Promising Areas for Future Research

Throughout this chapter's discussion of factors affecting the dissemination of fastidious prokaryotes, we occasionally alluded to areas needing further research. Many of these areas are interrelated and progress in one area may be dependent on progress in another. Thus, the development and improvement of techniques for isolating fastidious prokaryotes into pure culture may provide a means for following the progress of infection in plant hosts. Characterization of the pathogens should clarify which diseases are caused by the same or similar pathogens, and understanding the relationship between disease organisms should open the door for more work on vector specificity.

Few researchers have attempted to quantify the factors involved in the dissemination of fastidious prokaryotes. Numerous vector trapping studies have been made (Rice and Jones, 1972; Rosenberger and Jones,

1978; Tabooda *et al.*, 1975), but little effort has been given to relating numbers of vectors trapped to numerical populations of vectors per unit area in the field or even to the incidence of disease. Rates of disease spread vary greatly from site to site (McCoy *et al.*, 1976; Rosenberger and Jones, 1977a) because of the great variation in factors affecting disease spread. Purcell (1981) has outlined a theoretical model to account for the rate of spread of Pierce's disease, but until more accurate estimates are available for all of the variables in the model, the model will be of limited usefulness in predicting disease spread in the field.

Another potentially profitable area for future research involves new approaches to vector control. Weires and Straub (1980) have reported that periodical cicada avoided trees sprayed with the synthetic pyrethroid permethrin and Highwood (1979) suggested the repellent action of pyrethroids may have contributed to reduction in aphid-transmitted viruses. Whether other insects or leafhopper vectors would behave similarly has not been determined. Systemic insecticides such as aldicarb and carbofuran are being tested for use in nonbearing orchards, and these materials might also prove useful in reducing inoculation by insect vectors.

Throughout our discussion we have used examples from only a few disease systems because relatively little is known about the epidemiology of the majority of other diseases caused by fastidious prokaryotes. No vectors have been identified for many diseases, and only one or two vectors have been found for other diseases. These diseases provide innumerable opportunities for further epidemiological research on fastidious prokaryotes.

References

Adlerz, W. C., and Hopkins, D. L. (1979). *J. Econ. Entomol.* **72,** 916–919.
Alderz, W. C., and Hopkins, D. L. (1981). *Phytopathology* **71,** 856.
Anthon, E. W., and Wolfe, H. R. (1951). *Plant Dis. Rep.* **35,** 345–346.
Banko, T. J., and Helton, A. W. (1974). *Phytopathology* **64,** 899–901.
Banttari, E. E. (1965). *Phytopathology* **55,** 838–843.
Beckman, C. H. (1964). *Annu. Rev. Phytopathol.* **2,** 231–52.
Black, L. M. (1940). *Phytopathology* **30,** 2.
Calavan, E. C., and Oldfield, G. N. (1979). *In* "The Mycoplasmas—Plant and Insect Mycoplasmas" (R. F. Whitcomb and J. G. Tully, eds.), Vol. III, pp. 37–64. Academic Press, New York.
Carter, W. (1939). *U.S. Dep. Agric. Tech. Bull.* 206.
Cation, D. (1941). *Plant Dis. Rep.* **25,** 406–407.
Chiykowski, L. N. (1962). *Can. J. Bot.* **40,** 779–801.
Chiykowski, L. N. (1963). *Can. J. Bot.* **41,** 669–672.
Chiykowski, L. N. (1977). *Phytopathology* **67,** 522–524.

Chiykowski, L. N. (1981). *In* "Plant Diseases and Vectors: Ecology and Epidemiology" (K. Maramorosch and K. F. Harris, eds.), pp. 105–159. Academic Press, New York.
Chiykowski, L. N., and Chapman, R. K. (1965). *Univ. Wis., Madison, Res. Bull.* **261,** 23–45.
Chiykowski, L. N., and Sinha, R. C. (1969). *J. Econ. Entomol.* **62,** 883–886.
Davis, M. J., Purcell, A. H., and Thomson, S. V. (1978). *Science* **199,** 75–77.
Davis, M. J., Stassi, D. L., French, W. J., and Thomson, S. V. (1979). *Proc. Int. Conf. Plant Pathog. Bact., 4th, 1978, Angers* pp. 311–315.
Davis, M. J., Thomson, S. V., and Purcell, A. H. (1980). *Phytopathology* **70,** 472–475.
Davis, M. J., French, W. J., and Schaad, N. W. (1981). *Phytopathology* **71,** 869.
Davis, R. E. (1978). *Can. J. Microbiol.* **24,** 954–959.
De Long, D. M. (1948). *Ill. Natl. Hist. Survey Bull.* **24** (Article 2).
Doi, Y., Terenaka, M., Yora, K., and Asuyama, H. (1967). *Ann. Phytopathol. Soc. Jpn.* **33,** 259–266.
Dorst, H. E., and Davis, E. W. (1937). *J. Econ. Entomol.* **30,** 948–954.
Drake, D. C., and Chapman, R. K. (1965). *Univ. Wisc., Madison, Res. Bull.* **261,** 5–20.
Esau, K. (1948). *Hilgardia* **18,** 423–482.
Esau, K., and Cheadle, V. I. (1959). *Proc. Natl. Acad. Sci. U.S.A.* **45,** 156–162.
Fletcher, J., Schultz, G. A., Davis, R. E., Eastman, C. E., and Goodman, R. M. (1981). *Phytopathology* **71,** 1073–1080.
Frazier, N. W. (1965). *Proc. Int. Conf. Virus Vector Perennial Hosts, Univ. Calif. Div. Agric. Sci., Davis* pp. 91–99.
Freitag, J. H. (1951). *Phytopathology* **41,** 920–934.
Freitag, J. H., and Frazier, N. W. (1954). *Phytopathology* **44,** 7–11.
Gilmer, R. M., and Blodgett, E. C. (1976). *U.S. Dep. Agric. Handbook* **437,** pp. 145–155.
Gilmer, R. M., Moore, J. D., and Keitt, G. W. (1954). *Phytopathology* **44,** 180–185.
Gilmer, R. M., Palmiter, D. H., Schaffers, G. A., and McEwens, F. L. (1966). *N.Y. State Agric. Exp. Sta. (Geneva) Bull.* 813.
Goheen, A. C., Nyland, G., and Lowe, S. K. (1973). *Phytopathology* **63,** 341–345.
Granett, E. L., and Gilmer, R. M. (1971). *Phytopathology* **61,** 1036–1037.
Hagel, G. T., and Landis, B. J. (1967). *Ann. Entomol. Soc. Am.* **60,** 591–595.
Hampson, M. C., and Sinclair, W. A. (1973). *Phytopathology* **63,** 676–681.
Harris, K. F. (1979). *In* "Leafhopper Vectors and Plant Disease Agents" (K. Maramorosch and K. F. Harris, eds.), pp. 217–308. Academic Press, New York.
Hearon, S. S., Sherald, J. L., and Kostka, S. J. (1980). *Can. J. Bot.* **58,** 1986–1993.
Hewitt, W. B. (1939). *Phytopathology* **29,** 10.
Hewitt, W. B. (1958). *Plant Dis. Rep.* **42,** 211–215.
Hewitt, W. B. (1970). *In* "Virus Diseases of Small Fruits and Grapevines" (N. W. Frazier, ed.), pp. 192–200. Univ. of Calif., Div. of Agric. Sci., Berkeley.
Hewitt, W. B., Frazier, N. W., Jacob, H. E., and Freitag, J. H. (1942). *Calif. Agric. Exp. Sta. Circ.* **353,** 1–32.
Hewitt, W. B., Houston, B. R., Frazier, N. W., and Freitag, J. H. (1946). *Phytopathology* **36,** 117–128.
Highwood, D. P. (1979). *Proc. Br. Crop Protect. Conf. Pests Dis., November* pp. 361–369.
Hildebrand, E. M. (1953). *Cornell Univ. Agric. Exp. Sta. Mem.* **323,** 24.
Hildebrand, E. M., and Palmiter, D. H. (1942). *N.Y. State Hortic. Soc. Proc.* **87,** 34–40.
Hopkins, D. L. (1976). *Am. Wine Soc. J.* **8,** 26–27.
Hopkins, D. L. (1977). *Annu. Rev. Phytopathol.* **17,** 277–294.
Hopkins, D. L. (1981). *Phytopathology* **71,** 415–418.
Hopkins, D. L., and Mollenhauer, H. H. (1973). *Science* **179,** 289–300.
Hopkins, D. L., Mollenhauer, H. H., and French, W. J. (1973). *Phytopathology* **63,** 1422–1423.

Hopkins, D. L., Adlerz, W. C., and Bistline, F. W. (1978). *Plant Dis. Rep.* **62,** 442–445.
Houston, B. R., Esau, K., and Hewitt, W. B. (1947). *Phytopathology* **37,** 247–253.
Hutchins, L. M. (1933). *Office State Entomol., Ga. Bull.* **78.**
Hutchins, L. M., and Rue, J. L. (1949). *Phytopathology* **39,** 661.
Jensen, D. D. (1957). *J. Econ. Entomol.* **50,** 668–672.
Jensen, D. D. (1959). *Virology* **8,** 164–175.
Jensen, D. D. (1962). *Proc. Int. Congr. Entomol., 11th, Vienna, Aug. 1960* pp. 790–791.
Jensen, D. D. (1969). *J. Econ. Entomol.* **62,** 1147–1150.
Jensen, D. D. (1971). *J. Invertebr. Pathol.* **17,** 389–394.
Jensen, D. D., Frazier, N. W., and Thomas, H. E. (1952). *J. Econ. Entomol.* **45,** 335–337.
Jensen, D. D., Griggs, W. H., Gonzales, C. Q., and Schneider, H. (1964). *Phytopathology* **54,** 1346–1351.
Jones, A. L. (1981). *Am. Fruit Grower* **101,** 16.
Jones, A. L., Hopper, G. R., and Rosenberger, D. A. (1974). *Phytopathology* **64,** 755–756.
Kaloostian, G. H., Pollard, H. N., and Turner, W. F. (1962). *Plant Dis. Rep.* **46,** 292.
KenKnight, G. (1961). *Phytopathology* **51,** 345.
Kunkel, L. O. (1926). *Am. J. Bot.* **13,** 646–705.
Kunkel, L. O. (1936). *Phytopathology* **26,** 809–830.
Kunkel, L. O. (1955). *Adv. Virus Res.* **3,** 251–273.
Littau, V. C., and Maramorosch, K. (1956). *Virology* **2,** 128–30.
Littau, V. C., and Maramorosch, K. (1960). *Virology* **10,** 482–500.
Lukens, R. J., Miller, P. M., Walton, G. S., and Hitchcock, S. W. (1971). *Plant Dis. Rep.* **55,** 645–647.
MacBeath, J. H., Nyland, G., and Spurr, A. R. (1972). *Phytopathology* **62,** 935–937.
McClure, M. S. (1980). *Environ. Entomol.* **9,** 668–672.
McCoy, R. E. (1979). *NSC Symp. Ser.* **1,** 15–19.
McCoy, R. E., Carroll, V. J., Poucher, C. P., and Gwin, G. H. (1976). *Phytopathology* **66,** 1148–1150.
Magie, R. O., Smith, F. F., and Brierley, P. (1953). *In* "The Gladiolus," p. 93. New England Gladiolus Society, Boston, Massachusetts.
Maramorosch, K. (1979). *Am. Soc. Microbiol. Abstr. Annu. Meet., 79th* p. 85.
Maramorosch, K. (1981). *Bioscience* **31,** 374–380.
Maramorosch, K., Granados, R. R., and Hirumi, H. (1970). *Proc. Natl. Acad. Sci. U.S.A.* **45,** 156–162.
Markham, P. G., and Towsend, R. (1979). *In* "Leafhopper Vectors and Plant Disease Agents" (K. Maramorosch and K. F. Harris, eds.), pp. 413–445. Academic Press, New York.
Martinez, A. L., and Wallace, J. M. (1967). *Plant Dis. Rep.* **51,** 692–695.
Martsolf, J. D., Ritter, C. M., and Hatch, A. H. (1975). *J. Am. Soc. Hortic. Sci.* **100,** 122–129.
Mollenhauer, H. H., and Hopkins, D. L. (1976). *Physiol. Plant Pathol.* **9,** 95–100.
Nasu, S., Jensen, D. D., and Richardson, J. (1970). *Virology* **41,** 583–595.
Nielson, M. W. (1979). *In* "Leafhopper Vectors and Plant Disease Agents" (K. Maramorosch, and K. F. Harris, eds.), pp. 3–27. Academic Press, New York.
Nielson, M. W., and Jones, L. S. (1954). *Phytopathology* **54,** 218–219.
Nyland, G., and Schlocker, A. (1951). *Plant Dis. Rep.* **35,** 33.
Olson, E. O., and Rogers, B. (1969). *Plant Dis. Rep.* **53,** 45–49.
Osborn, H. (1912). *U.S. Dep. Agric. Bur. Entomol. Bull.* 108.
Parker, K. G., Palmiter, D. H., Gilmer, R. M., and Hickey, K. D. (1963). *N.Y. State Agric. Ext. Bull.* 1100.
Pierce, N. B. (1892). *U.S. Dep. Agric. Div. Veg. Pathol. Bull.* **2,** 1–22.

Purcell, A. H. (1974). *Am. J. Enol. Viticult.* **25,** 162–167.
Purcell, A. H. (1975). *Environ. Entomol.* **4,** 745–752.
Purcell, A. H. (1976). *Pan-Pac. Entomol.* **52,** 33–37.
Purcell, A. H. (1977). *Plant Dis. Rep.* **61,** 514–518.
Purcell, A. H. (1979a). *In* "Leafhopper Vectors and Plant Disease Agents" (K. Maramorosch and K. F. Harris, eds.), pp. 603–625. Academic Press, New York.
Purcell, A. H. (1979b). *Plant Dis. Rep.* **63,** 549–552.
Purcell, A. H. (1980). *Plant Dis.* **64,** 388–390.
Purcell, A. H. (1981). *Phytopathology* **71,** 429–435.
Purcell, A. H., and Finlay, A. H. (1979). *Phytopathology* **69,** 393–395.
Purcell, A. H., Latorre-Guzman, B. A., Kado, C. I., Goheen, A. C., and Shalla, T. A. (1977). *Phytopathology* **67,** 298–301.
Purcell, A. H., Finlay, A. H., and McLean, D. L. (1979). *Science* **206,** 839–841.
Purcell, A. H., Raju, B. C., and Nyland, G. (1981a). *Phytopathology* **71,** 108.
Purcell, A. H., Nyland, G., Raju, B. C., and Heringer, M. R. (1981b). *Plant Dis.* **65,** 365–368.
Raju, B. C., Nome, S. F., Docampo, D. M., Goheen, A. C., Nyland, G., and Lowe, S. K. (1980). *Am. J. Enol. Viticult.* **31,** 144–148.
Raju, B. C., Nyland, G., Goheen, A. C., Nome, S. F., Wells, J. W., Weaver, D. J., and Lee, R. F. (1981). *Phytopathology* **71,** 108.
Rawlins, T. E., and Horne, W. T. (1931). *Phytopathology* **21,** 331–335.
Rawlins, T. E., and Thomas, H. E. (1941). *Phytopathology* **31,** 916–925.
Reeves, E. L., Blodgett, E. C., Lott, T. B., Milbrath, J. A., Richards, B. L., and Zeller, S. M. (1951). *U.S. Dep. Agric. Handbook* No. 10, pp. 43–52.
Rice, R. E., and Jones, R. A. (1972). *Environ. Entomol.* **1,** 726–730.
Richards, R. L., and Cochran, L. C. (1957). *Utah Agric. Exp. Sta. Bull.* **384.**
Rosenberger, D. A., and Jones, A. L. (1977a). *Plant Dis. Rep.* **61,** 830–834.
Rosenberger, D. A., and Jones, A. L. (1977b). *Plant Dis. Rep.* **61,** 1022–1024.
Rosenberger, D. A., and Jones, A. L. (1978). *Phytopathology* **68,** 782–790.
Saglio, P., Lafleche, D., Bonissol, C., and Bove, J. M. (1971). *C.R. Acad. Sci. Paris Ser. D* **272,** 1387–1390.
Severin, H. H. P. (1929). *Hilgardia* **3,** 543–583.
Severin, H. H. P. (1934). *Hilgardia* **8,** 339–361.
Severin, H. H. P. (1945). *Hilgardia* **17,** 22–60.
Severin, H. H. P. (1946). *Hilgardia* **17,** 141–153.
Severin, H. H. P. (1947a). *Hilgardia* **17,** 197–212.
Severin, H. H. P. (1947b). *Hilgardia* **17,** 511–523.
Severin, H. H. P. (1948). *Hilgardia* **18,** 203–217.
Severin, H. H. P. (1949). *Hilgardia* **19,** 190–203.
Severin, H. H. P. (1950a). *Hilgardia* **19,** 357–382.
Severin, H. H. P. (1950b). *Hilgardia* **19,** 544–545.
Sinha, R. C., and Chiykowski, L. N. (1967). *Virology* **31,** 461–466.
Smith, A. J., McCoy, R. E., and Tsai, J. H. (1981). *Phytopathology* **71,** 819–822.
Smith, R. E. (1902). *Hatch Exp. Sta. Mass. Agric. Coll. Bull.* **79.**
Stearns, L. A., and MacCreary, D. (1938). *J. Econ. Entomol.* **31,** 226–229.
Steyskal, G. (1945). *Brooklyn Entomol. Soc. Bull.* **40,** 86.
Stoddard, E. M. (1947). *Conn. (State) Agric. Exp. Sta. Bull.* **506.**
Stoner, W. N. (1953). *Phytopathology* **43,** 611–615.
Storey, H. H. (1933). *Proc. R. Soc. London Ser. B* **113,** 463.
Taboada, O., Rosenberger, D. A., and Jones, A. L. (1975). *J. Econ. Entomol.* **68,** 255–257.

Thomas, H. E., Rawlins, T. E., and Parker, K. G. (1940). *Phytopathology* **30**, 322–328.
Timmer, L. W., Brlansky, R. H., Raju, B. C., and Lee, R. F. (1981). *Phytopathology* **71**, 909.
Townsend, R., and Markham, P. G. (1976). *Soc. Gen. Microbiol. Proc.* **3**, 156.
Townsend, R., Markham, P. G., Plaskitt, K. A., and Daniels, M. J. (1977). *J. Gen. Microbiol.* **100**, 15–21.
Turner, W. F. (1949). *Science* **109**, 87–88.
Turner, W. F., and Pollard, H. N. (1955). *J. Econ. Entomol.* **48**, 771–772.
Turner, W. F., and Pollard, H. N. (1959a). *U.S. Dep. Agric. Tech. Bull.* 1188.
Turner, W. F., and Pollard, H. N. (1959b). *U.S. Dep. Agric. Tech. Bull.* 1193.
Ulrychova, M., and Petru, E. (1980). *Biol. Plant.* **22**, 358–362.
Wallis, R. L. (1960). *U.S. Dep. Agric., Agric. Res. Serv. Bull.* 33–55.
Weires, R. W., and Straub, R. W. (1980). *J. Econ. Entomol.* **73**, 515–519.
Wells, J. M., Weaver, D. J., and Raju, B. C. (1980). *Phytopathology* **70**, 817–820.
Wells, J. M., Raju, B. C., Lowe, S. K., Feeley, J. C., and Nyland, G. (1981). *Phytopathology* **71**, 912.
Whitcomb, R. F., Jensen, D. D., and Richardson, J. (1967). *Virology* **31**, 539–549.
Whitcomb, R. F., Jensen, D. D., and Richardson, J. (1968a). *Virology* **34**, 69–78.
Whitcomb, R. F., Jensen, D. D., and Richardson, J. (1968b). *J. Invertebr. Pathol.* **12**, 192–201.
Whitcomb, R. F., Shapiro, M., and Richardson, J. (1968c). *J. Invertebr. Pathol.* **12**, 202–221.
Winkler, A. J., Hewitt, W. B., Frazier, N. W., and Freitag, J. H. (1949). *Hilgardia* **19**, 207–264.
Wolfe, H. R., and Anthon, E. W. (1953). *J. Econ. Entomol.* **46**, 1090–1092.
Wolfe, H. R., Anthon, E. W., and Jones, L. S. (1951a). *Science* **113**, 558.
Wolfe, H. R., Anthon, E. W., Kaloostian, G. H., and Jones, L. S. (1951b). *J. Econ. Entomol.* **44**, 616–619.

Part **II**

Host Coevolution with the Pathogen

This section elaborates on the dynamic nature of host–pathogen interactions and it emphasizes methods by which hosts have evolved to minimize damages caused by phytopathogenic prokaryotes. In Chapter 5, A. H. Ellingboe develops a logical basis for understanding host–parasite interactions and presents methods for determining which host and pathogen genes are involved in those interactions. The first barriers to infection and colonization of plants by prokaryotes are physical and/or chemical. A. J. Anderson discusses these passive systems for defense in Chapter 6. Chemical defenses induced by plant recognition of prokaryotes are discussed by J. L. McIntyre (Chapter 7). He also presents an hypothesis for systemic resistance. The hypersensitive response of nonhost plants to incompatible bacteria is described and contrasted with necrosis development in compatible host–pathogen interactions by Z. Klement in Chapter 8. Recognition of bacterial pathogens by plants is prerequisite for induced resistance and hypersensitive responses. N. T. Keen and M. J. Holliday review concepts for recognition mechanisms in Chapter 9.

Chapter **5**

Host Resistance and Host–Parasite Interactions: A Perspective

ALBERT H. ELLINGBOE

I. INTRODUCTION

The intent of this chapter is to present a perspective not just of host resistance but of host–parasite interactions. The reasons for including host–parasite interactions is my belief that it is essentially impossible to

Phytopathogenic Prokaryotes, Vol. 2

Copyright © 1982 by Academic Press, Inc.
All rights of reproduction in any form reserved.
ISBN 0-12-509002-1

examine resistance without consideration of the pathogen, that much of what we know of resistance was obtained by analyses of pathogens, and, most importantly, much, if not most, of what is yet to be learned will come from analyses with the pathogens. The basic assumptions are that interactions are determined by both partners, and that the interactions are predominantly dynamic. Another reason for the emphasis on the pathogen is that bacterial pathogens are now, or can be made, amenable to genetic analyses. Genetic analyses are considered, for all practical purposes, absolutely essential for studies of host–parasite interactions, particularly if the primary interests are the early interactions that are crucial to successful development of the parasitic relationship, or the functions necessary to prevent the successful development of that relationship.

II. GENE-FOR-GENE INTERACTIONS

It has been suggested that there are at least two kinds of genes involved in interactions between host and parasite (Ellingboe, 1976). Almost all of the naturally occurring genetic variability involving one host species and one pathogen species involves genes whose behavior is consistent with the gene-for-gene pattern. Though the pattern has been unequivocally established for interactions between fungal pathogens and plants, it has not, to my knowledge, been established unequivocally with bacterial pathogens and plants. It is known that single genes in plants can give resistance to particular strains of bacteria, and that the pattern of interactions of many host genotypes (of one species) and many strains of bacteria is consistent with the gene-for-gene hypothesis. The interaction between soybean [*Glycine max* (L.) Merr.] and *Rhizobium japonicum* (Kirchner) Buchanan best illustrates the pattern. Caldwell (1966) and Vest (1970) reported two host genes (*Rj*2 and *Rj*4) which prevented nodulation by certain strains of *R. japonicum.* Other strains were unaffected by those host genes. The pattern which emerged was identical to the pattern of a gene-for-gene interaction. The unfortunate aspect is that the detailed genetic analysis of the ability of the *R. japonicum* strains to infect and produce functioning nodules on the plants with different *Rj* genes has not been undertaken.

A. Development of Gene-for-Gene Relationships

The simplest explanation of the gene-for-gene relationship is that the specific recognition is for incompatibility. This conclusion was drawn from several observations. One is that only one parasite–host gene pair

(*P*/*R*) specifies incompatibility, whereas the other three parasite–host gene pairs (*P*/*r*, *p*/*R*, and *p*/*r*) (one locus in each organism and two alleles at each locus) give compatibility. A second is that it usually is the incompatible parasite–host genotype that is temperature-sensitive. A third is the pattern observed with alleles and intragenic recombinants. A fourth is the ease with which mutations in the host to susceptibility and mutations in the pathogen to increased virulence are obtained. A fifth is the pattern of epistasis. And there are other reasons.

The evolution of the gene-for-gene relationship is best explained if the assumption is made that the first mutation affecting interaction was made by the host to go from susceptibility to resistance followed by a mutation in the pathogen that rendered the host *R* gene ineffective (Person, 1959). The pattern fits the data nicely, whether the host and parasite genes are described in the sense of classical genetics as dominant or recessive. If the gene-for-gene interactions evolved as a genetic mechanism to go from compatibility to incompatibility to compatibility, then how did the initial compatibility evolve? It has been suggested that there first evolved a basic compatibility between host and parasite and then there evolved a gene-for-gene system superimposed on the basic incompatibility (Ellingboe, 1976). The basic compatibility evolved first. The gene-for-gene interactions evolved second. What types of genetic patterns would be expected of the postulated basic compatibility?

B. Development of Basic Compatibility

Basic compatibility was assumed to be made up of two types of interactions. One was the evolution of similar regulatory sensitivities between the two interacting organisms. For example, the two organisms would have similar sensitivities between the two interacting organisms. The two organisms would have similar sensitivities to end product inhibition and repression or derepression in the biosynthesis of an amino acid, such as tryptophan. If a relatively free movement of small molecules occurs between the two organisms, any perturbation of the regulatory machinery could lead to a degree of incompatibility in the relationship. It might be very detrimental to a pathogen if a host mutation led to a change in sensitivity to feedback inhibition and/or repression that had a net effect of the parasite spending 50% of its energy making one amino acid, or some other compound. The problem with this type of postulated interaction is that it is not seen as being readily testable in any definitive manner.

An organism like *Escherichia coli* (Migula) Castellani & Chalmers has all the necessary machinery for life. Its basic metabolism is similar to plant pathogens like *Pseudomonas solanacearum* (Smith) Smith. Yet *P.*

solanacearum can incite disease on potato, a trait that *E. coli* lacks. *P. solanacearum* could either have some capability to interact with the plant and be able to grow, or be missing some function that would render the host plant capable of restricting its growth. In the first case, *P. solanacearum* would be considered as having a positive function to continue its growth in the host plant and eventually produce disease. In the second case, there would be a positive function to be unable to grow. The second case is consistent with the gene-for-gene interaction, and that interaction does not provide a satisfactory explanation for the evolution of what is termed basic compatibility. It has been postulated, therefore, that there are genes in the parasite whose functions are necessary for growth in the environment of the host tissue. Evidence of genes whose function is necessary for successful development of the parasite in the host tissue has come from studies of toxins such as the one produced by *Helminthosporium victoriae* Meehan & Murphy. The fungus must produce the toxin and the host must have the *Vb* gene to permit a reasonable amount of growth of the fungus in the host tissue, and the production of the disease of the host plant (Litzenberger, 1949). The examples where bacteria appear to have a positive function to alter the host plant to grow are *Agrobacterium tumifaciens* (Smith & Townsend) Conn and *Rhizobium* spp. Both appear to have to stimulate host cell changes, hypertrophy and hyperplasia, for continued growth and development of the bacteria. The bacteria, in effect, have to make an environment acceptable to them. There must be a positive function on the part of the bacterium for growth, and an ability of the host to respond to be susceptible. The DNA of *Pseudomonas syringae* pv. *savastanoi* (Smith) Young *et al.* that codes for the increased production of indole acetic acid has been identified and cloned (Comai and Kosuge, 1982). Does that mean that a difference between host lines in their susceptibility to develop galls is the receptor of indole acetic acid? Or a regulator of the synthesis of IAA? The difficulty that I see in attempting to answer that question is the dearth of information about genetic variability in reaction within any one host species to *P. s.* pv. *savastanoi*.

III. IDENTIFICATION OF GENES FOR PARASITISM

A. Locating Genes for Parasitism

How can genes of a parasite whose functions are necessary for successful development in a host be identified? One approach with fungi has been to produce temperature-sensitive mutations in a pathogen.

The first experiments were performed with fungi that would grow on a synthetic medium as well as on the host. The objective was to get mutations of genes that would permit growth at the normal temperatures for those organisms, but not at a higher temperature at which the wild-type cultures would continue to grow. The basic assumption with these NTG-produced mutants was that the temperature sensitivity was the result of missense mutations which affected the temperature stability of the tertiary structure of the gene products. Three classes of mutants were produced (Ellingboe and Gabriel, 1977). Class I mutants were temperature-sensitive on both agar media and in the host. Class II mutants were temperature sensitive on agar media but not in the host. Class III mutants were not temperature-sensitive on agar media, but were in the host. Class III mutants were considered to be the result of mutations of genes whose functions were not crucial to basic life processes, because they were not temperature-sensitive on either minimal or fully supplemented media, but were crucial to parasitism. Since these mutants could produce disease at the normal temperature but not at the higher temperature, they are considered to be the result of mutations of genes whose functions are necessary for successful parasitism and pathogenesis. What is not known is how many loci in the pathogens will give this pattern, and whether there is any within-host-species variability in response to these mutants. If there was variability within a host species in response to these mutants, it might provide a way to identify host genes that respond to the mutated pathogen genes.

B. How Many Genes Are Important for Parasitism?

One question to ask is, "How many genes are there whose functions are necessary for successful development of a pathogen in a host?" One approach is to induce many independent mutations that affect interactions between host and parasite. If 500 independent mutations of the Class III mutants, described above, were induced in a pathogen, intercrosses between these mutants should have given an indication of the number of loci whose functions were necessary for successful parasitism and pathogenesis. Suppose that the 500 mutations mapped at 20 loci. The indications would be that perhaps only 25 loci were necessary for successful development of the parasite. If, on the other hand, the 500 mutations mapped at 300 loci, the possibility of getting a reasonably accurate estimate of the number of genes by the saturation procedure might be very slim.

A basic assumption in this approach is that the difference between a compatible and a noncompatible parasite–host relationship is not due to one protein, one toxin (no matter how host specific), one hormone, one glycoprotein, one polysaccharide, etc. Chances are many interactions are crucial to a compatible interaction (successful development of the parasitic relationship), and that they can be sorted out, one at a time, by the use of the appropriate genetic mutants. It also seems reasonable to expect that there will be certain interactions in common with all combinations of compatible host and parasite species, that certain interactions will be common only across a limited number of host and/or parasite species, that very few interactions will be very specific to one species of host and one species of parasite, that certain interactions are in common with specific stages of development of host and/or parasites, though not species specific, etc.

One result of the development of procedures to genetically manipulate bacterial pathogens is the realization that there are fewer species of phytopathogenic bacteria than previously thought to exist. Witness, for example, the consolidation of many species into a few species of *Corynebacterium*, *Pseudomonas*, and *Xanthomonas* with the designation of pathovars to designate the host affected by each pathovar (Dye *et al.*, 1980). How many genes differentiate the race of *P. solanacearum* that attacks potatoes (*Solanum tuberosum* L.) from the race that produces disease on bananas [*Musa paradisiaca* subsp. *saplentum* (L.) Kuntze], or the race on peppers (*Capsicum frutescens* L.), etc.? How many genes are in common? Are the genes which give variability within a host species to a series of strains of the pathogen races of that host species also involved in giving resistance to the other pathovars? With the ability to make the genetic crosses among plant pathogenic bacteria it becomes possible to answer these questions. If the limited observations with fungal pathogens also holds for bacterial pathogens, then genes which give within-host-species variability in resistance also give resistance across species designations. Once wheat (*Triticum aestivum* L.) was bred for susceptibility to rye rust, it was determined that the genes which gave wheat resistance to wheat rust also gave resistance to rye rust. Also, *Secalis* and *Agropyron* genes transferred into wheat gave resistance to wheat rust. But these are genes which follow the gene-for-gene pattern! Are there no genes for basic compatibility which differentiate these grass hosts? They certainly do not have all their pathogens in common. I believe these examples reemphasize the need to ask the questions in a manner so that experiments can be designed to critically distinguish between hypotheses, and not to continually add data that are consistent with but do not prove or disprove a hypothesis. The critical segregation tests can now be done with several plant pathogenic bacteria.

IV. HOST GENES IN PARASITIC INTERACTIONS

Thus far I have discussed the genetics of interactions between host and pathogen from the view of the genetics of the pathogen. Most of the work that has been done on the genetics of the host has been derived from breeding for disease resistance. With only a relatively small number of hosts has the inheritance of resistance to a given pathogen been analyzed in any great detail. A few of the host genes that have a major effect have been characterized. Genes that have small effects have usually not been analyzed systematically so they could be identified one at a time.

A. Functions for Host Genes

Several approaches have been made with pathogens. One was to make mutants of pathogens whose ability to grow in the host plant is reduced. An example is the research on transposon-induced mutations in *Rhizobium meliloti* Dangeard (Long *et al.*, 1982). I have also stated that it is easy to make mutations in pathogens from avirulence to virulence on host plants with single *R* genes. The mutations to avirulence, whether they be constitutive or temperature-sensitive, and the mutations to increase in virulence, suggest that there are at least two types of genes in the pathogen. If there are two types of genes in the pathogen, then we would predict that there are also at least two types of genes in the host. There are the genes in the host that follow the gene-for-gene relationship between the host and the pathogen. It is predicted that there are genes in the host which act in response to genes in the pathogen which have a positive function for virulence. It also seems probable that there should be genes in the host that respond to that positive parasite gene function. An example of positive function of host genes for successful development of the pathogen is with some of the pathogens that produce host-specific toxins. *Helminthosporium victoriae* produces a disease in oats (*Avena sativa* L.), but only those oat lines with a dominant *Vb* gene. This suggests that not only must the pathogen produce the toxin, but there must be a gene in the host that codes for the hypothetical receptor site. That means there must be a positive function on the part of the host to be susceptible to *H. victoriae.* The product of the dominant *Vb* gene must be present. The host plant must have a gene product to be susceptible. The host has a positive function to be susceptible. Similarly, then, with other systems we might expect to find at least two types of genes in the host: those genes for which the production of a gene product is necessary to be resistant, and those genes for which the production of a gene product is necessary for the host to be susceptible.

Almost all genes in the host that have been studied fit the pattern expected of the gene-for-gene relationship. It is estimated that more than 95% of the genes in the host that have been identified fit the pattern expected of the gene-for-gene relationship. In the gene-for-gene relationship, the simplest explanation is that the positive interaction is between the products of the dominant *R* gene in the host and the product of the dominant *P* gene in the pathogen to give an incompatible relationship. The pattern suggests a positive function for resistance and a positive function for avirulence. The products of the *P* and *R* genes, according to one hypothesis, form a dimer, and it is the dimer that is active in determining the fate of the interaction between the host and the parasite (Ellingboe, 1982). If this argument is true, then one should be able to make mutations in the host from resistance to susceptibility. Let's make an argument with host genes that is analogous to the argument with the pathogen genes. Whereas it has been found that it is easy to make mutations from avirulence to virulence on host lines with single *R* genes, it should be relatively easy to make mutations in the host from resistance to susceptibility to pathogens having single *P* genes. That argument should hold for the host genes because the change is from a condition where a gene product has a specific recognition of a *P* gene to any change that will lead to the absence of recognition of that *P* gene. Mutations from resistance to susceptibility have been obtained. I know of no example of mutations in the host from susceptibility to resistance which would be specific for a single *P* gene in the pathogen. It does not mean that such mutations do not exist; it is an observation that, thus far, we have not found them.

B. Identifying Host Genes

It should be possible to induce mutations in the host from susceptibility to resistance. Such mutations would be comparable to the mutations of what were considered to be affecting basic compatibility when the discussion was made earlier with the pathogen. If two different kinds of genes can be found in the pathogen, it should be entirely possible to find two different kinds of genes in the host: those genes which are active for resistance and those genes which are active for susceptibility. To go back to the example of *H. victoriae* and oats, oat plants that contained the dominant *Vb* gene were susceptible. It was possible to find mutations from susceptibility to resistance (Wallace *et al.*, 1967). Mutations to resistance are interpreted as being those leading to alleles that did not have the same affinity for the host-specific toxin produced by *H. victoriae*.

It should be very interesting to determine if mutations from susceptibility to resistance to other pathogens could be induced. It would be interesting to know if constitutive mutations from susceptibility to resistance could be recovered, or, to use the analogy with the parasite, if the induction and selection of conditional (temperature-sensitive) mutations in the host would be a means to identify genes whose products were necessary for susceptibility. The latter mutants would be expected to be susceptible at the normal temperature but be resistant at the higher temperature. They would be resistant at the higher temperature because, at the elevated temperature, the temperature-sensitive gene product would be unable to interact with the product of the gene from the parasite.

With the mutations from susceptibility to resistance, would there be corresponding genes in the pathogen? Will there be a pattern similar (but reciprocal) to the gene-for-gene relationship for the host genes for basic compatibility which interact with the genes in the pathogen? These genes in the host would be genes whose functions are necessary for basic compatibility with the pathogen. They would interact with the genes in the pathogen that have a positive function for successful growth of the parasite in the host.

C. Host Genes for "Low Levels" of Resistance

Plant breeders have successfully used the naturally occurring genetic variability in host lines to successfully breed plants that are resistant to plant pathogenic organisms. In the beginning, plant breeders used primarily those genes which had a major effect. Where and when they found a single gene that had a major effect in that it gave a high level of resistance to a pathogen, those were the genes which were used. After surveying the world collections of host genotypes, they frequently found that there was a limited number of genes which would give total immunity. What was commonly found was that there were many host lines which had lower levels of resistance, but levels which were certainly acceptable for commercial use. The initial genetic analyses had shown that the high levels of resistance followed the gene-for-gene pattern as discussed by Flor (1946, 1947, 1955). There has also been the suggestion that there were genes that did not follow the gene-for-gene pattern (Thurston, 1971). They gave what was known as "field resistance" or "generalized resistance." VanderPlank (1963) coined the term "horizontal resistance."

Genes that gave low levels of resistance were more difficult to handle in genetic crosses. The appearance, in the beginning, was that the low levels of resistance were controlled by many genes and that their expression was not dependent on the presence of *P* genes in the pathogens. More recent research has shown that the genes which give low levels of resistance follow essentially the same pattern as those genes which give high levels of resistance (Hare and McIntosh, 1980). It has been found that genes which give low levels of resistance are usually simply inherited and that they are specific to certain strains of the pathogen. It appears, therefore, in the naturally occurring genetic variability affecting host–parasite interactions, that the host genes which give low levels of resistance follow the same patterns as those which give high levels of resistance. Almost all naturally occurring genetic variability seems to follow the pattern of the gene-for-gene relationship. In fact, there is evidence that the same genes can give both high or low levels of resistance, depending upon the strain of the pathogen (Martin and Ellingboe, 1976). In the gene-for-gene relationship there seems to be a specific interaction for incompatibility. Compatibility represents those genotypes in which specific interaction of gene products does not occur.

The ability to control a disease depends, in part, on what the norm of the host species is in relation to a pathogen species. With some pathogens we find that it is easy to find resistance. If a hundred lines of a host species were evaluated for reaction to inoculation with a pathogen, a fairly high proportion of those might have some resistance to the pathogen. There are other examples where breeders and pathologists have had to screen thousands of different lines of a host genus before they would find a few genotypes which gave some resistance. What this implies to me is that there is a great difference in terms of the compatibility of a particular host species with a particular pathogen species. In some cases the individual mean of the host population may have a fairly high level of resistance. The genes which give low levels of resistance as well as those which give high levels may show that the average of the host population is fairly resistant. The average individual of the host species may be very susceptible in other host–parasite systems. This has a decided effect on how one would program the use of host genes in developing practical control measures. Such analyses can give an estimate of the possibility that the disease can be controlled by plant breeding. It also gives one an estimate of the numbers of genes in the host that are available to be used to affect the interactions with that pathogen.

D. How Many Host Genes Are Important for Parasitism?

In an earlier section of this chapter, I dealt with the idea that it is possible to get an estimate of the number of genes in a pathogen which are necessary for successful development in a host. If a large number of mutations to inability to grow in a host are made, and if those individual mutations are mapped, an estimate can be obtained of the number of loci which are crucial for successful development of that parasite in that host line. This same argument can be used to get an estimate of the number of host genes whose activity is necessary to support the development of the pathogen. The procedure would be to make a large number of mutations from susceptibility to resistance—not resistance to susceptibility—and map those genes to get an estimate of how many loci are involved in an interaction with a particular pathogen. A minor modification of this procedure was used by Wallace when he studied the mutants of the *Vb* locus in oats. He obtained lines of oats, following mutagenesis, that were more resistant to the host-specific toxin than was the susceptible parent. When he mapped these mutations, they all mapped at the *Vb* locus. If several hundred mutations all map at the *Vb* locus, that fact is very good evidence that the *Vb* locus is the only locus of any importance in interactions with that pathogen. If several hundred mutations were induced to resistance in a host to a given pathogen, and if all these mutations then mapped to a relatively small number of loci—let us say they mapped at 10, for example—that would be an indication that the total number of host loci involved in interactions with that pathogen was probably going to be something less than 15. If, on the other hand, the 200 independent mutations from susceptibility to resistance mapped at 50 loci, the estimate of the numbers of genes which were involved in interaction between the host and the pathogen would probably be more in the range of something like 75. One can make an exact calculation to get such an estimate. Such calculations have been made to get estimates of the numbers of alleles for sexual incompatibility factors in fungi (Raper *et al.*, 1960).

V. DIRECTION FOR FUTURE RESEARCH

A. Genetic Approaches

Most of the people to whom I have made the suggestion of using mutagenesis for obtaining particular types of mutations have immediately commented on the amount of work which would be involved in inducing several hundred independent mutations from susceptibility to resistance. And this is true. It would be a considerable amount of work to induce and select for either constitutive mutations from susceptibility to resistance or for temperature-sensitive mutations from susceptibility to resistance. It is also important to emphasize that complete immunity is not necessary to identify these genes. It is only necessary that the change in reaction from susceptibility to resistance be a recognizable difference in phenotype and that it be a reproducibly scoreable difference. The amount of work that would be involved to accomplish this goal does not seem to be very great when one considers the total effort that has already been expended in plant pathology to identify "the biochemical basis of resistance," and the little success that has been achieved toward that goal. For all the studies over three-fourths of a century—since the genetic variability in host–parasite relations was first shown to follow the same Mendelian rules as other genetic traits—we still do not know the product of a single host gene which gives resistance to a pathogen, and we do not know the product of a single *P* gene in the pathogen. Put into the context of the efforts of the approach of comparative biochemistry and comparative physiology and the limited success of that approach, the idea of maybe a half a dozen people spending a lifetime to make a genetic analysis of the numbers of genes which would help to explain the complexity of the interaction does not seem to be unreasonable. In fact, considering the failure to be able to identify the products of the genes for disease resistance by the standard procedure, the approach of making a genetic analysis via genetic mutations seems, at least to me, very reasonable. It may well represent the only way in which we will eventually get some idea of how many genes are involved in host–parasite interactions, and what the primary products of those genes are. Efforts to identify the primary products of genes involved in host–parasite interactions will obviously have to use genetic mutants.

Comparative biochemistry, physiology, cytology, etc., as procedures have given many suggestions on the mechanisms by which a host resists the development of the pathogen. We do know that some pathogens produce host-specific toxins, and it has been postulated that there are receptor sites for those toxins in the hosts. The hypothetical receptor sites have not been isolated, either by genetic means or by biochemical procedures. Most of the studies on the biochemistry of host–parasite interactions have begun by comparing the differences between resistant and susceptible hosts. Usually the comparisons are made beginning several days after inoculation when symptoms were obvious. From these studies, the biochemists and physiologists have tried to get to earlier and earlier stages of interaction. They have tried to determine when the crucial biochemical changes take place by looking at the phenotype at various times after inoculation. Many of the differences in protein profiles of infected and noninfected plants do not appear until several days after inoculation. Usually changes in the rates of respiration change 1, 2, or more days after the inoculation, long after a compatible or an incompatible relationship was obvious by microscopic examination. The genetic approach provides the opportunity to begin the study with the genes which control the processes. These genes were identified based upon the effect they had on the phenotype of the interaction between the host and the pathogen. What seems obvious to me is that top priority should be to determine the primary product of those genes and to determine what role those products play in the interaction between host and parasite.

B. Gene-for-Gene Interactions and Basic Compatibility

The genetic analyses that have been done to date suggest that the specific interactions are for an incompatible relationship. If the products of the *P* and the *R* genes interacted to regulate a series of other genes, we would expect to see a deviation from the one-gene-to-one-gene relationship in the formal genetics of interaction. It has been pointed out that if the products of the *P* and the *R* genes were really regulatory genes, then it should be possible to see variability of the genes that were regulated. In that example, as has been presented before (Ellingboe, 1982), deviations such as one gene in the parasite to five genes in the host would be observed if there was one host gene for recognition of the *P* gene product, and four genes that were regulated by the *P* and *R* genes. These deviations from the one-to-one relationship are not seen in the naturally occurring genetic variability.

I think it will become exceedingly important to determine whether genes which are involved in what has been called basic compatibility have corresponding genes in host and parasite. Assuming that mutations in the host which fit the expected pattern for basic compatibility can be found, it should be possible to identify the primary products of these genes. If genetic variability of those genes can be obtained—even if they have to be conditional mutants—a genetic analysis can begin which should eventually lead to the ability to identify the primary products of these genes.

C. Priorities for Future Research

In the past, studies of the host–parasite relations have been geared toward making the comparison between resistant and susceptible plants. It has been possible to identify the genes for naturally occurring variability by their effect on the phenotype. These have been manipulated in practical plant breeding. They have been used very little, however, for study of the basic interaction between host and parasite. To make progress, it is my opinion that we now need to make the necessary mutational analyses to find and identify genetic variants of the predicted different kinds of genes which are involved in interactions between host and parasite. The major thrust must now be to identify the primary products of the genes which control that interaction. We must determine the numbers of genes which are involved in interaction, the kinds of interactions, whether they fit the patterns expected for the gene-for-gene relationship, or whether they fit the patterns of interaction expected for basic compatibility. There are still very basic questions to ask. Is there a gene-for-gene relationship for genes involved in basic compatibility? Is the concept of basic compatibility an acceptable one that is experimentally testable? It is my feeling that it does have usefulness in that it provides an opportunity for selecting or designing experiments to screen for particular mutants which have a particular pattern of interaction. It should be possible to select for mutations at a given locus and get the necessary genetic variants which are required to identify primary gene products. It is now a matter for the pathologists to make the decision that they are going to go for the primary gene products, and to design their experiments and to establish the appropriate genetic material so that they can, in fact, clone these genes. Cloning of the genes, in my opinion, is a necessity to unequivocally identify the primary gene products. It is necessary to identify the products to know how they can be manipulated and used for practical control of plant diseases.

References

Caldwell, B. F. (1966). *Crop. Sci.* **6,** 427–8.

Comai, L., and Kosuge, T. (1982). *J. Bacteriol.* **149,** 40–46.

Dye, D. W., Bradbury, J. F., Goto, M., Hayward, A. C., Lelliott, R. A., and Schroth, M. N. (1980). *Rev. Plant Pathol.* **59,** 153–168.

Ellingboe, A. H. (1976). *In* "Encyclopedia of Plant Physiology, Vol. 4: Physiological Plant Pathology" (R. Heitefuss and P. H. Williams, eds.), pp. 761–778. Springer-Verlag, Berlin and New York.

Ellingboe, A. H. (1982). *In* "Active Defence Mechanisms in Plants" (R. K. S. Wood, ed.). Plenum, New York.

Ellingboe, A. H., and Gabriel, D. W. (1977). *In* "Use of Induced Mutations for Improving Disease Resistance in Crop Plants" (A. Micke, ed.). I.A.E.A., Vienna.

Flor, H. H. (1946). *J. Agric. Res.* **73,** 335–357.

Flor, H. H. (1947). *J. Agric. Res.* **74,** 241–262.

Flor, H. H. (1955). *Phytopathology* **45,** 680–685.
Hare, R. A., and McIntosh, R. A. (1980). *Z. Pflanzenzucht* **83,** 350–367.
Litzenberger, S. C. (1949). *Phytopathology* **39,** 300–18.
Long, S. R., Meade, H. M., Brown, S. E., and Ausebel, F. M. (1982). *In* "Genetic Engineering in the Plant Sciences." Praeger, New York.
Martin, W. J., and Ellingboe, A. H. (1976). *Phytopathology* **66,** 1435–8.
Person, C. (1959). *Can. J. Bot.* **37,** 1101–30.
Raper, J. R., Baxter, M. G., and Ellingboe, A. H. (1960). *Proc. Natl. Acad. Sci.* **46,** 833–842.
Thurston, H. D. (1971). *Phytopathology* **61,** 620–6.
VanderPlank, J. (1963). "Plant Diseases: Epidemics and Control." Academic Press, New York.
Vest, G. (1970). *Crop. Sci.* **10,** 34–5.
Wallace, A. T., Singh, R. M., and Browning, R. M. (1967). *In* "Induced Mutations and Their Utilization." Erwin-Baur Gedaechtnisvorlesungen IV. Academic-Verlag, Berlin.

Chapter **6**

Preformed Resistance Mechanisms

ANNE J. ANDERSON

I. INTRODUCTION

Plants have highly efficient defenses against the incessant challenges of microbial organisms. Preformed resistance mechanisms discourage entry of bacteria into the internal tissues and may restrict their growth when ingress has been gained. Both physical barriers and chemical deterrents are implicated in these passive systems of defense. The environment, however, can dramatically alter the effectiveness of the resistance mechanisms.

Phytopathogenic Prokaryotes, Vol. 2

Copyright © 1982 by Academic Press, Inc.
All rights of reproduction in any form reserved.
ISBN 0-12-509002-1

II. PHYSICAL BARRIERS: THE EPIDERMIS

The primary event in a challenge of any plant by a potentially pathogenic bacterium is contact between microbial and host cell surfaces. The complexity of the outer layers of a healthy plant's epidermal cells provides an absolute barrier to bacterial penetration. Bacterial pathogens do not synthesize the required array and amounts of enzymes necessary to destroy these outer layers of plant cells in the time frame involved in pathogenesis.

The membrane of the epidermal cell is protected by the crystalline lattice–gel complex of the plant cell wall, which consists of defined polysaccharides and protein components linked covalently and through hydrogen bonding (Albersheim, 1976). Its structural strength is provided by cellulose fibers. Neutral polysaccharides, protein, and the acidic pectin fraction constitute the gel matrix.

The cell wall, in turn, is coated with the plants' outermost layer, the cuticle (Campbell *et al.*, 1980; Kolattukudy, 1970, 1980). Cuticles of aerial parts of angiosperms and gymnosperms contain a polyester polymer of hydroxy and epoxy fatty acids termed cutin. The cutin deposit may be interspersed with waxes, possibly in a layered arrangement. The thickness and composition of the cutin layer varies between plant species and between plant tissues. In underground parts of a plant, and in certain cells of internal tissues, cutin is replaced with another polyester polymer, suberin. Suberin also contains aromatic components, and it is more intimately associated with the plant cell walls than is cutin.

It is the plant's cuticular layers that prevent direct penetration by pathogenic bacteria (Campbell *et al.*, 1980). Unlike certain fungi, the bacterial pathogens apparently have not evolved enzyme systems that can effectively degrade the polyester mixtures of cutin or suberin in sufficiently short time periods. Other properties of the cuticular layers may enhance their protective capacities. Cutin or suberin may contribute a negative charge to the plant surface (Schonherr and Huber, 1977) and thus repel or retain microbial cells according to their charges. A waxy layer may limit the degree of cohesiveness between bacterial and plant cell surfaces. The hydrophobic nature of a waxy cuticle may impede the accumulation of water on the plants surface (Campbell *et al.*, 1980). Because free water is required for bacterial survival the dryness of a waxy cuticle would constitute a hostile environment. Restriction in diffusion of water-soluble nutrients from the epidermal cells through the cuticle layer would also reduce colonization of the plant surface by bacteria (Tukey, 1970).

Topography of the plant surface could play an important role in resistance. A smooth surface would provide fewer crevices in which bacteria, nutrients, and water could lodge. Surface hairs could suspend bacterial cells above available free water and enhance desiccation of the microorganisms. Chemicals in the cuticular layers could exert antibacterial effects. Antifungal activity has been claimed for a variety of types of molecules present in the cuticular layers (Campbell *et al.*, 1980; Weinhold and Hancock, 1980). Studies of the antibacterial nature of cuticular components have not been reported.

The second physical barrier to penetration by certain bacterial pathogens is the plant cell wall. Its gel–lattice structure prevents diffusion of bacterial cells, thereby necessitating enzymic degradation before passage can be achieved. Only some bacterial pathogens, however, produce the required complement and amounts of enzymes needed to loosen cell wall structures. Seemuller and Beer (1976) have reported that *Erwinia amylovora* (Burrill) Winslow *et al.* does not degrade the cell walls of its host. In contrast, the soft rot bacteria produce enzymes that degrade pectin components so effectively that host plant tissues are macerated (Bateman and Basham, 1976). It is intriguing that no bacterial pathogens have evolved the fine precision that characterizes interactions of rhizobia with their hosts. In establishing their symbiotic relationships, these gain ingress through root-hair cell walls. Evidence summarized by Bauer (1981) suggests an intricate control of the synthesis of the rhizobial enzymes that degrade root-hair wall structures.

The plant also has "preexisting" defense systems that may limit enzymic degradation of the wall polysaccharides. Such systems include chemical modification of the structures by lignification and suberization. Enclosing the wall polysaccharides with these phenolic and polyester polymers sterically hinders the action of macerating enzymes (Schlosser, 1980). Lignification, and in certain tissues suberization, occur naturally as the cell walls mature from primary to secondary character (Esau, 1962). Both processes are also associated with wound healing (Akai and Fukutomi, 1980). The importance of suberization as a defense response has been elegantly demonstrated by studies of lenticel structure in potatoes (*Solanum tuberosum* L.) (Audi *et al.*, 1962; Fox *et al.*, 1971). Lenticel walls normally become suberized as they are formed. If the potato tuber is exposed to high humidity, however, growth of the phelloderm cells is stimulated, but the new walls are formed without suberization. These unsuberized tissues are prime points for attack by *Erwinia carotovora* (Jones) Bergey *et al.* (Fox *et al.*, 1971).

An ability to inhibit macerating enzymes has also been demonstrated for other plant factors. Tannins present in healthy plant tissues and the polyphenols generated in wound responses are potent inhibitors of pectic enzymes (Schlosser, 1980). Proteinaceous inhibitors of pectic enzymes have been detected in extracts of unchallenged sweet potato [*Ipomea batatas* (L.) Lam.] (Uritani and Stahmann, 1961), bean (*Phaseolus vulgaris* L.), and tomato (*Lycopersicon esculentum* Mill.) tissues (Anderson and Albersheim, 1971). These phenomena constitute general defense mechanisms of a preformed nature which could limit bacterial infection.

III. BACTERIAL ENTRY

The coatings on the epidermal surface are so effective that bacterial pathogens can gain ingress only through wounded tissues or natural openings in which the cuticular layers are breached or are only sparsely present. The effectiveness of these external coatings can be demonstrated by referring to the harsh conditions needed to initiate lesions in soybean leaves. No infection of soybean [*Glycine max* (L.) Merr.] leaves occurred upon wetting with *Pseudomonas syringae* pv. *glycinea* (Coerper) Young *et al.* unless the moisture was accompanied by wind (Daft and Leben, 1972). The wind–moisture combination established the water-soaked conditions needed for infection.

A. Natural Openings

The natural openings that permit bacterial entry include stomata, lenticels, hydathodes, and nectaries (Campbell *et al.*, 1980; Goodman, 1976). Morphological aspects of these natural openings may contribute to resistance mechanisms. The upper surfaces of peach [*Prunus persica* (L.) Batsch] leaves resist aerosols of *Xanthomonas campestris* pv. *pruni* (Smith) Dye because they lack stomata. Inoculation of the lower surfaces, where the stomates are located, produced a high infection rate (Rolfs, 1915). Resistance of Mandarin orange (*Citrus reticulata* Blancs) leaves to *X. c.* pv. *citri* (Hasse) Dye has been attributed to their having broad cuticular ridges around the stomatal pores (McLean, 1921). Grapefruit (*C. paradisi* Maef.) leaves lack these lip structures and are more susceptible to *P. s.* pv. *citri.* It is speculated that the smaller pores of the Mandarin orange stomates enhance closure of the pore by water films, thereby reducing its capacity to admit bacterial inoculum. Wide stomatal pores would promote disease because they would enhance the ease of water congestion in intercellular spaces. Size of stomatal aperture has also been implicated in the differential resistance of peach cultivars to *X. c.* pv. *pruni* (Matthee and Daines, 1969). The less susceptible

Red Haven has a smaller pore aperture than the more susceptible Sunhigh cultivar.

Other examples of morphological parameters that promote resistance to bacterial invasion are observed with nectary arrangements. Nectaries in apple (*Malus sylvestris*) blossoms are protected from bacterial inoculation by visiting insects because they have a closed receptacle (Hildebrand, 1937). In quince (*Cydonia oblonga* Mill.) the receptacle is lined by hairs, which also help reduce the amount of bacterial inoculum reaching the nectary (Goodman, 1976). The physical adaptions of the plants that hinder bacterial ingress through natural openings can be highly effective. Their nature is absolute and not subject to mutational adaptions by bacteria. Thus, studies of such mechanisms for use in breeding programs seem to offer substantial advantage.

B. Wounds

Disruption of the epidermal layer through wounding is probably the most important method of access for bacterial pathogens. Wounds may occur as a consequence of a plant's environment. All of the following natural events, abrasion against rough surfaces, animal and insect herbivory, and effects of ice, wind, rain, and hail, can breach the epidermal layer. Bacteria can also utilize insect vectors to generate their wounds. Insect transmissions of *E. amylovora* (Thomson and Purcell, 1979) and of Pierce's disease bacteria (Purcell, 1975) have been demonstrated. A recent paper by Purcell (1981) failed to find correlation between resistance of grape (*Vitis* spp.) cultivars to Pierce's disease bacterium and the feeding preference of the vector, the blue green sharpshooter. Clearly disease management practices should attempt to optimize any resistance to bacterial penetration afforded by the native plant's surface.

Wounds also occur naturally during plant development. Lateral root initiation, proliferation of phelloderm in potato tuber lenticels under high relative humidity, sloughing off of root hairs, and leaf or branch abscission can expose walls that are not sufficiently lignified or suberized to prevent bacterial colonization. In the tomato industry, problems with bacterial infection during the washing stage have been attributed to entry of inoculum into fruits exposed to wash water at a temperature cooler than the tomatoes. Fruits with immature stem scars became more heavily inoculated (Bartz and Showalter, 1981).

The breaches in the cuticular layers caused by these natural events are generally repaired within 24–48 hr by lignification, suberization, or formation of wound periderm. Bacteria, however, may enter a plant during this vulnerable period.

C. Adaptions to Prevent Bacterial Entry and Growth

Various parts of a plant may have specific modifications that can contribute to preformed resistance systems. The importance of stomatal and nectary morphology has been mentioned. The seed coat protects against entrance of bacteria, and moisture, and against leakage of nutrients. Phenolic materials incorporated into the seed casing may have antibacterial properties. The epidermal layer frequently possesses hairs that contain glands which produce phenolic compounds (Beckman *et al.*, 1972). These compounds, which would be liberated by mechanical injury to the tissue, may have antibacterial effects. In young cotton (*Gossypium hirsutum* L.) plants, the epidermal cells themselves accumulate terpenoid compounds (Bell, 1981). Similarly, roots of banana [*Musa paradisiaca* subsp. *sapientum* (L.) Kuntze] develop phenol-storing cells just behind the zone of elongation (Mace, 1963). Again, epidermal damage would release these potentially toxic compounds.

A growing root tip is covered with mucilage that may shield against bacterial penetration as well as reduce wounding of this tissue by abrasion of soil particles. Roots are frequently associated with symbiotic fungi that establish mycorrhizal relationships (Schenck, 1981). The fungal sheath covering the root surface during ectomycorrhizal symbiosis provides another physical barrier to bacteria. Ecto- and endomycorrhizal roots may exude fewer nutrients because of utilization of these chemicals by the symbiotic fungus. Consequently, fewer nutrients may be available in the rhizosphere as a food source for potential bacterial pathogens or as a chemotaxic source (Schenck, 1981). Mycorrhizal roots may produce antibacterial agents, either directly by the fungus or from the plant tissue as a consequence of the fungal–plant interaction. Evidence for enhanced protection of roots against fungal infection by such schemes has been reported (Schenck, 1981). At present, similar data relative to bacterial pathogens have not been presented.

IV. PROTECTION OF INTERNAL TISSUES

Penetration of bacteria into the intercellular spaces and xylem elements of their hosts necessitates internal methods of protection. Again, lignification and suberization of internal wall tissue provide essential physical barriers. However, the internal plant tissues may be largely protected by chemical deterrents. Evidence that plant chemicals inhibit bacterial development is generally based on speculation that if a chemical has antibacterial properties *in vitro* it may function similarly *in planta*. Plant compounds called the "secondary products" are most often implicated as chemical control agents. Although many secondary compounds have been assayed for their potential as antifungal agents, relatively few have been tested against bacteria, especially the plant pathogenic species. Wood (1967) has suggested criteria to use in establishing whether a preformed chemical functions as a resistance factor. A proposed inhibitor must (1) be in the plant parts that are invaded by the pathogen, (2) occur in the tissues at a time and in a concentration sufficient to cause inhibition, (3) have a form that is active toward the pathogen, and (4) vary in concentration in response to changes in susceptibility of the pathogen.

These criteria have not been proven for any given bacterial–chemical interaction. However, studies with several classes of compounds that demonstrate antibacterial activity suggest that the chemicals could help determine the ecology of hosts colonized by bacteria.

A role for an amino acid, homoserine, in the limited infection of pea (*Pisum sativum* L.) by bacterial pathogens has been suggested (Hildebrand, 1973). Although homoserine occurs in low levels in many plants, in peas its level increases rapidly after seed germination to peak and then fall to a still appreciable level in the maturing plants. Hildebrand (1973) observed that of 15 species of pseudomonads, only isolates of the pea pathogen *P. s.* pv. *pisi* (Sackett) Young *et al.* could utilize this amino acid for growth. Homoserine was toxic to the other pseudomonad species. The elevated levels of homoserine in pea plants may thus restrict growth of bacteria that have not evolved mechanisms to cope with its toxicity.

Secondary products that have antibacterial activity are frequently wide-spectrum toxins, so that the plant has to protect itself from their action. Protection may be achieved by compartmentalizing the chemical in vacuoles or by producing inactive derivatives (Schonbeck and Schlosser, 1976). Glycosylation of the potential toxin is a common strategy. The enzymes needed to generate the active inhibitor are present in the plant tissues, but are rendered inactive by compartmentalization away from their substances. Enzymes and the inhibitor precursors contact each other following cellular disruption. Enzymes of pathogen origin may also aid in liberating active inhibitor.

Glycosides of at least 18 different structures have been detected in over 1000 plant species as precursors of hydrogen cyanide. Rust *et al.* (1980) have demonstrated that growth of bacterial pathogens in liquid media was inhibited by HCN with ED_{50} levels of about 0.1 m*M*. This level of HCN could be generated in wounded cyanogenic tissues. Xanthomonads and pseudomonads pathogenic on cyanogenic hosts had little more tolerance to HCN than species that cause disease on noncyanogenic plants. Thus, in contrast to fungi (Fry and Evans, 1977), the bacterial pathogens of cyanogenic plants appear not to have mechanisms whereby they can adapt to HCN or metabolize it to nontoxic compounds. Clearly, HCN has the potential to act as a deterrent against bacterial growth. However, the metabolism of cyanogenic precursors in a resistant as well as a susceptible host–pathogen interaction awaits elucidation.

The putative antibacterial agents in the genus *Cruciferaceae* are the mustard oils, isothiocyanic acids (R—N=C=S), which are present in healthy tissues as glycosides. Upon cellular disruption these glycosides are converted to isothiocyanates by enzymes of the myrosinase complex, which are synthesized in separate cells to those containing the glycosides (Gaines and Goering, 1962; Schonbeck and Schlosser, 1976). Isothiocyanates possess bacteriostatic activity although no plant pathogenic species were used in the bioassays (McKay *et al.*, 1959). Consequently, the role of the mustard oils in restricting bacterial growth in plants remains speculative.

The genera *Lilaceae, Ranuculaceae,* and *Rosae* produce glycosides of unsaturated lactones, some of which have five- or six-membered cyclic ring structures (Haynes, 1948). Antibiotic effect of lactones has been demonstrated, although no plant pathogenic bacteria were assayed (Haynes, 1948). Localization of lactone derivatives to specific plant tissues has been observed (Schonbeck and Schlosser, 1976). Consequently, the distribution of the lactone compounds must correlate with any proposed role of lactones in resistance to bacterial infection.

In pear (*Pyrus communis* L.) and walnut (*Juglans regia* L.) the suspected antibacterial compounds are the hydroquinones obtained from the glycosides, arbutin and juglone, respectively. Powell and Hildebrand (1970) demonstrated that the pear pathogen, *E. amylovora,* was inhibited by the hydroquinone from arbutin, and that oxidation products from arbutin would complex with hydroquinone to give additional antibacterial compounds. The oxidation products were generated by polyphenoloxidases and peroxidases in pear extracts (Powell and Hildebrand, 1970). Thus, several constitutive enzymes from pear tissue along with the secondary compounds are implicated in this possible resistance scheme.

Benzoxazolinone derivatives have been suggested as factors contributing to resistance in rye (*Secale cereale* L.), wheat (*Triticum aestivum* L.), and corn (*Zea mays* L.) (Hartman *et al.*, 1975; Lacy *et al.*, 1979; Whitney and Mortimer, 1961). In healthy plants, the compounds are present as glycosides. The aglycone methoxy benzoxazolinone, obtained from field and sweet corn [*Z. mays* var. *saccharata* (Sturtev.) Bailey], inhibited growth of the causal agent of Stewarts disease, *Erwinia stewartii* (Smith) Dye (Whitney and Mortimer, 1961). Corcuera *et al.* (1978) assayed 2,4-dihydroxy-7-methoxy-benzoxazinone (DIMBOA), purified from corn extracts, for growth inhibition of pathogenic and nonpathogenic strains of *Erwinia* on corn. The majority of the strains pathogenic on corn were more tolerant of DIMBOA than were those pathogenic on the other hosts. The sensitivity of the non-corn pathogens to DIMBOA suggests that presence of DIMBOA at wound sites could screen against their initial colonization of wounded material. However, DIMBOA appears not to be a primary determinant for corn resistance against *Erwinia*. Lacy *et al.* (1979) demonstrated that seven of the DIMBOA-sensitive strains were highly pathogenic on DIMBOA-producing corn lines. Furthermore, corn lines lacking DIMBOA were no more susceptible to *Erwinia* pathogenesis than were DIMBOA-producing plants (Lacy *et al.*, 1979). These authors did not examine the role of DIMBOA in plant to plant dissemination. Since DIMBOA increases the lag phase of exposed bacteria (Corcuera *et al.*, 1978), it may slow successful colonization of new tissue by cells from infected plants.

Another class of secondary compounds that have antibacterial activity are the leek oils ($R{-}S{-}R^1$), thioesters found in the genera *Allium* and *Cruciferaceae*. Unlike the previous examples, the precursor of the leek oil in garlic (*Allium vineale* L.), alliin, is not glycosylated. Its conversion to the active component allicin involves the specific plant enzyme alliin lyase (Schonbeck and Schlosser, 1976). Allicin has been associated with the antibacterial activity detected in garlic extracts (Cavallito and Bailey, 1944), but no reported studies indicate a function of this, or other leek oils, in bacterial resistance.

Other wound-stimulated reactions that may participate in restricting pathogen development involve the production of polyphenols. Following cellular disruption, phenols previously stored in vacuoles contact the plants polyphenoloxidase and peroxidase enzymes (Eric, 1976). The resulting polyphenols have been demonstrated to be potent inhibitors of enzymes such as the macerating pectinases (Hunter, 1974). Consequently, the production of polyphenols after wounding may limit the spread of bacteria by inhibiting enzymes vital to pathogenesis. Polyphenol induction is also believed to be a key function in the hypersensitive response, an induced defense mechanism of a plant against bacterial challenge. These aspects are discussed more fully by Klement (this volume, Chapter 8).

The secondary compounds discussed in these examples are preformed and are converted into inhibitors of bacterial development upon disruption of plant tissue. Bell (1981) describes these components as wound antibiotics; their synthesis is not directly triggered by the bacterial challenge. Indeed these systems supplement the wound repair achieved by lignification and suberization of the cell walls. Because these preformed components have a broad range of activity, they are unlikely to be the only factors in determining resistance. Rather they provide another hurdle for virulent bacteria to overcome, or to which less aggressive pathogens may succumb. Clearly, we do not understand the avoidance mechanisms used by virulent bacteria. Indeed, studies to date primarily provide the stimulus for needed experimentation. The role of the preformed chemical inhibitors in bacterial resistance remains only vaguely perceived.

V. THE RESISTANT STATE

Bacteria that penetrate resistant hosts experience only limited multiplication and spread. The passive defense systems here discussed may be augmented by active resistance mechanisms initiated by the bacterial challenge. The recognition processes that determine whether or not these resistance systems are triggered probably involve other preformed structures in the plant.

A. Resistance and Water Soaking

A plant may resist bacteria that have invaded the intercellular spaces by restricting their access to an essential requirement, water. Indeed, susceptibility can be induced in a normally resistant plant if water congestion is artificially maintained at the inoculation site (Cook and Stall, 1977; Stall and Cook, 1979; Young, 1974). The saprophytic bacterium *P. fluorescens* Migula has produced disease symptoms in inoculated tobacco (*Nicotiana tabacum* L.) leaf tissue that has maintained in the dark at 100% relative humidity (Lovrekovich and Lovrekovich, 1970).

Rudolf and co-workers (1980, 1981) have suggested that virulence of the xanthomonads and pseudomonads, which are intercellular pathogens, involves the ability of their extracellular polysaccharides to preserve a water-congested state. By themselves, the purified extracellular polysaccharides will produce and maintain water-soaking symptoms, but only in leaves of plants that are susceptible to the pathogen. Intercellular fluids from plant leaves caused degradation of the extracellular polysaccharides from bacteria avirulent on the plant, but less degradation occurred with the complex from virulent bacteria (El Banoby *et al.*,

1981). Resistance to this type of pathogen may thus require that the plant's intercellular space contains enzymes that will prevent maintenance of the water-congested state. Since the polysaccharide-degrading enzymes were detected in unchallenged plant tissues, their synthesis is independent of bacterial challenge. The degradative enzymes are therefore another facet of the plants' preformed defense systems.

B. Preformed Factors in Hypersensitivity and Immobilization Responses

Resistance to bacteria has been associated with the induced responses of hypersensitivity and immobilization, which are discussed more fully by McIntyre, Klement, and Keen and Holliday (this volume, Chapters 7, 8, and 9). These responses are initiated by bacterial challenge and presumably involve specific recognition events between bacterial and plant cell surfaces. It is pertinent to suggest, however, that initial recognition by the plant depends upon certain preformed entities.

The physiological changes characteristic of the hypersensitive response can be produced by treating plant tissues with pathogen-produced components, termed elicitors. The elicitors isolated from *P. s.* pv. *glycinea* by Bruegger and Keen (1979) are active upon soybean tissues previously unchallenged by bacteria. The receptors for these elicitors are therefore synthesized in the absence of the bacterial cells.

In the immobilization process, preformed factors in the plant may be responsible for the initial attachment of the bacteria to the plant cell wall. Preparations from a variety of plant tissues have the ability to agglutinate bacterial cells. Extracts from potato tubers possess lectins that agglutinate avirulent but not virulent isolates of *Pseudomonas solanacearum* (Smith) Smith. Preliminary studies show that similar lectins are also present on the cell walls of foliar parts of the plant (Sequeira, 1980). A factor extracted from Red Mexican bean seed preferentially agglutinated cells of the race of *P. s.* pv. *phaseolicola* (Burkholder) Young *et al.* that is avirulent on this cultivar, rather than cells of the virulent race (Slusarenko and Wood, 1981). Lectins from corn seed will cause cells of *E. stewartii*, *E. carotovora*, and *E. chrysanthemi* Burkholder *et al.* (Sequeira, personal communication) to agglutinate. A high-molecular-weight glycoprotein complex, extracted from a variety of plant sources, caused agglutination of cells of saprophytic pseudomonads but not species of pseudomonads that have plant pathogenic potential (Jasalavich and Anderson, 1981). Each of these agglutinins is the product of unchallenged plant tissues. Their agglutinating abilities suggest that they could function in the immobilization response.

Thus, preliminary evidence indicates that preformed factors may be involved in the initial recognition processes that occur during the active defense response of immobilization.

C. Resistance and Environment

Resistance of a plant to a pathogen is frequently not an absolute state. Rather, many factors may influence the outcome of this interaction. The aggressiveness of the pathogen may determine the degree of resistance that a given cultivar displays. Resistance often varies with plant age, and such time-related factors have recently been discussed by Bell (1980). The age of the plant could influence the physical defense systems afforded by the cuticle and plant cell wall layers. The hydrophobicity of the leaf surface decreases with maturation (Martin and Juniper, 1970; Tukey, 1970), and this could alter the degree of its cohesion with microbial cells. Other possible consequences include increased water deposition and leaching of plant metabolites on the leaf surface. All of these events could promote bacterial colonization on the leaf surface. Indeed an increase in pseudomonad population on beetroot leaves as they age has been correlated to an increasing nutrient exudation (Blakeman, 1972). The maturation of primary to secondary walls as plants age involves an increase in the resistance of those walls to macerating enzymes. Thus, aging of the wall structures could increase the resistance of a plant to a pathogen.

Seasonal fluctuations in resistance to bacterial pathogens are reported. Crosse (1956) observed that leaf abscission scars produced in cherry (*Prunus avium* L.) early in the season were more easily invaded by *P. s.* pv. *morsprunorum* (Wormald) Young *et al.* than those occurring in autumn. One explanation for these observations is that leaf scars become suberized concomitant with abscission in autumn but that suberization is delayed earlier in the season. Another possibility is that the greater transpirational pull in the summer than in the autumn causes introduction of more inoculum into the exposed xylem elements.

The environment clearly can alter the host–pathogen relationship. Plant resistance is dependent upon nutritional status and thus is influenced by the environmental variables of light, temperature, water, and nutrient availability. Higher temperature and light intensity and lower humidity increase wax production by plants, thereby enhancing the penetration barrier (Kolattukudy, 1970). In peaches, better nutrition raised susceptibility to *X. c.* pv. *pruni* (Matthee and Daines, 1969). This nutrition-related decrease in field resistance may be connected to an enlargement in the aperture of the foliar stomates, which would promote inoculum entry.

Light may affect resistance when a limitation in photosynthate restricts the metabolite flow into the biosynthetic pathways for suberin and lignin. If low light conditions do reduce the extent of suberization and lignification, increased susceptibility of the plant cell walls to enzyme maceration would result, and this could explain the reduced resistance levels. Increased disease severity in tomato plants infected with *P. solanacearum* was observed under low light (Gallegy and Walker, 1949). Low light combined with high nutritional levels decreased resistance of guar [*Cyamopsis tetragonoloba* (L.) Taub.] to *X. c.* pv. *cyaniopsidis* (Patel *et al.*) Young *et al.* (Orellana and Thomas, 1968) and of sesame (*Sesamum indicum* L.) to *P. s.* pv. *sesami* (Malkoff) Young *et al.* and *X. c.* pv. *sesami* (Sabet & Dowson) Dye (Thomas, 1965). No resistance was observed in dark-grown pepper (*Capsicum frutescens* L.) plants challenged with *X. c.* pv. *phaseoli* (Smith) Dye (Sasser *et al.*, 1974). In contrast, however, no symptoms developed in soybean plants inoculated with *P. s.* pv. *glycinea* that had previously been grown in darkness (Smith and Kennedy, 1970). Thus the effect of any given environmental factor may vary with the host–pathogen interaction in question.

Air pollutants markedly affect the severity of the disease responses of plants to bacterial pathogens. In general, the physiology of these responses is not understood, but the preformed resistance mechanisms could be altered. Exposure of soybean to ozone prior to and during inoculation with *P. s.* pv. *glycinea* gave a protectant effect (Lawrence and Wood, 1978a). Ozone treatments reduced lesion size in wild strawberry *Fragaria virginiana* Duchesne infected with *Xanthomonas fragariae* Kennedy & King (Lawrence and Wood, 1978b). Ozone may restrict pathogen ingress by reducing stomatal apertures. The ability of ozone to stimulate stomatal closure varies among plant species (Hill and Littlefield, 1969; MacKnight, 1968). In some cases, ozone may stimulate the production of secondary products that have an antibacterial activity. Keen and Taylor (1975) reported that ozone treatment of soybean plants enhanced synthesis of such compounds as daidzein, coumestrol, and sajagol. Phytoalexins, associated with the hypersensitivity response, were not produced following ozone treatment.

Shriner (1978) observed that simulated acid rain on bean plants increased or decreased the severity of disease caused by *P. s.* pv. *phaseolicola* according to the stage in the disease cycle when treatments were applied. Acid rain has been observed to cause an increased leakage of nutrients (Wood and Bormann, 1975), and this phenomenon could promote bacterial colonization. A major factor however could be the effect of the acidity rating of the rain directly on bacterial growth. Indeed, growth of *P. s.* pv. *phaseolicola* is inhibited below pH 5 (Shriner, 1978).

Corn and soybean plants were protected against inoculations with *Corynebacterium nebraskense* (Schuster *et al.*) emend. Vidaver & Mandel or *X. c.* pv. *phaseoli*, respectively, by various treatments with SO_2 (Lawrence and Aluisio, 1981). Whether the passive defense mechanisms were being altered is unknown. Cuticle abrasion, epidermal cell damage, and stomatal closure, however, are consequences of SO_2 exposure (Kimmerer and Kozlowski, 1981; Rist and Davis, 1979).

Environmental factors clearly alter the surface characteristics of plants, and thus could influence the establishment of bacterial colonies on the host surface prior to infection. Aerosol inoculation of prewetted soybean leaves with *P. s.* pv. *glycinea* resulted in the establishment of epiphytic populations upon the leaf surfaces (Surico *et al.*, 1981). It is intriguing that the numbers of cells of *P. s.* pv. *morsprunorum* that could be washed from the leaf surfaces of a susceptible cherry variety were consistently higher than those washed from a resistant variety (Crosse, 1963). Daub and Hagedorn (1981) reported similar observations with snap bean and *P. s.* pv. *syringae* van Hall, in that epiphytic populations were higher on leaves of susceptible than resistant cultivars. About 10^6 cells per gram of fresh weight were isolated from leaves of the susceptible cultivar, compared to 10^3 cells per gram fresh weight from leaves of a resistant line. The reduced population of the resistant line did not appear to be due to the presence of antagonistic microflora.

It is tempting to speculate that resistance systems of a plant extend beyond its physical boundaries into the phylloplane and the rhizosphere. Could the lower levels of colonization in resistant varieties be due to the presence of antibacterial agents or different nutrient levels in the leaf exudates? More involved studies of the chemistry of leaf and root exudates relative to nutrients and bacterial deterrents are necessary to resolve this point.

Bacterial pathogens are aware of the external aura of their hosts. Chemotaxis toward root and leaf exudates has been demonstrated and the phenomenon generally attributed to the presence in the exudates of certain amino acids, organic acids, or sugars. Studies with *P. s.* pv. *lachrymans* (Smith & Breyan) Young *et al.* showed leaf exudates from resistant plants were no less chemotaxic than exudates from susceptible roots (Chet *et al.*, 1973). Specialization, however, has been demonstrated. Cells of *X. c.* pv. *oryzae* (Ishiyama) Dye were more attracted to exudates from susceptible than resistant rice (*Oryza sativa* L.) plants (Feng and Kuo, 1975). The colonization of bean by *X. c.* pv. *phaseoli* var. *fuscans* (Burkholder) Starr & Burkholder may be promoted by biologically active peptides in the bean root exudates (Vancura *et al.*, 1969). Raymundo and Ries (1980) have reported that *E. amylovora* is attracted to organic acids and aspartate but not to sugars or other amino acids. Taxis of *E. amylovora* toward organic acids such as malate is an intriguing idea because these acids accumulate in vacuoles of cells in apple tissues and could be available on cellular damage. Apple nectar was also chemotaxic.

Exudates from leaves and roots probably help establish microflora antagonistic to bacterial pathogens in the phylloplane and rhizosphere. Current research has demonstrated phylloplane and rhizosphere pseudomonads that will reduce disease severity caused by fungal pathogens (Kloepper *et al.*, 1980). *Erwinia herbicola* (Löhnis) Dye is a saprophytic bacterium that occupies the same ecological niche as *E. amylovora* and is antagonistic to this pathogen (Erskine and Lopatecki, 1975; Thomson *et al.*, 1976). The antagonism of certain isolates of *Agrobacterium radiobacter* (Beijerinck & van Delden) Conn against the crown gall organism *A. tumefaciens* (Smith & Townsend) Conn is so effective that it has gained worldwide field usage as a biological control agent (Cooksey and Moore, 1979; Kerr, 1980). The methods by which these antagonists achieve control over the pathogen may be independent of the plant. However, as the antagonist may be largely nurtured by nutrients in the plant exudates, this method of control can be broadly regarded as another scheme by which resistance involves factors that are a normal part of the plant's structure.

VI. SUMMARY

Plants have evolved defense systems to thwart bacterial penetration, spread, and reproduction. The systems described in this chapter are an integral part of each plant's functions; they exist before bacterial challenge occurs. Many of these factors also work against other pathogens such as fungi and insects. The exact stimulus for their evolution remains unknown, as does the potential for their exploitation in pest management programs.

The passive defenses discussed here constitute primary attempts to avert bacterial growth. Three zones of defense are proposed. In the rhizosphere and phylloplane the supply of nutrients and water along with the presence of antagonistic microflora or antibacterial compounds may limit colonization of the host surface. The second zone involves the physical barriers to prevent penetration: the cuticular layer and the plant cell wall. The third zone for internal protection relies again on physical barriers but also upon bizarre chemicals that have antibacterial properties. In each zone, bacteria that have not evolved with these defense systems may be screened out.

Increased understanding of the passive systems involved in resistance needs research to couple physiology of the plant to the pathogenic process. The role of the cuticular layer in controlling establishment of epiphytic colonies which can act as an inoculum source is in special need of clarification. The significance of the chemical deterrents to bacterial disease resistance could provide direction to plant breeders. The effects of environment on resistance are highly significant as we try to maximize our crop yields from minimum energy inputs. Meanwhile, until we learn more, we can be greatful that evolution has provided us with plants that are thick skinned.

References

Akai, S., and Fukutomi, M. (1980). *In* "Plant Disease" (J. G. Horsfall and E. B. Cowling, eds.), Vol. 5, pp. 139–159. Academic Press, New York.

Albersheim, P. (1976). *In* "Plant Biochemistry" (J. Bonner and J. E. Varner, eds.), Vol. 3, pp. 226–277. Academic Press, New York.

Albersheim P., and Anderson, A. J. (1971). *Proc. Natl. Acad. Sci. U.S.A.* **68,** 1815–1819.

Audia, W. V., Smith, W. L., and Craft, C. C. (1962). *Bot. Gaz.* **123,** 255–258.

Bartz, A., and Showalter, R. K. (1981). *Phytopathology* **71,** 515–518.

Bateman, D. F., and Basham, H. G. (1976). *In* "Physiological Plant Pathology" (R. Heitefuss and P. H. Williams, eds.), pp. 316–355. Springer-Verlag, Berlin and New York.

Bauer, W. D. (1981). *Annu. Rev. Plant Physiol.* **32,** 406–449.

Beckman, C. H., Mueller, W. C., and McHardy, W. E. (1972). *Physiol. Plant Pathol.* **2,** 69–74.

Bell, A. (1980). *In* "Plant Disease" (J. G. Horsfall and E. B. Cowling, eds.), Vol. 5, pp. 53–73. Academic Press, New York.

Bell, A. (1981). *Annu. Rev. Plant Physiol.* **32,** 21–81.

Blakeman, J. P. (1972). *Physiol. Plant Pathol.* **2,** 143–152.

Bruegger, B. B., and Keen, N. T. (1979). *Physiol. Plant Pathol.* **15,** 43–51.

Campbell, C. L., Huang, J., and Payne, G. A. (1980). *In* "Plant Disease" (J. G. Horsfall and E. B. Cowling, eds.), Vol. 5, pp. 103–118. Academic Press, New York.

Cavallito, J., and Bailey, J. (1944). *J. Am. Chem. Soc.* **66,** 1950–1951.

Chet, I., Zilberstein, Y., and Henis, Y. (1973). *Physiol. Plant Pathol.* **3,** 473–479.

Cook, A. A., and Stall, R. E. (1977). *Phytopathology* **67,** 1107–1193.

Cooksey, D. A., and Moore, L. W. (1979). *Phytopathology* **70,** 506–509.

Corcuera, L. J., Woodward, M. D., Helgeson, J. P., Kelman, A., and Upper, C. D. (1978). *Plant Physiol.* **61,** 791–795.

Crosse, J. E. (1956). *J. Hortic. Sci.* **31,** 212–224.

Crosse, J. E. (1963). *Ann. Appl. Biol.* **52,** 97–104.

Daft, G. C., and Leben, C. (1971). *Phytopathology* **62,** 57–62.
Daub, E., and Hagedorn, D. J. (1981). *Phytopathology* **71,** 547–550.
El-Banoby, F. E., Rudolph, K., and Huttermann, A. (1980). *Physiol. Plant Pathol.* **17,** 291–301.
El-Banoby, F. E., Rudolph, K., and Mendgen, K. (1981). *Physiol. Plant Pathol.* **18,** 91–98.
Eric, F. (1976). *In* "Physiological Plant Pathology" (R. Heitefuss and P. H. Williams, eds.), Vol. 4, pp. 617–631. Springer-Verlag, Berlin and New York.
Erskine, J. M., and Lopatecki, L. E. (1975). *Can. J. Microbiol.* **21,** 35–41.
Esau, K. (1977). *In* "Anatomy of Seed Plants," pp. 43–60. Wiley, New York.
Feng, T. Y., and Kuo, T. T. (1975). *Acad. Sin. Inst. Bot. Bull.* **16**(2), 126–236.
Fox, R. T. V., Manners, J. G., and Myers, A. (1971). *Potato Res.* **14,** 61–73.
Gaines, R. D., and Goering, K. J. (1962). *Biophysics* **96,** 13–19.
Gallegy, M. E., and Walker, J. C. (1949). *Phytopathology* **39,** 936–946.
Goodman, R. N. (1976). *In* "Physiological Plant Pathology" (R. Heitefuss and P. H. Williams, eds.), pp. 173–196. Springer-Verlag, Berlin and New York.
Hartman, R., Kelman, A., and Upper, C. D. (1975). *Phytopathology* **65,** 1082–1088.
Haynes, L. J. (1948). *Q. Rev. Chem. Soc.* **2,** 46–72.
Hildebrand, E. M. (1937). *Phytopathology* **27,** 850–852.
Hildebrand, D. C. (1973). *Phytopathology* **63,** 301–302.
Hill, A. C., and Littlefield, N. (1969). *Environ. Sci. Tech.* **3,** 52–56.
Hunter, R. E. (1974). *Physiol. Plant Pathol.* **4,** 151–159.
Jasalavich, C. A., and Anderson, A. J. (1981). *Can. J. Bot.* **59,** 264–271.
Keen, N. T., and Taylor, O. C. (1975). *Plant Physiol.* **55,** 731–733.
Kerr, A. (1980). *Plant Dis.* **64,** 25–30.
Kimmerer, T. W., and Kozlowski, T. T. (1981). *Plant Physiol.* **67,** 990–995.
Kloepper, J. W., Leong, J., Teintze, M., and Schroth, M. N. (1980). *Curr. Microbiol.* **4,** 317–320.
Kolattukudy, P. E. (1970). *Annu. Rev. Plant Pathol.* **21,** 163–192.
Kolattukudy, P. E. (1980). *Science* **208,** 990–1000.
Lacy, G. H., Hirano, S. S., Victoria, J. I., Kelman, A., and Upper, C. D. (1969). *Phytopathology* **69,** 757–763.
Laurence, J. A., and Aluisio, A. L. (1981). *Phytopathology* **71,** 445–448.
Laurence, J. A., and Wood, F. A. (1978a). *Phytopathology* **68,** 441–445.
Laurence, J. A., and Wood, F. A. (1978b). *Phytopathology* **68,** 689–692.
Lovrekovich, L., and Lovrekovich, H. (1978). *Phytopathology* **60,** 1279–1280.
Mace, M. E. (1963). *Physiol. Plant.* **16,** 915–925.
MacKnight, M. (1968). MS thesis, University of Utah.
McKay, A. F., Garmaise, D. L., Guadry, R., Baker, H. A., Paris, G. Y., Kay, R. W., Just, G. E., and Schwartz, R. (1959). *J. Am. Chem. Soc.* **81,** 4328–4335.
McLean, R. T. (1921). *Bull. Torrey Bot. Club* **48,** 101–106.
Martin, J. T., and Juniper, B. E. (1970). *In* "The Cuticles of Plants," pp. 248–251. St. Martin's Press, New York.
Matthee, F. N., and Daines, R. H. (1969). *Phytopathology* **59,** 285–287.
Orellana, R. G., and Thomas, C. A. (1968). *Phytopathology* **58,** 250–251.
Powell, C. C., Jr., and Hildebrand, D. C. (1970). *Phytopathology* **60,** 337–340.
Purcell, A. H. (1975). *Environ. Entomol.* **4,** 745–752.
Purcell, A. H. (1981). *Phytopathology* **71,** 429–435.
Raymundo, A. K., and Ries, S. M. (1980). *Phytopathology* **70,** 1066–1069.
Rist, D. L., and Davis, D. D. (1979). *Phytopathology* **69,** 231–235.
Rolfs, R. M. (1915). *Cornell Univ. Agric. Exp. Sta. Mem.* **8,** 377–436.

Rust, L. A., Fry, W. E., and Beer, S. V. (1980). *Phytopathology* **70**, 1005–1008.
Sasser, M., Andrews, A. K., and Doganay, Z. U. (1974). *Phytopathology* **64**, 770–772.
Schenck, N. C. (1981). *Plant Dis.* **65**, 230–234.
Schlosser, E. W. (1980). *In* "Plant Disease" (J. G. Horsfall and E. B. Cowling, eds.), Vol. 5, pp. 161–176. Academic Press, New York.
Schonbeck, F., and Schlosser, E. (1976). *In* "Physiological Plant Pathology" (R. Heitefuss and P. H. Williams, eds.), pp. 653–678. Springer-Verlag, Berlin and New York.
Schonherr, J., and Huber, R. (1977). *Plant Physiol.* **59**, 145–149.
Seemuller, E. A., and Beer, S. V. (1976). *Phytopathology* **66**, 433–436.
Sequeira, L. (1980). *In* "Plant Disease" (J. G. Horsfall and E. B. Cowling, eds.), Vol. 5, pp. 179–200. Academic Press, New York.
Shriner, D. S. (1978). *Phytopathology* **68**, 213–218.
Shriner, D. S., Decot, M. E., and Cowling, E. B. (1974). *Proc. Am. Phytopathol. Soc.* **1**, 112.
Slusarenko, A. J., and Wood, R. K. S. (1981). *Physiol. Plant Pathol.* **18**, 187–193.
Smith, M. A., and Kennedy, B. W. (1970). *Phytopathology* **60**, 723–725.
Stall, R. E., and Cook, A. A. (1979). *Physiol. Plant Pathol.* **14**, 77–84.
Surico, G., Kennedy, B. W., and Ercolani, G. L. (1981). *Phytopathology* **71**, 532–536.
Thomas, C. A. (1965). *Plant Dis. Rep.* **49**, 119–120.
Thomson, S. V., and Purcell, A. H. (1979). *Phytopathology* **69**, 8.
Thomson, S. V., Schroth, M. N., Moller, W. J., and Reil, W. O. (1976). *Phytopathology* **66**, 1457–1459.
Tukey, H. B. (1970). *Annu. Rev. Plant Physiol.* **21**, 305–324.
Uritani, I., and Stahmann, M. A. (1961). *Phytopathology* **51**, 277–285.
Vancura, V., Stanek, M., and Hanzlikova, A. (1969). *Folia Microbiol.* **14**, 23–27.
Weinhold, A. R., and Hancock, J. G. (1980). *In* "Plant Disease" (J. G. Horsfall and E. B. Cowling, eds.), Vol. 5, pp. 121–134. Academic Press, New York.
Whitney, N. J., and Mortimore, C. G. (1961). *Nature (London)* **189**, 596–597.
Wood, R. K. S. (1967). *Physiol. Plant Pathol.* 570.
Wood, T., and Bormann, R. H. (1975). *Ambio* **4**, 169–171.
Young, J. M. (1974). *N.Z. J. Agric. Res.* **17**, 115–119.

Chapter **7**

Induced Resistance

JOHN L. MCINTYRE

I. INTRODUCTION

The observation that the cowpox virus immunized humans against the causal agent of chicken pox not only permitted its use for disease control, but led to a basic understanding of certain diseases. It seems that the development and ultimate use of the plant "immune system" (induced resistance) is presently at the "cowpox" stage. Numerous reports indicate that treatment of a plant with inducing agents such as living, killed, or subcellular components of microorganisms, or abiotic agents may protect the plant against disease incited by certain phytopathogens (challengers). Exploitation of this phenomenon for practical disease control has yet to be achieved.

Although our understanding of the mechanisms of induced resistance is incomplete, research to date has led to the development of several

Phytopathogenic Prokaryotes, Vol. 2

Copyright © 1982 by Academic Press, Inc.
All rights of reproduction in any form reserved.

ISBN 0-12-509002-1

concepts. Protection may occur because the inducer blocks host cell sites required by the challenger. The inducer may also trigger resistant responses in the plant that are effective against the challenger. Alternatively, the inducer may predispose the host plant such that it rapidly undergoes defensive reactions, but the actual defensive mechanisms may not become activated until the plant is challenged. The latter in particular suggests a plant "immune system," and its potential use for plant disease control appears immense. This, of course, does not reduce the potential and practical importance of any interaction that results in crop protection.

Recent reviews (Goodman, 1980; Hamilton, 1980; Kuc, 1981; Matta, 1980; McIntyre, 1980; Sequeira, 1979; Suzuki, 1980) provide insight into the phenomenon of induced plant resistance against phytopathogens. In this chapter we will explore several aspects of induced resistance. Special attention will be given to current results and opportunities for future research and application. The emphasis will be on induced resistance against prokaryotes, especially bacteria, since this author is unaware of reports on induced resistance against mycoplasma-like organisms or similar prokaryotes. The number of studies concerning induced resistance against bacteria seems scant when compared to induced resistance against fungi or viruses. Recent results from several laboratories, however, indicate that induced resistance is a general phenomenon against diverse challengers, including bacteria. Thus, to best indicate what induced resistance is and its potential for practical disease control, it becomes necessary to discuss also induced resistance as a general phenomenon rather than one specific to a particular group of pathogens.

II. INDUCED RESISTANCE AGAINST BACTERIA

A. Bacteria as Inducers

Mixed inoculations of plants with virulent and nonvirulent bacterial cells may result in protection, while in other cases the inducer must precede the challenger for protection to occur. Coinoculation of tobacco (*Nicotiana tobacum* L.) with virulent and avirulent cells of *Pseudomonas solanacearum* (Smith) Smith results in reduced levels of disease (Averre and Kelman, 1964). The disease severity caused by *Pseudomonas syringae* pv. *morsprunorum* (Wormald) Young *et al.* on cherries (*Prunus avium* L.) is also reduced when coinoculated with an *Erwinia*-like epiphyte (Crosse, 1965), and mixed infections of rice (*Oryza sativa* L.) with the epiphyte *Erwinia herbicola* (Löhnis) Dye and the rice pathogen *Xanthomonas campestris* pv. *oryzae* (Ishiyama) Dye result also in protection (Hsieh and Buddenhagen, 1974).

Although induced resistance might be inferred from the coinoculation data, other factors must also be considered. Averre and Kelman (1964) suggest that the avirulent isolates of *P. solanacearum* cause a hypersensitive response in the host, and thereby sequesters the virulent cells within the area of the necrotic tissue. In a culture medium, *E. herbicola* reduces both pH (Farabee and Lockwood, 1958) and nitrogen levels (Riggle and Klos, 1972), thus establishing an environment unsuitable for growth of the fire blight pathogen, *Erwinia amylovora* (Burrill) Winslow *et al.*

In other cases the avirulent bacteria, especially when given the advantage in cell numbers, may attach to host cell sites also required by the virulent cells. Lippincott and Lippincott (1969) demonstrate this to be the case in protection of pinto bean (*Phaseolus vulgaris*) against *Agrobacterium tumefaciens* (Smith & Townsend) Conn, and Ercolani (1970) indicates a similar interaction in tomato (*Lycopersicon esculentum* Mill.) using avirulent cells of *Corynebacterium michiganense* (Smith) Jensen to protect against virulent cells of this pathogen.

In some studies, a time period is required between inducer and challenger inoculations for protection to occur. Although this does not preclude competition as a factor in protection, it does infer that a host response is required. Goodman (1967) reports that inoculation of apple (*Malus sylvestris* Mill.) stems with avirulent *E. amylovora, E. herbicola,* or *Pseudomonas syringae* pv. *tabaci* (Wolf & Foster) Young *et al.* 30 min prior to inoculation with virulent *E. amylovora* results in protection. This protection, however, was transient and may be due to competition. Protection, however, reoccurs 7 to 10 hr later, suggesting initiation of a host response.

In a similar study, McIntyre *et al.* (1972) demonstrate that prior inoculation of pear shoots (*Pyrus communis* L.) with avirulent *E. amylovora, E. herbicola,* or *P. s.* pv. *tabaci* protects against virulent *E. amylovora.* In this study, a time period of 24 hr was necessary between inducer and challenge inoculations. Similar results were obtained using immature pear fruit (Wrather *et al.,* 1973).

B. Bacterial Components and Other Agents as Inducers

As we have discussed already, living bacteria may induce resistance against bacterial pathogens. Other evidence, however, indicates that heat-killed bacterial cells, cell-free bacterial sonicates, bacterial components, and abiotic agents also induce resistance against bacterial pathogens.

Lovrekovich and Farkas (1965) report that heat-killed cells of *P. s.* pv. *tabaci* protect tobacco against the virulent pathogen when the challenger follows the inducer by 24 to 48 hr. Likewise, heat-killed cells of *A. tumefaciens* protect against virulent *A. tumefaciens* (Lippincott and Lippincott, 1969).

In the fire blight of pear system, McIntyre *et al.* (1972) found that cell-free sonicates of virulent or avirulent *E. amylovora* induce resistance against virulent *E. amylovora.* For protection to occur, a time period was required between inducer and challenge inoculations, indicating an activation of host resistance mechanisms. In further studies, purified deoxyribonucleic acid (DNA) but not ribonucleic acid from the virulent or avirulent *E. amylovora* cells induced resistance (McIntyre *et al.*, 1975). In fact, as the purity and native conformation of the DNA preparation were improved, the level of resistance not only increased, but systemic resistance developed. The practical role of bacterial DNA as an inducer of plant resistance has yet to be determined.

Novacky and Hanchy (1976) report that tobacco leaves injected with water or rubbed with cotton swabs or carborundum are protected against the hypersensitive response evoked by *P. s.* pv. *pisi* (Sackett) Young *et al.* Tobacco is protected also against *P. s.* pv. *pisi* by kinetin or other compounds with cytokinin activity (Novacky, 1972). Agents such as polyacrylic acid (Gianinazzi and Kassanis, 1974) and acetylsalicylic acid (White, 1979) have been used also as inducers against viruses. Although the mode of action is unknown, these results indicate the diversity of agents capable of inducing plant resistance, thereby increasing the opportunities to use this phenomenon for practical disease control.

III. THE *Pseudomonas solanacearum* STORY

One of the most complete efforts to describe a host–parasite system for induced resistance against a bacterium comes from the laboratory of L. Sequeira. For more than a decade, this group has studied induced resistance of tobacco against the hypersensitive response caused by *P. solanacearum.* These studies, with corroborative evidence from other host–parasite systems, provide not only a better understanding of induced resistance against bacteria, but insights into both the nature of the bacterial inducing factors and induced host resistance responses.

Sequeira and his colleagues report initially that heat-killed cells of *P.*

solanacearum induce resistance of tobacco against living cells of this bacterium (Lozano and Sequeira, 1970). Heat-killed cells of *P. s.* pv. *lachrymans* (Smith & Bryan) Young *et al.* and *X. axonopodis* (Starr & Garces) but not *Escherichia coli* (Migula) Castellani & Chalmers had a similar effect. This response is both light and time dependent, suggesting that a host resistance response is required for protection to occur. Under certain conditions, this resistance becomes systemic (Sequeira, 1979).

A. Inducing Factors

Further studies were performed to identify both the bacterial inducing factor and the host resistance mechanisms. Sequeira *et al.* (1972) report that a proteinaceous constituent of *P. solanacearum* is the inducing factor. The component was obtained from both soluble and insoluble bacterial cell wall fractions. Inducing activity was associated with a major protein peak obtained after partial purification. Upon gel electrofocusing, however, only partial protection was associated with a major protein band, and results were inconsistent.

In recent studies (Graham *et al.*, 1977) it was found that a protein-free lipopolysaccharide (LPS) fraction isolated from cell walls of *P. solanacearum* had a high inducer activity and the factor could be isolated from both virulent and avirulent forms of the bacterium. The evidence indicates that the core lipid A section of the LPS molecule was the active portion.

There is additional evidence that bacterial LPS acts as an inducer. Mazzuchi and Pupillo (1976) report that protein–LPS from *Erwinia chrysanthemi* Burkholder *et al.* protects tobacco against hypersensitive necrosis caused by the same bacterium. In contrast to the studies of Graham *et al.* (1977), the protein component was required for protection to occur in this system.

The discrepancy between these reports in the requirement for LPS to have an associated protein for inducer activity suggests that the chemical nature of inducers may vary among the systems. This point is further exemplified in the study of McIntyre *et al.* (1975), where bacterial DNA was identified as the inducer.

B. Host Resistance Responses

Several host mechanisms are associated with induced resistance against *P. solanacearum*. First, heat-killed bacterial cells, when introduced into the host, attach to host cell sites, and the bacterial cells become enveloped (Sequeira *et al.*, 1977). Purified LPS, upon introduction, likewise attaches to tobacco mesophyll cell walls and causes host changes similar to those initiated by the heat-killed cells (Graham *et al.*, 1977). When the host is challenged, the challenger bacteria do not attach and are not enveloped by the host cell walls, indicating that HR prevention may be due to this lack of attachment.

Agglutination of bacteria is demonstrated in several incompatible host–parasite interactions, and this topic has been reviewed recently (Sequeira, 1980, 1981). Additional evidence that bacterial agglutination is a factor in induced resistance comes from a study by G. Bergstrom (University of Kentucky, Lexington, personnel communication). In the cucumber (*Cucumis sativus* L.) system (see Section IV), extracts from plants induced with either *P. s.* pv. *lachrymans* or tobacco necrosis virus show increased agglutination of *E. tracheaphila* (Smith) Bergey *et al.* and rabbit red blood cells. This effect is systemic, and indicates further the role of bacterial agglutination as a host defensive mechanism. Although agglutination in several incompatible host–parasite systems is related with host lectins (Sequeira, 1980, 1981), the agglutinating factor from cucumber has yet to be described.

It has been noted also that growth and survival of *P. solanacearum* in the intercellular spaces of protected tobacco tissues is reduced (Rathmell and Sequeira, 1975). Fluids from protected leaves reduce bacterial growth *in vitro*, and introduction of these fluids into leaves, at times, results in protection. The active components fractionated from protecting fluids are heat-stable, low-molecular-weight molecules, and do not appear to be phenols.

Other studies show also that plants may accumulate antibacterial metabolites when the HR is incited by bacteria (Chen *et al.*, 1969; Stall and Cook, 1968). Keen and Kennedy (1974) provide evidence that several phytoalexins, including hydroxyphaseollin, coumestrol, daidzein, and sojagol accumulate in soybean tissue inoculated with HR inciting strains of *P. s.* pv. *glycinea* (Coerper) Young *et al.* or the nonpathogen *P. s.* pv. *lachrymans*. Further, inoculation of plants with compatible races of *P. s.* pv. *glycinea* leads to a delayed appearance of these metabolites, and the levels are 10% less than in resistant leaves. Both hydroxyphaseollin and coumestrol are shown to have antibacterial activity at levels that accumulate in the plant tissues.

Introduction of heat-killed cells or LPS from *P. solanacearum* also causes increases in host peroxidase activity, and the appearance of an additional isozyme (Nadolny and Sequeira, 1980). Unfortunately, similar peroxidase activities were caused by noninducing agents. Thus this increased activity appears related to but not responsible for induced resistance in this system.

Increases in peroxidase activity, of course, have been implicated as a factor involved with disease resistance in several host–parasite systems. The studies, however, are inconclusive and reports such as those by Nadolny and Sequeira (1980) and Seevers and Daly (1970) indicate its role to be secondary in conferring disease resistance to plants.

IV. INDUCED RESISTANCE AGAINST DIVERSE CHALLENGERS

The studies discussed thus far might suggest that induced resistance against bacteria is a specific phenomenon. Other studies, however, demonstrate that once a plant is induced, it may develop resistance against diverse challengers including fungi, bacteria, viruses, and insects.

That bacteria can induce resistance against diverse challengers, or vice versa, is shown in several studies. Heat-killed cells of *Pseudomonas syringae* pv. *syringae* van Hall interfere with tobacco mosaic virus local lesion formation in tobacco (Loebenstein and Lovrekovich, 1966). Caruso and Kuc (1979) show that inoculation of a cucumber leaf with either *P. s.* pv. *lachrymans* or *Colletotrichum lagenarium* (Pass.) Ell. & Hals protects susceptible cultivars against subsequent challenge with either pathogen. The elicitation of this immune response is time dependent, systemic, and lasts up to 37 days. In further studies (Jenns and Kuc, 1980; Kuc, 1981) infection with *P. s.* pv. *lachrymans, C. lagenarium,* or tobacco necrosis virus induces resistance of cucumber against each of these three organisms and *Cladosporium cucumerinum* Ell. & Arth.

McIntyre *et al.* (1981) demonstrate that localized infections of tobacco with tobacco mosaic virus (TMV) induce systemic and persistent resistance against diverse challengers including *P. s.* pv. *tabaci, Phytophthora parasitica* Dast. var. *nicotianae* (Breda de Haan) Tucker, *Peronospora tabacina* Adam, TMV, and the green peach aphid, *Myzus persicae* (Sulz.). Localized infections of tobacco with TMV also induce resistance against the tobacco hornworm, *Manducca sexta* (Johan.) (Hare and McIntyre, unpublished). Again, the development of resistance requires a time period between inducer and challenger inoculations.

V. THE NATURE OF INDUCED RESISTANCE— AN HYPOTHESIS

We have discussed already that several different bacterial components may induce plant resistance, and that several different host mechanisms may relate to the expression of resistance against bacteria. Thus it is not surprising that additional elicitors of induced resistance and potential host defensive mechanisms are described for other systems utilizing fungi and viruses (Hamilton, 1980; Sequeira, 1979). In fact, considering the phylogenetic differences between fungi, bacteria, and viruses, it would seem that each may possess a different means to induce resistance, and that host defenses against these pathogens would differ. We might still, however, expect some commonality in induced resistance and its expression.

To explore what may be similarities between induced resistance in different host–parasite systems, let us examine why induced resistance may occur, and why systemic induced resistance may develop.

A. Why Resistance Occurs

Several studies indicate that protection results from competition for host cell sites, or that the inducer activates host defensive mechanisms that are also effective against the challenger. That these interactions result in protection is not surprising and, in fact, it might be argued that these types of interactions are not "induced resistance." Other results, however, suggest that the host has the genetic capability for resistant responses, but that they are not activated rapidly enough in the noninduced plant. Upon induction, and given adequate time to respond, these systems are "activated" and capable of warding off the challenge by the pathogenic microbe. This may be more aptly termed induced resistance.

This aspect of induced resistance has been discussed recently by Kuc (1981). Further evidence for the activation of host defenses is discussed by McIntyre and Dodds (1979) and McIntyre *et al.* (1981). When systemic resistance against diverse challengers is induced in tobacco by TMV, the TMV particles are localized to a few cells around the lesion (Israel and Ross, 1967). Thus, for systemic resistance to occur, a direct interaction between TMV and the challengers is precluded. Likewise, the biochemical changes thus far detected after TMV inoculation probably do not directly confer resistance to the challengers. These biochemical changes include altered levels of peroxidase and catalase activity (Simons and Ross, 1971a), indoleacetic acid (Van Loon and Berbee, 1978), cytokinins (Balasz *et al.*, 1977), and several proteins (Van Loon, 1976). When challenged with TMV, however, the induced plant responds more rapidly than does the noninduced plant (Simons and Ross, 1971b). This indicates that the plant is genetically capable of resistant responses to both TMV and presumably other types of pathogens, but that these responses occur too slowly in the susceptible plant for resistance to be realized.

When induced, the resistance responses may occur more rapidly, and resistance is expressed.

McIntyre *et al.* (1981) have hypothesized an evolutionary advantage to this type of induced resistance, whereby resistance genes are conserved but not necessarily expressed. When pathogen attack is spurious, the synthesis of metabolites used for host defenses can be "turned off." Thus the energy saved may be used for increased reproduction while a pool of resistance genes could be conserved by the plant. It is these genes that are then "turned on" when the plant is induced, and the products of which are expressed when the plant is challenged. If exploited, the potential of induced resistance for disease control is obvious. Rather than using conventional breeding procedures to incorporate resistance into agronomic crops, it permits activation of genes for disease resistance that are possessed already by the agronomically acceptable plant.

B. How Systemic Resistance Develops

Kuc (1977) and McIntyre *et al.* (1981) have hypothesized a translocated signal, moving from the induced leaf throughout the plant. This signal is not an inhibitory metabolite but rather activates the potential of host resistance responses to occur when the plant is challenged.

Jenns and Kuc (1979) demonstrate in the cucumber system that the signal is graft-transmissible, but not cultivar-, genus-, or species-specific. This suggests that the signal could be a common factor in induced resistance.

McIntyre (1981) provides evidence that the signal in the tobacco system is translocated in the phloem. Local but not systemic resistance develops if the phloem but not xylem transport from the induced leaf is blocked. Likewise, if the phloem transport is blocked into a systemically located leaf, the entire plant, except for the phloem-blocked leaf, develops resistance. Identification of this signal could provide both a further insight into the biochemical nature of induced resistance, and an agent for the controlled induction of resistance in agronomic crops.

VI. FROM THE LABORATORY TO THE FIELD

Although induced resistance is a widely recognized interaction, most of the research effort has been devoted to the development of a basic understanding of the phenomenon. Since induced resistance may be systemic, persistent, and effective against diverse challengers, its potential for practical disease control seems great.

At present, however, induced resistance remains as a laboratory curiosity, with only limited efforts to test its widespread utility in the field. New methods for disease control are needed and the results to date indicate that induced resistance is a logical candidate. We should, therefore, utilize the available information to determine if induced resistance can be exploited in the field. If successful, further improvements in both the levels of induced resistance and its use for many crops and against different types of phytopathogens can be achieved through additional basic studies.

References

Averre, C. W., and Kelman, A. (1964). *Phytopathology* **54,** 779–783.

Balasz, E., Sziraki, S., and Kiraly, Z. (1977). *Physiol. Plant Pathol.* **11,** 29–37.

Caruso, F., and Kuc, J. (1979). *Physiol. Plant Pathol.* **14,** 191–201.

Chen, S. C., Stall, R. E., and Cook, A. A. (1969). *Phytopathology* **589,** 112 (Abstr.).

Crosse, J. E. (1965). *Ann. Appl. Biol.* **56,** 149–160.

Ercolani, G. L. (1970). *Phytopathol. Mediterr.* **9,** 151–159.

Farabee, G. J., and Lockwood, J. L. (1958). *Phytopathology* **48,** 209–211.

Gianinazzi, S., and Kassanis, B. (1974). *J. Gen. Virol.* **23,** 1–9.

Goodman, R. N. (1967). *Phytopathology* **57,** 22–24.

Goodman, R. N. (1980). *In* "Plant Disease" (J. G. Horsfall and E. B. Cowling, eds.), Vol. 5, pp. 305–317. Academic Press, New York.

Graham, T. L., Sequeira, L., and Huang, T. R. (1977). *Appl. Environ. Microbiol.* **34,** 424–432.

Hamilton, R. I. (1980). *In* "Plant Disease" (J. G. Horsfall and E. B. Cowling, eds.), Vol. 5, pp. 279–303. Academic Press, New York.

Hsieh, S. P. Y., and Buddenhagen, I. W. (1974). *Phytopathology* **64,** 1182–1185.

Israel, H. W., and Ross, A. F. (1967). *Virology* **33,** 272–286.

Jenns, A. E., and Kuc, J. (1979). *Phytopathology* **69,** 753–756.

Jenns, A. E., and Kuc, J. (1980). *Physiol. Plant Pathol.* **17,** 81–91.

Keen, N. T., and Kennedy, B. W. (1974). *Physiol. Plant Pathol.* **4,** 173–185.

Kuc, J. (1977). *Neth. J. Plant Pathol.* **83,** 463–471.

Kuc, J. (1981). *In* "Plant Disease Control" (R. C. Staples and G. H. Toenniessen, eds.), pp. 259–272. Wiley, New York.

Lippincott, B. B., and Lippincott, J. A. (1969). *J. Bacteriol.* **97,** 620–628.

Loebenstein, G., and Lovrekovich, L. (1966). *Virology* **30,** 587–591.

Lovrekovich, L., and Farkas, G. L. (1965). *Nature (London)* **205,** 823–824.

Lozano, J. C., and Sequeira, L. (1970). *Phytopathology* **60,** 875–879.

McIntyre, J. L. (1980). *In* "Plant Disease" (J. G. Horsfall and E. B. Cowling, eds.), Vol. 5, pp. 333–343. Academic Press, New York.

McIntyre, J. L. (1981). *Phytopathology* **71,** in press (Abstr.).

McIntyre, J. L., and Dodds, J. A. (1979). *Physiol. Plant Pathol.* **15,** 321–330.

McIntyre, J. L., Kuc, J., and Williams, E. B. (1972). *Phytopathology* **63,** 872–877.

McIntyre, J. L., Kuc, J., and Williams, E. B. (1975). *Physiol. Plant Pathol.* **7,** 153–170.

McIntyre, J. L., Dodds, J. A., and Hare, J. D. (1981). *Phytopathology* **71**, 297–301.
Matta, A. (1980). *In* "Plant Disease" (J. G. Horsfall and E. B. Cowling, eds.), Vol. 5, pp. 345–361. Academic Press, New York.
Mazzuchi, V., and Pupillo, P. (1976). *Physiol. Plant Pathol.* **9**, 101–112.
Nadolny, L., and Sequeira, L. (1980). *Physiol. Plant Pathol.* **16**, 1–8.
Novacky, A. (1972). *Physiol. Plant Pathol.* **2**, 101–104.
Novacky, A., and Hanchy, P. (1976). *Acta Phytopathol. Acad. Sci. Hung.* **11**, 217–222.
Rathmell, W. G., and Sequeira, L. (1975). *Physiol. Plant Pathol.* **5**, 65–73.
Riggle, J. H., and Klos, E. J. (1972). *Can. J. Bot.* **50**, 1077–1083.
Seevers, P. M., and Daly, J. M. (1970). *Phytopathology* **60**, 1642–1647.
Sequeira, L. (1979). *In* "Recognition and Specificity in Plant Host—Parasite Interactions" (J. M. Daly and I. Uritani, eds.), pp. 231–251. Japan Science Society Press, Tokyo.
Sequeira, L. (1980). *In* "Plant Disease" (J. G. Horsfall and E. B. Cowling, eds.), Vol. 5, pp. 179–200. Academic Press, New York.
Sequeira, L. (1981). *In* "Plant Disease Control" (R. C. Staples and G. H. Toenniessen, eds.), pp. 143–152. Wiley, New York.
Sequeira, L., Aist, S., and Ainslie, V. (1972). *Phytopathology* **62**, 536–541.
Sequeira, L., Gaard, G., and DeZoeten, G. A. (1977). *Physiol. Plant Pathol.* **10**, 43–50.
Simons, T. J., and Ross, A. F. (1971a). *Phytopathology* **61**, 293–300.
Simons, T. J., and Ross, A. F. (1971b). *Phytopathology* **61**, 1261–1265.
Stall, R. E., and Cook, A. A. (1968). *Phytopathology* **58**, 1584–1587.
Suzuki, H. (1980). *In* "Plant Disease" (J. G. Horsfall and E. B. Cowling, eds.), Vol. 5, pp. 319–332. Academic Press, New York.
Van Loon, L. C. (1976). *J. Gen. Virol.* **36**, 375–379.
Van Loon, L. C., and Berbee, A. Th. (1978). *Z. Pflanzen Physiol.* **89**, 373–375.
White, R. F. (1979). *Virology* **99**, 410–412.
Wrather, J. A., Kuc, J., and Williams, E. B. (1973). *Phytopathology* **63**, 1075–1076.

Chapter **8**

Hypersensitivity

ZOLTAN KLEMENT

Phytopathogenic Prokaryotes, Vol. 2

Copyright © 1982 by Academic Press, Inc.
All rights of reproduction in any form reserved.
ISBN 0-12-509002-1

I. INTRODUCTION

Plants, like other living systems, have several ways of protecting themselves from invasion by microorganisms. Hypersensitivity is thought to be one type of defense reaction of plants to pathogens which occurs only in an incompatible host–pathogen relationship. A rapid cell collapse is induced in nonhost or resistant plants by pathogens, often associated with the localization of the pathogen near its entry point.

Hypersensitivity is a universal phenomenon in the plant kingdom and is operative whether the pathogen be a fungus (Stakman, 1915), a virus (Holmes, 1929), or a bacterium (Klement *et al.*, 1964). Almost half a century had to pass before the hypersensitive reaction (HR) was recognized in plant diseases caused by bacteria (Klement, 1963; Klement *et al.*, 1964; Klement and Lovrekovich, 1961, 1962). This may have been due to the fact that with diseases caused by fungi and viruses the symptoms of HR appear in the form of small local necroses so they are easily recognized, whereas the host response evoked in plants by a few incompatible bacteria is normally not readily discernible.

In a few instances, however, the HR necrosis appears in the form of local necroses. For example, small necrotic spots on leaves of stone-fruit trees in early spring are certainly an HR to *Pseudomonas syringae* van Hall. According to D. C. Sands (personal communication), leaf necrosis and bleaching of leaves of cereals are due to high levels of *P. syringae* pv. *syringae* van Hall on the leaf surface during cool moist periods, resulting in bacterial entry and subsequent HR. Gross and DeVay (DeVay, personal communication) found that black streak of sugar beet (*Beta vulgaris* L.) leaves caused by *P. s.* pv. *aptata* (Brown & Jamieson) Young *et al.* rarely occurs, but when it does, the leaves are predisposed to the disease by cold injury. In all respects the disease resembles HR. It seems that in these instances HR symptoms are viewed as disease symptoms.

The application of the injection–infiltration method for studying HR has opened new possibilities for studying host–parasite relationships (Hagborg, 1970; Klement, 1963). With this method, a large number of bacterial cells can be introduced into the plant's intercellular spaces, thereby exposing more plant cells to the bacteria, which results in the HR becoming visible.

II. DETERMINATION AND CHARACTERIZATION OF HYPERSENSITIVITY

Hypersensitivity has originally been characterized as the defense reaction of the plant which is accompanied by rapid tissue necrosis. The reaction is often also accompanied by phytoalexin production in the incompatible host–parasite relationship which appears to result in the localization of the pathogen. Reducing the HR to tissue necrosis and phytoalexin production is an oversimplification as they constitute only the consequences of "hypersensitivity," namely, the syndrome of "hypersensitive reaction." This is why the role of the HR as a defense mechanism came to be questioned (Section VIII).

Therefore, in defining the term HR it is necessary to enumerate all the facets of its development including recognition of the pathogen by the plant, induction of the reaction, development of the necrosis, formation of antimicrobial substances, and localization of the pathogen. Accordingly, it is more precise to characterize HR as being a subtle defense mechanism wherein the plant and pathogen are able to recognize each other in the early stages of infection. This leads to the autolysis of some plant cells and, consequently, characteristic metabolic changes occur and the pathogen is localized at the infection site.

III. SPECIFICITY OF THE HYPERSENSITIVE REACTION (HR)

Numerous investigations have indicated that most phytopathogenic bacteria have HR-inducing properties but that saprophytic microorganisms do not (Klement, 1963; Klement and Goodman, 1967). From perusal of the literature, it is apparent that among phytopathogenic bacteria only pseudomonads and xanthomonads, that induce local lesions, and pathogens belonging to other genera, which cause necrosis of plant tissue, cause HR in incompatible hosts. Thus, for example tumor-inducing agrobacteria and some soft-rot *Erwinia* spp. do not induce HR (Schroth and Hildebrand, 1967). For example, *P. s.* pv. *savastanoi* (Smith) Young *et al.* causes galls in olive (*Olea europaea* L.) and oleander (*Nerium oleander* L.) that become necrotic, and is also able to cause HR in tobacco (*Nicotiana tabacum* L.) (Smidt and Kosuge, 1978). All phytopathogenic pseudomonads can induce HR except *P. marginalis* (Brown) Stevens, which causes leaf rot in lettuce (*Lactuca sativa* L.) and soft-rotting in the tissues of other plants (Schroth and Hildebrand, 1967). Generally it could be established that those pathogens which induce HR are rather host-specific, whereas those not inducing HR tend to be polyvirulent bacteria.

HR is a general defense mechanism in the plant kingdom. It occurs in many incompatible host–pathogen relationships (Table I). HR can exist in relationships between pathogens and nonhost species, host species,

Table I. Host–Parasite Relationships

Combinations	HR	Typical disease symptom
Susceptible host–virulent bacteria species[a]	–	+
Normally susceptible host–bacteria lose their virulence[b]	+	–
Nonhost species–species-nonvirulent bacteria[b]	+	–
Resistant cultivars–cultivar-nonvirulent bacteria[b]	+	–
Plants (all)–saprophytic bacteria	–	–

[a] Compatible host–pathogen relationship.
[b] Incompatible host–pathogen relationship.

and nonvirulent bacteria, or between resistant cultivars and virulent bacteria.

The ability of tissue necrotizing bacteria to induce HR in incompatible host–pathogen combinations has revealed some important features of pathogenicity. Hence, the establishment of a host–pathogen relationship leads to spot or blight disease development only if a pathogen is unable to induce HR in a particular host. This has recently been shown since the inhibition of HR with blasticidin S in an incompatible soybean [*Glycine max* (L.) Merr.]–*P. s.* pv. *glycinea* (Coerper) Young *et al.* combination allowed multiplication of the bacterium and development of typical water-soaked disease symptoms (Keen *et al.,* 1981).

IV. INFLUENCE OF ENVIRONMENTAL CONDITIONS ON HR

A. Temperature

Confluent HR necrosis induced by most phytopathogenic *Pseudomonas* spp. in tobacco develops well at laboratory temperatures. However, the HR-inducing ability of some xanthomonads in tobacco leaves varies greatly even within one bacterial species under laboratory conditions. Schroth and Hildebrand (1967) and Hildebrand and Riddle (1971) found that temperatures of 30–32°C prior to the inoculation favored HR development by xanthomonads and *P. solanacearum* (Smith) Smith and most xanthomonad strains induced confluent HR necrosis. In contrast, lower temperatures reduced the number of *P. s.* pv. *syringae*, *P. s.* pv. *phaseolicola* (Burkholder) Young *et al.*, and *P. s.* pv. *savastanoi* cells required for induction of confluent HR. However, when tobacco plants were kept at a relatively high temperature (37°C) for 1–3 days before inoculation with *P. solanacearum*, tissue necrosis was delayed (Hevesi and Király, 1977).

Temperature does not influence the development of HR after inoculation within the range of 16–35°C, but at/or above 37°C, HR does not occur since most phytopathogenic bacteria are unable to multiply at these high temperatures. Pathogens which can multiply at higher temperatures, such as *P. solanacearum*, are able to cause HR (Durbin and Klement, 1977).

B. Light

The effect of light on HR was investigated in detail by Sasser *et al.* (1974) and Lyon and Wood (1976). They found that HR developed as readily in the dark as in the light. Smith and Kennedy (1970) also reported that pre- and postinoculation dark treatments did not alter HR development. However, some non-HR-inducing bacteria like virulent and avirulent *Agrobacterium tumefaciens* (Smith & Townsend) Conn or saprophytic *P. fluorescens* Migula cause confluent necrosis in tobacco similar to HR necrosis when they were kept continuously in the dark with high humidity (Hildebrand and Riddle, 1971; Lovrekovich and Lovrekovich, 1970). It is difficult to distinguish this type of necrosis from HR symptoms. I believe that this symptom is caused by the nonspecific toxicity of autolyzing bacterial cells.

C. Humidity

Continuous high humidity, which can prevent the evaporation of water from infiltrated water-soaked leaves, delays HR symptoms (Klement and Goodman, 1967; Lyon and Wood, 1976). HR does in fact occur and membranes are destroyed. However HR appears to be arrested only because plant cell water cannot diffuse into the already saturated atmosphere (Goodman, 1972).

D. Physiological State of the Plant

It has been observed that tobacco leaves, at various positions on the vertical axis of the plant, exhibited HR necrosis at different times following inoculation with incompatible bacteria. On upper and younger leaves, the necrosis appeared 1–1.5 hr earlier than on lower and older ones (Klement, unpublished work). It seems a paradox, however, that old senescent leaves require a lower inoculum concentration than young leaves to induce confluent HR necrosis (Hevesi and Király, 1977; Süle, 1973). Studies of Oguchi and Patil (1979) found that mature leaf tissue of a susceptible bean cultivar becomes resistant to *P. s.* pv. *phaseolicola*. Ho and Patil (1981) found that when primary leaves of a resistant cultivar were inoculated within 24 hr after unfolding they developed typical susceptible water-soaked symptoms and had higher bacterial multiplication rates compared to the HR of older leaves. Probably a similar situation exists in the spring on very young leaves of stone fruits after the infection of *P. s.* pv. *syringae* or *P. s.* pv. *morsprunorum* (Wormald) Young *et al.*

V. DEVELOPMENT OF HR

Investigations of HR development created considerable interest since it was thought that they would help reveal the cause and basis of resistance. When more than 5×10^6 cells ml^{-1} of *P. s.* pv. *pisi* (Sackett) Young *et al.* are injected into the intercellular spaces of nonhost tobacco leaves, the infiltrated tissue collapses as early as 6 hr after inoculation and forms a desiccated light brown lesion within 18 hr. The sequence of events defining HR development has been divided into three stages by Klement (1971) and four stages by Roebuck *et al.* (1978); they are induction time, latent period, collapse, and desiccation of host tissue. The length of induction time and appearance of HR necrosis depend on the host–pathogen combination. For instance in the nonhost tobacco–*P. s.* pv. *pisi* combination, induction time is 1.5–2 hr and the appearance of tissue collapse is about 6–8 hr. With *P. s.* pv. *phaseolicola* these periods are longer, 4 and 12–14 hr, respectively. Apparently, in an incompatible race-specific system, the appearance of HR requires more time. In the following sections the sequence of events relating to HR development will be presented in detail (Fig. 1).

A. Induction

1. *Induction Time*

The induction time is that period during which the bacterium triggers the HR irreversibly. The time required for induction of HR was determined by injecting leaves with antibiotics at hourly intervals after in-

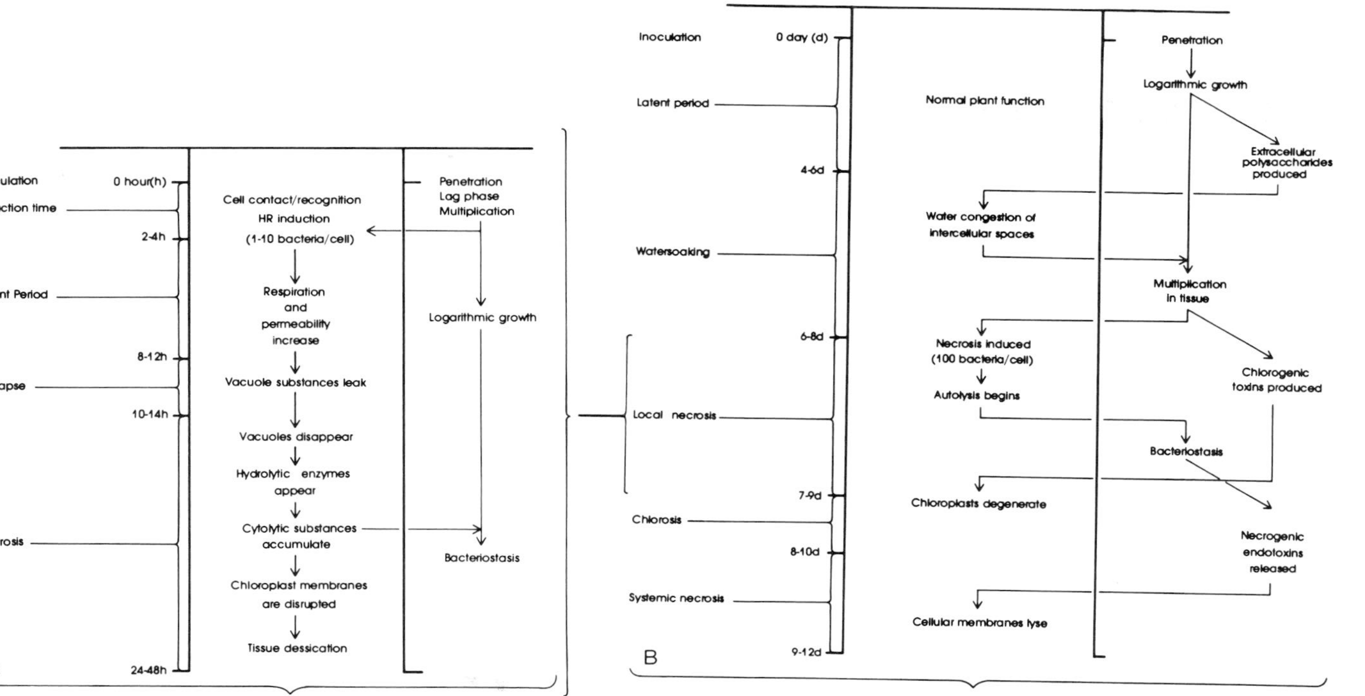

Figure 1. Scheme for bacterial blight disease development in resistant (A) and susceptible (B) host plant, emphasizing the similarity of hypersensitive necrosis in the incompatible (A) interaction to local necroses in the compatible (B) interaction.

oculation. The period between inoculation and the antibiotic application that stopped cell collapse was designated as the induction time (Klement, 1971; Klement and Goodman, 1967). Once the induction is effected, HR development is not prevented by killing the inoculated bacteria. The length of induction time was investigated in many host–bacteria combinations (Keen *et al.*, 1981; Klement, 1981; Klement and Goodman, 1967; Lyon and Wood, 1976; Meadows and Stall, 1981, and others). The approximate induction times, for instance, in tobacco leaves are 1.5–2, 3–4, and 3–5 hr for *P. s.* pv *pisi*, *P. s.* pv. *phaseolicola*, and *X. campestris* pv. *vesicatoria* (Doidge) Dye, respectively.

2. *Inoculum Concentration*

Inoculum concentration does not influence the time of induction and the appearance of the HR, the lowest inoculum concentration of *P. s.* pv. *pisi* required to induce confluent necrotic lesions in tobacco leaves is 5×10^6 cells ml^{-1}. However, visible necrotic lesions are not produced when low concentrations of pathogenic bacteria are introduced into nonhost tissue. Some researchers, however, have found that HR also occurs at the cellular level, in leaves containing only a few incompatible bacteria. Individual, selectively stained dead plant cells were detected in symptomless leaves inoculated with incompatible bacteria at concentrations lower than those required to give confluent HR necrosis (Essenberg *et al.*, 1979; Holliday *et al.*, 1979; Turner and Novacky, 1974).

Only one *P. s.* pv. *pisi* cell was required to induce HR or produce one dead tobacco cell (Turner and Novacky, 1974). A similar 1 : 1 ratio was observed in a *P. s.* pv. *morsprunorum*–bean leaf combination (Lyon and Wood, 1976). In a compatible relationship, however (Section VI), a higher number of bacterial cells is required to induce cell necrosis [50–100 *P. s.* pv. *tabaci* (Wolf & Foster) Young *et al.* cells per tobacco cell] (Klement *et al.*, 1978).

3. *Is HR Induced by Bacterial Toxins?*

Several hypotheses have been proposed to explain the crucial first step of HR development. If a single bacterium can cause the death of a large plant cell ($<1\ \mu m^3$ versus $50{,}000\ \mu m^3$), the mechanism involved must reflect the action of one or more products of the bacterium that come in contact with the host cell wall membrane (Goodman and Plurad, 1971). Numerous attempts have been made to isolate a bacterial product from several species of bacteria that induce HR. However, all efforts have failed (Klement and Goodman, 1967; Lyon and Wood, 1976). According to Gardner and Kado (1972) a compound isolated from *E. rubrifaciens* Wilson *et al.* reproduced HR symptoms. Similarly, Sequeira and Ainslie

(1969) reported that a cell fraction of *P. solanacearum* caused necrosis similar to HR in tobacco leaves. The latter report has since been revised (Sequeira, 1976). Others also suggested that certain products or toxins of bacteria might be associated with HR (Cook and Stall, 1969). The problem is complicated as it is difficult to distinguish typical HR necrosis from the nonspecific toxicity of high concentrations of bacterial components or their metabolites. When these preparations are diluted to concentrations similar to those of cell populations causing HR, necrosis is not obtained (Sequeira, 1976). On the basis of several investigations, Sequeira (1976) supposed that the bacterium produces a highly unstable toxin that damages host membranes only when released in close proximity to the cell wall. This hypothesis, however, was not supported by an experiment of Klement (1977). Flushing a previously inoculated leaf into the adjacent tissue at different periods during the induction time failed to reveal the presence of toxic metabolites responsible for HR induction. It seems, from these experiments, that toxic bacterial metabolites are not responsible for HR induction.

4. *The Role of Living and Multiplying Bacteria*

HR is induced only by living or metabolically active bacterial cells (Klement and Goodman, 1967). The generation times of most plant pathogenic bacteria coincide with the HR induction time, so it is very difficult to demonstrate multiplication of bacteria during this short time interval. However, the age of bacterial cultures determined the length of induction time but not the time of the latent period (Süle and Klement, 1971). O'Brien and Klement (unpublished) have shown that either bacteria lysed by bacteriophages or bacteriophage-infected bacterial cells were unable to induce HR. Ercolani (1970) did not observe HR on tomato (*Lycopersicon esculentum* Mill.) plants inoculated with a histidine-requiring mutant of *P. s.* pv. *syringae* because this strain was unable to multiply in the leaves unless histidine was added. However, this mutant could induce HR when histidine was added. Similarly, histidine- and arginine-deficient auxotrophs of *P. s.* pv. *pisi* did not cause HR unless supplemented with the required amino acid (Sasser, 1978). It was also demonstrated that HR did not occur when nonpermissive temperatures inhibited the multiplication of incompatible bacteria (see Section IV,A). To determine if cell division is an important factor in HR induction, nalidixic acid was mixed with an *X. c.* pv. *vesicatoria* inoculum. Multiplication of the bacterium stopped but HR development was not inhibited (Meadows and Stall, 1981). It may be concluded that cell division is not important for HR development but active metabolism of the pathogen is essential for HR induction.

Inhibition of bacterial protein synthesis by protein synthesis-inhibiting antibiotics completely prevents induction of the HR (Meadows and Stall, 1981; Sasser, 1978). Antibiotic-resistant mutants induced the HR in the presence of antibiotics, indicating that their effect was upon the bacteria, rather than the plant (Sasser, 1978). The fact that restricted bacterial protein synthesis prevents HR is strong evidence that this synthesis is implicit to the reaction. It does not follow that the HR inducer is a protein, because the effect of inhibition of bacterial protein synthesis on HR may be indirect. When proteolytic enzymes were added to the inoculum, HR did not develop. However, the enzymes did not inhibit the multiplication of bacteria *in vitro*, nor did they prevent HR in enzyme pretreated plants. This result may suggest the participation of an extracellular protein(s) synthesized during the interaction of bacteria and host cells in the induction of HR (Sasser, 1980).

5. *Cell Contact Recognition*

Specificity of HR, time dependency of induction, necessity for live and metabolically active cells, and sufficiency of a single bacterial cell for induction all infer a proximally close connection between the host and the bacterial cell. Since Ercolani proposed his attractive hypothesis (1970) on cell-contact recognition, much evidence has indicated attachment of bacteria to the cell walls of the host. Goodman *et al.* (1976) and Sequeira *et al.* (1977) recorded the attachment and the envelopment of cells of incompatible bacteria, but not compatible ones, by plant cell wall components. The attachment of nonvirulent bacteria to the cell wall in the plant during the induction time was suggested to be an essential step in HR. However, these and other investigations indicated that binding, per se, does not initiate HR, since saprophytic bacteria were also bound to the cell wall without initiation of HR (Goodman *et al.*, 1976; Sing and Schroth, 1977). Recently, Burgyán and Klement (1979) recognized a defense mechanism occurring at an early stage of infection (3–6 hr after inoculation or after the HR induction period but before the appearance of HR-associated necrosis). Since this early induced resistance and the development of HR coincide, the role of binding and encapsulation of bacteria in HR remains uncertain (Section V,D,2,a). According to Atkinson *et al.* (1981), efficient adsorption of the incompatible bacterium is not essential for the induction of HR. However, surface contact between the host and pathogen cell walls may contribute to recognition of the pathogen and HR induction. This idea is strongly supported by the observation of Cook and Stall (1977) that HR did not develop in pepper (*Capsicum frutescens* L.) leaves kept continuously water-soaked after inoculation with bacteria. When HR was prevented in water-soaked leaves, a susceptible reaction occurred with electrolyte leakage. Young (1974) reported that compatible and incompatible bacteria multiplied equally well in water-soaked bean leaves. Stall and Cook (1979) immobilized *X. c.* pv. *vesicatoria* cells in water–agar in intercellular spaces of leaves of resistant and susceptible cultivars of tomato. Bacteria immobilized in the intercellular spaces of leaves did not induce HR, but caused typical disease symptoms. Evidently the contact or attachment in the hypersensitive system is different from the immobilization process supposed earlier which may be indicative of more than one type of contact or attachment for bacteria in leaf tissue. The attachment and encapsulation of bacteria may be related to early selective inhibition of bacteria (Burgyán and Klement, 1979) but the contact between the bacterial cell and the plant cell seems to be essential for recognition or triggering of HR and for induction of HR (Stall and Cook, 1979).

As can be seen, recognition of the pathogen which leads to either the susceptible or resistant reaction is determined in the early stage of interaction. Most observations indicate that contact between the bacterium and plant cell is necessary to initiate the rapid cell collapse associated with HR. If this contact is prevented, the reaction fails to take place, and the bacteria multiply vigorously causing disease or the susceptible reaction. Two hypotheses have emerged related to regulation of this reaction. According to the first, the induction of HR in the compatible relationship is suppressed. This idea was supported by the observation that phaseotoxin suppressed the HR and phytoalexin synthesis in bean cultivars (Gnanamanicham and Patil, 1977). According to the second hypothesis, in a compatible relationship the failure of the bacterium to induce HR may not be connected with the lack of an HR inducer per se or with the failure of the bacterium to bind to a susceptible plant cell (Roebuck *et al.*, 1978). The latter model presupposes the existence of special receptor sites on the cell wall surface of the host. However, this has not yet been demonstrated.

The massive plant cell wall prevents bacteria from direct contact with the host plasmalemma. The host cell wall contains lectin-like compounds which may play a role as receptor sites on the cell wall surface. In the induction of HR in tobacco by *P. solanacearum*, recognition between host and pathogen was thought to involve an interaction between plant lectins and bacterial lipopolysaccharides (LPS). The outer membrane of Gram-negative bacteria contains LPS which may play the major role in the recognition phenomenon. This idea was based on the results of Whatle *et al.* (1980) which indicated differences in sugar composition between the HR-inducing and non-HR-inducing strains of *P. sol-*

anacearum. However, in light of their most recent investigation, the interactions of LPS and the hydroxyproline-rich proteins in the tobacco cell wall are not specific and, therefore, not dependent on lectins as they had thought initially. The interaction takes place, but is ionic in nature and dependent on the charge at the surface of the bacterium (Sequeira, personal communication).

B. Latent Period

The duration of the latent period is from the start of plant reaction up to the appearance of the tissue collapse. This period is symptomless and usually requires 4–6 hr. The development of the host response during the latent period is independent of the presence of the pathogen. Specifically, if bacterial cells are inhibited or killed by antibiotics after the induction of the HR, the cell collapse will nevertheless occur. Consequently, if the "controlling factors" are activated in the host tissue during induction, HR proceeds without living bacterial cells. Unfortunately, very little is known about the initial biochemical processes which trigger the development of the HR. During this symptomless period some physiological and biochemical changes occur. For instance, development of the HR was accompanied by a significant increase in the intensity of respiration (Németh and Klement, 1967). Maximal rate of respiration was observed about 30 min before the appearance of the tissue collapse. Intensity of respiration induced by the incompatible pathogen was higher than that obtained with the compatible or saprophytic bacteria. Changes in enzyme activity associated with the rapid tissue collapse during the latent period were measured by Németh *et al.* (1969). Increased activities of ribonuclease, G-6P-dehydrogenase, 6-P-G-dehydrogenase, and shikimate dehydrogenase were detected. The level of peptidase, polyphenoloxidase, peroxidase, phenylalanine, ammonia lyase, and cytochrome oxidase remained unchanged. Most probably the speed of the development of HR is the reason why an increase in polyphenoloxidase or peroxidase activity (the most widespread biochemical symptom of many other hypersensitive host–parasite complexes) was not observed in bacterial systems. The significance of enzyme changes associated with the development of HR is not clear, but some of these changes occur in infected susceptible tissue as well.

Only negligible ultrastructural changes in this phase can be detected. Cytoplasm accumulation was observed in spongy mesophyll cells of bean leaf adjacent to attached bacteria. Accumulated cytoplasm occasionally contained osmiophyllic droplets (Roebuck *et al.* 1978).

An increased, irreversible permeability of plant cell membranes is one of the most significant and important changes of this period which begins at the end of the latent period and reaches its peak in the tissue collapse phase (Cook and Stall, 1968; Goodman, 1968). Increase in cell permeability was followed by electrolyte leakage in all instances when plants were inoculated with incompatible bacteria. However, only a gradual increase of electrolyte leakage was measured in susceptible combinations at the same time. *Pseudomonas fluorescens,* a saprophyte, caused little or no change in permeability. Maximal electrolyte loss occurred before the first signs of tissue collapse appeared (Cook and Stall, 1968).

C. Tissue Collapse

The most dramatic phase in the development of HR is tissue collapse. The rapid biochemical and physiological changes in this stage are expressed visibly. This sudden collapse, depending on the specific host–parasite relationship, appears 7–18 hr after inoculation. The tissue loses it turgor and collapses but the green color remains in this phase. If the inoculum concentration is less than 10^{6-7} cell ml^{-1}, then tissue collapse cannot be seen (Essenberg *et al.*, 1981; Holliday *et al.*, 1981; Turner and Novacky, 1974). In this case, the rate of cell collapse is proportional to the concentration of the inoculum.

The cell vacuole is generally assumed to be the main storage organ for phenols present usually as glycosidic derivatives. The sudden rise in cell membrane permeability mentioned above causes an increase in tonoplast permeability and, as a consequence, vacuole contents flow into the cytoplasm. It is possible that autolysis of plant cells undergoing HR may result from the activity of hydrolytic enzymes such as protease, esterase, phosphatase, and ribonuclease, contained in the vacuole and these enzymes may interact with phenolic glycosides or free phenols to form antimicrobial compounds (Sequeira, 1976). This idea seems to contradict the results of Németh *et al.* (1969) since there are no significant increases of protease, polyphenoloxidase, peroxidase, and phosphatidase activities. However, in these experiments enzyme activities were measured before tissue collapse at the end of the latent period when these enzymes may not have been released. Direct evidence for HR-linked denaturation of membrane proteins is supplied by Huang and Goodman (1972). They reported that structural proteins of chloroplast membranes isolated from tissues undergoing HR were altered in their physicochemical properties 3 hr after bacterial infiltration.

These biochemical and physiological alterations during the self-destruction of the host cell have been followed by ultrastructural investigations. In mesophyll cells, extensive deposits appear on the tonoplast. Later, similar deposits appear in the vacuoles (Lyon and Wood, 1970). Finally, cytoplasmic invasion of the vacuolar region appears to take place and the vacuole breaks into a series of large membrane-bound vesicles (Roebuck *et al.*, 1978). Many cells undergo alterations in ultrastructure such as vesiculation and accumulation of osmiophylic droplets. These droplets may represent localized accumulation of phytoalexins or other antibacterial compounds (Guanamanicham and Patil, 1977; Lyon and Wood, 1975). Perhaps most profound is the complete destruction of all organellar membranes, plasmalemma, tonoplast, chloroplast, mitochondria, and microbody within 6 hr after infiltration of tobacco by *P. s.* pv. *pisi* (Goodman and Plurad, 1971).

D. Necrotization of Host Tissue and Bacteriostasis

Hypersensitive tissue which has lost its turgor, depending on environmental conditions, becomes necrotized 2–4 hr after the appearance of cell collapse, and later desiccates. In this stage the tissue turns white or light brown and the necrotized area becomes parchment-like. When the inoculum concentration is low and only localized patches of cells have undergone HR, then these cells turn brown and die but there is no desiccation.

A different point of view in connection with tissue necrosis has been published by Lovrekovich *et al.* (1970) who reported that increases in pH and ammonia, resulting from bacterial multiplication in tissue, were sufficient to cause cellular collapse. However, Goodman (1972) and others concluded that neither ammonia accumulation nor increased pH was causally related to the HR.

Phenolic compounds and their oxidation products, formed during cell collapse as a result of invasion of cytoplasm by vacuolar contents, are likely to have profound effects on both the necrotization of tissue and the inhibition of bacteria. Essenberg *et al.* (1981) described four inhibitory sesquiterpenoid phytoalexins produced during HR in cotton (*Gossypium hirsutum* L.) plants resistant to *X. c.* pv. *malvacearum* (Smith) Dye. Their preliminary observations by fluorescent microscopy indicated a connection between phytoalexin production and hypersensitive necrosis. A yellow-green fluorescence was localized in the brown host cells that had responded hypersensitively to inoculation. In inoculated susceptible leaves, the fluorescence was less brilliant. However, it was also localized in certain host cells. These cells were not brown, although they appeared irregular in shape. These observations suggest that high concentrations of phytoalexins are the cause of host cell necrosis (Essenberg, personal communication).

1. Inhibition of Bacteria in Hypersensitive Tissue

During the necrotization process, antimicrobial compounds (phytoalexins) may accumulate and diffuse into the intercellular spaces and, in turn, inhibit bacterial multiplication or cause bacteriostasis. Bacteriostasis in living plant tissue may be detected by the agar-plate-count method (Klement, 1970, 1974).

Before bacterial HR had been discovered, it was known that the trend of bacterial multiplication in resistant cultivars differed from that observed in the susceptible plants (Allington and Chamberlain, 1949; Diachun and Troutman, 1954). Since then, many studies indicated that plant pathogenic bacteria start to multiply in intercellular space, whether or not they are normally able to infect that particular plant. Multiplication of virulent bacteria in their susceptible host (compatible combination) goes on at a high rate, whereas multiplication of incompatible pathogens stops in nonhost or resistant plants during HR development. Saprophytic pseudomonads are unable to multiply in plants, although they freely multiply in pressed juice or the intercellular fluid of leaves (Klement, 1965).

The multiplication rate of various incompatible, compatible, and saprophytic bacteria has been investigated in many laboratories. The multiplication rates of *X. c.* pv. *malvacearum* in susceptible and resistant cotton cultivars were related to inoculum concentrations (Essenberg *et al.*, 1979). In the susceptible cotton cultivar, the upper limit of the population of *X. c.* pv. *malvacearum* was approximately 5×10^8 bacteria per cm^2 attained after 10^3 to 10^6-fold increases in cell members. The length of time from inoculation to the appearance of the first water-soaked symptom depended on the concentration of the inoculum. In the resistant host, the upper limit was 5×10^6 cells per cm^2 and the time required for the host to inhibit bacterial growth was 4 days during which the bacteria multiplied about 2×10^3-fold. The constancy of the time of inhibition in the host suggests that the bacteriostatic response is local and independent of initial population density. Essenberg and her coworkers (1979) calculated the diameter of the inhibitory zone around colonies of *X. c.* pv. *malvacearum.* They found that this zone in hypersensitive cotton leaf tissue was 440 μm or approximately 20 pallisade cell widths.

2. *In Vitro Bacteriostasis in Intercellular Fluid*

Since pathogenic bacteria multiply in the fluid of intercellular spaces, the bacteriostatic effect of this substance was investigated during HR development (Klement, 1965). Fluid from the intercellular spaces of incompatible tobacco leaves was sampled at 2-hr intervals for 24 hr after inoculation with *P. solanacearum* and assayed for bacteriostatic activity. An inhibitory effect was observed in the fluid 12–18 hr after the infection (Lozano, 1969). Inhibition of *X. c.* pv. *vesicatoria* in fluids from pepper occurred in extracts from hypersensitive leaves after 8 hr of incubation, but only after 48 hr was a similar inhibitory activity detected in susceptible leaves (Stall and Cook, 1968). Since the inhibitory effect in the extract and in the tissue appeared about the same time, it was presumed that the inhibitor was the same in both cases. The inhibitors of bacterial growth in the hypersensitive plant have not been described completely, because the compounds are difficult to extract.

a. Immobilization of Bacteria by Host Cell Surface Components. In the last 5 years, several plants have been reported to immobilize incompatible (Cason *et al.*, 1978; Goodman *et al.*, 1976; Sequeira *et al.* 1977) and saprophytic bacteria (Sing and Schroth, 1977) but not virulent compatible pathogens.

The first step of immobilization is the attachment of bacteria to the plant cell wall. However, Hildebrand *et al.* (1980) suggest that the attachment of bacteria is not an active process, instead it may be related to evaporation of intercellular water. In contrast, Goodman *et al.* (1976), Politis and Goodman (1978), and Sequeira *et al.* (1977) observed cell wall swelling and fibrillar apposition and vesicular transport of fibrils opposite encapsulated bacteria. The second step of the immobilization process after attachment is the envelopment of bacterial cells. The bacteria are surrounded by a thin, fibrillar mass, that separates from the host cell wall surface within 2–3 hr. By 7 hr, the bacteria become surrounded by granular and fibrillar materials (Cason *et al.*, 1978; Goodman *et al.*, 1976; Sequeira *et al.*, 1977).

No difference in encapsulation was detected between compatible and incompatible pathogens or saprophytes (Hildebrand *et al.*, 1980). However, compatible pathogens appeared to multiply and break free of the entrapping structures but incompatible and saprophytic bacteria did not. Immobilization develops prior to the occurrence of the HR necrosis but after the induction of HR. The coincidence of HR immobilization process makes separate examination of these phenomena difficult (Sequeira, 1981; Sequeira *et al.*, 1977). The immobilization processes, on the basis of coincidence in time, may be related to early selectively induced resistance rather than to HR (Burgyán and Klement, 1979). Furthermore, in both host responses, pathogens and saprophytes induce these reactions, but compatible bacteria are not inhibited. These observations leads us to conclude that immobilization is the appearance of early induced resistance rather than the HR.

Lectin-like compounds may be responsible for immobilization since they agglutinate incompatible bacteria *in vitro* (Huang *et al.*, 1973; Romeiro *et al.*, 1981). According to El-Banoby and Rudolph (1980), lectin extracts from the resistant breeding lines agglutinated bacteria of race 1 and 2 of *P. s.* pv. *phaseolicola*, whereas lectin extracts from the susceptible cultivar did not cause agglutination. Érsek *et al.* (1981) isolated a material from the intercellular spaces of soybean leaves which specifically agglutinated incompatible but not compatible races of *P. s.* pv. *glycinea*. The *in vitro* agglutination test of Fett and Sequeira (1980), in contrast with their previous findings, could not show a correlation between pathogenicity of *P. solanacearum* and agglutination.

b. Phytoalexins and Other Antimicrobial Compounds. Hypersensitivity of some plants to bacterial inoculation leads to the production and accumulation of a number of phenolics. Certain phenolic compounds which are present in healthy plants in the form of inactive precursors are activated in the course of necrobiosis and become antimicrobial. Antimicrobial compounds having postinfectional origin include phytoalexins. In most cases, production of phytoalexins is correlated with HR. Accumulation of these compounds in some host plants may be induced not only with fungi and viruses but also with bacteria. Phytoalexins are produced in nonhost plants as well as in resistant cultivars. However, phytoalexins often form in susceptible hosts also.

Production of phytoalexins was observed after bacterial infection in only a few cases. The best known antibacterial isoflavanoids (phaseollin, glyceollin, etc.) are produced by resistant cultivars of bean or soybean inoculated with *P. s.* pv. *phaeolicola* or *P. s.* pv. *glycinea*, respectively. These antibiotics may be responsible for bacteriostatic effects in these plants (Gnanamamichan and Patil, 1977; Keen and Kennedy, 1974).

Four sesquiterpenoids identified by Essenberg *et al.* (1981) and produced during HR of genetically resistant cotton plants inoculated with *X. c.* pv. *malvacearum* may have a role in inhibiting the bacterium. Several studies indicated that antifungal phytoalexins are also inhibitory to plant pathogenic bacteria *in vitro*. However, Wyman and VanEtten (1978) were unable to confirm this, and have suggested that the apparent bacteriostatic activity may depend on bioassay conditions.

The accumulation of phytoalexins can be observed during the appearance of cell collapse at the site of infection by inoculation at low concentrations. Fluorescent microscopy suggests that compounds exhibiting irregularly distributed yellow autofluorescence in leaf tissue are localized in cells undergoing collapse. According to Holliday *et al.* (1981), autofluorescence of necrotic cells of soybean leaves inoculated with *P. s.* pv. *glycinea* may be attributed to the accumulation of the phytoalexin glyceollin. In resistant leaves, glyceollin accumulates during the period of cell collapse (9–24 hr). According to Essenberg and her co-workers (personal communication), cells with yellow fluorescence in immune cotton leaves inoculated with *X. c.* pv. *malvacearum* appeared abnormal in shape. Their study provided an exact determination of the site and time of phytoalexin production around colonies of the pathogen.

One can surmise from these findings that phytoalexin accumulation occurs during or just after the disappearance of the vacuole in the period following degradation of the tonoplast and other cell membranes. Phytoalexins formed in the degenerated plant cells diffuse into the intercellular spaces through damaged plasma membranes where they may exert a bacteriostatic effect. *In planta* bacteriostatic effects of phytoalexins have not been unequivocally demonstrated.

VI. SIMILARITY OF NECROSIS DEVELOPMENT IN HYPERSENSITIVE AND NORMOSENSITIVE HOSTS

In bacterial spot diseases, four phases of symptom development are discernible in susceptible hosts: water-soaked spots appear, become necrotic lesions, chlorotic halos develop around the lesions, and, finally, secondary necroses form between local lesions. A scheme for defining compatible and incompatible host and pathogen combinations is summarized in Table I.

After bacterial penetration into the plant, multiplication begins in the intercellular spaces. Intercellular spaces of the mesophyll are normally air-filled, but the pathogen can reach high population levels only when the intercellular spaces are water-filled. Many phytopathogenic bacteria produce extracellular polysaccharides (ESP) (Ayers *et al.*, 1979; El-Banoby and Rudolph, 1979; Politis and Goodman, 1980) or lipomucopolysaccharides (Keen and Williams, 1971) during the logarithmic phase of multiplication. When environmental conditions are suitable, these compounds induce permanent water soaking in the intercellular spaces (El-Banoby and Rudolph, 1979). This corresponds to the appearance of water-soaked spots characteristic of bacterial blight diseases. Extracellular polysaccharides from *P. fluorescens* did not induce water-soaked spots in plants. Only the susceptible cultivars of the host, but not the resistant ones, were affected by the polysaccharide of the corresponding bacterial species. The mechanisms which lead to persistent watersoaking are not known but it has been shown that ESP completely loses its watersoaking activity when it is incubated with intercellular fluid from resistant leaves. This evidence has raised additional questions concerning the nature of host–pathogen specificity (El-Banoby, 1980).

Water congestion of intercellular spaces produces an ideal medium for vigorous multiplication of bacterial cells. When the cell number rises to a critical level, the compatible pathogen can induce local necroses and thus the symptoms of bacterial spot disease develop.

The causal factor of "normosensitive" necroses, in contrast to HR-related necroses, is not clearly defined but it has generally been accepted that host cells are killed as a result of the action of toxic substances liberated by the pathogen. An opposing viewpoint was expressed by Klement *et al.* (1978) who found that the development of necroses in both susceptible and hypersensitive tobacco is the same in many respects. Their results indicated that the only difference in necrogenesis was to be found in the number of bacterial cells necessary to induce plant cell collapse. Only one cell of *P. s.* pv. *pisi* was necessary to induce one tobacco mesophyll cell to respond hypersensitively, whereas, in the compatible combination, 50–100 *P. s.* pv. *tabaci* cells per tobacco cell are necessary to cause necrosis.

With low inoculum levels, resembling the natural infection process, bacteria form colonies in the intercellular spaces of infected susceptible tissue, hence, a few individual plant cells are surrounded by hundreds of bacteria while many other plant cells are not in contact with enough bacteria to induce cell collapse. The pathogen multiplies in the intercellular fluid until it reaches the numbers necessary for induction of necrosis. Thus, the necrotization process spreads laterally from cell to cell of the host and is the reason why necrosis starts at the middle of the water-soaked spot. Water congestion of intercellular spaces thus promotes multiplication of bacteria in the tissue and hinders the contact of bacteria and plant cells necessary for inducing HR-type necrosis. This results in a delayed collapse of plant cells and provides the pathogen with more time to multiply and produce toxic bacterial metabolites. This may explain why high concentrations of bacteria introduced into tissue cause rapid necrosis with minimal water-soaking. In such a case, the symptoms resemble HR necrosis.

After the appearance of localized brown spots, the bacterial number decreases in the necrotized tissue. During and after necrotization, chlorosis-inducing toxins penetrate into the adjoining tissues causing a halo to develop around the local necrotic spot. Finally necrotoxins, like syringomycin, syringotoxin, or others, are released from dead bacterial cells. These endotoxic compounds diffuse from local necrotic spots into adjacent areas causing secondary (confluent) necrosis and total destruction of infected tissues.

The development of hypersensitive and normosensitive necroses was compared in tobacco leaves (Klement *et al.*, 1978). Those features which resemble or are the same in the two necrotic reactions include (1) compatible bacteria in an amount higher than the critical cell number (namely, more than about 100 bacterial cells per each plant cell) induce necroses just as quickly as incompatible bacteria cause the HR. (2) With high bacterial populations, the induction time for both reactions is almost identical. (3) All the conditions required for the induction of HR are also necessary for induction of normosensitive necrosis (i.e., live, metabolically active bacterial cells). (4) During the development of both types of necroses, almost identical physiological and biochemical changes occur in the plant except that they develop more slowly in the normosensitive necrosis. (5) There is no characteristic difference in quantity and quality of phytoalexins at the time of the appearance of the necrosis. However, during slow normosensitive necrosis, qualitative and quantitative changes may take place. (6) The development of normosensitive necroses may be inhibited by those manipulations which protect against HR (Section VII).

These similarities are, however, only superficial. In a normosensitive relationship, in which the necrosis spreads from cell to cell, these biochemical processes are delayed and merge at the tissue level. The biochemical and physiological changes in resistant and susceptible plants may only be comparable when high bacterial cell numbers are used to induce confluent necrosis. In the tobacco–*P. s.* pv. *pisi* combination, this concentration must be more than 5×10^6 cells ml^{-1}. In the compatible combination (*P. s.* pv. *tabaci*–tobacco) however, at least 2×10^8 cells ml^{-1} are required. In this case we are ensured that the induction takes place in all plant cells of both combinations at the same time, so that the biochemical and physiological changes of necrobiosis are synchronized.

There are transitional stages between the immune and susceptible reactions. With *X. c.* pv. *malvacearum*–cotton or *P. s.* pv. *glycinea*–soybean combinations, immune, resistant, intermediate, and susceptible relationships are known. These reactions depend on the time needed for the pathogen to multiply to the induction level required for each response.

VII. SUPPRESSION OF HR DEVELOPMENT

A. Inhibition of Bacterial Growth

If the active metabolic processes of the bacterial cell are blocked, the cell is unable to induce HR. Therefore, HR can be inhibited with different antibiotics, bacteriophages, or by heat treatment. For example, 37°C does not inhibit the necrosis itself but, rather, bacterial multiplication (Durbin and Klement, 1977). Antibacterial compounds or heat treatment influence the development of HR only if the bacteriostatic or bacteriolytic effect is affected during the induction period.

B. Induced Resistance

Plants pretreated with heat-killed bacteria or with cell-free extracts of bacteria become resistant to subsequent infection (Goodman, 1967; Lovrekovich and Farkas, 1965; Mazzucchi and Pupillo, 1976; Wacek and Sequeira, 1973). This induced or acquired resistance also plays a role in prevention of HR by the inhibition of bacterial growth (Lozano and Sequeira, 1970). This type of "induced resistance" is a time- and light-dependent reaction of plants. An "early selective induced resistance" which is light-independent, can also inhibit HR 3–6 hr after pretreatment (Burgyán and Klement, 1978). Both types of induced resistance inhibit bacterial growth and thereby the induction of HR. It is likely that early induced resistance caused by a low inoculum concentration may prevent HR induction since bacterial inhibition will not allow multiplication to the required levels (Novacky *et al.*, 1973).

C. Inhibition of Cell Contact Recognition

Cell contact between bacteria and host cells seems to be an important factor in inducing HR. If physical contact is prevented, for instance, by immobilization of bacteria in water–agar, the induction of HR does not occur. Thus, bacteria are allowed to multiply vigorously and cause the water soaking typical of the susceptible reaction (Stall and Cook, 1979). Environmental conditions may prevent cell contact recognition. At 31°C, in soybean leaves inoculated with an incompatible race of *P. s.* pv. *glycinea,* no HR necrosis developed but compatible water soaking symptoms occurred. When the plants were incubated at 22°C, however, HR was observed. Keen *et al.* (1981) speculated that higher temperature may have affected the bacterium, rather than the host metabolism, to interfere with HR.

D. Unknown Mechanisms

Several years ago Gnanamanicham and Patil (1977) reported that the toxin produced by *P. s.* pv. *phaseolicola* suppressed HR in bean cultivars incompatible with *P. s.* pv. *phaseolicola.* To investigate whether or not the toxin acts as a general suppressor for HR, they inoculated the resistant toxin-treated bean seedlings with several bacterial phytopathogens. Their results showed that only *P. s.* pv. *phaseolicola* caused a susceptible reaction but others induced HR. Gantotti and Patil (personal communication) found that protein inhibitors such as blasticidin S and cycloheximide also suppress HR induced by all bacteria tested including *P. s.* pv. *phaseolicola*. Thus, the toxin appears to specifically suppress HR induced by *P. s.* pv. *phaseolicola*.

Suppression of electrolyte loss from hypersensitive and susceptible leaf tissue infiltrated with calcium prior to or simultaneous with bacterial inoculation was reported by Cook and Stall (1971). It has been known that substances that reduce permeability also affect development of HR. Cycloheximide suppresses the leakage of electrolytes and tissue collapse in both hypersensitive and susceptible plants. As in the case of calcium, cycloheximide did not affect permeability changes resulting from treatment with ammonia, which is necrotoxic for plants. The effect of these substances is difficult to interpret but it may be correlated with stabilization of host cell membranes either during the induction process or during the development of cell collapse.

From the discussion above, it may be concluded that if bacterial multiplication is inhibited then not only HR but, in addition, the development of susceptible symptoms is also inhibited (Sections VII,A and B). In most cases, however, where bacterial multiplication is not inhibited but inhibition occurs in another way (Sections VII,C and D), the susceptible reaction develops. The susceptible reaction may occur only if the bacterium is a potential pathogen for that plant species.

VIII. IS THE HYPERSENSITIVE NECROTIC LESION A CONSEQUENCE OF BACTERIOSTASIS?

To assess this, several questions have to be discussed. The first of these is whether or not confluent HR necrosis caused by a high inoculum concentration is a defense mechanism of the plant. In this case, HR has been interpreted as an artifact produced by unnaturally high inoculum concentrations (Ercolani, 1973). Since only a small number of bacteria penetrate the plant tissue under natural conditions, the validity of the concept of HR as a possible disease resistance mechanism appeared to be only hypothetical (Rudolph, 1976). In recent years, however, many data have indicated that HR also occurs at the cellular level. Therefore, under natural conditions, HR may be induced in individual plant cells by very small numbers of bacteria (Essenberg *et al.*, 1979; Roebuck *et al.*, 1978; Turner and Novacky, 1974).

The second question is whether HR is the cause or the consequence of resistance. This question presupposes the existence of a defense mechanism hitherto unknown, whose consequence is rapid necrosis and in certain cases phytoalexin accumulation. To reply to this question we must first study what is meant by HR (Section II). According to an older definition, HR is a defense reaction of the plant accompanied by rapid tissue necrosis and, often, phytoalexin accumulation in the incompatible host–parasite relationship. In this connotation HR is identified with rapid tissue necrosis which in itself is not correct because HR necrosis is in reality only a symptom of hypersensitivity and perhaps not the cause of bacteriostasis (Király, 1980). It appears that necrosis itself does not have a direct role in bacterial inhibition, rather it influences the accumulation of antimicrobial materials in the inoculated tissues. These compounds are formed as a consequence of bacterially induced autolysis of host cells. If, however, we mean by hypersensitivity the whole process of defense—from recognition of the foreign pathogen to the induction of HR through the self-destruction of host cells and finally to inhibition of the pathogen—then HR is not only a symptom but is indeed an "active defense mechanism."

Apparent contradictions often occur when HR necrosis is suppressed artificially and bacterial multiplication stops. HR may be suppressed in diverse ways as we have already discussed (Section VII). Where induction of HR is inhibited through bacteriostasis (for instance by antibiotics or induced resistance), further multiplication of either bacteria or the appearance of susceptible symptoms is not expected.

By contrast, when HR suppression takes place without inhibition of bacterial multiplication, then the failure of HR may lead to a compatible reaction. This idea was strongly supported by the data of Stall and Cook (1979) who prevented HR induction by cell contact inhibition and, thus, also caused a compatible reaction to develop in the resistant cultivar.

Another question often debated is whether or not HR actually has a primary role in resistance. A basic misunderstanding about the role of HR is that it is often regarded as the only resistance factor. If we consider that pathogens express their pathogenicity in different ways, then we should not be surprised that plants resort to a variety of defense mechanisms. The situation is aggravated by the fact that several defense mechanisms coincide in time. Recently we have found that "early selective induced resistance" develops in parallel with HR. Therefore, it is difficult to differentiate the bacteriostatic effects of the two defense mechanisms (Burgyán and Klement, 1978).

Another common source of misunderstanding occurs when necroses caused by HR as well as by toxic metabolites of bacteria or inorganic materials are assumed to be the same thing. Although the external appearance of these necroses may be identical, their induction and development are different.

IX. PRACTICAL ASPECTS FOR HR USE

Knowledge of HR induced by bacteria has provided us with methods facilitating selection of breeding material. Using HR we also have rapid methods for detecting pathogenicity of plant-associated bacteria and studying their host ranges. Application of HR in plant breeding programs has been often reported (Cook, 1973; Cross *et al.*, 1966; Essenberg *et al.*, 1979; Omer and Wood, 1969), therefore, only the two latter topics will be dealt with.

A. Rapid Detection of Pathogenicity

Pathogenicity is the most important feature of phytopathogenic bacteria. Determination of pathogenicity remains a complicated and time-consuming procedure. Primarily, the problem was that infected tissue is frequently contaminated with numerous saprophytic bacteria which are difficult to differentiate from pathogens. This is especially true for the pseudomonads. Pathogenicity of a bacterial isolate could be verified only after the appearance of the typical disease symptoms on the homologous host plant. A further complication is that homologous host plants are not always available. This aspect causes even greater problems with woody plants. Therefore, verification of pathogenicity took weeks or, in the case of woody plants, months. After introduction of the tobacco infiltration method for detection of HR, verification of the pathogenicity of an unknown bacterial isolate was reduced to 8–10 hr (Klement, 1963).

B. Host Range Determination

In the past, when bacteria of unknown pathogenic characteristics were introduced in large quantities into the experimental plant species, visible necrotic spots appeared. In such cases, HR necrosis was often mistaken for typical disease symptoms. Hence, several investigators, prior to the discovery of HR, were misled by the appearance of HR necroses and inadvertently published incorrect host ranges for some phytopathogenic bacteria. In many texts, the host ranges of phytopathogenic bacteria may not correspond to the situation in nature. As a consequence, reported host ranges reflect the inoculation method used and the number of plant species included in the experiment (Klement, 1968). Clearly, the host ranges of phytopathogenic bacteria require redefinition.

X. CONCLUSION

As we have mentioned in the introduction, HR induced by phytopathogenic bacteria was discovered almost half a century later than fungi-induced HR and 30 years after the virus-induced HR. Comparison of HR caused by viruses, fungi, and bacteria has already been accomplished by Király (1980) and will not be discussed here. From his account and this chapter it is obvious that this lag of half a century has been made up even though only a few laboratories have dealt with the question. In fact, in many respects we have made considerable advances. In our review (Klement and Goodman, 1967) over a decade ago, we summed up those advantages and methodological possibilities which have enhanced our work with bacteria in studying the host–parasite relationships. Without doubt these simplified methodological procedures promoted rapid progress. A brief summary of our knowledge and discussion of the gaps in our information about HR induction and development is necessary.

We know that one or several bacterial cells are adequate for initiating an autolytic process in a single mesophyll cell (Turner and Novacky, 1974). In an indirect way, it has also been demonstrated that cell contact between the pathogen and host cell is an important precondition for recognition and for the induction of HR (Stall and Cook, 1979). Numerous attempts have been made to isolate the material responsible for HR induction; thus far all have failed. We know also that induction requires live bacteria (Klement and Goodman, 1967). Another aspect worth considering is that the factor responsible for induction can only be transferred to the plant by metabolically active cells (Durbin and Klement, 1977). The plant's recognition of incompatible bacteria takes place in 1–3 hr depending on the bacterial species (Klement, 1972). The biochemical and physiological processes of host cells undergoing HR are not known. These reactions take place during the latent phase but before symptoms are produced. Beginning at the end of the latent period, the physiological changes in the plant cell suddenly become visible. Early signs of this are total membrane disruption and rapid cell collapse. The most characteristic physiological change during this phase is an irreversible increase in permeability of cell membranes and, consequently, an increase of electrolyte leakage into intercellular spaces (Cook and Stall, 1968; Goodman, 1968). Electron microscopy has verified membrane disintegration in hypersensitive cells including loss of vacuoles followed by mixture of the vacuolar contents with the cytoplasm (Goodman and Plurad, 1971; Lyon and Wood, 1976; Sigee and Epton, 1976; Roebuck *et al.*, 1978). Phenolic contents of the vacuole may react with substances in the cytoplasm resulting in the formation of cytolytic compounds that may be toxic to both host and bacterial cells. After HR necrosis occurs, the multiplication of surrounding bacteria stops whether the cell collapse entails only a few plant cells or a larger region of tissue (Essenberg *et al.*, 1979). It has not been clarified exactly whether these compounds are responsible for *in planta* bacteriostasis. Although major progress has been made with respect to the appearance and accumulation of certain phytoalexins, clarification of an active role for these *in planta* has not been proved unequivocally (Essenberg *et al.*, 1981; Keen *et al.*, 1981).

As we can see there are gaps in our knowledge of hypersensitivity. To remedy this deficiency, new hypotheses and experiments should help in promoting a better understanding of the development of HR as a total process. Experimental methods have a major role in the advance of all natural science. Development ceases when the methods at our disposal prove to be inadequate for solving the problems next in line. No doubt we detour around areas of research where our present methodological procedures are not adequate. For further progress, more refined genetic and molecular biological methods are needed.

To summarize this chapter, I would like to stress the most general conclusions of our recent knowledge as follows: (1) HR, as a mechanism connected to resistance, occurs in the resistant plant host only if the bacterial cell (but not its toxic product or enzymes) is capable of initiating necrosis. (2) The development of hypersensitive and normosensitive necroses must be considered as being similar processes. Their induction, however, requires different numbers of bacterial cells and their development proceeds at different rates. (3) During the development of HR, but independent of it, other types of defense mechanisms are also in progress. The parallel development of these various host responses has, to date, caused difficulties in distinguishing the bacteriostatic effect of HR. (4) The biochemical nature of the inducer of this reaction remains unknown.

Acknowledgments

The author expresses his appreciation to Drs. Z. Király, T. Érsek, and R. N. Goodman for their critical appraisal of the manuscript.

References

Allington, W. B., and Chamberlain, D. W. (1949). *Phytopathology* **39**, 656–660.

Atkinson, M. M., Huang, J., and Van Dyke, C. G. (1981). *Physiol. Plant Pathol.* **18**, 1–5.

Ayers, A. R., Ayers, S. B., and Goodman, R. N. (1979). *Appl. Environ. Microbiol.* **38**, 659–666.

Burgyán, J., and Klement, Z. (1978). *Acta Phytopathol. Acad. Sci. Hung.* **13**, 369–374.

Burgyán, J., and Klement, Z. (1979). *Phytopathol. Mediterr.* **18**, 153–161.

Cason, E. T., Jr., Richardson, P. E., Essenberg, M. K., Brinkenhoff, J. A., Johnson, W. M., and Venére, R. J. (1978). *Phytopathology* **68**, 1015–1021.

Cook, A. A. (1973). *Phytopathology* **63**, 915–918.

Cook, A. A., and Stall, R. E. (1968). *Phytopathology* **58**, 617–619.

Cook, A. A., and Stall, R. E. (1969a). *Plant Dis. Rep.* **53**, 617–619.

Cook, A. A., and Stall, R. E. (1969b). *Phytopathology* **59**, 259–260.

Cook, A. A., and Stall, R. E. (1971). *Phytopathology* **61**, 484–487.

Cook, A. A., and Stall, R. E. (1977). *Phytopathology* **67**, 1101–1103.

Cross, J. E. (1966). *Annu. Rev. Phytopathol.* **4**, 291–310.

Cross, J. E., Kennedy, B. W., Lambert, Y. W., and Cooper, R. L. (1966). *Plant Dis. Rep.* **50**, 557–560.

Diachun, S., and Troutman, J. (1954). *Phytopathology* **44**, 186–187.

Durbin, R. D., and Klement, Z. (1977). *In* "Current Topics in Plant Pathology" (Z. Király, ed.), pp. 239–242. Akadémiai Kiadó, Budapest.

El-Banoby, F. E. (1980). D.S. thesis, Georg-August-University, Göttingen.

El-Banoby, F. E., and Rudolph, K. (1979). *Physiol. Plant Pathol.* **15**, 341–349.

El-Banoby, F. E., and Rudolph, K. (1980). *Phytopathol. Z.* **98**, 91–95.

Ercolani, G. L. (1970). *Phytopathol. Mediterr.* **9**, 151–159.

Ercolani, G. L. (1973). *J. Gen. Microbiol.* **75**, 83–95.

Érsek, T., Sarhan, A. R. T., and Pongor, S. (1981). *Acta Phytopathol. Acad. Sci. Hung.* **16**, (in press).

Essenberg, M., Cason, E. T., Jr., Hamilton, B., Brinkerhoff, L. A., Gholson, R. K., and Richardson, R. E. (1979). *Physiol. Plant Pathol.* **15**, 53–68.

Essenberg, M., Doherty, M. D., Hamilton, B. K., Henning, V. T., Cover, E. C., McFaul, S. J., and Johnson, W. M. (1981). *Phytopathology* (in press).

Fett, W. F., and Sequeira, L. (1980). *Plant Physiol.* **66**, 853–858.

Gáborjányi, R., O'Brien, F., and Klement, Z. (1974). *Acta Phytopathol. Acad. Sci. Hung.* **9**, 31–33.

Gardner, J. M., and Kado, C. I. (1972). *Phytopathology* **62**, 759 (Abstr.).

Gnanamanicham, S. S., and Patil, S. S. (1977). *Physiol. Plant Pathol.* **10**, 169–179.

Goodman, R. N. (1967). *Phytopathology* **57**, 22–24.

Goodman, R. N. (1968). *Phytopathology* **58**, 872–875.

Goodman, R. N. (1971). *Phytopathology* **61**, 893 (Abstr.).

Goodman, R. N. (1972). *Phytopathology* **62**, 1327–1331.

Goodman, R. N., and Plurad, S. B. (1971). *Physiol. Plant Pathol.* **1**, 11–16.

Goodman, R. N., Huang, P. Y., and White, J. A. (1976). *Phytopathology* **66**, 754–764.

Hagborg, W. A. F. (1970). *Can. J. Bot.* **48**, 1135–1137.

Hevesi, M., and Király, Z. (1977). *In* "Current Topics in Plant Pathology" (Z. Király, ed.), pp. 243–248. Akadémiai Kiadó, Budapest.
Hildebrand, D. C., and Riddle, B. (1971). *Hilgardia* **41,** 33–43.
Hildebrand, D. C., Alosi, M. C., and Schroth, M. N. (1980). *Phytopathology* **70,** 98–109.
Ho, G. Kan-hwa, and Patil, S. S. (1981). *Phytopathology* **71** (in press).
Holliday, M. J., Keen, N. T., and Long, M. (1979). *Int. Congr. Plant Protect., 9th, Washington D.C.* (Abstr.).
Holliday, M. J., Keen, N. T., and Long, M. (1981). *Physiol. Plant Pathol.* **18** (in press).
Holmes, F. O. (1929). *Bot. Gaz. (Chicago)* **87,** 39–55.
Huang, J. S., and Goodman, R. N. (1972). *Phytopathology* **62,** 1428–1434.
Huang, J. S., Huang, P.-Y., and Goodman, R. N. (1973). *Am. J. Bot.* **60,** 80–85.
Keen, N. T., and Kennedy, B. W. (1974). *Physiol. Plant. Pathol.* **4,** 173–185.
Keen, N. T., and Williams, P. H. (1971). *Physiol. Plant Pathol.* **1,** 247–264.
Keen, N. T., Érsek, T., Long, M., Bruegger, B., and Holliday, M. (1981). *Physiol. Plant Pathol.* **18** (in press).
Király, Z. (1980). *In* "Plant Disease" (J. G. Horsfall and E. B. Cowling, eds.), Vol. 5, pp. 201–224. Academic Press, New York.
Klement, Z. (1963). *Nature (London)* **199,** 299–300.
Klement, Z. (1965). *Phytopathology* **55,** 1033–1034.
Klement, Z. (1968). *Phytopathology* **58,** 1218–1221.
Klement, Z. (1970). *In* "Methods in Plant Pathology" (Z. Király, ed.), pp. 201–202. Akadémia Kiadó, Budapest, and Elsevier, Amsterdam.
Klement, Z. (1971). *Acta Phytopathol. Acad. Sci. Hung.* **6,** 115–118.
Klement, Z. (1972). *Proc. Int. Conf. Plant Pathol. Bact., 3rd, Wageningen, 1971.*
Klement, Z. (1974). *In* "Methods in Plant Pathology" (Z. Király, ed.). Akademia Kiado, Budapest.
Klement, Z. (1977). *Acta Phytopathol. Acad. Sci. Hung.* **12,** 257–261.
Klement, Z., and Goodman, R. N. (1967). *Annu. Rev. Phytopathol.* **5,** 17–44.
Klement, Z., and Lovrekovich, L. (1961). *Phytopathol. Z.* **41,** 217–227.
Klement, Z., and Lovrekovich, L. (1962). *Phytopathol. Z.* **45,** 81–88.
Klement, Z., Farkas, G. L., and Lovrekovich, L. (1964). *Phytopathology* **54,** 474–477.
Klement, Z., Hevesi, M., and Sasser, M. (1978). *Proc. Int. Conf. Plant Pathog. Bact., 4th* pp. 679–685.
Lovrekovich, L., and Farkas, G. L. (1965). *Nature (London)* **205,** 823–824.
Lovrekovich, L., and Lovrekovich, H. (1970). *Phytopathology* **60,** 1279–1280.
Lovrekovich, L., Lovrekovich, H., and Goodman, R. N. (1970). *J. Can. Bot.* **48,** 167–171.
Lozano, J. C. (1969). M.S. thesis, University of Wisconsin, Madison.
Lozano, J. C., and Sequeira, L. (1970). *Phytopathology* **60,** 875–879.
Lyon, F. W., and Wood, R. K. S. (1975). *Physiol. Plant Pathol.* **6,** 117–124.
Lyon, F. W., and Wood, R. K. S. (1976). *Ann. Bot.* **40,** 479–491.
Mazzucchi and Pupillo (1976). *Physiol. Plant Pathol.* **9,** 101–112.
Meadows, M. E., and Stall, R. E. (1981). *Phytopathology* **70** (in press).
Németh, J., and Klement, Z. (1967). *Acta Phytopathol. Acad. Sci. Hung.* **2,** 303–308.
Németh, J., Klement, Z., and Farkas, G. L. (1969). *Phytopathol. Z.* **65,** 267–278.
Novacky, A., Acedo, and Goodman, R. N. (1973). *Physiol. Plant Pathol.* **3,** 133–136.
Oguchi, T., and Patil, S. S. (1979). *Phytopathology* **69,** 1040.
Omer, M. E., and Wood, R. K. S. (1969). *Ann. Appl. Biol.* **63,** 103–116.
Politis, D. J., and Goodman, R. N. (1980). *Appl. Environ. Microbiol.* **40,** 596–607.
Roebuck, P., Sexton, R., and Mansfield, J. W. (1978). *Physiol. Plant Pathol.* **12,** 151–157.
Romeiro, R. de., Karr, A., and Goodman, R. N. (1981). *Plant Physiol.* **68,** 772–777.

Rudolph, K. (1976). *In* "Specificity in Plant Diseases" (R. K. S. Wood and A. Graniti, eds.), pp. 109–130. Plenum, New York.
Sasser, M. (1978). *Phytopathology* **68,** 361–363.
Sasser, M. (1980). *Phytopathology* **70,** 692 (Abstr.).
Sasser, M., Andrews, A. K., and Doganay, Z. V. (1974). *Phytopathology* **64,** 770–772.
Sequeira, L. (1976). *In* "Specificity in Plant Diseases" (R. K. S. Wood and A. Granity, eds.), pp. 289–310. Plenum, New York.
Sequeira, L. (1981). *In* "Plant Disease Control" (R. C. Staples, ed.). Wiley, New York.
Sequeira, L., and Ainslie, V. (1969). *Int. Bot. Congr., 11th* p. 195 (Abstr.).
Sequeira, L., Gaard, G., and De Zoeten, G. A. (1977). *Physiol. Plant Pathol.* **10,** 43–50.
Schroth, M. N., and Hildebrand, D. C. (1967). *Proc. Int. Conf. Phytopathog. Bact., 2nd, Oeiras, Portugal* p. 23.
Sigee, D. C., and Epton, H. A. S. (1976). *Physiol. Plant Pathol.* **9,** 1–8.
Sing, V. O., and Schroth, M. N. (1977). *Science* **197,** 759–761.
Smidt, M., and Kosuge, T. (1978). *Physiol. Plant Pathol.* **13,** 203–214.
Smith, M. A., and Kennedy, B. W. (1970). *Phytopathology* **60,** 723–725.
Stakman, E. C. (1915). *J. Agric. Res.* **4,** 139–200.
Stall, R. E., and Cook, A. A. (1968). *Phytopathology* **58,** 1584–1587.
Stall, R. E., and Cook, A. A. (1979). *Physiol. Plant Pathol.* **14,** 77–84.
Süle, S. (1973). C.S. dissertation, Hungarian Academy of Sciences.
Süle, S., and Klement, Z. (1971). *Acta Phytopathol. Acad. Sci. Hung.* **6,** 119–122.
Turner, J. G., and Novacky, A. (1974). *Phytopathology* **64,** 885–890.
Wacek, T. J., and Sequeira, L. (1973). *Physiol. Plant Pathol.* **3,** 363–369.
Whatley, M. H., Hunter, N., Cantrell, M. A., Hendrick, C., Keegstra, K., and Sequeira, L. (1980). *Plant Physiol.* **65,** 557–559.
Wyman, J. G., and VanEtten, H. D. (1978). *Phytopathology* **68,** 583–589.
Young, J. M. (1974). *N. Z. J. Agric. Res.* **17,** 115–119.

Chapter **9**

Recognition of Bacterial Pathogens by Plants

N. T. KEEN *and* **M. J. HOLLIDAY**

Visitor, are you friend or foe?
How useful it would be to know.

I. INTRODUCTION

Specific recognition of pathogens by plants may, in theory, lead to establishment of compatible host–parasite interactions (susceptible plant reactions) or to incompatible relationships (resistant plant reac-

Phytopathogenic Prokaryotes, Vol. 2

Copyright © 1982 by Academic Press, Inc.
All rights of reproduction in any form reserved.
ISBN 0-12-509002-1

tions). As Ellingboe (1976) and Nelson (1979) have outlined, however, evolution of plants and their parasites would eventually be expected to result in the occurrence of specific surveillance mechanisms in the host which tend to reduce colonization by the pathogen to some level that is consistent with the continued survival of both partners. This process may be extrapolated to the point where a commensal relationship exists.

The bacterial–plant relationships occurring at this point in time represent various evolutionary stages. In some, such as those involving soft-rotting bacteria, specific recognitional mechanisms do not appear to have yet evolved in plant hosts, and such associations might therefore be considered relatively primitive. In others, involving certain leaf-spotting pseudomonads and xanthomonads, specific resistance genes may occur in host plants which condition a reduction in bacterial multiplication. One of the most highly evolved systems is the interaction of rhizobia with legume hosts. In these symbiotic associations, specific recognition mechanisms have evolved which tend to promote host infection by the bacteria (Bauer, 1981; Dazzo, 1980; Solheim and Paxton, 1981). There are several analogous examples in which positive recognition is associated with successful infection of animal tissues by bacteria (Beachey, 1980; Ellwood *et al.*, 1979; Ofek *et al.*, 1978; Smith, 1977) but there is little evidence indicating that such events occur between plants and compatible pathogenic bacteria. One exception may be the interaction of *Agrobacterium tumefaciens* (Sm. & Town.) Conn with dicotyledenous plant cells, discussed in Section V. Generally, however, specific recognition of pathogenic bacteria by plants leads to the occurrence of incompatible host reactions; the corollary to this is that failure of specific recognition to occur may be associated with the expression of compatibility. In this review we will discuss some of the recognition mechanisms occurring between bacteria and their hosts. Much of the terminology and theory is from Keen (1982a). Authorities will be noted for bacterial names when they are first introduced except for pathovars of *Pseudomonas syringae* and *Xanthomonas campestris* which will uniformly follow the nomenclature of Dye *et al.* (1980). Common names of host plants will be used throughout.

II. MECHANISMS CONFERRING BASIC COMPATIBILITY

Successful plant pathogens possess varied mechanisms permitting multiplication in their hosts. These factors constitute what has been called "basic compatibility" (Ellingboe, 1976). As indicated in the last section, specific recognition systems controlling active defense mechanisms in the plant may be superimposed on basic compatibility factors, and render the plant resistant to certain races or pathovars of the pathogenic species. Before such specific surveillance mechanisms can function, however, the pathogen species in question must possess the machinery accounting for basic compatibility.

The nature of mechanisms accounting for the basic compatibility of bacterial pathogens is considered in detail in Volume 1 by Stacey and Brill (Chapter 9), Mills and Gonzalez (Chapter 5), Goodman (Chapter 3), Sands *et al.* (Chapter 4), and Durbin (Chapter 17) and will consequently only be summarized here. In certain soft-rotting *Erwinia* spp., it has been conclusively shown that production of pectate lyases is required for pathogenicity (Beraha and Garber, 1971; Chatterjee and Starr, 1977; Mount *et al.*, 1979). The work of Rudolph and co-workers (El-Banoby and Rudolph, 1979) similarly suggests that extracellular polysaccharides (EPS) are important in the production of water-soaking in hosts by leaf-spotting pathovars of *Pseudomonas syringae.* Extracellular polysaccharides have also been shown to be important in the prevention of host recognition of *P. solanacearum* E. F. Smith (Sequeira and Graham, 1977) and *Erwinia amylovora* (Burrill) Wins. (Ayers *et al.*, 1979; Bennet and Billing, 1978). Accordingly, EPS can be considered a factor contributing to basic compatibility in these cases. Toxins appear to be important factors in the parasitism of plants by certain bacteria (e.g., Gonzalez *et al.*, 1981; Gross and DeVay, 1977; Husain and Kelman, 1958; Ries and Strobel, 1972; Sinden *et al.*, 1971). There are also indications that the phytotoxin phaseotoxin (phaseolotoxin), produced by *P. syringae* pv. *phaseolicola*, may contribute to basic compatibility by blocking active host defense (Gnanamanickam and Patil, 1977b). The latter conclusion is confounded, however, by observations that toxin-deficient strains of the bacterium appear to multiply as well as the wild-type in inoculated host tissues, but do not produce local or systemic chlorotic halo-blight symptoms (Jamieson *et al.*, 1981; Patil *et al.*, 1974). Pathogenic *P. s.* pv. *savastanoi* (E. F. Smith) Young *et al.* isolates produce indoleacetic acid that is required for gall formation on oleander stems (Smidt and Kosuge, 1978). It has also recently been established that plasmid-borne genes are responsible for indoleacetic acid synthesis by the bacterium (Comai and Kosuge, 1982). Finally, common antigenic relationships between certain pathogenic bacteria and their host plants have been demonstrated (DeVay and Adler, 1976), and this may have more general significance in the establishment of basic compatibility. There are doubtless many additional factors contributing to the parasitic success of bacterial plant pathogens. The mechanisms now known, however, are constitutive requirements for the pathogenicity of a certain bacterial species or pathovar on a plant species but are not directly related to cultivar-specific pathogenicity. As such, mechanisms conferring basic compatibility overcome what has been called general plant resistance.

III. MECHANISMS CONFERRING PLANT RESISTANCE

Bacteria lacking one or more factors required for basic compatibility with a plant will be nonpathogenic, and the unbreached host barrier consequently constitutes a defense mechanism. In addition to such preformed defense barriers (see Anderson, this volume, Chapter 6) plants also possess inducible or active mechanisms such as the hypersensitive reaction. Some suggested host resistance mechanisms against bacterial pathogens are listed in Table I, many of which are discussed in other chapters in these volumes. Only those defense mechanisms that are

Table I. Some Suggested Defense Mechanisms in Plants against Bacterial Pathogens[a]

Mechanism	Type of resistance	Examples	Reference
Structural and morphologic barriers	General-preformed	Cell walls, stomates	Wood (1967)
Cell wall lectins	General-preformed	Tobacco	Sequeira (1979)
Toxin insensitivity	General or specific-preformed	Alfalfa	Ries and Strobel (1972)
Agglutinins	General or specific-preformed	Several plants	Anderson (1980b)
Preformed antibiotic compounds	General-preformed	Green bean	Klement and Lovrekovich (1962)
Liberation of anti-bacterial compounds from preformed compounds	General-induced	Pears	Hildebrand and Schroth (1964)
Protective response	General-induced	Solanaceous plants	Sequeira (1979)
Hypersensitive response	General or specific-induced	Many plants	Klement and Goodman (1967)
Phytoalexins	General or specific-induced	Many plants	Keen (1982a)

[a] Mechanisms denoted as general are effective within an entire plant species to an entire parasite species or pathovar. Specific mechanisms function against some but not all strains or races of a pathogen and are present in some but not all plant cultivars. Preformed mechanisms occur before infection while inducible mechanisms occur following infection.

inducible and appear to be modulated by specific recognition mechanisms will be considered in detail here.

A. Protective Response

The occurrence of this induced resistance response has been most studied in members of the Solanaceae but does not appear to function in certain other plant species (e.g., Keen and Kennedy, 1974; Lyon and Wood, 1977; Smith and Mansfield, 1981). The protective response confers resistance in leaves to the multiplication of normally compatible or incompatible bacteria following treatment by various nonspecific agents. These include inoculation with low numbers of compatible bacteria, dead bacterial cells, or infiltration with bacterial lipopolysaccharides (LPS). The protective response has been thoroughly reviewed by Goodman (1980) and Sequeira (1979). Graham *et al.* (1977) identified the inducing agent for the protective response elicited by *P. solanacearum* in tobacco as the lipid A portion of bacterial LPS (for a summary of LPS structure, see Section V). Protected plant tissues appear to have acquired the ability to immobilize subsequently inoculated bacteria, perhaps functionally explaining the response. Rathmell and Sequeira (1975), however, extracted low-molecular-weight bacterial growth inhibitors from protected tobacco leaves which might also be functionally important.

B. Hypersensitive Reaction

1. *General Characteristics*

The occurrence of the hypersensitive reaction (HR) as a wide-spread higher plant defense mechanism to bacterial pathogens was first recognized by the classic research of Klement *et al.* (1964). This work is thoroughly reviewed by Klement and Goodman (1967) and by Klement in this volume (Chapter 8). Compatible pathovars of *P. syringae* multiplied in the normal host plant but did not elicit the HR; however, all heterologous (pathogenic to hosts other than the one studied) *P. syringae* pathovars and nonpathogenic isolates of several other bacterial genera elicited necrotic hypersensitive responses in tobacco, green bean, pepper, and cowpea plants, but did not multiply appreciably. It was noted that the HR occurred within a few hours after inoculation with an incompatible pathogen, but pathogenic isolates produced water-soaking symptoms after 48–72 hr, typical of a compatible interaction. An additional important discovery was the observation that infiltration of streptomycin into leaves inoculated with an incompatible bacterium completely blocked expression of the HR, providing that it was introduced within a few minutes or hours following inoculation. If infiltrated later, streptomycin did not block expression of the HR. This demonstrates that the HR is an inducible process and that, once elicited, it is irreversible.

The HR of leaves to incompatible bacteria is generally studied by infiltrating concentrations of bacteria ($\geq 10^7$ cells ml^{-1}) which elicit "confluent" hypersensitive necrosis (Klement and Goodman, 1967). When cell concentrations of 10^5 ml^{-1} or less are infiltrated, no visible hypersensitive necrosis results. This raises the question of whether the same mechanism functions as when high cell densities are inoculated. The microscopic studies of Turner and Novacky (1974) with the *P. s.* pv. *pisi*-tobacco interaction, of Essenberg *et al.* (1979) with the *Xanthomonas campestris* pv. *malvacearum*–cotton system, and of Holliday *et al.* (1981a) with the *P. s.* pv. *glycinea*–soybean interaction demonstrated that host cell death was also observed in response to low concentrations of bacteria when microscopic observation was used. In the latter system, it was further noted that the race-specificity of several *P. s.* pv. *glycinea* isolates was the same on a range of differential soybean cultivars, irrespective of inoculum concentration (Keen and Kennedy, 1974). These observations indicate that the HR functions the same regardless of inoculum density, but that the number of host cells participating in the reaction is different.

2. *Mechanisms by Which Bacterial Multiplication Is Restricted in Hypersensitive Host Tissue*

In solanaceous plants, hypersensitive reactions to incompatible bacteria are typified by rapid electrolyte loss, followed by the death and desiccation of host cells (see Sequeira, 1979). It is uncertain, however, whether host cell death and tissue desiccation are directly responsible for inhibiting bacterial multiplication, especially in response to low inoculum concentrations.

Goodman *et al.* (1976a) and Sequeira *et al.* (1977) observed that incompatible bacteria became "attached" to tobacco leaf cell walls almost immediately after inoculation and later became enveloped by a fibrillar pellicle of host origin. Since similar results were not observed with virulent strains of bacteria, it is possible that attachment and engulfment of incompatible bacteria accounts for the inhibition of their multiplication. The mechanism does not appear to have general applicability for conferral of the higher plant HR, since attachment of incompatible bacteria has not been convincingly demonstrated to occur in several other plants (e.g., Daub and Hagedorn, 1980; Fett and Jones, 1981). Furthermore, Hildebrand *et al.* (1980) have criticized the observed attachment of bacterial cells in plants as a possible artifact resulting from the drying of intercellular water films onto plant cell walls following inoculation. It is also puzzling that, in tobacco, infiltration of dead bacterial cells results in their attachment, but no HR is produced as with living cells (see Sequeira, 1979). Instead, the "protective response" is elicited which protects plants against subsequent hypersensitive resistant or susceptible responses when reinoculated with the appropriate bacteria.

A role for phytoalexins in the conferral of hypersensitive resistance to certain fungal pathogens of plants has been firmly established (Bailey, 1982; Keen, 1982b). However, the evidence linking the production of such inducibly formed plant antibiotic compounds with the expression of resistance to bacterial pathogens is inconclusive. Suggestive evidence pointing to a possible causal role has been obtained with a few bacterial–plant systems (Essenberg *et al.*, 1981; Gnanamanickam and Patil, 1977a; Keen and Kennedy, 1974; Lyon and Wood, 1975; Stall and Cook, 1968; Webster and Sequeira, 1977). More recent experiments pertaining to the possible role of phytoalexins in the conferral of hypersensitive resistance in soybeans to incompatible races of *P. s.* pv. *glycinea* will be considered later.

IV. SPECIFIC RECOGNITION OF PATHOGENS

A. Differentiation of Pathogens by Phages, Bacteriocins, Antibodies, and Lectins

Since bacteriophages, bacteriocins, antibodies, and plant lectins frequently are used to distinguish bacteria depending on their surface carbohydrate structures, these agents are of potential use in attempts to relate such differences with pathogenic specificity. If, for instance, races or pathovars of phytopathogenic bacteria could be reliably differentiated by one of the above agents with known receptor specificity, this would offer a strong suggestion that the receptor was related to pathogenic specificity.

A few cases are recognized in which sensitivity to certain phages is related to pathogenicity (see Civerolo, 1972; Jindal and Patel, 1981; Lindberg, 1973). Anderson (1980a) confirmed earlier work indicating that phage 12P specifically lyses cells of *P. s.* pv. *phaseolicola*, but not other tested pseudomonads. Isolated LPS or EPS from *P. s.* pv.

phaseolicola but not the other pseudomonads competed with phage attachment, thus suggesting that some unique feature of the surface carbohydrates of *P. s.* pv. *phaseolicola* is recognized by the phage. Further, Anderson (1980a) demonstrated that mutants of *P. s.* pv. *phaseolicola* which were resistant to the phage had greatly altered polysaccharide compositions. This work therefore raises the possibility that *P. s.* pv. *phaseolicola* has evolved so that its surface carbohydrate structure does not elicit defense in its normal host, bean, but that the surface carbohydrates of other *P. syringae* pathovars have different compositions which are recognized by green bean. Garrett (1978) and Quirk *et al.* (1976) reported two phages, each specific for either race 1 or race 2 of *P. s.* pv. *morsprunorum*, which also have LPS attachment sites. Finally, Whatley *et al.* (1980) observed that phage CH154 generally differentiated avirulent isolates of *P. solanacearum*, containing incomplete LPS and eliciting HR in tobacco, from virulent strains which have complete O-side chains and do not elicit a hypersensitive reaction.

There are a few cases where bacteriocin specificity shows a relationship to pathogenic specificity (Vidaver, 1976). Vidaver *et al.* (1972) examined several bacteriocins from three *P. syringae* pathovars, and although different specificities were observed in bacteriocin production and sensitivity, none of these correlated well with race or pathovar specificity. The best defined example of a specific bacteriocin is agrocin 84, which has been shown to only affect strains of *Agrobacterium tumefaciens* carrying the Ti plasmid (Tate *et al.*, 1979).

Serology has been used extensively for typing bacterial pathogens of animals (see Jann and Westphal, 1975; Rudbach and Baker, 1977). With plant pathogenic bacteria, antisera specific for narrow taxa have generally not been obtained (see Schaad, 1979, for a review). Lovrekovich and Klement (1961), however, reported that antisera prepared to thermostable antigens of *P. syringae* pathovars *tabaci* or *angulata* differentiated these two pathogens of tobacco from other *P. syringae* pathovars. Other serologic investigations have also suggested that phytopathogenic bacteria may be differentiated by serologic methods. For instance, Lucas and Grogan (1969a,b) classified *P. syringae* pathovars *lachrymans* and *phaseolicola* into serotypes and observed that serotype was correlated with the sugar composition of LPS from the various bacterial isolates. This may also indicate that alterations in surface carbohydrate structure are related to host specificity of the various *P. syringae* pathovars. In view of the elegant association of serotypes of certain enterobacteria with LPS structure (Jann and Westphal, 1975), more extensive efforts to prepare whole antisera or monoclonal antibodies specific for certain pathovars or races of plant pathogenic pseudomonads and xanthomonads should be fruitful.

B. Levels of Recognition by Plants

Specific recognition mechanisms function at several taxonomic levels between plants and bacterial pathogens (Table II). As discussed in Section III, wide-spectrum recognition occurs in plants such as tobacco to heterologous *P. syringae* pathovars (Table IIB; Klement and Goodman, 1967). Heterologous *P. syringae* pathovars and other plant pathogenic bacteria produced hypersensitive reactions in inoculated leaves; however, the tested saprophytic and soft-rotting pseudomonads did not multiply in tobacco leaves, despite the fact that the hypersensitive defense reaction was not invoked (Table IIA). Similar findings have been made on the behavior of various pseudomonads and xanthomonads in green bean (Klement and Lovrekovich, 1961) and soybean (Keen *et al.*, 1981). These observations suggest that plants have evolved broad-spectrum recognition mechanisms which modulate the HR against heterologous pseudomonads and other plant pathogens but not against

Table II. Levels of Recognition Specificity Occurring in Plants against Incompatible Bacteria

Type of interaction	Type of resistance	Level of recognition	Examples
A. Bacteria lack one or more mechanisms needed for basic compatibility, but do not initiate active defense	General	None known	Saprophytic bacteria
B. Heterologous plant pathogens elicit host hypersensitive reactions	General	Species or pathovar specificity	Heterologous pseudomonads on tobacco
C. Avirulent isolates of a single species or pathovar	Specific	Strain specific	*P. solanacearum* strains on potato and tobacco
D. Protective host response	General	Nonspecific	Dead bacterial cells in tobacco
E. Incompatible races of a single bacterial pathovar elicit a hypersensitive reaction	Specific	Race specific	*Xanthomonas campestris* pv. *malvacearum* on cotton

saprophytic bacteria or compatible pathogenic species. It is likely, therefore, that the saprophytic bacteria lack one or more factors required for basic compatibility, and plants have consequently not evolved recognitional mechanisms which invoke active defense against them (Table IIA). This interpretation is supported by demonstrations that saprophytic bacteria indeed multiply in plant tissues if coinoculated with a compatible phytopathogenic bacterium (Keen *et al.*, 1981; Young, 1974b).

Another level of host–bacterium recognition is that occurring to avirulent but not virulent isolates of the same bacterium (Table IIC). As discussed in Section II, avirulent mutants but not pathogenic isolates of *P. solanacearum* and *E. amylovora* elicit host HR.

The protective response of tobacco plants (Table IID) represents another level of recognition specificity, in which low levels of living or dead phytopathogenic bacteria or their LPS elicit the subsequent resistance of plant tissue to inoculation with compatible or incompatible bacteria (see Goodman, 1980; Sequeira, 1979; Sequeira and Graham, 1977).

Highly specific recognition mechanisms also occur in plants to some but not all races or strains of a single bacterial species or pathovar and invoke the HR (Table IIE). As is the case with fungus, nematode, and virus pathogens, this recognition is frequently modulated by single dominant resistance genes in the plants. Although certain bacterial pathogens have evolved virulent races which "overcome" the effects of resistance genes, genetic data have not been obtained to adequately assess whether gene-for-gene complementarity (Day, 1974) exists in their interactions with host plant resistance genes. Despite this, assembly of the proper bacterial strains and host resistance genotypes allows construction of the quadratic check (Fig. 1A), a cardinal feature of gene-for-gene interactions (Day, 1974; Keen, 1982a). In addition, several bacterial–plant systems exhibit reciprocal specificities (Fig. 1B), also characteristic of gene-for-gene plant–parasite interactions, but not of simple specificities involving general resistance (Fig. 1C). Host and pathogen strains representing the interactions in Fig. 1A and B constitute systems for testing hypotheses on the identity of recognition systems conferring such specificites.

C. Hypotheses for Recognition Mechanisms

Research in the last few years has disclosed that plant hypersensitive responses may be divided into two chronologically and functionally distinct phases. Recognition of an incompatible pathogen by host cells

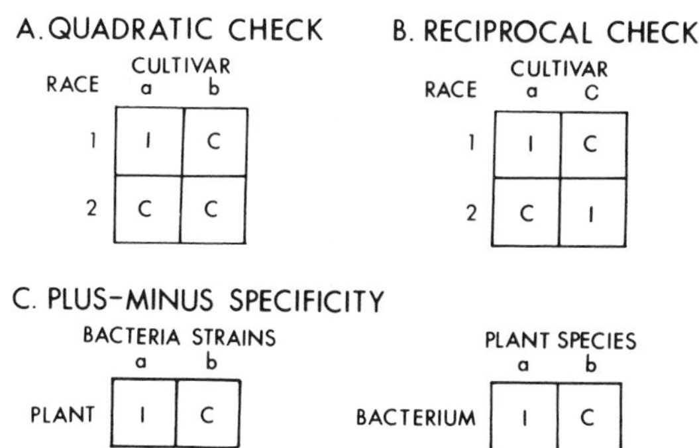

Figure 1. Features of gene-for-gene host–parasite complementarity and simple specificities. "I" denotes an incompatible plant reaction, "C" denotes a compatible reaction.

occurs within a few hours following inoculation, but the events that actually restrict parasite multiplication occur later. Keen and Bruegger (1977) employed the term "determinative phase" for the period when recognitional events occur and "expressive phase" for the later executional events associated with the expression of resistance. The existence of the two phases can be most clearly demonstrated by the use of agents which block one phase or the other. With bacterial–plant systems, for example, the expressive phase of the HR may be blocked by plant protein synthesis inhibitors (Keen *et al.*, 1981; Pinkas and Novacky, 1971), cytokinins (Lyon and Wood, 1977; Novacky, 1972), photosynthetic inhibitors (Sasser *et al.*, 1974), or agents which directly block phytoalexin biosynthesis (Holliday, 1981). The determinative phase may be blocked by agents affecting only bacterial metabolism (Keen *et al.*, 1981; Klement and Goodman, 1967) or by incubation of inoculated plants at an elevated temperature (Holliday *et al.*, 1981b; Klement and Goodman, 1967). Sasser (1978) demonstrated that protein synthesis inhibitors specific for bacteria blocked their ability to cause the HR in a heterologous plant. More recently, Sasser (1980) observed that proteolytic enzymes added to incompatible bacteria blocked the HR in tobacco and cowpea plants. This may indicate that an extracellular or surface protein of the host or parasite is involved in induction of the HR.

Research with fungus–plant and bacterial–plant systems involving hypersensitive reactions points to the probable importance of surface molecules on host and parasite cells in the conferral of specific recognition (see Keen, 1982a). Stall and Cook (1979) demonstrated that occurrence of the HR in pepper leaves inoculated with an incompatible race of *X. c.* pv. *vesicatoria* was blocked if the inoculated leaves were kept water-soaked after inoculation. Bacteria immmobilized in water agar in the leaves also did not elicit the HR, but multiplied like a compatible race. Neither treatment affected multiplication or symptom production by a compatible bacterial race. The results were interpreted to indicate that at least transient bacterium–host cell contact is necessary for the HR to occur in response to an incompatible race. It should be noted, however, that excess water in the leaf intercellular spaces would also be expected to dilute possible extracellular bacterial elicitors of the HR such that they might no longer be effective. Also, the possibility cannot be discarded that water-soaking interferes with gas exchange in leaf cells so that metabolism is impaired and the HR cannot occur. It should further be noted that hypersensitive reactions occurred when incompatible bacteria were maintained in water-soaked leaves of green bean (Lyon and Wood, 1976; Young, 1974b) and soybean (Keen, unpublished; Kennedy and Mew, 1971).

Klement (1977) arrived at similar conclusions to those of Stall and Cook, above, based on experiments in which tobacco leaves inoculated with incompatible bacteria were later infiltrated with a streptomycin solution. It was assumed that the streptomycin solution would disperse bacteria outside of the initial inoculation zone but prevent their multiplication in the newly colonized tissue. Since no subsequent HR was observed outside the zone of the initial inoculation as was produced within the zone, it was concluded that a soluble HR elicitor was probably not produced, but that surface contact of bacteria and host cells was instead required. The interpretation is, however, prone to some of the reservations mentioned in the last paragraph. Nevertheless, these indirect experiments offer some support for the possible role of bacterial surface molecules in determining the HR.

In bacteria–plant systems involving general or specific resistance (Fig. 1), mixture of incompatible and compatible races or strains of bacteria results in an incompatible reaction, even when the compatible cells are in a 10- or 100-fold excess (Averre and Kelman, 1964; Garrett and Crosse, 1975; Keen and Kennedy, 1974; Stall *et al.*, 1972). This argues that the incompatible race is specifically recognized, that the compatible race does not effectively suppress this recognition, and that once elicited, the HR inhibits the multiplication of both races. As discussed more fully by Keen (1982a), such findings are also consistent with the generally observed dominant inheritance of resistance genes in plants and of avirulence genes in fungal pathogens.

As noted previously, inoculation of high concentrations of incompatible bacteria is required to elicit confluent hypersensitive necrosis and bacterial multiplication after inoculation is necessary in all cases for induction of the HR. Klement and Goodman (1967) suggested therefore that high concentrations of HR-eliciting bacterial factors were required in inoculated leaves. Since the investigators were unable to produce the HR by injecting heat-killed bacteria, culture fluids, bacterial sonicates, or extracts from leaves undergoing the HR into plant tissue, the identity of such factors was uncertain.

Research in the last 10 years has disclosed the wide-spread biological importance of cell-surface carbohydrates in the conferral of many processes involving specific cellular recognition (see Ashwell and Morell, 1977; Ballou, 1976; Frazier and Glaser, 1979; Gibson *et al.*, 1980; Sharon and Lis, 1981; Talmadge and Burger, 1975; Turner, 1980). These findings and the realization that relatively small changes in the structure of complex cell surface carbohydrates may lead to large effects on recognition specificity (e.g., Stanley and Sudo, 1981) and that more structural variation can be contained in complex carbohydrates, on a weight basis, than in either proteins or nucleic acids (Sharon and Lis, 1981) have stimulated considerable interest in cell surface carbohydrates. Since plant–parasite interactions represent well-defined examples of specific recognition, it has been suspected that surface carbohydrates on the cells of plant pathogens and/or their hosts may be functionally involved.

Based on these considerations and a small amount of direct evidence, several authors have proposed elicitor–receptor models to explain the recognition of incompatible but not compatible pathogen races or strains by plant cells (Albersheim and Anderson-Prouty, 1975; Callow, 1977; Ercolani, 1970; Hadwiger and Schwochau, 1969; Keen, 1982a; Keen and Bruegger, 1977). The models generally propose that incompatible pathogen races or strains possess surface molecules, probably complex carbohydrates, which interact with surface receptors on plant cells and thereby lead to invocation of active plant defense mechanisms. Compatible pathogen races or strains are postulated to have structurally altered surface molecules that are not efficiently recognized by the plant receptors. Some experimental evidence supports the occurrence of this model with fungus–plant systems (Anderson, 1980b; Keen, 1981, 1982b; Keen and Legrand, 1980; Wade and Albersheim, 1979), but it is as yet inconclusive. The model may also have applicability to plant recognition of incompatible bacteria, and tests of its occurrence in bacterial systems would be desirable. The required first steps are to determine if (1) incompatible bacterial races and pathovars possess surface molecules which specifically elicit active defense systems in plants and (2) if plants contain molecules which specifically interact with them. The following sections will assess progress in this direction. For comparative purposes, bacterial systems in which positive recognition leads to compatibility will be examined initially.

V. PLANT RECOGNITION SYSTEMS

A. Compatibility

1. *Rhizobium–Legume Interactions*

The selective infection of legume roots by certain soil-borne rhizobia results in the formation of an intricate symbiotic relationship characterized by the presence of nitrogen-fixing nodules on the legume root. Varying degrees of host–symbiont specificity are observed in these interactions as exemplified by the taxonomic grouping of rhizobia into cross-inoculation groups according to the host plants which they can infect. It appears, therefore, that legumes have acquired the advantageous ability to specifically recognize and form a symbiotic relationship with certain infective rhizobia while excluding noninfective rhizobia and other soil inhabiting microorganisms. Although it is acknowledged that many molecular events are critical to the successful development of effective nitrogen-fixing root nodules (Bauer, 1981; Stacey and Brill, Vol. 1, Chapter 9) the processes controlling infection specificity are thought to occur during the early stages of interaction prior to formation of the infection thread. One process, the adsorption or attachment of infective rhizobia to legume root surfaces, has received much attention as a potential mechanism for conferral of specificity. Since our current knowledge of attachment and the specificity of the infection process is covered in several excellent reviews (Bauer, 1981; Broughton, 1978; Dazzo, 1980; Schmidt, 1979; Solheim and Paxton, 1981; Stacey and Brill, Vol. 1, Chapter 9) our coverage will emphasize only those aspects which may have analogy to host plant recognition of plant pathogenic bacteria.

After having become established in the legume rhizosphere, infective rhizobia are observed to adhere to the root surface (see Broughton, 1978). Selective attachment of infective rhizobial strains but not noninfective strains has been proposed to explain infection specificity in the symbiotic interaction between *Rhizobium japonicum* (Kirch.) Buchanan and soybeans (Bohlool and Schmidt, 1974) *R. trifolii* Dangeard and white clover (Dazzo and Hubbell, 1975) and others (see Stacey and Brill, Vol. 1, Chapter 9). Models advanced to explain the attachment process involve, with some minor modifications, the specific binding of infective *Rhizobium* strains to legume root lectins. In one model (Dazzo and Hubbell, 1975), bacterial attachment is envisioned to occur through polyvalent lectin cross-bridging between lectin-specific sites on the host root and bacterial cell surface carbohydrates.

In their landmark paper, Bohlool and Schmidt (1974) reported a strong correlation between the *in vitro* binding of soybean seed lectin to *R. japonicum* cells and the ability of such strains to infect soybean roots. These observations were independently confirmed by Bhuvaneswari *et al.* (1977) who also demonstrated that the soybean lectin haptens, *N*-acetyl-D-galactosamine and D-galactose (Lis *et al.*, 1970), reversed lectin binding to *R. japonicum* cells. It was later demonstrated by Stacey *et al.* (1980) that the soybean lectin haptens specifically inhibited attachment of *R. japonicum* cells to soybean roots. In early studies, a few infective strains of *R. japonicum* were found that did not bind soybean lectin (Bohlool and Schmidt, 1974; Bhuvaneswari *et al.*, 1977), but later work by Bhuvaneswari and Bauer (1978) demonstrated that the few non-lectin-binding *R. japonicum* strains in fact possessed lectin binding properties when cultured in a soybean root exudate medium.

Lectin-mediated attachment has also been implicated in clover–*R. trifolii* interactions and perfect correlations between *in vitro* lectin binding and strain infectivity were demonstrated (Dazzo and Hubbell, 1975). The hapten, 2-deoxyglucose, was shown to specifically prevent lectin binding to bacterial cells (Dazzo *et al.*, 1978) and also prevented the attachment of *R. trifolii* cells to clover root surfaces (Dazzo *et al.*, 1976). Significantly, the clover seed lectin originally used in binding studies has been shown to be present on the root hair surfaces where *Rhizobium* attachment occurs (Dazzo *et al.*, 1978). Similarly, soybean seed lectin has recently been localized to the site of *Rhizobium* attachment to roots (Stacey *et al.*, 1980; Stacey and Brill, Vol. 1, Chapter 9).

In spite of the mounting evidence indicating lectin involvement in specific attachment, some evidence argues against this mechanism for conferring host range specificity (see Bauer, 1981; Stacey and Brill, Vol. 1, Chapter 9). Recent models deemphasize the lectin hypothesis and instead propose that some plant receptor, which may or may not be lectin, recognizes a specific component on the bacterial cell surface, possibly resulting in receptor-induced responses in one or both members of the symbiotic pair. This concept, in several forms, is discussed in a recent review by Bauer (1981). Stacey and Brill (Vol. 1, Chapter 9) present the additional possibility that lectins may function to increase the affinity of a host recognition process that does not itself involve lectin.

Whether involved in lectin binding or not, *Rhizobium* cell surface carbohydrates are being scrutinized closely to determine whether they are specifically recognized by legume cell-surface receptors (see Bauer, 1981). The structure and biological activity of *Rhizobium* exopolysaccharides, capsular polysaccharides, lipopolysaccharides, and unique bacterial glucans have been examined. The biological importance of any particular carbohydrate component remains a subject of controversy, but current indications suggest a role for EPS in the soybean–*R. japonicum* interaction (Bauer, 1981). The study of *Rhizobium* carbohydrates has increased our knowledge of bacterial cell surface architecture and will continue to provide important insight for the question of how bacteria are recognized by host plants. Recent reports that the host range of *Rhizobium* spp. may be determined by plasmid-borne factors (Beynon *et al.*, 1980; Brevin *et al.*, 1980; Prakash *et al.*, 1980) indicate that detailed genetic analysis of host range specificity will be forthcoming.

2. *Agrobacterium tumefaciens*–Dicot Interactions

The only acknowledged case in which positive host recognition is associated with compatibility to a plant pathogenic bacterium is *Agrobacterium tumefaciens*. Tumor induction by virulent strains requires the physical binding of bacterial cells to wounded plant cells (Lippincott and Lippincott, 1969). This attachment appears to be required for the subsequent transfer of the bacterial Ti plasmid to host cells. Lippincott and Lippincott (1980) have thoroughly reviewed the available information on factors mediating the attachment process and accordingly only the salient features are summarized here. The carbohydrate portion of the lipopolysaccharide of *A. tumefaciens* has been implicated as the factor involved in specific binding of the bacteria to plant cells (Banerjee *et al.*, 1981; Liao and Heberlein, 1979; Matthysse *et al.*, 1978; Whatley *et al.*, 1976). This conclusion is consistent with the finding that attachment competency in the bacteria is mediated by both plasmid-borne and chromosomal genes (Whatley *et al.*, 1978) which may code for glycosyl transferase enzymes contributing to the structure of bacterial LPS.

Pectic substances in the cell walls of dicot plants appear to be the receptors which mediate bacterial attachment (Lippincott and Lippincott, 1977; Peuppke and Benny, 1981). Significantly, the more highly methylated pectic substances of several monocots were relatively poor receptors for the bacteria, and this may explain the failure of *Agrobacterium* to induce galls on these plants in nature.

The work with *Agrobacterium* points to the importance of specific recognition of bacterial surface carbohydrates by crown gall susceptible higher plants. This poses the possibility that similar mechanisms may also account for the incompatibility of certain plants to pathogenic bacteria.

B. Incompatibility

1. *Agglutinins and Lectins*

Lectins are proteins or glycoproteins that specifically bind to certain carbohydrate structures (Callow, 1977; Liener, 1976; Sequeira, 1978). Their high degree of hapten specificity has made lectins very useful in the study of bacterial cell surface carbohydrates (e.g., Lotan *et al.*, 1975). It has also been proposed that lectins present on the cell walls and plasma membranes of higher plant cells may function as recognition elements for avirulent strains of phytopathogenic bacteria (Goodman, 1978; Sequeira, 1978, 1979, 1981). Certain plant lectins have been reported to agglutinate bacterial cells *in vitro*. For example, Anderson and Jasalavich (1979) reported that phytopathogenic and saprophytic pseudomonads were hapten-specifically agglutinated by wheat germ agglutinin, phytohemagglutinin, and concanavalin A, but not by ricin. Lectins have been used in the same way with other bacteria (Ahamed *et al.*, 1980; Gilboa-Garber and Mizrahi, 1981; Stacey *et al.*, 1980), but the significance of the observations to recognition of phytopathogens by plant cells is uncertain since lectin-binding specificities have not generally been correlated with pathogenic specificities. One exception is the preferential binding by potato lectin of the LPS from rough, nonpathogenic isolates of *P. solanacearum*; in contrast, less binding occurred with the complete LPS from smooth pathogenic strains (Sequeira, 1981).

In addition to studies with lectins of known hapten specificity, factors with unknown specificities have been prepared from several plant tissues that will agglutinate bacteria *in vitro* (e.g., Fett and Sequeira, 1980; Jasalavich and Anderson, 1981; Romeiro *et al.*, 1981b). It is noteworthy that some of the plant agglutinins and lectins are effective only against acapsular bacteria and not against encapsulated isolates of the same bacterium (Bradshaw-Rouse *et al.*, 1981; Romeiro *et al.*, 1981b; Sequeira and Graham, 1977). In these cases it is suspected that the agglutinin receptors may be lipopolysaccharides (LPS) and that extracellular polysaccharide (EPS) capsules prevent recognition and attachment of bacterial cells to agglutinins on host cell walls (Ayers *et al.*, 1979; Sequeira, 1979). If this is true, the EPS could be viewed as virulence factors important for escaping plant defenses.

El-Banoby and Rudolph (1980) and Slusarenko and Wood (1981) extracted factors from green bean leaves and seeds, respectively, that specifically agglutinated cells of *P. s.* pv. *phaseolicola in vitro*. The extracts agglutinated cells of an incompatible race of the bacterium but not those of a compatible race. Further, extracts from a cultivar that was susceptible to both bacterial races did not agglutinate cells of either race. Based on sensitivity to periodate, the seed agglutinin was thought to be carbohydrate (Slusarenko and Wood, 1981). The results may accordingly indicate that bean plants possess relatively specific receptors for certain incompatible but not compatible races of bacteria. It will be of interest to see if further research supports the hypothesis that the agglutinins are associated with the expression of single gene resistance to *P. s.* pv. *phaseolicola*. The work also encourages investigation of the possibility that similar agglutinins are present in bacteria–plant systems exhibiting reciprocal specificities (Fig. 1B), a relationship currently unavailable in the bean–*P. s.* pv. *phaseolicola* system.

In addition, recent research has added to our knowledge of the mechanisms responsible for bacteriostasis in plant defense reactions to incompatible bacteria and offers important clues to the identity of the recognitional mechanisms involved in the conferral of specificity. In the following sections we will explore two of these systems in detail.

2. *The Apple–Erwinia amylovora System*

Although resistance occurs in certain apple cultivars to the bacterium, the majority of research has centered on the general resistance of apple tissues to avirulent strains of the bacterium. The system accordingly is an example of plus/minus specificity (Table IC). The failure of avirulent strains of *E. amylovora* to colonize apple stem tissue was attributed by Huang *et al.* (1975) to the occurrence of three inducible host defense mechanisms. Avirulent bacteria which contacted parenchymatous host cells elicited a hypersensitive reaction, while bacteria within xylem parenchyma cells were engulfed and destroyed. Avirulent cells which entered petiolar xylem vessels were agglutinated. Unlike avirulent strains, virulent *E. amylovora* cells did not elicit the above responses and were characterized by the production of a galactose-rich capsular polysaccharide called amylovorin, which is also exuded in infected host tissue. The suggestion that the capsular EPS functions as a host-specific toxin (Goodman *et al.*, 1978) has been disputed (Sjulin and Beer, 1978), but it appears to be an essential pathogenic requirement of virulent bacteria since it is not produced by avirulent strains (Ayers *et al.*, 1979; Bennett, 1980; Bennett and Billing, 1978, 1980; Goodman *et al.*, 1978). The current concept is that the capsular EPS blocks recognition of underlying bacterial polymers by host cells, thus preventing invocation of the active defense mechanisms (Goodman, 1980).

Goodman *et al.* (1976b) observed that extracts from apple stem tissue infiltrated with an avirulent strain of *E. amylovora* agglutinated avirulent cells *in vitro*. Concentrations of the agglutinin also appeared to increase after inoculation. Hsu and Goodman (1978) subsequently showed that apple cell suspension cultures produced a similar factor which also agglutinated avirulent cells.

Romeiro *et al.* (1981b) extracted a low-molecular-weight, heat-stable protein from apple tissues which agglutinated avirulent, noncapsular cells of *E. amylovora* at less than 1 μg ml^{-1}, but was much less active against virulent cells. The failure to observe substantial agglutination with virulent cells was ascribed to the fact that a significant portion of the capsular EPS of these cells is loosely bound (Politis and Goodman, 1980), and associates with the precipitin, thus sequestering it and leaving the bacterial cells nonagglutinated. Confirming this interpretation, isolated EPS from virulent cells was precipitated by the agglutinin and addition of EPS from virulent cells to reaction mixtures containing avirulent cells decreased their agglutination. The apple agglutinin was thought not to be a classical plant lectin since no specific sugar hapten was found, and instead it appeared to bind nonspecifically to polyanions. For example, agglutination of avirulent cells was also inhibited by carboxymethyl cellulose and sodium polygalacturonate. This and the fact that poly-L-lysine also agglutinated the avirulent cells led to the suspicion that polyanions on the surface of these cells might function as a receptor for the apple agglutinin.

Romeiro *et al.* (1981a) obtained data supporting the polyanion binding idea when they prepared LPS from the avirulent *E. amylovora* strain and demonstrated that it was bound by the apple agglutinin. Following mild acid hydrolysis and fractionation, the LPS core carbohydrates but not the O-chains were precipitated by the agglutinin. The agglutinin was accordingly concluded to be specific for the core region of LPS, which in Gram-negative bacteria is highly polyanionic. The results are therefore consistent with the idea that avirulent cells are agglutinated by interaction of the apple agglutinin with the core region of LPS and that virulent *E. amylovora* cells are not similarly agglutinated because of the production of soluble EPS which masks cell-bound LPS and ties up the agglutinin. Some uncertainties, such as the relatively low pH optimum observed for agglutination *in vitro*, remain to be investigated before this mechanism can be fully accepted. However, the results of Romeiro *et al.* (1981a,b) will be seen to readily explain the plus/minus specificity (Fig. 1C) observed with the interaction of avirulent and virulent cells of *E. amylovora* with apple tissues.

3. *The Soybean–Pseudomonas syringae pv. glycinea System*

Single gene resistance occurs in several plants to phytopathogenic bacteria, especially members of the *P. syringae* and *X. campestris* groups. As indicated in a previous section, phytoalexin production by the host has been proposed as a conferral mechanism for the bacteriostatic environment created in certain hypersensitive resistant reactions. One of the better studied of these systems is the soybean–*P. s.* pv. *glycinea* interaction. In addition to its apparent association with specific resistance, the hypersensitive response also occurs in soybean leaves following inoculation with several heterologous phytopathogenic bacteria (Keen *et al.*, 1981; Giddix *et al.*, 1981). Thus, the HR may also be involved in the general resistance of soybeans to bacteria.

Cross *et al.* (1966) defined seven races of *P. s.* pv. *glycinea* based on the occurrence of differential reactions with several soybean cultivars. The number of described races of the bacterium is currently 10 (Fett and Sequeira, 1981; Gnanamanickam and Ward, 1981; Thomas and Leary, 1980), but Mitchell *et al.* (1982) concluded that isolates previously defined as race 9 are in fact *P. s.* pv. *phaseolicola.* Nevertheless, several quadratic checks (Fig. 1A) and reciprocal checks (Fig. 1B) can be constructed with the appropriate host cultivars and bacterial races. The system therefore represents a probable gene-for-gene interaction, despite the fact that only two dominant resistance genes have been defined in the host by crossing (Mukherjee, 1965, 1966) and the inheritance of virulence genes has not been investigated in the bacteria.

Although race-specific reactions of *P. s.* pv. *glycinea* are generally studied in soybean leaves, germinating seeds (Laurence and Kennedy, 1974) and cotyledons (Bruegger and Keen, 1979) also express a degree of race-specific resistance. This implies that the relevant recognitional molecules must be associated with cells of several soybean tissues.

Certain isolates of *P. s.* pv. *glycinea* produce local and systemic toxemia symptoms in soybean leaves (Gulya and Dunleavy, 1979), and this has been shown to result from production of the phytotoxin, coronatine (Mitchell and Young, 1978). However, as in the previously discussed case of phaseolotoxin, there is no indication that coronatine contributes directly to bacterial multiplication in soybean leaves or is involved in race specificity.

Fett and Jones (1982) performed an ultrastructural study on hypersensitive incompatible and compatible reactions of soybean leaves to various *P. s.* pv. *glycinea* races and did not observe specific attachment of incompatible bacteria to host cell walls. Occasional envelopment of some compatible or incompatible bacteria cells was observed at 4 and 24 hr after inoculation, but the magnitude of the response was not related to the host reaction. Attachment of incompatible cells to host cell walls accordingly does not appear to be involved with the expression of hypersensitive resistance.

As discussed above, incompatible host reactions to *P. s.* pv. *glycinea* involve hypersensitive responses and the cessation of bacterial multiplication occurs concomitantly with accumulation of the soybean phytoalexin glyceollin in the hypersensitive tissue (Cross *et al.*, 1966; Keen and Kennedy, 1974; Keen, 1978). Significant accumulation has not been observed in leaves inoculated with any investigated compatible race. These considerations and the fact that mixed inocula of incompatible and compatible bacterial races result in the full expression of incompatibility and phytoalexin accumulation (Keen and Kennedy, 1974) suggest a priori that glyceollin accumulation may be associated with the restriction of bacterial populations that occurs in incompatible plants. They also indicate that resistant soybean cultivars possess recognition mechanisms that specifically detect the presence of incompatible *P. s.* pv. *glycinea* races. Recent investigations have further assessed the possible role of glyceollin in resistance expression.

Soybean produces three major isomers of glyceollin (Lyne *et al.*, 1976) which possess antibiotic activity toward fungi, bacteria, and nematodes (Fig. 2). Partial information is also available on the biosynthetic enzymes leading to these compounds (Ingham *et al.*, 1981; Zähringer *et al.*, 1981). Isomer III is the major compound produced by soybean leaves, but isomer I is the predominant component produced by roots, hypocotyls, and cotyledons. As is the case with other plant phytoalexins (see Keen, 1981), glyceollin levels in healthy soybean tissues are below detection limits, and its accumulation is strictly localized in hypersensi-

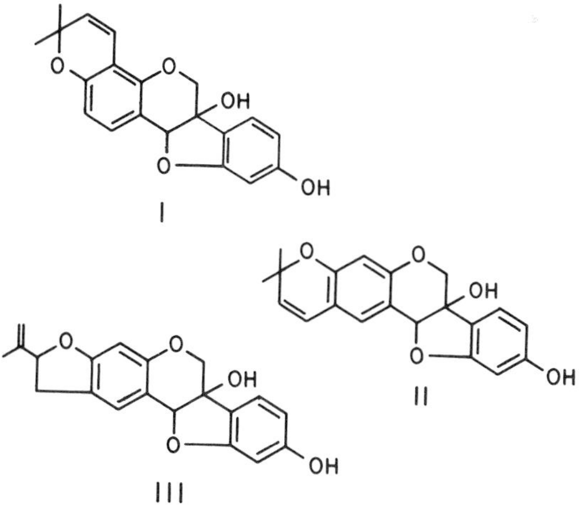

Figure 2. Structures of the major glyceollin isomers (I–III) produced by the cultivated soybean, *Glycine max*. Two additional isomers are produced by other *Glycine* spp. (Lyne *et al.*, 1981).

tive tissues. The production of glyceollin in soybean involves the initial recognition of metabolites called elicitors (Keen and Bruegger, 1977), *de novo* DNA transcription, and messenger RNA translation (Yoshikawa *et al.*, 1977, 1978) and the inducible synthesis of enzymes in the terminal biosynthetic pathway (Zähringer *et al.*, 1978, 1981).

The antibiotic activity of glyceollin toward *P. s.* pv. *glycinea* was initially reported by Keen and Kennedy (1974), who observed that it completely inhibited colony formation by bacterial cells in solid media at 100 $\mu g\ ml^{-1}$. No significant differences were noted in the sensitivity of different bacterial races to the phytoalexin. Albersheim and Valent (1978) and Weinstein *et al.* (1981) confirmed the antibacterial activity and observed that bacterial multiplication was inhibited in liquid medium by glyceollin concentrations as low as 25 $\mu g\ ml^{-1}$. Fett and Osman (1982), however, did not observe glyceollin toxicity using certain bioassays, and ca. 400 $\mu g\ ml^{-1}$ concentrations were required to significantly inhibit the growth of one strain. It was also concluded that glyceollin was bactericidal rather than static at high concentrations. Some of the above inconsistencies concerning the *in vitro* toxicity of glyceollin may be accounted for by the relative insolubility of the highly purified chemical in water. Even when aliquots of dimethyl sulfoxide or ethanol solutions of glyceollin are added to media, the phytoalexin rapidly precipitates out of solution. Effective concentrations therefore are lower than the initial. To minimize this problem, bacteria must be applied to solid media plates immediately after the incorporation of glyceollin. The above experimental uncertainties notwithstanding, it appears that glyceollin concentrations of 100–400 $\mu g\ ml^{-1}$ are required to completely inhibit the growth of *P. s.* pv. *glycinea in vitro*. An important consideration, therefore, is to inquire if sufficient concentrations of the phytoalexin are produced in incompatible soybean leaves at the time inhibition of bacterial growth occurs.

The precise concentration of glyceollin to which individual bacteria are exposed in an incompatible reacting soybean leaf is difficult to determine and a firm conclusion on this point is not currently possible. Bacterial multiplication occurs in incompatible soybean leaves for at least 24 hr after inoculation, inhibition is first observed at 24–30 hr, and populations do not increase after 48 hr (Holliday *et al.*, 1981b; Keen *et al.*, 1981; Keen and Kennedy, 1974). The efficiency of glyceollin extraction from soybean leaves is uncertain and only ca. one-half of the primary leaf is infiltrated with bacteria. Correcting the recovered glyceollin levels for the amount of tissue extracted, concentrations of 400 $\mu g\ g^{-1}$ or greater have been observed at 30 hr after inoculation, when bacteriostasis is first observed (Holliday *et al.*, 1981b). Although there is ambiguity concerning the localized distribution of glyceollin within the hypersensitive leaf tissue and in the *in vivo* sensitivity of the bacteria to glyceollin, it appears that sufficient phytoalexin is present in the hypersensitive soybean tissues during bacteriostasis to explain host resistance.

Fett and Zacharius (1982) demonstrated that soybean cell suspension cultures produced low levels of glyceollin in response to living *P. s.* pv. *glycinea* cells, but race specificity was not observed. This is not unexpected since difficulty was previously observed in reproducing the phytoalexin specificity observed in intact soybean tissues with cultured cells (Holliday and Klarman, 1979; Keen and Horsch, 1972; Kennedy *et al.*, 1972). Significantly, however, Fett and Zacharius (1982) reported that hypersensitive cell death did not occur in cultured cells producing glyceollin in response to an incompatible *P. s.* pv. *glycinea* race or to a fungal glucan elicitor. This may indicate that glyceollin production by soybean cells is a process that is independent from hypersensitive cell death.

Insight into problems with suspension cultured soybean cells was obtained recently by Holliday (1981). Glyceollin accumulation and biosynthesis in leaf cells responding hypersensitively were compared with surrounding healthy cells. Unchallenged cells did not exhibit significant glyceollin accumulation or biosynthetic activity, based on feeding experiments with [^{14}C]phenylalanine. Glyceollin accumulation and biosynthetic activity also did not occur in the hypersensitive area unless it was surrounded by adjacent unchallenged cells. Further, radioactivity supplied as [^{14}C]phenylalanine but not [^{14}C]leucine and fed to leaves through the petioles accumulated in the hypersensitive areas. Therefore it was concluded that healthy leaf cells surrounding those in the hypersensitive area export biosynthetic intermediates of glyceollin into the hypersensitive area where the phytoalexin is synthesized. These experiments emphasize that hypersensitive resistance and glyceollin accumulation are whole tissue responses and accordingly may explain some of the difficulties noted with cell culture systems.

Holliday (1981) determined glyceollin biosynthetic rates by pulse feeding [^{14}C]phenylalanine to leaves at various times after inoculation with an incompatible race of *P. s.* pv. *glycinea.* The observed rates correlated well with the kinetics of glyceollin accumulation in leaves, with a peak of synthetic activity occurring at 25–30 hr, when the rate of glyceollin accumulation was highest, followed by a decline until 48 hr, when glyceollin did not accumulate further. The evidence also indicated that degradation of glyceollin did not occur in the hypersensitive tissue, a conclusion previously suggested by the kinetics of glyceollin accumulation (Keen and Kennedy, 1974). The work of Holliday (1981) is therefore consistent with that obtained in other phytoalexin studies indicating that the most important event modulating phytoalexin accumulation is activation of the biosynthetic pathway (Zähringer *et al.*, 1978, 1981).

Holliday *et al.* (1981a) used the uptake of sodium fluorescein as an indicator of hypersensitive cell death in inoculated soybean leaves. Normal host cells accumulated the vital stain but hypersensitive cells did not. Hypersensitive necrosis first occurred at 9 hr after inoculation, glyceollin was first detected by extraction of leaves at about 16 hr, and inhibition of bacterial multiplication occurred at about 30 hr. Following the initial appearance of single or small clusters of hypersensitive host cells in the incompatible reaction, the areas of dead cells increased and coalesced, forming a large mass of confluent hypersensitive necrotic cells at 16 hr, when macroscopic symptoms were first observed. In a compatible reaction, rapid host cell death did not occur, but considerable necrosis was observed at about 36 hr when visible symptoms appeared. Significantly, Holliday *et al.* (1981a) also observed host cell death in leaves inoculated with low concentrations of incompatible bacteria that did not produce macroscopically visible symptoms. Isolated areas of necrotic host cells were first detected only after 24 hr incubation, presumably because bacterial multiplication was required before the HR occurred. The results therefore indicated that the mechanism operating in confluent HR was identical to that occurring in response to low cell densities except that more host cells were involved in the former reaction.

Hypersensitive resistance in cv. Harosoy soybeans to race 1 of *P. s.* pv. *syringae* is temperature sensitive (Keen *et al.*, 1981). A hypersensitive resistant reaction occurred when inoculated plants were incubated at 22°C, but a completely compatible reaction and little glyceollin accumulation occurred when plants were incubated at 31°C. Further observations disclosed (1) irreversible expression of resistance occurred at 31°C in plants previously incubated at 22°C for at least 18 hr after inoculation, intermediate levels of resistance were subsequently observed when the temperature shifts were made at 8 and 12 hr and completely compatible reactions resulted when the temperature shift was made at 0–4 hr after inoculation; (2) compatible reactions which occurred at 31°C were always converted to completely incompatible reactions when plants were shifted from 31 to 22°C at all times after inoculation; (3) glyceollin accumulation was consistently correlated with resistance expression in the temperature shift experiments (Holliday *et al.*, 1981b). These results strongly support the contention that incompatibility is the specifically determined character in soybean leaves and that glyceollin accumulation is involved with restriction of bacterial multiplication in incompatible interactions. The results also offer clues concerning the informational system conferring specific recognition of incompatible bacterial races.

Data from the temperature-shift experiments corroborated the conclusions of previous work (Keen *et al.*, 1981) in suggesting that incompatible bacteria are first recognized at about 8 hr after inoculation and that recognition is complete by about 18 hr. This is of interest since bacterial multiplication in the host is required until 4–8 hr after inoculation (Fett and Jones, 1982; Keen *et al.*, 1981) before recognition occurs, even when 8×10^7 cells ml^{-1} are infiltrated into the leaves. It is also noteworthy that, although initial host cell recognition of bacteria occurs at ca. 8 hr, hypersensitive cell death is first observed microscopically at 9 hr, glyceollin is not initially detected until 16 hr, and inhibition of bacterial multiplication does not occur until ca. 30 hr, when glyceollin concentrations reach ca. 400 $\mu g\ g^{-1}$ leaf tissue. As noted in other host–parasite systems (Keen and Bruegger, 1977), these observations clearly indicate that recognition events occur chronologically before the events which confer bacteriostasis.

Glyceollin accumulation in soybean leaves inoculated with an incompatible race of *P. s.* pv. *glycinea* was inhibited 90% by treating plants with the herbicide glyphosate (Holliday, 1981). Glyphosate has been reported to inhibit the conversion of shikimate to chorismate in higher plants (Amrhein *et al.*, 1980a,b). Significantly, however, glyphosate treatment did not block the occurrence of hypersensitive host cell necrosis in leaves inoculated with an incompatible bacterial race (Holliday, 1981). Glyphosate therefore is the first known inhibitor which selectively inhibits phytoalexin accumulation but not the occurrence of hypersensitive host cell death. Populations of the incompatible bacteria in glyphosate-treated leaves were twofold higher than in untreated leaves, but similar increased bacterial multiplication was not observed in glyphosate-treated leaves when glyceollin accumulation was restored by feeding plants phenylalanine and tyrosine. This indicates that the effect of glyphosate on phytoalexin production and resistance to *P. s.* pv. *glycinea* was due to an inhibition of phenylalanine biosynthesis. Inhibition of glyceollin accumulation by glyphosate did not, however, result in a completely susceptible plant reaction since incompatible bacterial populations were still eightfold lower than those of a compatible race in the glyphosate-treated leaves. It is possible that hypersensitive cell death per se or desiccation of the hypersensitive tissue may contribute to resistance or that glyphosate may have some unknown inhibitory effects on the incompatible bacteria in leaves. This uncertainty notwithstanding, the experiments with glyphosate indicate that glyceollin accumulation is responsible for at least part of the bacteriostasis observed in the resistant soybean leaves.

The preceding evidence supports the hypothesis that glyceollin accumulation is causally related to the inhibition of bacterial multiplication which occurs in incompatible soybean leaves, but we do not consider the case proven. An independent avenue for assessing the role of glyceollin is afforded by investigation of the recognition system conferring race-specific resistance. If the pathogen factor(s) which are specifically recognized by incompatible plant genotypes are isolated and shown to exhibit the same relative specificity for elicitation of glyceollin in various soybean cultivars as the living bacterial races from which they are obtained, this would constitute strong evidence linking glyceollin production with resistance expression. We have investigated the possible occurrence of such factors.

4. *Bacterial Elicitors of Phytoalexins and the Hypersensitive Reaction*

Phytoalexin production may be initiated in plant tissues by agents called elicitors, many of them obtained from plant pathogens (Albersheim and Valent, 1978; Keen and Bruegger, 1977; West, 1981). Some observations suggest that elicitors inciting phytoalexin synthesis also invoke hypersensitive cell necrosis (e.g., Doke and Tomiyama, 1980). With bacterial–plant systems, there is little information concerning the nature of elicitors of host phytoalexins or hypersensitive responses. Fractions from incompatible bacterial pathogens caused responses interpreted as the HR in tobacco (Gardner and Kado, 1976; Hoitink and Bradfute, 1972; Lozano and Sequeira, 1970; Sequeira and Ainslie, 1969) and pepper (Crosthwaite and Patil, 1978). Purified pectic enzymes from bacterial pathogens have been shown to elicit necrotic responses similar to the HR (Hopper *et al.*, 1975; Gardner and Kato, 1976) and also to function as phytoalexin elicitors (Lyon and Albersheim, 1980). However, it has not been established that these factors are physiologically functional in the induction of the HR by living bacteria. As noted in prior sections, soft-rotting bacteria are copious producers of pectic enzymes, but do not generally elicit plant hypersensitive reactions.

Cell envelope fractions prepared from several races of *P. s.* pv. *glycinea* elicited glyceollin production in cotyledons of two soybean cultivars with the same relative specificity as the living bacteria (Bruegger and Keen, 1979). The envelope fractions were solubilized with sodium dodecyl sulfate (SDS) and these also yielded race-specific elicitor activity. Highly concentrated preparations were required for activity, however, and the elicitor-active molecules were not isolated from the solubilized membrane preparations. Nevertheless, the fact that the observed elicitor activity was race specific suggested that components of the bacterial cell envelope might be recognized specifically by soybean cells to account for disease resistance. The elicitor activity in SDS-solubilized envelope preparations was consistently associated with carbohydrates when these were fractionated by column chromatography, but crude LPS and EPS fractions prepared from culture fluids, whole cells and envelope fractions of *P. s.* pv. *glycinea* did not yield detectable elicitor activity. The solubility of the crude LPS preparations was very low, however. Since carbohydrates from fungal plant pathogens have been demonstrated to possess elicitor activity (Albersheim and Valent, 1978; Keen, 1982a; West, 1981), we recently reinvestigated the possible role of LPS and EPS from *P. s.* pv. *glycinea* as phytoalexin elicitors in soybean.

Phenol-extracted LPS possessed elicitor activity in soybean cotyledons, providing that the LPS was converted to the highly soluble triethylamine (TEA) salt form. Crude TEA–LPS preparations were purified on BioGel A-15m columns equilibrated with triethylamine and EDTA (Carlson *et al.*, 1978) and recovered as included polydisperse peaks containing carbohydrate and ketodeoxyoctonate, a specific marker for LPS, but no protein or nucleic acid. These purified LPS migrated on SDS polyacrylamide slab gels as a series of closely spaced carbohydrate bands, interpreted by Palva and Mäkelä (1980) and Goldman and Leive (1980) to represent homologous series of LPS molecules with varying numbers of repeating units in the O-chains. The purified TEA–LPS preparations also gave glyceollin elicitor activity in cv. Harosoy soybean cotyledons and preparations from race 1 (incompatible) were about fourfold more active than those from race 5 (compatible), indicating a degree of race specificity. The significance of the observations is unclear, however, since elicitor activity was detected only when the LPS were bioassayed at 1 mg ml^{-1} or greater concentrations.

In contrast to the earlier report of Bruegger and Keen (1979), we recently observed that crude EPS preparations from *P. s.* pv. *glycinea* exhibited elicitor activity in soybean cotyledons. When purified by gel filtration and passage through a mixed-bed ion exchange column, the preparations were active at a minimum concentration of about 100 μg ml^{-1} in the cotyledon bioassay. The relevance of these observations remains uncertain, but they encourage the further examination of purified bacterial surface polysaccharides to see if they are the bacterial factors which are recognized by incompatible soybean cells to elicit race-specific resistance.

Recent experiments by Ersek *et al.* (1981) suggest the occurrence of surface molecules on soybean leaf cells that specifically recognize incompatible races of *P. s.* pv. *glycinea*, as discussed in Section IV,C. A factor was extracted from leaves of cv. Harosoy by infiltrating intercellular spaces with a NaCl solution and subsequently recovering the intercellular fluids by centrifuging. The solutions thus obtained agglutinated cells of *P. s.* pv. *glycinea* race 1 (incompatible on cv. Harosoy), but not those of compatible race 2. The extracts also agglutinated erythrocytes, but the activity was concluded not to reside in soybean seed lectin (SBA) since agglutination was not inhibited by *N*-acetyl galactosamine, a specific hapten for SBA. It will be of interest to see if the agglutinins discovered by Ersek *et al.* (1981) generally function as specific recognitional molecules for incompatible but not compatible races of *P. s.* pv. *glycinea* in soybean leaves and if they are responsible for eliciting glyceollin accumulation in response to incompatible bacterial races.

C. Cell Surface Polysaccharides and Recognition

If the incomplete body of evidence discussed in the previous sections is not leading us astray, bacterial surface carbohydrates may play a central role in plant recognition leading to resistant reactions. More critical testing of this possibility is clearly needed.

Several factors should be considered in assessing the possible role of LPS or EPS as elicitors of the HR and phytoalexin accumulation in plants: (1) as previously noted, bacterial multiplication is required in an incompatible plant before recognition and resistance expression occur. This implies that a threshold local population of bacterial cells is necessary in the host cell environment for the HR to be elicited. Concentrations of LPS or EPS presented to host cells, either associated with bacteria or eluted from them, may accordingly be relatively high. It is noteworthy in this regard that phytopathogenic bacteria have been reported to lose vesicular material in host tissue which has been assumed to be LPS and/or EPS (Passmore and Epton, 1979; Sigee and Epton, 1975); (2) the phage research discussed in Section IV indicates that surface carbohydrate structure may determine pathovar and/or race specificity; (3) the structures of the O-chains of Gram-negative bacterial LPS are highly variable in closely related bacterial strains (Jann and Westphal, 1975). This plasticity makes the O-chains immediate candidates for the elements which are specifically recognized by plants that have gene-for-gene interactions with bacterial pathogens. With certain fungal plant pathogens, analogous surface glycoconjugates appear to be involved with gene-for-gene specificity (Keen, 1982a,b; Wade and Albersheim, 1979). Variation in the structure of these complex carbohydrates as well as bacterial LPS or EPS could account theoretically for the reciprocal specificities observed in gene-for-gene interactions (Fig. 1B; Keen, 1982a).

Can the structure of a single bacterial surface glycoconjugate such as LPS confer both race-specific recognition (Table IIE) in a certain plant species and also nonspecific recognition (Table IIB and C) of heterologous bacteria in other plants? The answer is unclear but the factors previously discussed in this paper suggest that plants may possess two distinct kinds of receptors for bacterial surface carbohydrates, each leading to a hypersensitive defense reaction. One class includes several relatively nonspecific receptors for conserved features of bacterial surface molecules such as the core carbohydrate and perhaps certain EPS. This would permit the recognition of a large number of heterologous bacteria (and perhaps other types of pathogens) by a single receptor molecule. Successful pathogens, however, must have evolved altered structural elements in order to escape such general receptors. Alternatively, successful bacteria may physically mask the recognition element(s) by production of capsular EPS (Ayers *et al.*, 1979) or by production of complete LPS O-chains (Whatley *et al.*, 1980). By either means, the bacterial species or pathovar which successfully avoids detection by the postulated general plant receptors is capable of causing disease on a particular plant species.

A pathogenic bacterium may, however, also be detected by the second, more specific type of plant receptors, which have evolved to detect discrete structural features of the pathogenic bacterium, perhaps LPS O-chains, and again invoke active defense. These specific receptors are hypothesized to be the products of plant resistance genes (Keen, 1982a), and virulent parasite races may have evolved surface carbohydrate structures which are not efficiently recognized. The elicitor–receptor model holds that the various specific and nonspecific plant receptors all modulate a common active defense mechanism, such as the HR/phytoalexin system. It is not yet understood whether some of the bacterial agglutinins and lectins described from higher plants are in fact these receptors. It should, however, be possible in the near future to test whether the elicitor–receptor model operates in bacterial–plant interactions.

In order to critically test the elicitor–receptor model, we need more detailed chemical characterization of the surface carbohydrates from various races and strains of phytopathogenic bacteria. Does the O-side chain chemotype correlate with pathogenic specificity as is the case in the enterobacteriaceae (Galanos *et al.*, 1977)? Do various pathovars and races of *P. syringae*, for example, possess unique surface carbohydrate structures as suggested by the indirect experiments of the preceding sections? The elucidation of complex carbohydrate structures remains a technically difficult area, but recent advances (e.g., Valent *et al.*, 1980) encourage the thought that considerable progress should be realized with the cell surface carbohydrates from phytopathogenic bacteria.

Considerable information is available on the structure of lipopolysaccharides from several Gram-negative bacteria (for recent reviews see Clark and Richmond, 1975; Galanos *et al.*, 1977, 1979; Nikaido, 1973; Wilkinson, 1977). Wild type LPS is composed of three regions, called lipid A, the core carbohydrate, and the O-polysaccharide side chains (Fig. 3). The structure of the lipid A region varies only slightly among various bacterial taxa. The core carbohydrate region is more variable, but is nevertheless relatively conserved, especially within closely related bacteria. The O-chains, however, are the site of considerable structural diversity, even among very closely related bacteria. This and the fact that they are usually the major somatic antigens of Gram-negative bacteria account for the existence of a large number of distinct serotypes in bacteria such as *Salmonella* spp. The O-carbohydrate chains are variable in length, and are composed of repeating units of sugar oligomers, generally with four to six residues in each repeating unit (Fig. 3).

A substantial literature exists on the nature of biosynthetic enzymes which add the sugar residues to EPS and LPS (see Nikaido, 1973). As in eukaryotes, the structure of complex bacterial polysaccharides is determined by the complement of glycosyl transferases, enzymes catalyzing the addition of specific sugars in specific linkage and anomeric config-

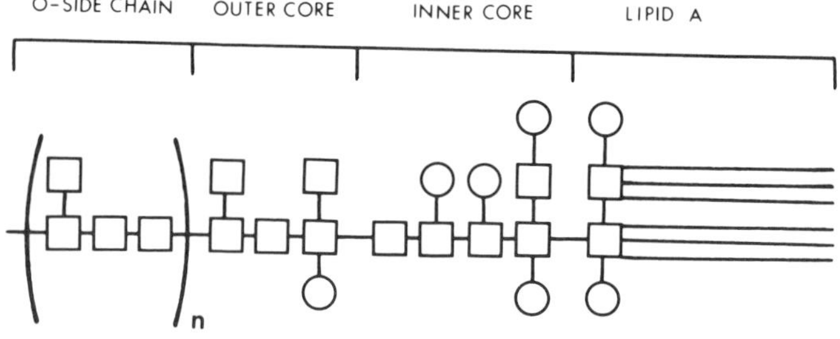

Figure 3. Generalized schematic structure of the lipopolysaccharides of Gram-negative bacteria. The boxes represent the sugar moieties, the long straight lines represent the fatty acid moieties, and the circles represent charged groups, including carbonyl, phosphoethanolamine, or phosphate.

urations to carrier-linked carbohydrates destined to appear in the bacterial surface carbohydrates. Mutations in these genes result in altered surface carbohydrate structures and altered serotypes. In *Salmonella* spp., a series of mutations in these genes are responsible for rough mutants in which LPS lacks the O-chain carbohydrates and various portions of the core carbohydrate (Wilkinson, 1977). Genes coding for the glycosyl transferase enzymes of the O-chains are clustered in *Salmonella*, while those coding for glycosyl transferases of the core region are also clustered but occur on a different part of the chromosome (Nikaido, 1973).

With few exceptions (e.g., Huang, 1980), the glycosyl transferases of plant pathogenic bacteria have not been studied. They may be important, however, in producing unique surface carbohydrate structures which are specifically detected by certain plant resistance genotypes to invoke active host defense. With gene-for-gene plant–parasite systems, Albersheim and Anderson-Prouty (1975) proposed the hypothesis that glycosyl transferases are precisely the products of pathogen avirulence genes. The same proposition may be true with bacterial pathogens involved in such interactions with their hosts, but this possibility has not been tested.

VI. GENETIC APPROACHES TO THE STUDY OF RECOGNITION

Unambiguously assessing the role of surface carbohydrates such as LPS in plant recognition of pathovars or races of phytopathogenic bacteria requires the use of genetic techniques. To decisively test whether structural features of LPS molecules are associated with the recognition of a certain bacterial race, for example, it is necessary to develop a near-isogenic line of the bacterium which gives an altered reaction in the appropriate differential host cultivar but is otherwise identical. This has been done successfully with two pathovars of *X. campestris* by selecting virulent mutants of normally incompatible bacterial races (Dahlbeck and Stall, 1979; Schnathorst, 1970). It would appear straightforward to compare the biological and chemical properties of surface glycoconjugate molecules from such paired bacterial strains in order to assess whether unique chemical features were in fact the basis of race-specific host reactions. It should also be possible to use such lines to directly test the hypothesis proposed in the previous section that virulent races lack glycosyl transferase enzymes contributing to the structure of a glycoconjugate molecule.

It is ironic that bacterial pathogens which are not involved in race-specific recognition by host plants, such as members of *Erwinia*, are those in which useful conjugational systems are available for genetic analysis and mapping. However, systems in which a higher degree of host specificity is exhibited, including pseudomonads and xanthomonads, do not at present have usable conjugational systems. As a result, we do not yet have conclusive genetic proof that gene-for-gene complementarity exists in the interaction of these bacteria with specific resistance genes in their host plants. Consequently, one must consider alternative approaches to mapping bacterial genes conferring race specificity and studying their function.

An immediate approach is the use of transposon insertion mutations. Transposons are translocatable DNA elements of characteristic structure which may enter prokaryote cells and physically insert into chromosomal or plasmid DNA sequences, thus inducing mutation of the inserted cistron (Foster and Kleckner, 1980; Kleckner, 1977; Kopecko, 1980a,b). It would seem feasible to screen for transposon mutations of bacterial genes conferring specific incompatible responses in host plants. Because they carry drug resistance markers, transposon insertions are easy to detect and the mutants could be screened for altered host reactions by inoculating differential cultivars. It should be possible in this way to determine whether single bacterial genes are responsible for incompatible host reactions (viz. whether such genes are the precise equivalent of avirulence genes in fungal pathogens) and also to attempt the use of restriction mapping to determine their location on the bacterial chromosome. It is probable that such loci could be cloned, introduced into a normally compatible race of the bacterium, and these recipients inoculated into an appropriate differential plant cultivar to see if they would then respond in an incompatible manner. The decisive final steps would involve comparison of the surface carbohydrate structure of the wild-type compatible race with its incompatible transformant and assay of their glycosyl transferase enzymes. If the hypotheses discussed in this chapter are correct, the introduced avirulence gene would code for a glycosyl transferase enzyme, lacking in the wild-type compatible race, which would produce a unique surface carbohydrate structure.

VII. EPILOGUE

Bacterial–plant systems represent several evolutionary stages of recognitional specificity. Complex systems which exhibit species, pathovar, or race specificity are a consequence of the occurrence of plant surveillance mechanisms which have evolved for defensive purposes or to promote symbiotic associations. The available research points to bacterial surface carbohydrates as the molecules which are specifically detected by plant cells in these cases. We know little, however, about the chemistry of the surface molecules or of the nature of the plant receptors. It is likely that the latter are plasma membrane proteins or glycoproteins which are similar to classical seed lectins and function by signaling either the invocation of active host defense or the complex reactions associated with symbiosis. Despite our current ignorance of these mechanisms in bacterial–plant systems, the foregoing constitutes a plausible biochemical model for such recognitional specificities which can be directly tested experimentally. The inherent experimental advantages of bacteria over eukaryote plant pathogens encourage the thought that considerable progress in the biochemistry and molecular biology of specific plant recognition of bacteria will occur in the following years.

Acknowledgments

We thank Drs. R. Goodman, M. Essenberg, and W. Fett for supplying manuscripts before their publication and to several authors in these volumes for sending outlines or manuscripts of their chapters. The ideas on uses of transposons are largely those of Drs. N. Panopoulos and B. Staskawicz. The authors' research was supported by NSF grant PCM 7724346.

References

Ahamed, N. M., Radziejewska-Lebrecht, J., Widemann, C., and Mayer, H. (1980). *Abl. Bakt. Hyg., I. Abt. Orig. A* **247,** 468–482.

Albersheim, P., and Anderson-Prouty, A. J. (1975). *Annu. Rev. Plant Physiol.* **26,** 31–52.

Albersheim, P., and Valent, B. (1978). *J. Cell Biol.* **78,** 627–643.

Amrhein, N., Schab, J., and Steinrücken, H. C. (1980a). *Naturwissenschaften* **67,** 356–357.

Amrhein, N., Deus, B., Gehrke, P., and Steinrücken, H. C. (1980b). *Plant Physiol.* **66,** 830–834.

Anderson, A. J. (1980a). *Can. J. Microbiol.* **26,** 1422–1427.

Anderson, A. J. (1980b). *Can. J. Microbiol.* **26,** 1473–1479.

Anderson, A. J., and Jasalavich, C. (1979). *Physiol. Plant Pathol.* **15,** 149–159.

Ashwell, G., and Morell, A. G. (1977). *Trends Biochem. Sci.* **2,** 76–78.

Averre, C. W., III, and Kelman, A. (1964). *Phytopathology* **54,** 779–783.

Ayers, A. R., Ayers, S. B., and Goodman, R. N. (1979). *Appl. Environ. Microbiol.* **38,** 659–666.

Bailey, J. A. (1982). *In* "Active Defense Mechanisms in Plants" (R. K. S. Wood, ed.), pp. 39–65. Plenum, New York.

Ballou, C. (1976). *Adv. Microbiol. Physiol.* **14,** 93–158.

Banerjee, D., Basu, M., Choudhury, I., and Chatterjee, G. C. (1981). *Biochem. Biophys. Res. Commun.* **100,** 1384–1388.

Bauer, W. D. (1981). *Annu. Rev. Plant Physiol.* **32,** 407–449.

Beachey, E. H. (1980). "Bacterial Adherence." Receptors and Recognition, Ser. B, Vol. 6. Chapman & Hall, London.

Bennett, R. A. (1980). *J. Gen. Microbiol.* **116**, 351–356.

Bennett, R. A., and Billing, E. (1978). *Ann. Appl. Biol.* **89**, 41–45.

Bennett, R. A., and Billing, E. (1980). *J. Gen. Microbiol.* **116**, 341–349.

Beraha, L., and Garber, E. D. (1971). *Phytopathol. Z.* **70**, 335–344.

Beynon, J. L., Beringer, J. E., and Johnston, A. W. B. (1980). *J. Gen. Microbiol.* **120**, 421–429.

Bhuvaneswari, T. V., and Bauer, W. D. (1978). *Plant Physiol.* **62**, 71–74.

Bhuvaneswari, T. V., Pueppke, S. G., and Bauer, W. D. (1977). *Plant Physiol.* **60**, 486–491.

Bohlool, B. B., and Schmidt, E. L. (1974). *Science* **185**, 269–271.

Bradshaw-Rouse, J. J., Whatley, M. H., Coplin, D. L., Woods, A., Sequeira, L., and Kelman, A. (1981). *Appl. Environ. Microbiol.* **42**, 344–350.

Brewin, N. J., Beringer, J. E., and Johnston, A. W. B. (1980). *J. Gen. Microbiol.* **120**, 413–420.

Broughton, W. J. (1978). *J. Appl. Bacteriol.* **45**, 165–194.

Bruegger, B. B., and Keen, N. T. (1979). *Physiol. Plant Pathol.* **15**, 43–51.

Callow, J. A. (1977). *Adv. Bot. Res.* **4**, 1–49.

Carlson, R. W., Sanders, R. E., Napoli, C., and Albersheim, P. (1978). *Plant Physiol.* **62**, 912–917.

Chatterjee, A. K., and Starr, M. P. (1977). *J. Bacteriol.* **132**, 862–869.

Civerolo, E. L. (1972). *Proc. Int. Conf. Plant Pathog. Bact., 3rd* pp. 25–37.

Clarke, P. H., and Richmond, M. L. H. (1975). "Genetics and Biochemistry of Pseudomonas." Wiley, New York.

Comai, L., and Kosuge, T. (1982). *J. Bacteriol.* **149**, 40–46.

Cross, J. E., Kennedy, B. W., Lambert, J. W., and Cooper, R. L. (1966). *Plant Dis. Rep.* **50**, 557–560.

Crosthwaite, L. M., and Patil, S. (1978). *Phytopathol. Z.* **91**, 80–90.

Dahlbeck, D., and Stall, R. E. (1979). *Phytopathology* **69**, 634–636.

Daub, M. E., and Hagedorn, D. J. (1980). *Phytopathology* **70**, 429–436.

Day, P. R. (1974). "Genetics of Host-Parasite Interactions." Freeman, San Francisco, California.

Dazzo, F. B. (1980). *In* "Nitrogen Fixation" (W. E. Newton and W. H. Orme-Johnsen, eds.), Vol. II, pp. 165–187. Univ. Park Press, Baltimore, Maryland.

Dazzo, F. B., and Hubbell, D. H. (1975). *Appl. Microbiol.* **30**, 1017–1033.

Dazzo, F. B., Napoli, C. A., and Hubbell, D. H. (1976). *Appl. Environ. Microbiol.* **32**, 166–171.

Dazzo, F. B., Yanke, W. E., and Brill, W. J. (1978). *Biochim. Biophys. Acta* **539**, 276–286.

DeVay, J. E., and Adler, H. E. (1976). *Annu. Rev. Microbiol.* **30**, 147–168.

Doke, N., and Tomiyama, K. (1980). *Physiol. Plant Pathol.* **16**, 169–176.

Dye, D. W., Bradbury, J. F., Goto, M., Hayward, A. C., Lelliott, R. A., and Schroth, M. N. (1980). *Rev. Plant Pathol.* **59**, 153–168.

El-Banoby, F. E., and Rudolph, K. (1979). *Physiol. Plant Pathol.* **15**, 341–349.

El-Banoby, F. E., and Rudolph, K. (1980). *Phytopathol. Z.* **98**, 91–95.

Ellingboe, A. H. (1976). *In* "Physiological Plant Pathology" (R. Heitefuss and P. H. Williams, eds.), pp. 761–778. Springer-Verlag, Berlin and New York.

Ellwood, D. C., Melling, J., and Rutter, P. (1979). "Adhesion of Microorganisms to Surfaces." Academic Press, New York.

Ercolani, G. L. (1970). *Inst. Patol. Veg. Dell Univ.* pp. 151–160.

Ersek, T., Sarhan, A. R. T., and Pongors, S. (1981). *Acta Phytopathol. Acad. Sci. Hung.* **16**, 137–138.

Essenberg, M., Cason, E. T., Hamilton, B., Brinkerhoff, L. A., Gholson, R. K., and Richardson, P. E. (1979). *Physiol. Plant Pathol.* **15**, 53–68.

Essenberg, M., Doherty, M. D., Hamilton, B. K., Henning, V. T., McFaul, S. J., and Johnson, W. M. (1982). *Phytopathology* (in press).

Fett, W. F., and Jones, S. B. (1982). *Phytopathology* **72**, 488–492.

Fett, W. F., and Osman, S. F. (1982). *Phytopathology* **72**, 755–760.

Fett, W. F., and Sequeira, L. (1980). *Plant Physiol.* **66**, 847–852.

Fett, W. F., and Sequeira, L. (1981). *Can. J. Bot.* **59**, 283–287.

Fett, W. F., and Zacharius, R. M. (1982). *Plant. Sci. Lett.* **24**, 303–309.

Foster, T. J., and Kleckner, N. (1980). *In* "Plasmids and Transposons" (C. Stuttard and K. R. Rozee, eds.), pp. 207–224. Academic Press, New York.

Frazier, W., and Glaser, L. (1979). *Annu. Rev. Biochem.* **48**, 491–523.

Galanos, C., Lüderitz, O., Rietschel, E. T., and Westphal, O. (1977). *Int. Rev. Biochem.* **14**, 239–335.

Galanos, C., Freudenberg, M. A., Lüderitz, O., Reitschel, E. T., and Westphal, O. (1979). *Prog. Clin. Biol. Res.* **29**, 321–332.

Gardner, J. M., and Kado, C. I. (1976). *J. Bacteriol.* **127**, 451–460.

Garrett, M. E. (1978). *Proc. Int. Congr. Plant Pathog. Bact., 4th, Angers* **2**, 889–890.

Garrett, C. M. E., and Crosse, J. E. (1975). *Physiol. Plant Pathol.* **5**, 89–94.

Gibson, R., Kornfeld, S., and Schlesinger, S. (1980). *Trends Biochem. Sci.* **5**, 290–293.

Giddix, L. R., Lukezic, F. L., and Pell, E. J. (1981). *Phytopathology* **71**, 111–115.

Gilboa-Garber, N., and Mizrahi, L. (1981). *J. Appl. Bacteriol.* **50**, 21–28.

Gnanamanickam, S. S., and Patil, S. S. (1977a). *Physiol. Plant Pathol.* **10**, 159–168.

Gnanamanickam, S. S., and Patil, S. S. (1977b). *Physiol. Plant Pathol.* **10**, 169–179.

Gnanamanickam, S. S., and Ward, E. W. B. (1981). *Proc. Can. Phytopathol. Soc.* (Abstr.).

Goldman, R. C., and Leive, L. (1980). *Eur. J. Biochem.* **107**, 145–153.

Goodman, R. N. (1978). *Mycopathologia* **65**, 107–113.

Goodman, R. N. (1980). *In* "Plant Disease" (J. Horsfall and E. Cowling, eds.), Vol. 5, pp. 305–317. Academic Press, New York.

Goodman, R. N., Huang, P.-Y., and White, J. A. (1976a). *Phytopathology* **66**, 754–764.

Goodman, R. N., Huang, P.-Y., Huang, J. S., and Thiapanich, V. (1976b). *In* "Biochem. Cytol. Plant-Parasite Interaction" (K. Tomiyama *et al.*, eds.), pp. 35–42. Kodansha, Tokyo.

Goodman, R. N., Huang, J. S., and Huang, P.-Y. (1978). *Science* **183**, 1081–1082.

Gonzalez, C. F., DeVay, J. E., and Wakeman, R. J. (1981). *Physiol. Plant Pathol.* **18**, 41–50.

Graham, T. L., Sequeira, L., and Huang, T.-S. R. (1977). *Appl. Environ. Microbiol.* **34**, 424–432.

Gross, D. C., and DeVay, J. E. (1977). *Physiol. Plant Pathol.* **11**, 1–11.

Gulya, T., and Dunleavy, J. M. (1979). *Crop Sci.* **19**, 261–264.

Hadwiger, L. A., and Schwochau, M. E. (1969). *Phytopathology* **59**, 223–227.

Hildebrand, D. C., and Schroth, M. N. (1964). *Phytopathology* **54**, 640–645.

Hildebrand, D. C., Alosi, M. C., and Schroth, M. N. (1980). *Phytopathology* **70**, 98–109.

Hoitink, H. A. J., and Bradfute, O. E. (1972). *Proc. Int. Conf. Plant Pathog. Bact., 3rd* pp. 55–58.

Holliday, M. J. (1981). Ph.D. thesis, University of California, Riverside.

Holliday, M. J., and W. L. Klarman (1979). *Phytopathology* **69**, 576–578.

Holliday, M. J., Keen, N. T., and Long, M. (1981a). *Physiol. Plant Pathol.* **18**, 279–287.

Holliday, M. J., Long, M., and Keen, N. T. (1981b). *Physiol. Plant Pathol.* **19,** 209–216.
Hopper, D. G., Venere, R. J., Brinkerhoff, L. A., and Gholson, R. K. (1975). *Phytopathology* **65,** 206–213.
Hsu, S-T., and Goodman, R. N. (1978). *Phytopathology* **68,** 355–360.
Huang, J. S. (1980). *Physiol. Plant Pathol.* **17,** 73–80.
Huang, P.-Y., Huang, J.-S., and Goodman, R. N. (1975). *Physiol. Plant Pathol.* **6,** 283–287.
Husain, A., and Kelman, A. (1958). *Phytopathology* **48,** 155–165.
Ingham, J. L., Keen, N. T., Mulheirn, L. J., and Lyne, R. L. (1981). *Phytochemistry* **20,** 795–798.
Jamieson, A. F., Bielski, R. L., and Mitchell, R. E. (1981). *J. Gen. Microbiol.* **122,** 161–165.
Jann, K., and Westphal, O. (1975). *In* "The Antigens" (M. Sela, ed.), Vol. 3, pp. 1–125. Academic Press, New York.
Jasalavich, C. A., and Anderson, A. J. (1981). *Can. J. Bot.* **59,** 264–271.
Jindal, J. K., and Patel, P. N. (1981). *Phytopathol. Z.* **100,** 97–110.
Keen, N. T. (1978). *Phytopathology* **68,** 1237–1239.
Keen, N. T. (1982a). *In* "Advances in Plant Pathology" (P. H. Williams and D. Ingram, eds.), Vol I. Academic Press, New York.
Keen, N. T. (1982b). *In* "The Physiological and Biochemical Basis of Plant Infection" (Y. Asada, W. R. Bushnell, S. Ouchi, and C. P. Vance, eds.). Japan Scientific Soc. Press (in press).
Keen, N. T., and Bruegger, B. (1977). *Am. Chem. Soc. Symp. Ser.* **62,** 1–26.
Keen, N. T., and Horsch, R. (1972). *Phytopathology* **62,** 439–442.
Keen, N. T., and Kennedy, B. W. (1974). *Physiol. Plant Pathol.* **4,** 173–185.
Keen, N. T., and Legrand, M. (1980). *Physiol. Plant Pathol.* **17,** 175–192.
Keen, N. T., Ersek, T., Long, M., Bruegger, B., and Holliday, M. (1981). *Physiol. Plant Pathol.* **18,** 325–337.
Kennedy, B. W., and Mew, T. W. (1971). *Phytopathology* **61,** 879–880.
Kennedy, B. W., Mew, T. W., and Olson, L. (1972). *Proc. Int. Conf. Plant Pathog. Bact., 3rd* pp. 201–202.
Kleckner, N. (1977). *Cell* **11,** 11–23.
Klement, Z. (1977). *Acta Phytopathol. Acad. Sci. Hung.* **12,** 257–261.
Klement, Z., and Goodman, R. N. (1967). *Annu. Rev. Phytopathol.* **5,** 17–44.
Klement, Z., and Lovrekovich, L. (1961). *Phytopathol. Z.* **41,** 217–227.
Klement, Z., and Lovrekovich, L. (1962). *Phytopathol. Z.* **45,** 81–88.
Klement, Z., Farkas, G. L., and Lovrekovich, L. (1964). *Phytopathology* **54,** 474–477.
Kopecko, D. J. (1980a). *Prog. Mol. Subcell. Biol.* **7,** 135–234.
Kopecko, D. J. (1980b). *In* "Plasmids and Transposons" (C. Suttard and K. R. Rozee, eds.), pp. 165–205. Academic Press, New York.
Laurence, J. A., and Kennedy, B. W. (1974). *Phytopathology* **64,** 1470–1471.
Liao, C. H., and Heberlein, G. T. (1979). *Can. J. Microbiol.* **25,** 185–191.
Liener, I. E. (1976). *Annu. Rev. Plant Physiol.* **27,** 291–319.
Lindberg, A. A. (1973). *Annu. Rev. Microbiol.* **27,** 205–241.
Lippincott, B. B., and Lippincott, J. A. (1969). *J. Bacteriol.* **97,** 620–628.
Lippincott, J. A., and Lippincott, B. B. (1977). *In* "Cell Wall Biochemistry Related to Specificity in Host-Plant Pathogen Interactions" (B. Solheim and J. Raa, eds.), pp. 439–451. Universitetsforlaget, Oslo.
Lippincott, J. A., and Lippincott, B. B. (1980). *In* "Bacterial Adherence. Receptors and Recognition" (E. H. Beachey, ed.), Ser. B, Vol. 6, pp. 375–398. Chapman & Hall, London.

Lis, H., Sela, B., Sachs, L., and Sharon, N. (1970). *Biochim. Biophys. Acta* **211,** 582–585.

Lotan, R., Sharon, N., and Mirelman, D. (1975). *Eur. J. Biochem.* **55,** 257–262.

Lovrekovich, L., and Klement, Z. (1961). *Acta Microbiol.* **8,** 303–310.

Lozano, J. C., and Sequeira, L. (1970). *Phytopathology* **60,** 833–838.

Lucas, L. T., and Grogan, R. G. (1969a). *Phytopathology* **59,** 1908–1912.

Lucas, L. T., and Grogan, R. G. (1969b). *Phytopathology* **59,** 1913–1917.

Lyne, R. L., Mulheirn, L. J., and Leworthy, D. P. (1976). *J. Chem. Soc. Chem. Commun.* pp. 497–498.

Lyne, R. L., Mulheirn, L. J., and Keen, N. T. (1981). *Tetrahedron Lett.* **22,** 2483–2484.

Lyon, F. M., and Wood, R. K. S. (1975). *Physiol. Plant Pathol.* **6,** 117–124.

Lyon, F., and Wood, R. K. S. (1976). *Ann. Bot.* **40,** 479–491.

Lyon, F., and Wood, R. K. S. (1977). *Ann. Bot.* **41,** 359–367.

Lyon, G., and Albersheim, P. (1980). *Plant Physiol. Suppl.* **65,** 137.

Matthysse, A. G., Wyman, P. M., and Holmes, K. V. (1978). *Infect. Immun.* **22,** 516–522.

Mitchell, R. E., and Young, H. (1978). *Phytochemistry* **17,** 2028–2029.

Mitchell, R. E., Hale, C. N., and Shanks, J. C. (1982). *Physiol. Plant Pathol.* **20,** 91–98.

Mount, M. S., Berman, P. M., Mortlock, R. P., and Hubbard, J. P. (1979). *Phytopathology* **69,** 117–120.

Mukherjee, D. (1965). *Diss. Abstr.* **26,** 43.

Mukherjee, D., Lambert, J. W., Cooper, R. L., and Kennedy, B. W. (1966). *Crop Sci.* **6,** 324–326.

Nelson, R. R. (1979). *In* "Host-Parasite Interfaces" (B. B. Nickol, ed.), pp. 17–25. Academic Press, New York.

Nikaido, H. (1973). *In* "Bacterial Membranes and Walls" (L. Leive, ed.), pp. 131–208. Dekker, New York.

Novacky, A. (1972). *Physiol. Plant Pathol.* **2,** 101–104.

Ofek, I., Beachey, E. H., and Sharon, N. (1978). *Trends Biochem. Sci.* **3,** 159–160.

Palva, E. T., and Mäkelä, P. H. (1980). *Eur. J. Biochem.* **107,** 137–143.

Passmoor, M., and Epton, H. A. S. (1978). *Proc. Int. Conf. Plant Pathog. Bact., 4th, Angers* **2,** 675–678.

Patil, S. S., Hayward, A. C., and Emmons, R. (1974). *Phytopathology* **64,** 590–595.

Pinkas, Y., and Novacky, A. (1971). *Phytopathology* **61,** 906–907 (Abstr.).

Politis, D. J., and Goodman, R. N. (1980). *Appl. Environ. Microbiol.* **40,** 596–607.

Prakash, R. K., Hooykaas, P. J. J., Ledeboer, A. M., Kijne, J. W., Schilperoort, R. A., Nuti, M. P., Lepidi, A. A., Casse, F., Boucher, C., Julliot, J. S., and Dénarié, J. (1980). *In* "Nitrogen Fixation" (W. E. Newton and W. H. Orme-Johnson, eds.), Vol. II, pp. 139–163. Univ. Park Press, Baltimore, Maryland.

Pueppke, S. G., and Benny, U. K. (1981). *Physiol. Plant Pathol.* **18,** 169–179.

Quirk, A. V., Sletten, A., and Hignett, R. C. (1976). *J. Gen. Microbiol.* **96,** 375–381.

Rathmell, W. G., and Sequeira, L. (1975). *Physiol. Plant Pathol.* **5,** 65–73.

Ries, S. M., and Strobel, G. A. (1972). *Physiol. Plant Pathol.* **2,** 133–142.

Romeiro, R., de Karr, A. L., and Goodman, R. N. (1981a). *Physiol. Plant Pathol.* **19,** 383–390.

Romeiro, R., Karr, A., and Goodman, R. (1981b). *Plant Physiol.* **69,** 772–777.

Rudbach, J. A., and Baker, P. J. (1977). *In* "Immunobiology of Bacterial Polysaccharides" (J. A. Rudbach and P. J. Baker, eds.), Developments in Immunol. Vol. 2, pp. 1–17. Elsevier, Amsterdam.

Sasser, M. (1978). *Phytopathology* **68,** 361–363.

Sasser, M. (1980). *Phytopathology* **70,** 692 (Abstr.).

Sasser, M., Andrews, A. K., and Doganay, Z. U. (1974). *Phytopathology* **64**, 770–772.
Schaad, N. W. (1979). *Annu. Rev. Phytopathol.* **17**, 123–147.
Schmidt, E. L. (1979). *Annu. Rev. Microbiol.* **33**, 355–376.
Schnathorst, W. C. (1970). *Phytopathology* **60**, 258–260.
Sequeira, L. (1978). *Annu. Rev. Phytopathol.* **16**, 453–481.
Sequeira, L. (1979). *In* "Host-Parasite Interfaces" (B. B. Nickol, ed.), pp. 71–84. Academic Press, New York.
Sequeira, L. (1981). *In* "Plant Disease Control" (R. C. Staples and G. Toeniessen, eds.), pp. 143–153. Wiley, New York.
Sequeira, L., and Ainslie, V. (1969). *Proc. Int. Bot. Congr., 11th* (Abstr.).
Sequeira, L., and Graham, T. L. (1977). *Physiol. Plant Pathol.* **11**, 43–54.
Sequeira, L., Gaard, G., and De Zoeten, G. A. (1977). *Physiol. Plant Pathol.* **10**, 43–50.
Sharon, N., and Lis, H. (1981). *Chem. Eng. News* pp. 21–44.
Sigee, D. C., and Epton, H. A. S. (1975). *Physiol. Plant Pathol.* **6**, 29–34.
Sinden, S. L., DeVay, J. E., and Backman, P. A. (1971). *Physiol. Plant Pathol.* **1**, 199–213.
Sjulin, T. M., and Beer, S. V. (1978). *Phytopathology* **68**, 89–94.
Slusarenko, A. J., and Wood, R. K. S. (1981). *Physiol. Plant Pathol.* **18**, 187–193.
Smidt, M., and Kosuge, T. (1978). *Physiol. Plant Pathol.* **13**, 203–214.
Smith, H. (1977). *Bacteriol. Rev.* **41**, 475–500.
Smith, J. J., and Mansfield, J. W. (1981). *Physiol. Plant Pathol.* **18**, 345–356.
Solheim, B., and Paxton, J. (1981). *In* "Plant Disease Control" (R. C. Staples and G. H. Toenniessen, eds.), pp. 71–83. Wiley, New York.
Stacey, G., Paau, A. S., and Brill, W. J. (1980). *Plant Physiol.* **66**, 609–614.
Stall, R. E., and Cook, A. A. (1968). *Phytopathology* **58**, 1584–1587.
Stall, R. E., and Cook, A. A. (1979). *Physiol. Plant Pathol.* **14**, 77–84.
Stall, R. E., Bartz, J. A., and Cook, A. A. (1972). *Phytopathology* **62**, 791 (Abstr.).
Stanley, P., and Sudo, T. (1981). *Cell* **23**, 763–769.
Talmadge, K. W., and Burger, M. M. (1975). *Biochem. Sci.* **5**, 43–93.
Tate, M. E., Murphy, P. J., Roberts, W. P., and Kerr, A. (1979). *Nature* (*London*) **280**, 697–699.
Thomas, M. D., and Leary, J. V. (1980). *Phytopathology* **70**, 310–312.
Turner, J. G., and Novacky, A. (1974). *Phytopathology* **64**, 885–890.
Turner, M. (1980). *Nature* (*London*) **284**, 13–14.
Valent, B. S., Darvill, A. G., McNeil, M., Robertsen, B. K., and Albersheim, P. (1980). *Carbohydr. Res.* **79**, 165–192.
Vidaver, A. K. (1976). *Annu. Rev. Phytopathol.* **14**, 451–465.
Vidaver, A. K., Mathyus, M. L., Thomas, M. E., and Schuster, M. L. (1972). *Can J. Microbiol.* **18**, 705–713.
Wade, M., and Albersheim, P. (1979). *Proc. Natl. Acad. Sci. U.S.A.* **76**, 4433–4437.
Webster, D. M., and Sequeira, L. (1977). *Can. J. Bot.* **15**, 2043–2052.
Weinstein, L. I., Hahn, M. G., and Albersheim, P. (1981). *Plant Physiol.* **68**, 358–363.
Whatley, M. H., Bodwen, J. S., Lippincott, B. B., and Lippincott, J. A. (1976). *Infect. Immun.* **13**, 1080–1083.
Whatley, M. H., Margot, J. B., Schell, J., Lippincott, B. B., and Lippincott, J. A. (1978). *J. Gen. Microbiol.* **107**, 395–398.
Whatley, M. H., Hunter, N., Cantrell, M. A., Hendrick, C., Keegstra, K., and Sequeira, L. (1980). *Plant Physiol.* **65**, 557–559.
Wilkinson, S. G. (1977). *In* "Surface Carbohydrates of the Procaryotic Cell" (I. Sutherland, ed.), pp. 97–175. Academic Press, New York.
West, C. A. (1981). *Naturwissenschaften* **68**, 447–457.

Wood, R. K. S. (1967). "Physiological Plant Pathology." Blackwell, Oxford.
Yoshikawa, M., Masago, H., and Keen, N. T. (1977). *Physiol. Plant Pathol.* **10**, 125–138.
Yoshikawa, M., Yamauchi, K., and Masago, H. (1978). *Plant Physiol.* **61**, 314–317.
Young, J. M. (1974a). *N. Z. J. Agric. Res.* **17**, 105–113.
Young, J. M. (1974b). *N. Z. J. Agric. Res.* **17**, 115–119.
Zähringer, U., Ebel, J., and Grisebach, H. (1978). *Arch. Biochem. Biophys.* **188**, 450–455.
Zähringer, U., Schaller, E., and Grisebach, H. (1981). *Z. Naturforsch.* **36**, 234–241.

Part **III**

Pathogen Coevolution with the Host

Coevolution with plants requires phytopathogenic prokaryote counteraction of host resistance—or, host evolutionary developments that would serve to exclude the pathogens. The basis for coevolution resides in the ability of pathogens to add, subtract, recombine, and change their heritable characteristics in response to selective pressures exerted by the environment and their hosts. Therefore, the study of genetics of pathogens is important for understanding inheritance, pathogenicity, and, in turn, pathogenesis. G. H. Lacy and S. S. Patil (Chapter 10) reason that genetic tools can probe host–pathogen interactions in a manner unbiased by our preconceived concepts. J. V. Leary and D. W. Fulbright discuss in Chapter 11 progress in and methods for developing chromosomal genetic systems of phytopathogenic bacteria. They also present possible roles for genetic isolation and genetic acquisition in the development of pathogenicity. Plasmids are widespread in phytopathogenic prokaryotes and constitute up to 25% of the DNA present in some strains. D. L. Coplin describes how plasmids are or may be related to pathogenicity and discusses research methodologies (Chapter 12). The most intensively studied plasmids associated with plant disease are agrobacteria plasmids involved with tissue proliferation diseases. D. J. Merlo (Chapter 13) reviews this area of research from the perspective of bacterial DNA transfer to plant cells and the integration of this DNA into the plant genome. The potential use of this transfer system for genetic modification of plants for increased agronomic usefulness is presented by C. I. Kado and P. F. Lurquin in Chapter 14.

Chapter **10**

Why Genetics?

GEORGE H. LACY *and* SURESH S. PATIL

I. INTRODUCTION

The most important tool in understanding control of heritable characteristics in biological systems, including prokaryotes pathogenic for plants, is genetics. Genetics deals with the determinants of these characteristics which reside in ordered sequences of deoxyribonucleic acid (DNA) in living organisms. Therefore, the study of the structure of DNA and the regulation of its transcription and translation into biological products is important for understanding the control of heritable characteristics related to plant pathogenesis.

In recent years, fundamental advances in the genetics of living organisms have been made. In particular, the advances made in genetics of prokaryotes have been spectacular and have resulted in the development of new and powerful genetic tools for analyzing existing genotypes and constructing new ones. Such tools, based on recombi-

Copyright © 1982 by Academic Press, Inc.
All rights of reproduction in any form reserved.
ISBN 0-12-509002-1

nant DNA techniques, are now being used widely in the study of prokaryotes and, to a lesser extent, eukaryotes.

Generally, the progress made in genetics of prokaryotes has been extraordinary; until recently it has had little impact on the study of phytopathogenic prokaryotes (Mills and Gonzalez, Vol. 1, Chapter 5). Plant pathologists need to understand the bases for specificity between plants and their pathogens (Keen and Holliday, this volume, Chapter 9; Klement, this volume, Chapter 8; Stacey and Brill, Vol. 1, Chapter 9). The tools of modern genetics, properly used, should help dissect the pathogenic relationships on which specific plant host–bacterial combinations are based. In the following pages, we examine why genetic studies of prokaryotic phytopathogens have been neglected in the past, discuss briefly how the study of prokaryotic genetics is important in plant pathology, give some examples of recent progress in this area, and speculate on future advances.

II. GENETICS OF PATHOGENICITY

Genetics of pathogenesis may be divided into three parts: genetics of the host, agricorpus, and pathogen. The usefulness of host genetics is immediately evident through the results of breeding programs for improved agronomic characters, including resistance to disease (Hagedorn, this volume, Chapter 17). To this end, the genetically controlled interactions of host and pathogen, expressed as disease symptoms (genetics of the agricorpus), have been used for evaluation of pathogen races and host resistance genes (Ellingboe, this volume, Chapter 5).

The genetics of phytopathogenic prokaryotes has lagged behind the other areas. There are several reasons for this lag. One is that prokaryotes lack easily discerned morphological stages that have allowed "genetic dissection" or sequencing of events in penetration, infection, and colonization of host tissues by other pathogens. This morphological dissection of pathogenesis has been used successfully by fungal geneticists studying powdery mildews and rusts. However, a more important reason may be that, because of their economic importance, fungal and viral plant pathogens have been given more emphasis in the training of new plant pathologists. Therefore, fewer researchers work with prokaryotic plant pathogens as compared to other pathogens. Prokaryotic phytopathogens, however, make better models for studying the mechanisms for pathogenesis and bases for specificity between host and pathogen. This is because most prokaryotes are easy to culture and are more amenable to sophisticated genetic manipulations than are other pathogens. In addition, phytopathogenic prokaryotes share with their fungal and viral counterparts, gene-for-gene virulence and resistance systems, pathotypes, and relatively simple assays for virulence or pathogenicity.

In contrast to prokaryotic model systems, fungal and viral systems are more difficult to study. In fungal pathogens, their complex eukaryotic nature is a hindrance to the isolation and purification of molecular species and genetic material necessary for molecular studies. Further, many of the best fungal systems and all viral systems available for genetic analyses involve obligate parasites, whereas most important pathogenic prokaryotes are not nutritionally fastidious. Thus, prokaryotes offer us unique opportunities for deciphering the bases for host–pathogen specificity and, even though some may argue that the diseases caused by prokaryotes are not as economically important or as numerous as those caused by other classes of pathogens, the basic understanding of specificity in plant diseases is likely to be accomplished more easily with prokaryotic systems.

III. THE "NULL HYPOTHESIS" APPROACH

As plant pathologists, our ultimate goal is to alleviate crop losses caused by diseases. To this end, many pathologists study host–pathogen interactions to determine the nature of specificity between plants and their pathogens. If specificity is understood, intelligent strategies for control of plant diseases may be developed. However, studies of host–pathogen interactions have mostly uncovered the mechanisms by which the pathogen causes damage in the host. Thus, extensive work on toxins (Durbin, Vol. 1, Chapter 17), macerating enzymes (Collmer *et al.*, Vol. 1, Chapter 16), growth regulators (Kemp, Vol. 1, Chapter 18; Kosuge and Kimpel, Vol. 1, Chapter 15), wilt mechanisms (Van Alfen, Vol. 1, Chapter 19), and other factors produced by various pathogens, which induce damage in affected host plants, have been reported. However, two fundamental questions remain unanswered: The first question asks why a specific pathogen is able to establish itself in its compatible host, whereas it fails to do so in other closely related plant species? The second question asks why nonpathogenic prokaryotes, some equipped with enzymes, potential wilt-inducing extracellular polysaccharides, and growth regulators similar to pathogenic bacteria, are incapable of being pathogens? In other words, we now know more about how damage is caused by pathogens than why they are pathogens.

The reason for considering why an organism is a pathogen separately from the mechanism whereby a pathogen damages a plant goes back to how pathogenesis occurs. Penetration, infection, and colonization of host tissue by pathogens are generally accepted as stages of pathogenesis that precede the appearance of symptoms (Goodman, Vol. 1, Chapter 3). Penetration and the ability to infect and colonize have been studied from the points of view of wounds, water congestion, motility, vectors, hypersensitivity, and compounds and structures involved in resistance (Anderson, this volume, Chapter 6; Keen and Holliday, this volume, Chapter 9; Klement, this volume, Chapter 8; McIntyre, this volume, Chapter 7; Stacey and Brill, Vol. 1, Chapter 9). However, more subtle, but essential interactions probably have been missed, since it is difficult to formulate hypotheses to test when we cannot see or guess what might be important in host–pathogen interactions at the early infection stages.

Using genetics as a tool or probe for interactions between plants and their pathogens, we can eliminate the bias in our approach derived from "seeing or guessing." For instance, although we cannot "see" or even "guess" their purpose or mechanisms, genes for resistance to fungal diseases can be detected in flax (*Linum usitatissimum* L.) and wheat (*Triticum aestivum* L.) and corresponding genes for virulence can be found in their pathogens, *Melampsora lini* (Pers.) Lev. and *Puccinia graminis* Pers. However, determining how these genes function, what they produce, or how they relate to pathogenesis has not been generally successful because the eukaryotic or obligate parasitic natures of these fungal plant pathogens have, so far, prevented such studies.

These same analyses are potentially available for phytopathogenic prokaryotes and their hosts. Several systems come to mind: Pathovars or biotypes exist for *Pseudomonas syringae* van Hall, *P. solanacearum* (Smith) Smith, *Erwinia chrysanthemi* Burkholder *et al.*, *Xanthomonas campestris* (Pammel) Dowson, *Agrobacterium tumefaciens* (Smith & Townsend) Conn, *Corynebacterium michiganense* (Smith) Jensen, and others. Further, the prokaryotic nature of these bacterial plant pathogens should facilitate the molecular studies that are so difficult with fungal or viral pathogens.

IV. ACCOMPLISHMENTS INVOLVING PROKARYOTIC GENETICS

Until very recently, aspects of prokaryotic diseases were studied by relatively few plant pathologists and the concepts they developed were not stressed heavily in training programs. Times are changing. Some remarkable advances in genetics of prokaryotes indicate that the rest of the scientific world, in addition to plant pathologists, are now recognizing the potential contributions of phytopathogenic prokaryotes for studying molecular aspects of pathology. These advances are examined in detail in the following chapters. Briefly, they include spectacular advances in our knowledge about the molecular nature of the crown gall "caused" by *Agrobacterium tumefaciens* (Kemp, Vol. 1, Chapter 18; Merlo, this volume, Chapter 13; Mills and Gonzalez, Vol. 1, Chapter 5). Evidence that a lowly bacterium might have a mechanism to cross the evolutionary gulf between eukaryotes and prokaryotes and genetically alter its host plant has not been lost to plant geneticists. Using this mechanism, they have now been able to insert selected genes into plants and plan to introduce other genes for improvement of agronomic characters (Kado and Lurquin, this volume, Chapter 14).

Another impressive accomplishment in the understanding of the genomes of pathogenic prokaryotes has resulted from the work with mapping of the chromosomes of *Erwinia amylovora* (Burrill) Winslow *et al.* and *E. chrysanthemi* (Chatterjee and Starr, 1980; Leary and Fulbright, this volume, Chapter 11). This work sets the stage for comparison of the genomes of phytopathogens with animal and human pathogens in the Enterobacteriaceae (Starr and Chatterjee, 1972). This will be the basis for comparative pathology! It opens the gate for the development of unifying concepts of pathology, just as unifying concepts of biochemical genetics have been so useful for understanding the physiology of plants, animals, and prokaryotes.

Other areas of research in which exciting results have been obtained include studies concerning the plasmid nature of genetic elements mediating the ability of *Pseudomonas syringae* pv. *savastanoi* (Smith) Young *et al.* to produce indoleacetic acid (IAA) and incite gall formation (Comai and Kosuge, 1980; Coplin, this volume, Chapter 13).

Another interesting area of research has dealt with using plasmids to control disease. Specifically, a plasmid-encoded bacteriocin, agrocin 84, in *Agrobacterium radiobacter* (Beijerinck & van Delden) Conn has been used for crown gall control (Moore and Warren, 1979; Vidaver, this volume, Chapter 18). Thus, crown gall, a disease itself incited by a plasmid-borne agent (Merlo, this volume, Chapter 13) carried by *Agrobacterium tumefaciens*, is controlled by pitting one plasmid against another.

V. PROSPECTS

The prospects for the future are bright. More scientists than ever before are studying plant pathogenesis incited by prokaryotes. Further, more is known about the genetics of prokaryotes that are, or may be, related to genetics of pathogenesis (Mills and Gonzalez, Vol. 1, Chapter 5). Therefore, we expect to continue to see significant developments in determining the number and kinds of genes involved in pathogenesis and isolation and characterization of these genes. Altogether, this will result in greater insight into what pathogens are and how plants might be bred for resistance or altered genetically.

A. Chromosomal Mapping

Leary and Fulbright (this volume, Chapter 11) discuss the use of and impact of classical substitutive recombinational genetic studies on understanding the chromosomal genetics of phytopathogenic prokaryotes. Despite the tremendous impetus that plasmid genetics and recombinant DNA techniques have had, mapping the chromosomes of pathogens will be basic to understanding how bacteria associate with plants until pathogenesis occurs. The key to this development will be recognizing and mapping loci involved with pathogenesis. Until now, however, development has been slow, since few researchers have been working in this area. Now, however, classic genetic mapping techniques, including conjugal transfer, transformation, and transduction, will be aided and speeded by the use of new technologies developed for transposon mapping (Coplin, this volume, Chapter 12; Mills and Gonzalez, Vol. 1, Chapter 5) and the merozygote formation with plasmids or other genetic vehicles created by recombinant DNA techniques (Kado and Lurquin, this volume, Chapter 14).

B. Plasmids and Pathogenicity

The contribution of plasmids to pathogenicity, of course, cannot be overlooked since they are numerous and may make up 1–25% of the total genetic material of pathogens (Coplin, this volume, Chapter 12). However, their major role in pathogenicity will probably be determined to be in support of host damage or mechanisms giving nutritional or competitive advantages to the prokaryotic pathogen. In other words, plasmids will probably aid pathogenesis in their prokaryotic hosts already capable of associating with plants. *Agrobacterium tumefaciens* is an excellent example of this point of view. Since *A. radiobacter* is a plant-associated bacterium and must acquire a plasmid (Ti) before it can cause gall formation (or become *A. tumefaciens*), the plasmid only gives the bacterium the ability to form a more specialized plant association—

pathogenesis (Merlo, this volume, Chapter 13). In fact, we should consider that *A. tumefaciens* (or *A. radiobacter*/Ti) is not a plant pathogen at all, but a vector or vehicle for the Ti plasmid. The Ti plasmid, in turn, may be considered a vehicle for the T-DNA, which is the actual pathogen. This concept may be troubled by lack of evidence for a disease cycle that would return T-DNA from plant tissue to Ti and, hence, to the bacterium. We cannot overlook the possibility that T-DNA may be the first representative of a new group of pathogens, or, alternatively, the first viroid-like DNA agent described.

Correlating indigenous cryptic plasmids with their functions, if any, in plant pathogens has been a major stumbling block to this area of research. However, use of transposons to mark cryptic plasmids will speed their identification and the determination of their function (Coplin, this volume, Chapter 12). Further, development of transformation systems among phytopathogens (Gantotti *et al.*, 1979; Lacy and Sparks, 1979) will supplement conjugal transfer or plasmid mobilization systems already in use (Coplin, this volume, Chapter 12).

C. Gene Isolation

Recombinant techniques, already used to study the T-DNA of agrobacteria (Comai and Kosuge, 1982; Merlo, this volume, Chapter 13; Nester and Kosuge, 1981) have clearly demonstrated their usefulness for dissection and understanding the genetic bases for plant pathogenicity. The greatest benefits to plant pathology are yet to come. These techniques, used in combination with genetic mapping of loci involved in pathogenicity on chromosomes and plasmids, will reveal the structure, function, and regulation of genes involved with the subtle interactions that allow bacteria to associate with and colonize plants. Genes for association will also be interesting to the plant breeder, since they will provide clues for tactics useful in breeding resistant plants.

D. Plant Engineering

The potential impact of genetic and molecular studies of prokaryotes causing plant disease for genetically altering their eukaryotic hosts must again be mentioned. At present, the only successful insertions of foreign genes into plant genomes has been accomplished using the prokaryotic vector *Agrobacterium tumefaciens* and its indigenous Ti plasmid. Kado and Lurquin (this volume, Chapter 14) discuss in greater length the ramifications of these successes.

E. Biological Control

Genetic manipulations may allow the enhancement of or the creation of prokaryotes useful for biological control. Numerous bacteria associated with plant surfaces (Blakeman, Vol. 1, Chapter 13; Foster and Bowen, Vol. 1, Chapter 7; Lindow, Vol. 1, Chapter 14; Suslow, Vol. 1, Chapter 8; Vidaver, this volume, Chapter 18) have been shown to be antagonists of pathogens and to have some possible roles in biological control. The traits that cause antagonism to pathogens, competition for available substrates, chemical alteration of the environment, bacteriocin and antibiotic production, siderophore production, etc., may be genetically manipulated. Since effective biological control agents must be able to colonize plant surfaces, the key to success will be to engineer organisms that remain efficient colonizers. Therefore, knowledge of plant-association functions, as well as those characters useful in antagonism, will be needed. The important concept to understand about the mechanisms and genetics of plant-association genes is that simply adding genes for antagonism to engineered agents may cause bionomic energy shifts that may result in reduced effectiveness of the strains for plant colonization. One way this problem might be circumvented is by "disengaging," through genetic engineering, other energy-requiring processes of the bacterium not related to competitiveness on plant surfaces and antagonism toward pathogens.

The answer to the question "Why genetics?" should now be obvious. Until as recently as 1972 (Lacy and Leary, 1979), there were no formal genetics of phytopathogenic bacteria. In the last 10 years, we have witnessed an explosion of knowledge about the genetics of their pathogenicity and even possible methods for engineering plants. This progress, reviewed in the following chapters by D. L. Coplin, C. I. Kado and P. F. Lurqin, J. V. Leary and D. W. Fulbright, and D. J. Merlo and in Volume 1 by D. Mills and C. F. Gonzalez, should be convincing evidence that genetic analyses are the most important tools available for understanding pathogenicity and pathogenesis.

References

Chatterjee, A. K., and Starr, M. P. (1980). *Annu. Rev. Microbiol.* **34,** 645–676.
Comai, L., and Kosuge, T. (1980). *J. Bacteriol.* **143,** 950–957.
Comai, L., and Kosuge, T. (1982). *J. Bacteriol.* **149,** 40–46.
Gantotti, B. V., Patil, S. S., and Mandel, M. (1979). *Gen. Genet.* **174,** 101–103.
Lacy, G. H., and Leary, J. V. (1979). *Annu. Rev. Phytopathol.* **17,** 181–202.
Lacy, G. H., and Sparks, R. B., Jr. (1979). *Phytopathology* **69,** 1293–1297.
Moore, L. W., and Warren, G. (1979). *Annu. Rev. Phytopathol.* **17,** 163–179.
Nester, E. W., and Kosuge, T. (1981). *Annu. Rev. Microbiol.* **35,** 531–565.
Starr, M. P., and Chatterjee, A. K. (1972). *Annu. Rev. Microbiol.* **26,** 389–426.

Chapter **11**

Chromosomal Genetics of Pseudomonas spp. and Erwinia spp.

J. V. LEARY *and* D. W. FULBRIGHT

I. INTRODUCTION

A hypothetical conversation between a phytopathogenic pseudomonad (Sue) and a phytopathogenic *Erwinia* (Erv) might proceed as follows:

Sue: "Oh, how I wish I was normal, just like *E. coli*. How nice it would be and how happy I would make everyone."
Erv: "But *I* am just like *E. coli* and not very many people have been happy with me."
Sue: "What do you think the matter is?"
Erv: "I think it's them!"
Sue: "Could it be us?"

Phytopathogenic Prokaryotes, Vol. 2

Copyright © 1982 by Academic Press, Inc.
All rights of reproduction in any form reserved.
ISBN 0-12-509002-1

The subject matter to be discussed in this chapter is defined in the title of the chapter. The content of the text and our approach to writing this chapter are emphatically stated in the hypothetical conversation between the two phytopathogenic prokaryotes above.

Of course, we are being facetious in our description of the conversation. To more seriously describe what we are saying, we offer the following arguments that plant pathologists should, at the present time, know much, much more than we do about the chromosomal genetics of these two important genera of phytopathogenic bacteria, *Erwinia* and *Pseudomonas*.

First, the genus *Erwinia* is placed in the Enterobacteriaceae, which also includes *Escherichia coli* (Migula) Castellani & Chalmers, the bridgestone of prokaryote genetics. Also, included in this family are *Salmonella* spp. which have been very well-characterized genetically. Yet, disappointingly, to date only approximately 20 chromosomal genes have been mapped in *Erwinia chrysanthemi* Burkholder *et al.* and about 10 in *E. amylovora* (Burrill) Winslow *et al.* Equally, or even more disappointing, is the fact that in each species only one locus apparently involved in pathogenicity and virulence has been mapped. In contrast, in *E. coli* several hundred genes involved in almost every possible physiological function have been mapped.

The reasons for this disparity in genetic information between two closely related genera are not clear but we feel that the principal fault lies with the failure of many plant pathologists to appreciate the enormous value of formal genetics. The best evidence to support this view is the fact that almost all of the information on the chromosomal genetics of *Erwinia* spp. has been provided by a single research group consisting of M. P. Starr, A. K. Chatterjee, and colleagues. So, as *Erwinia* said in the hypothetical conversation above, "I think it's them."

Why then did the pseudomonad ask "Could it be us?" We have recent evidence that suggests that even a concerted effort to understand the chromosomal genetics of several phytopathogenic pseudomonads, particularly those in the *P. syringae* pv. *syringae* Van Hall group, might come to naught. We will discuss this in detail in Section II.

In this chapter we will discuss that which is known of the chromosomal genetics of the leaf-spotting pseudomonads and the genus *Erwinia*.

II. LEAF-SPOTTING PSEUDOMONADS

Those phytopathogenic pseudomonads considered to be leaf-spotting or blight organisms are given in Table I. We will restrict the majority of

Table I. The Leaf-Spotting Pseudomonads and the Diseases They Cause

Pseudomonas syringae pathovars	Common name of disease
angulata	Angular leafspot or wildfire of tobacco
coronafaciens	Halo blight of oats
delphinii	Black spot of delphinium
gardeniae	Bacterial leaf-spot of gardenias
glycinea	Bacterial blight of soybean
lachrymans	Angular leaf-spot of cucumber
mori	Bacterial blight of mulberry
phaseolicola	Halo blight of beans
pisi	Bacterial blight of peas
syringae	Citrus blast, pear blast, bean leaf spot
tabaci	Wildfire of tobacco

the discussion of the chromosomal genetics to those members of the genus *Pseudomonas.* However, we will also discuss the potential for mapping the chromosome of the phytopathogen *Pseudomonas syringae* pv. *morsprunorum* (Wormald) Young *et al.* utilizing a recently discovered indigenous conjugative plasmid (Errington and Vivian, 1981).

A. Genetic Techniques

1. *Mutation*

One frequently used means of probing the chromosomal genetics of bacteria is physical and/or chemical mutagenesis, with subsequent selection for mutants of traits presumed to be chromosomally transmitted. That presumption is a great one, since it is well known that many phenotypic characteristics are extrachromosomally (plasmid) conferred. It has recently become common practice to examine those strains to be mutagenized for the presence of indigenous, cryptic plasmids, and if such are found, to attempt to remove the plasmids from the bacterial cells by curing techniques (Coplin, this volume, Chapter 12). However, before the techniques necessary for rapid isolation and identification of indigenous plasmids became available, this "control" was not attempted. Thus, many traits for which mutants were obtained, such as virulence, were only presumed to be chromosomal.

Nevertheless, the earliest attempts to probe the chromosome of the phytopathogenic pseudomonads were those attempting to correlate mutations of chromosomal loci for such phenotypic traits as the failure to synthesize essential nutrients (auxotrophy), resistance/susceptibility to antibiotics, or production of capsular polysaccharides, with changes in virulence.

Such studies, especially the earlier ones, were prompted by the appearance of antibiotic-resistant strains in nature (Stall and Thayer, 1962; Thayer and Stall, 1961). Dye (1958) noted this phenomenon and reported that only 7 out of 60 mutants of *P. syringae* pv. *syringae* Van Hall resistant to streptomycin remained pathogenic, concluding that the appearance of the resistant mutants did not seriously affect the efficiency of utilizing the antibiotic for control. Russell (1975) reached the same conclusion with streptomycin-resistant mutants of *P. syringae* pv. *phaseolicola* (Burkholder) Young *et al.* These and other workers concluded that mutations of any type reduced the fitness of phytopathogens and therefore reduced the virulence/pathogenicity.

Such a conclusion was not without considerable support. The premise that the success of a pathogen in infecting and colonizing a plant host is possible only under conditions of adequate nutrition and ineffective inhibition was presented by Garber (1956) as the basis for his nutrition-inhibition hypothesis. Many reports, usually based on the reduction of virulence in a small number of induced, presumably chromosomal, auxotrophic mutants, have appeared. Support for the nutrition-inhibition hypothesis in the pseudomonads was also provided by studies on *P. s.* pv. *syringae* (Ercolani, 1970) and *P. s.* pv. *tabaci* (Wolf & Foster) Young *et al.* (Garber, 1959).

These results in support of the nutrition-inhibition hypothesis imply the primary means of regulating the virulence of pathogens is the nutrition provided by the host. The further implications are that (1) if the required nutrient is supplied exogenously in some manner, this regulation will be removed and the auxotrophs will become virulent, and (2) that no auxotrophic mutants will manifest wild-type virulence without an adequate supply of the required nutrients. Recently, however, we have presented data which demonstrate that neither of these implications is correct (Thomas and Leary, 1980). In this study, it was shown that, while many of the induced auxotrophic mutants were avirulent, fully virulent mutants requiring histidine, or adenine, or methionine could be recovered at reasonable frequencies. These data also indicate that the levels of nutrient available in the plant to the auxotrophic mutants had little influence on their virulence. Another observation of note was that in all cases where avirulent auxotrophs were reverted to prototrophy, virulence was restored.

We suggest that in view of these findings, it is possible that chromosomal genes responsible for the virulent phenotype may be included in, coincident with, or regulated by chromosomal genes which determine nutritional characteristics and are therefore directly selectable. It should be possible to extend these studies and to obtain information which would support or refute this hypothesis. For this purpose, the technique known as sequential mutagenesis (Cerda-Olmedo *et al.*, 1968), based on mutagenesis with *N*-methyl-*N'*-nitro-*N*-nitrosoguanidine (NTG) which produces higher mutation frequencies in the replication region or "replicating fork" of the bacterial chromosome, may be useful. Thus, if synchronized bacterial cultures are treated with a unit dose of NTG for varying times and subsequent selection is performed for specific mutations, selectable mutations appear sequentially in the order that they are replicated. Theoretically, one could thus obtain an estimate of the relative order of the genes on the chromosome, unless replication is bidirectional rather than unidirectional.

Regardless of the mode of replication once such an order of gene replication is established, the relative position of a gene or genes involved in pathogenicity could be determined. If a significant number of avirulent auxotrophic mutants which did not recover virulence when prototrophy was restored were obtained, one could assume that the avirulence was due to a mutation in a gene very closely linked to the gene for nutritional competency. The sequential mutagenesis could be repeated. Surviving cells selected at times after exposure to the mutagen flanking the time at which the auxotrophs appeared in greatest frequency could then be directly tested for loss of virulence. The time after mutagenesis at which such avirulent mutants appear would establish the relative position of the virulence gene on the chromosome and establish flanking nutritional markers that could be used for further analyses.

Such analysis would not produce a detailed, complete map of a pathogen genome but directed mutagenesis has the potential to probe the chromosome of the phytopathogenic pseudomonads for loci associated with virulence. A complete understanding of the chromosomal genetics of these organisms will require the use of the genetic procedures so successful in other systems including conjugation, transduction, and transformation.

2. *Conjugation*

The process of determining the genetics of any bacterium by conjugal transfer and recombination of chromosomal genes is dependent upon several conditions. These are that: (1) the conjugal event occurs by the establishment of a stable contact between the donor and recipient cells; (2) only cells which have the capacity to function as donors of chromosomal material are capable of forming such contacts with potential recipients; (3) stable conjugal contact is required before the chromosomal material can be transferred from the donor to the recipient cell; (4) the capacity to function as a donor, establish the conjugal contact or bridge, and transfer chromosomal material to the recipient cell is conferred by an extrachromosomal DNA element (plasmid) present only in the donor at the time of conjugation; (5) the plasmid functions as the vehicle for transfer of the chromosomal DNA across the conjugation bridge into the recipient; and (6) the recipient cell must be capable of stable genomic incorporation and expression of genes from the donor chromosomal DNA.

To satisfy all of the above conditions would appear to be a tall order and maybe not possible. However, in order to list such conditions it is obvious that there are bacterial systems in which these conditions are met. The earliest information on the capacity for conjugal gene transfer and recombination in bacteria was obtained from the study of the plasmid fertility factor (F)-mediated chromosomal gene transfer in *E. coli* (Lederberg *et al.*, 1952). The F plasmid functions strictly as a sex factor. Thus, its presence in certain strains confers the capacity to function as a donor of chromosomal DNA by coding for the development of conjugal bridges (pili), coding for the capacity to intimately associate with the donor chromosome and thus incorporate chromosomal DNA into the F plasmid DNA, and coding for the capacity to move across the pilus into the recipient, and function as a vehicle for the transfer of host chromosomal DNA into the recipient.

The use of the F plasmid and its variants (F′ and Hfr) was the means by which the early maps of the *E. coli* chromosome were produced. Plasmids which function solely as sex factors were discovered in a few other bacterial genera, such as the FP plasmids in *Pseudomonas aeruginosa* (Schroeter) Migula (Holloway and Fargie, 1960), but the existence of fertility plasmids was considered rare. This apparent absence of fertility plasmids in the majority of the bacterial species of interest to phytopathologists precluded attempts to map the chromosomes of phytopathogenic bacteria by "*E. coli* methods." However, Holloway and Richmond (1973) showed that some antibiotic resistance (R) plasmids found in *P. aeruginosa* and *E. coli* could also function as conjugative fertility plasmids. Since some of these plasmids had very broad host-ranges (Datta and Hedges, 1972) they became candidates as sex factors in phytopathogenic bacteria. Later studies showed that these plasmids could indeed be transferred to the leaf-spotting pseudomonads (Cho *et al.*, 1975; Guimaraes, 1976; Guimaraes *et al.*, 1979; Lacy and Leary, 1975; Panopoulos *et al.*, 1975).

To determine that an R plasmid may transfer chromosomal material depends on the construction of multiple auxotrophs and/or multiple drug-resistant mutants. We emphasize the need for multiply marked strains to be used as potential donors and recipients for reasons which will be explained later.

Using this approach we were able to demonstrate for the first time that the antibiotic resistance plasmids would mobilize portions of the *P. s.* pv. *glycinea* (Coerper) Young *et al.* chromosome which converted the multiply auxotrophic recipient cells to prototrophy at one or more *unselected* loci (Lacy and Leary, 1976). The transconjugant recipients were selected by including an antibiotic to which resistance is conferred by the R plasmid and excluding from the medium a nutrient required by the recipient. Crucial to the assumption that the antibiotic-resistant, partially prototrophic transconjugants had received a portion of the donor chromosome was the demonstration that prototrophy was also restored at one or more unselected chromosomal loci. Otherwise, the possibility that the transconjugant had merely received the plasmid and a reversion had occurred to restore prototrophy at the single selected locus could not be excluded. Thus, the need for multiply marked strains for use in such crosses. Only when coinheritance of unselected markers can be demonstrated at frequencies approaching the appearance of prototrophs for the selected marker can it be assumed that conjugative chromosomal gene transfer has occurred.

Since reversion of auxotrophic loci to prototrophy can occur at significant frequencies, it is necessary for the researcher to determine in advance the reversion frequency of each and every marker in potential donors and recipients. Only those strains in which the auxotrophs revert at low frequencies (10^{-8}–10^{-10} revertants/auxotroph) should be used in conjugations. Such mutants are readily obtainable. And since mutation/reversion frequencies in a single strain are additive, another reason for having multiply marked strains and for always assaying for coinheritance becomes obvious. Consider the following example: a donor strain is constructed *leu thr* RP1^{+} and a recipient strain is constructed *his met rif*. The histidine requirement reverts to prototrophy at a frequency of 10^{-8} (a bit high but useful for this example) and the methionine requirement reverts at a frequency of 10^{-9}. In any cross of these donors and recipients in which selection is for His^{+}, putative recombinants are recovered at a frequency of 10^{7} recipient cells, a frequency which is uncomfortably close to the reversion frequency. If, however, 1–5% of those His^{+} transconjugants are also shown to be Met^{+}, it can be assumed that these cells resulted from the conjugal transfer and recombination of these loci from the donor, because the chances of such cells appearing spontaneously due to a double reversion are 10^{-17}, an undetectable frequency.

In addition to the need to rule out reversion by using multiply marked strains and assaying for coinheritance of unselected markers, such strains and procedures also permit the researcher to circumvent a problem frequently encountered in genetic analyses. We refer to the phenomenon as "feeding off their dead brothers." This rather indelicate phrase refers to the observation that, frequently, colonies will appear on the selection media which appear to be prototrophic at the selected locus. If such colonies are transferred to new plates of selective media they will continue to grow, prompting the researcher to conclude that they represent stable recombinants. However, this is frequently not the case. We feel that what is actually occurring is that the colonies detected are the result of the intimate association of donor and recipient cells on the selection plate and the subsequent unknowing transfer of both types of cells to the new plates. The easiest means to determine if the original colonies represent true recombinants or are due to the phenomenon described above is to streak for isolated colonies on selective medium.

Frequently, very few single colonies will appear outside the secondary streak. If these are subsequently treated in the same way, no growth will result other than in the area of the initial streak and this growth will rarely be as single colonies. By the methodical streaking and the use of defined selection media, the intimate association between the cells has been broken and the putative recombinants which were actually the mixed donor and auxotrophic recipient cells cannot survive without the required nutrients.

Although this task is tedious, especially if a large number of "recombinants" must be tested, it is made much simpler and results are more conclusive if multiply marked recipients are used and if the researcher insists upon a significant frequency of coinheritance of unselected markers!

We do not mean to discourage attempts to elucidate the chromosomal genetics of phytopathogenic bacteria. But such efforts to gain increased knowledge of the genetics of pathogenicity, host range, and regulation must have a solid base in classical genetic procedures, and must be precise, and conclusive.

Once the genetic methods were developed which permitted successful conjugal crosses of complementing, multiply auxotrophic donors and recipients, we initiated attempts to produce a map of the *P. s.* pv. *glycinea* chromosome using three-factor crosses (Lacy and Leary, 1975, 1976). Plate matings were performed on media supplemented with all but one of the nutrients required by the recipient in order to select for single-locus recombinants. The frequency of coinheritance of unselected markers was determined by plating the putative single-locus recombinants onto medium lacking another of the recipients required nutrients and determining the number of recombinant single colonies which grew versus the number tested. The inheritance and stability of the R plasmid vehicle was assessed by determining the antibiotic resistance spectrum of the chromosomal recombinants through several transfers. Several recombinants were subsequently shown to function as donors, demonstrating the functionality of the plasmid vehicle.

These studies provided evidence for a linear linkage group comprising 10 auxotrophic loci and 1 antibiotic resistance locus (Fulbright and Leary, 1978). The order of the loci on this segment was determined by analysis of three-factor crosses. No other linkage groups have been described in leaf-spotting phytopathogenic pseudomonads.

Unfortunately, no loci for pathogenicity/virulence were located in these crosses, since the donor and recipient strains were determined to be nonpathogenic. This condition was most probably due to the multiple auxotrophy and/or the repeated mutagenesis used to develop the multiple mutants. Consequently, new strains were developed utilizing the mutants of the newly described Race 8 strain, PgB3, as the wild-type parent. Each mutant was screened for pathogenicity. Only those auxotrophs which maintained near wild-type pathogenicity/virulence were considered as possible donors. The experimental plan which was to be followed was (1) construct auxotrophic, virulent donors which contained R plasmids; (2) develop antibiotic-resistant, multiply auxotrophic avirulent recipients which would not revert to virulence when the auxotrophic loci were reverted; (3) perform matings and select for prototrophic recombinants at one locus; (4) analyze for coinheritance of the unselected prototrophic markers; and (5) screen the recombinants for the recovery of virulence.

Preliminary experiments designed to establish recombination frequencies in this new strain were performed, using a number of different donors and recipients. However, we were unable to obtain any stable recombinants. The crosses were repeated and expanded until a total of 26 auxotrophic loci in the recipients and 6 plasmid vehicles had been tested. In no instance were stable recombinants isolated. These results were totally unexpected. One possible explanation that occurred to us was that the recombination frequency was so low that it could not be detected. But this was rejected because of the large number of crosses made and the number of cells plated for each cross.

Subsequent research has provided considerable evidence that the strains used are recombination-deficient (Rec$^-$) and that this condition existed in the wild-type parent. The evidence and implications of the Rec$^-$ phenotype in the wild-type will be discussed in a later section.

There have been numerous other reports of conjugal transfer of chromosomal genes in the phytopathogenic pseudomonads. Although Currier (1981) reported chromosomal transfer, coinheritance of unselected markers was not assayed, and we cannot be sure that these are evidence of actual conjugal gene transfer.

It appears, however, that all is not bleak and that systems will be developed for the successful investigation of the chromosomal genetics of phytopathogenic pseudomonads. Recently, Errington and Vivian (1981) reported the discovery of fertility in *P. s.* pv. *morsprunorum,* the causal organism of bacterial canker in cherry and plum. These authors performed crosses between doubly auxotrophic donors and recipients and putative recombinants were selected on media selective for one marker in each parent, the remaining two markers being unselected. Coinheritance of unselected markers was scored by replica plating to appropriately supplemented minimal medium. Using the nitrocellulose filter mating technique and the analyses described above, they detected an approximate recombination frequency for all four markers of 3.5×10^{-7}. This frequency was quite a bit higher than the highest reversion frequency at a single locus (3.8×10^{-9} for *gly-1*), providing good evidence for conjugal recombination. More convincing are the data on the coinheritance of unselected markers by which the possible gene order and the closeness of linkage were deduced. These data apparently demonstrate conjugative transfer and recombination of chromosomal genes and not reversion or transformation. The authors also state, though data are not given, that "donor ability" segregates among recombinants, suggesting the involvement of a chromosomal element as the conjugal vehicle rather than a plasmid which nearly 100% of the recombinants should acquire. The authors also state, though again data are not presented, that agarose gel electrophoresis analysis has failed to reveal consistent differences in the plasmid profiles of "donor" and "recipient" strains. They do not suggest, as perhaps they should have, that this situation is what would be expected if the "plasmid" vehicle was integrated into the chromosome, Hfr style. If further studies reveal that this is the case, it would represent a very exciting development for the study of the chromosomal genetics of phytopathogenic pseudomonads.

3. *Transformation*

The process of transformation, in which exogenously applied naked DNA is acquired by recipient cells and subsequently incorporated into the transformant's genome, represents a powerful tool in the study of the formal genetics of bacteria. This process is of tremendous value in recombinant DNA research. Several researchers have presented evidence for transformation (Gantotti *et al.*, 1979; Twiddy and Liu, 1972). However, the most convincing evidence has been reported by Gross and Vidaver (1981) and Sato *et al.* (1981). A concerted effort is being made to define conditions for successful transformation and identify and/or construct transforming vehicles for this important group of phytopathogens (Gross and Vidaver, 1981; Sato *et al.*, 1981).

4. *Transduction*

Although numerous bacteriophages, both lytic (Fulton, 1950) and lysogenic (Sato, 1978), have been isolated and characterized, there is not a single report of the successful transduction of a phytopathogenic pseudomonad.

B. Recombination: Yes or No?

Here, then, we finally come to the question asked by Sue: "Could it be us?" It is obvious that the most critical process necessary for the study of the chromosomal genetics of any organism is recombination. It is the only method by which inheritable alterations in the relationship of genes on the chromosome can be produced. In generalized recombination, reciprocal exchange of largely homologous genome segments occurs when mediated by host recombination mechanisms. The host mechanism is enzymatic and involves more than one enzyme. Generalized recombination is best understood in *E. coli* and has been the subject of several excellent recent reviews (Catchside, 1977; Eisenstark, 1977; Kopecko, 1978; Muskavitch and Linn, 1981; Radding, 1973; Schwesinger, 1977). Therefore, the reader is directed to these sources for detailed information on recombination mechanisms. In this section recombination as generalized from *E. coli* will be compared to the situation in phytopathogenic pseudomonads based on studies with *P. s.* pv. *glycinea* Race 8, strain PgB3.

The majority of generalized recombination in *E. coli* and other bacteria takes place due to the activity of deoxyribonucleases (DNases) designated *rec* A protein and *rec* BC exonuclease 5 (Exo V) protein. The *rec* A protein has both low constitutive activity and high inducible activity, the latter occurring after the introduction of foreign DNA. The *rec* BC Exo V protein is constitutive and can be detected easily in vegetative cells. The *in vitro* assay for Exo V is straightforward and relies upon the fact that the enzyme activity is absolutely dependent upon ATP. The assay is equally valid for crude lysates or purified preparations.

The phenotypes of *rec A, rec BC,* and *rec A rec BC* mutants are drastically different from the wild type and include (1) increased sensitivity to ultraviolet irradiation (UV), (2) decreased frequency of ultraviolet light-induced mutations, (3) increased sensitivity to the chemical mutagen methyl-methane-sulfonate (MMS), (4) increased doubling time, (5) decreased viability of cultures over time, (6) inability to harbor lysogenic phages, and (7) resistance to antibiotics such as novobiocin.

The *P. s.* pv. *glycinea* wild-type strain PgB3 and its derivatives manifest all of the above phenotypic traits, in addition to failing to produce detectable, viable, stable recombinants after conjugation or transduction. However, an intergeneric comparison of such characteristics may be inappropriate. The most acceptable comparison would be to Rec$^+$ strains of *P. s.* pv. *glycinea* such as those used in earlier studies. Such comparisons have been made and indeed, PgB3 is markedly more sensitive to UV and MMS, resistant to novobiocin, and has a considerably greater doubling time than the PgR strains used by Fulbright and Leary (1978). Thus, there is supporting evidence for the Rec$^-$ phenotype of PgB3 and other wild-type strains of *P. s.* pv. *glycinea* Race 8.

1. *Reasons for Rec$^-$ Phenotype—Experimental Evidence*

a. Rec A, Rec BC-like Systems. The inability to detect recombination suggests the absence of this process and therefore the absence of such recombination systems. Up to this point all of the support for this hypothesis has been purely circumstantial. However, tests for direct proof are available and, in the case of the *rec* BC product, Exo V, rather simple. The test is based on the knowledge mentioned above that *E. coli* Exo V is absolutely dependent on ATP for activity. Thus, if radioactively labeled linear dsDNA is incubated in an appropriate reaction mixture containing crude lysates of the bacterium, the linear DNA molecules will be reduced to trichloroacetic acid (TCA)-soluble fragments only if exogenous ATP is added. In the absence of ATP, the enzymatic activity is reduced up to 90%. When crude lysates of strain PgB3 are assayed in this manner, no ATP-dependent Exo V-like nuclease activity is detected (Thomas and Leary, 1980). In fact, the nuclease activity which is detected is inhibited by the addition of ATP. Isolates of *P. s.* pv. *glycinea* races 1, 2, 4, and 5 assayed in similar tests all showed an absence of ATP-dependent Exo V-like activity while control lysates of *E. coli* K-12, *P. aeruginosa*, and *P. fluorescens* Migula all exhibited Exo V-like activity. From these data, we must conclude that the *P. s.* pv. *glycinea* isolates examined do not possess a nuclease with an activity similar to that of the *rec* BC protein considered essential for stable genetic recombination.

The assay for *rec* A protein nuclease activity is considerably more complex and depends upon induction. Immunological assay of PgB3 for the presence of *rec* A protein using monoclonal antibodies to *E. coli* K-12 *rec* A protein (graciously supplied by Dr. Alex Karu, Dept. of Biochemistry, University of California, Riverside) showed no cross-reactivity, indicating that, at least, there is no protein of *rec* A-like antigenic activity. This result, of course, does not rule out the presence of an antigenically dissimilar protein with recombination activity but the other data would make that situation appear unlikely.

b. Restriction Endonucleases and Exonucleases. In the attempts discussed earlier (Section II,A,2) to assess conjugal transfer and recombination of chromosomal genes with PgB3-derived donors and recipients, it was more difficult to isolate potential donors containing the R plasmids. The frequency of transfer appeared to be considerably lower, and the stability of the plasmid-conferred phenotype was much reduced. Frequently, one or more of the plasmid-conferred resistances was lost. When the plasmid DNA from those transconjugants which expressed the complete antibiotic-resistance plasmid phenotype was examined by agarose gel electrophoresis, the plasmids were reduced in size. These observations suggest that at least one explanation for the changes in the plasmid was restriction endonuclease activity in the PgB3 recipients.

Recently, we have identified and partially purified endonuclease activity from lysates of PgB3 (Leary, unpublished results). There appear to be two enzymes, which are site-specific having similar but not identical activities. The enzymes will cleave both circular and linear DNA molecules, with the greatest activity being on linear λ and adenovirus DNA. Interestingly, the enzymes cleave the R plasmids RP1 and R68 into numerous fragments but there is no cleavage of pBR322. Further, an exonuclease activity has been identified which may be associated with one of the restriction endonucleases. The exonuclease is particularly active on linear dsDNA molecules and is inhibited by the addition of ATP or tRNA to the reaction mixture.

2. *Implications, Real and Theoretical*

Failure to demonstrate the existence of recombination system enzymes in PgB3 and other wild-type strains of *P. s.* pv. *glycinea*, together with the demonstration of the restriction endonuclease and exonuclease activities, suggests very strongly that the strains examined are incapable of generalized recombination. It is possible that other enzyme systems mediating low levels of recombination exist in these strains but no evidence for such activity has been obtained.

If the above is true, it implies that the phytopathogenic pseudomonads are genetically isolated. Such a possibility is also suggested by the near-identity of the majority of the phytopathogenic pseudomonads to the type-species *P. syringae*. In fact, the only significant difference between the bacteria in this group is the primary host they attack. That combination of similarity of most taxonomic characteristics and the fact that the members of the oxidase-negative, green fluorescent phytopathogenic pseudomonads can be distinguished only by host range differences, prompted the change from species status to that of pathovars of a single species, *P. syringae*.

The existence of Rec⁻ mutants in other organisms demonstrates that recombination deficiency is an evolutionary option available to bacteria, providing that it does not put the strain at a selective disadvantage. Organisms which do not depend primarily on pathogenesis for continued existence, such as *E. coli*, have evolved toward diversification and it is clear that generalized recombination has been a selective advantage by providing a broad gene pool. Phytopathogenic pseudomonads, unlike other bacteria, have evolved toward strict specialization and, therefore, a limitation on recombination may be advantageous. These bacteria are thought to have coevolved with their hosts, developing complex host–pathogen relationships. It is possible that if a bacterial population colonizing a plant is too heterogeneous, the host plants' resistance response to bacteria may be triggered, whereas when a single pathovar is present, resistance does not operate.

C. Conclusions

The experimental evidence reported here does not represent conclusive proof that virulent wild-type strains of *P. s.* pv. *glycinea* are incapable of recombination. There is the strong suggestion that this possibility should be considered when planning research on the control of these bacteria. If the Rec⁻ phenotype is conclusively verified in *P. s.* pv. *glycinea* and other members of the *P. syringae* group, there is a good possibility that significant information may then be obtained on the nature and evolution of pathogenesis.

III. *Erwinia*

Within the past decade, genetic research on the genus *Erwinia* has made this genus the most genetically understood of the phytopathogenic prokaryotes. Initial studies on the genetics of the erwinias were begun to sort out the confusing taxonomic makeup of the genus (Chatterjee and Starr, 1980; Starr and Chatterjee, 1972). Only the pseudomonads and xanthomonads can match the diversification found in this heterogeneous listing of bacterial species. Such diversification was imposed in the early days of bacterial taxonomy when the genus

Erwinia was originally proposed by a committee for those phytopathogenic bacteria that fit into the Enterobacteriaceae (Starr and Chatterjee, 1972). Therefore, this genus exists as a result of the separate development of plant and animal bacteriology. Today it, not unlike *Pseudomonas,* includes not only plant pathogens but human and animal pathogens as well as soil and plant saprophytes (Starr and Chatterjee, 1972). Phytopathologists have commonly divided the erwinias into four natural groups based on their appearance in culture and their pathogenic capacity (Dye, 1968, 1969a,b,c). These are briefly defined as follows: (1) the "Herbicola Group" which includes yellow-pigmented species associated with saprophytic growth on plants and soil, and also includes a number of strains associated with animal clinical specimens; (2) the "Amylovora Group" which includes those species that are nonpigmented and cause wilt or necrotic symptoms on plants; (3) the "Carotovora Group" which consists of the plant tissue-macerating species; and (4) a collection of miscellaneous species. The Carotovora Group, by way of bacteriological traits, appears to be more closely related to the coliform enterobacteria than the other three groups (Brenner *et al.,* 1972; Chatterjee and Starr, 1978; Mount *et al.,* 1979).

The true relationship of all organisms is found in their genetic composition. A genetic understanding of the various species placed in each group would help us understand the biological processes that make these organisms different. Many years ago, Riker (1940) stated that many fundamental questions regarding virulence, infection, immunity, and epidemiology could be approached through phytopathogenic bacteria. The construction of genetic maps has been useful in determining the location, number, and role of genes thought to be important in the differing ecological roles of many organisms (Matsumoto and Tazaki, 1971). Once constructed, these maps provide a framework in which genes involved in disease production, host specificity, the parasitic nature of the organism, and initiation of host defense mechanisms may be located (Chatterjee, 1978; Dickson and Postgate, 1971). It would be attractive to remove the gene systems that increase genetic compatibility and by introducing these into other organisms increase host range for potentially beneficial organisms (Dickson and Cannon, 1976). With such goals in mind, it soon becomes apparent why such importance is placed on constructing genetic linkage maps. However, it is difficult to discover the genetic makeup of organisms whose biology is unknown. A better understanding of phytopathogens and the diseases they cause can emerge only from concerted genetic, biochemical, biophysical, and pathobiological studies—in which disciplinary barriers are breached by comparative approaches (Chatterjee and Starr, 1980).

Although some may question the validity of grouping such heterogeneous species into one genus called *Erwinia,* there can be no doubt that they are placed in the proper family (Chatterjee and Starr, 1980; Sanderson, 1976; Starr and Chatterjee, 1972). The morphological and serological characteristics, types of fermentation end products, DNA base ratios, and recombination systems provide sound evidence of the relatedness of *Erwinia* to the Enterobacteriaceae (Starr and Chatterjee, 1972). DNA homology studies have compared the segmented homology between species of *Erwinia* and other enterobacteria. This work is based on chromosome homology comparison from a limited number of strains (Brenner *et al.,* 1972). Such experiments have indicated that the amount of relatedness shown by *E. carotovora, E. amylovora,* and *E. coli* is nearly equivalent to the size of segments shared by *E. carotovora, E. amylovora,* and *E. herbicola* (Gardner and Kado, 1972; Murata and Starr, 1974). Further studies showed that *Erwinia* is hardly separable from *Escherichia, Salmonella,* and *Shigella* (Murata and Starr, 1974). The four recognized natural groups discussed above form clusters based on this DNA homology, lending credence to these unofficial divisions. However, the extent of common segments was not great enough to warrant official recognition of any of the groups as a new genus (Murata and Starr, 1974). This demonstrated relatedness lends credence to Erv's statement "But I am just like *E. coli.*"

A. Genetic Tools

With the obvious degrees of relatedness between *Erwinia* and other enterics, it should not be too surprising to find that many of the techniques used for mapping other enterobacteria have also been successful on various *Erwinia* species (Bachman and Low, 1980; Chatterjee, 1978; Chatterjee and Starr, 1980; Pérombelon and Boucher, 1978). Reviews of the genetic systems in *Erwinia* have recently been completed (Chatterjee and Starr, 1980; Lacy and Leary, 1978) and therefore only a brief description of these genetic tools will be given here.

Chatterjee and Starr (1973) were the first to map chromosomal genes of an *Erwinia* species by conjugation. Unstable donor strains were constructed by transferring F'*lac*$^+$ and F'*his*$^+$ from *E. coli* into genetically marked strains (*lac* and *his,* respectively) of *E. amylovora.* Stable strains were selected after treatment with acridine orange. These strains, thought to be carrying integrated F'*lac*$^+$ or F'*his*$^+$, were subsequently tested for the ability to mobilize chromosomal genes. Those strains able to transfer chromosomal genes were called Hfr strains (analogous to the *E. coli* system for high frequency of recombination) because they transferred chromosomal markers in a polarized manner. Therefore genes could be mapped using time of entry analysis (interrupted matings), gradient of marker transmission analysis, and linkage analysis (two- and three-factor crosses) (Bachman and Low, 1980; Chatterjee and Starr, 1973, 1977; Pugashetti and Starr, 1975; Pugashetti *et al.*, 1978). This type of donor strain has been isolated in *E. amylovora* as well as *E. chrysanthemi* (Chatterjee and Starr, 1977, 1978; Pugashetti *et al.*, 1978).

Techniques similar to those used in F′ plasmid transfer were utilized to transfer R plasmids to *Erwinia* species (Chatterjee and Starr, 1972; Pérombelon and Boucher, 1978). Plasmid genes conferring resistance to a variety of antibiotics were used to select transconjugants. Certain R plasmids (RP1, R68.45, RK2, Rts1) will mobilize chromosomal genes in *E. amylovora*, *E. carotovora*, and *E. chrysanthemi* (Boistard and Boucher, 1978; Chatterjee, 1978, 1980; Chatterjee *et al.*, 1981; Guimaraes *et al.*, 1978; Lacy, 1978; Pérombelon and Boucher, 1978). Plasmid R68.45, which has been commonly used to mobilize chromosomal genes in various bacteria (Holloway, 1978), has chromosome mobilization ability (Cma) in both *E. chrysanthemi* (Chatterjee, 1980) and *E. carotovora* but not in *E. amylovora* (Chatterjee and Starr, 1980). Using R plasmids, chromosomal genes have been mapped by analyzing coinheritance data (Chatterjee, 1980). The mechanism of R68.45 (or any other R plasmid)-mediated gene transfer is not known. Since gradients of marker transfer rarely appear in *Erwinia* spp., a mechanism of generalized gene transfer is suggested (Chatterjee and Starr, 1980). Although R prime plasmids have been found in other bacterial systems (Holloway, 1978), no integrated R primes equivalent to the Hfr state have been used to map phytopathogenic bacteria (Guimaraes *et al.*, 1978). R plasmid-mediated crosses transfer shorter pieces of the chromosome than the Hfr system (Chatterjee, 1980).

A temperate bacteriophage mediating generalized transduction in *E. chrysanthemi* was isolated by Chatterjee and Brown (1980). This is the first transducing phage found in a phytopathogenic bacterium. This phage, Erch-12, when grown on a wild-type prototrophic strain of *E. chrysanthemi*, was capable of transferring eight auxotrophic markers, one gene conferring antibiotic resistance, and one gene coding for pigment production. Linkage has been established between three pairs of markers indicating that most of the markers were not closely linked. Therefore, small fragments of DNA are transduced (Chatterjee and Brown, 1980, 1981).

Commutation techniques, discussed in Section II,A, and transpositional mutations are tools that have been used to obtain desired genetic constructs in *Erwinia* species (Chatterjee and Brown, 1980, 1981; Guerola *et al.*, 1971).

Transposons are segments of DNA often carried on antibiotic resistance plasmids that can move from one genome to another [plasmid to chromosome; plasmid to plasmid (Boistard and Boucher, 1978; Boucher *et al.*, 1981; Kleckner *et al.*, 1977)] and are another useful tool for obtaining and locating mutations in *E. chrysanthemi* (Chatterjee *et al.*, 1981). Such mutations are important because they can mark specific segments of the chromosomes (or cryptic plasmids) that may otherwise be unobservable due to the lack of selection procedures. Transposon insertion mutations create strong polar mutations that may eventually be important in fine-structure mapping (Kleckner *et al.*, 1977). Plasmids carrying transposons TN5 (kanamycin resistance), TN402 (trimethoprim resistance), and TN406 (carbenicillin resistance) were transferred to *E. chrysanthemi* (Chatterjee *et al.*, 1981). Due to the instability of these plasmids in the host bacterium, these workers were able to select those colonies that lost the plasmid markers yet maintained the phenotype of the transposon. It is assumed that the transposon inserted into the chromosome or another stable plasmid genome. TN5 insertions have been determined to be responsible for *arg, met, cys, gua, ura, pat,* and *lec* mutations in *E. chrysanthemi* (Chatterjee *et al.*, 1981; Chatterjee, personal communication). See Table II for the names of genetic loci mapped in *Erwinia* spp.

B. Linkage Maps of *E. amylovora* and *E. chrysanthemi*

1. *E. amylovora*

Development of linkage maps in the genus *Erwinia* began in 1972 with the demonstration that F'*lac*$^+$ and R plasmids could be transferred from *E. coli* to various *Erwinia* spp. (Chatterjee and Starr, 1972a,b). It became obvious that "*E. coli* genetics" could be performed in these phytopathogenic bacteria. The first donor strain isolated was an F'*lac*$^+$ harboring Hfr strain of *E. amylovora* (Chatterjee and Starr, 1973). The donor transferred *arg*$^+$, *cys*$^+$, *gua*$^+$, *ilv*$^+$, *met*$^+$, *pro*$^+$, *ser*$^+$, and *trp*$^+$ into a number of recipient strains (Chatterjee and Starr, 1973). The markers were found to transfer with specific frequencies. The results of interrupted matings demonstrated that *cys*$^+$ and *ser*$^+$ had different times of entry in the course of the 3 hr mating process (Chatterjee and Starr, 1972a,b). Pugashetti and Starr (1978) placed 11 loci in relative order on the chromosomal map of *E. amylovora* by analyzing interrupted matings and coinheritance data. They found the Hfr strain constructed by F'*his*$^+$ integration (Hfr99 F'*lac*$^+$) is different in terms of origin and direction of transfer from that derived from F'*lac*$^+$ integration (Hfr159 F'*his*$^+$). For

Table II. Genetic Loci Mapped in *Erwinia* Species

Gene symbol	Phenotypic trait
lac	Lactose utilization
gtu	D-Galacturonate utilization
gal	Galactose utilization
trp	Tryptophan synthesis
his	Histidine synthesis
pat	Polygalacturonic acid *trans*-eliminase synthesis
idg	Indigoidine synthesis (blue pigment)
arg	Arginine synthesis
mcu	Glycerol, arabinose, ribose, xylose, galacturonic acid, polygalacturonic acid utilization
ilv	Isoleucine and valine synthesis
rif	Rifampicin resistance
ade	Adenine synthesis
lys	Lysine synthesis
ser	Serine synthesis
thr	Threonine synthesis
leu	Leucine synthesis
tra	Chromosome transfer
rbs	Ribose utilization
vir	Restores virulence in *E. amylovora*
prt	Protease synthesis
plc	Phospholipase C

example, Hfr99 transferred *cys*$^+$ and *ser*$^+$ as proximal markers and *ilv*$^+$ as a distal marker, whereas, Hfr159 transferred *ilv*$^+$ as a proximal marker and *ser*$^+$ as a distal marker, suggesting that the F′ plasmid genes integrated into different regions of the *E. amylovora* chromosome. This integration appears to be site specific since F′*lac*$^+$ always transfers *cys*$^+$ and *ser*$^+$ as proximal markers while F′*his*$^+$ transfers *his*$^+$ as a proximal marker.

Times of entry of *his*$^+$, *ilv*$^+$, *rbs*$^+$, and *ser*$^+$ were determined by interrupted matings in *E. amylovora* (Boistard and Boucher, 1978; Pugashetti *et al.*, 1978). Log-phase cultures of the recipient and Hfr donor were mixed and collected on filter membranes. After 10 min the filters were transferred to nutrient broth and the cells gently dislodged by gentle shaking. Samples of the mating mixture were transferred to buffer containing streptomycin (to kill the donor), vortexed vigorously to break mating pairs, and plated on selective medium. Samples were removed at the initiation of the matings (after cells were dislodged from the filter) and at various times during the 3 hr mating. The number of recombinants per milliliter of mating mixture was plotted against time and times of entry were calculated by regression analysis. Precise locations, in minutes, of markers were therefore determined by these interrupted matings.

The chromosome map of *E. amylovora* (Fig. 1) was synthesized using all available information obtained from times of marker entry derived from interrupted matings, transfer frequencies, and linkage of unselected markers. The latter two methods are less precise and exact map locations are not yet certain (Pugashetti *et al.*, 1978).

A gene(s) conferring virulence was located on the chromosome. In crosses involving avirulent recipients and virulent Hfr donors, the resulting recombinants isolated were as virulent as the donor strain. The segment of the chromosome conferring virulence was transferred within 15 min after the start of mating. This virulence segment is linked to *ser* and *rbs* (Pugashetti and Starr, 1975; Pugashetti *et al.*, 1978). The gene product(s) of this segment is (are) not yet known.

2. *E. chrysanthemi*

Twenty loci have been ordered on the *E. chrysanthemi* linkage map (Fig. 2) by analysis of conjugation and transduction data (Chatterjee, 1978; Chatterjee *et al.*, 1981). In crosses, utilizing Hfr8 (F'*lac*$^+$), the kinetics of marker entry and transfer frequencies indicate that *thr*$^+$ and *leu*$^+$ enter the recipient as proximal markers and that *lac*$^+$ enters as a distal marker. It appears that F'*lac*$^+$ integrates into the chromosome at a region adjacent to *thr*$^+$ and *leu*$^+$ (Chatterjee and Starr, 1977).

Although the transducing phage Erch-12 was able to mobilize eight chromosomal genes only three pairs were linked (Chatterjee and Brown, 1980, 1981). The frequency of coinheritance between markers *rif* and *ade* in recombinants from transductional crosses ranged from 3 to 5% (Chat-

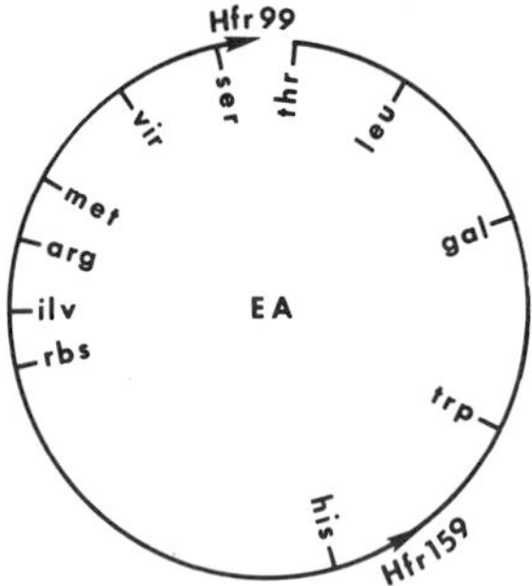

Figure 1. Linkage map of *Erwinia amylovora* strain EA 178. Genes have been mapped in relation to each other by time-of-entry analysis and coinheritance data. Circularity of the chromosome has not been established. The arrowheads indicate the direction of gene transfer. Hfr99 and Hfr159 indicate the sites of F'*lac*$^+$ and F'*his*$^+$ integration, respectively.

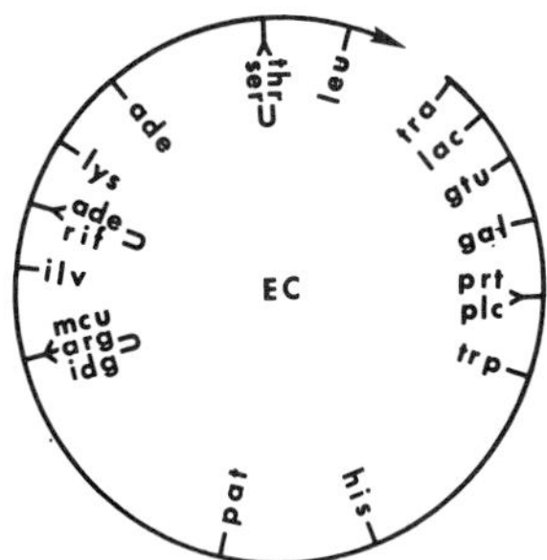

Figure 2. Linkage map of *Erwinia chrysanthemi* strain EC 16. Genes have been mapped in relation to each other by time-of-entry analysis and coinheritance data. Cotransduction of genes is indicated by ⊃. Unknown gene order is indicated by ≺. The arrowhead indicates the direction of gene transfer. A gene required for chromosome transfer is labeled *tra*.

terjee and Brown, 1980). In recombinants from R68.45-mediated conjugal crosses, the coinheritance of *rif* and *ade* was more frequent. Marker pairs *arg* and *idg* were also linked. Linkage between *arg* and *idg* was 72% during transduction but nearly 93% during R plasmid-mediated conjugation. This suggests smaller genomic fragments are transferred during transduction than during conjugation (Chatterjee and Brown, 1981).

As in *E. amylovora*, crosses between multiply marked avirulent recipients and virulent donors have located a virulence gene on the chromosome (Chatterjee and Starr, 1977, 1978). The gene, *pat*, codes for the production of polygalacturonic acid *trans*-eliminase (PATE). Transfer of pat^+ from virulent strains into pat^- avirulent strains restores virulence. This genetic evidence suggests that PATE plays an essential role in plant–tissue maceration (Chatterjee and Starr, 1980).

Although it may be premature to make many conclusions about gene order on chromosomal maps of *Erwinia* spp., it becomes evident that *trp*, *his*, *ser*, *thr*, *leu*, and *gal* appear to be similarly arranged on the maps of both *E. amylovora* and *E. chrysanthemi* (Chatterjee, 1978; Chatterjee and Starr, 1980). Furthermore, when *E. chrysanthemi* is compared with *E. coli*, 13 of the 20 known markers in *E. chrysanthemi* are arranged in an order similar to that in *E. coli*. In *E. amylovora*, 10 of the 11 known genes are in a similar, or near similar order (Chatterjee, 1978). Some gene segments may be inverted, but inversions have been noted between other enterobacteria (Chatterjee, 1978; Chatterjee and Starr, 1980). This knowledge has been useful in selecting mutants with close linkage (Chatterjee and Brown, 1980). For example, *thr* and *ser* and *rif* and *ade* are closely linked on both the *E. coli* and *Salmonella typhimurium* (Loeffler) Castellani & Chalmers chromosomes. Selecting for commutations in those genes provided evidence for cotransduction of closely linked genes. Therefore, it may be possible to use the *E. coli* map as a surrogate map when exact locations of genes are not known on the *Erwinia* spp. chromosome.

The evidence from DNA homology, recombination, F′ transfer and similarity in gene order suggest that *E. amylovora*, *E. chrysanthemi*, and *E. coli* may have a core of genetic material that is homologous. That F′*lac*$^+$ and F′*his*$^+$ from *E. coli* can produce gene products and complement metabolic defects in *Erwinia* further substantiates similarities (Chatterjee, 1978), although a variety of genes from different sources can produce functional products in bacteria (Mergeay and Gertis, 1978). Taken together it suggests that the enterobacteria have not been subjected to extensive genomic rearrangements and gene shuffling. Chatterjee and Starr (1980) theorize that the genetic information required for the evolutionary divergence in habitats in the enterobacteria was acquired later in their evolution, and that these changes were possibly superimposed on a core of genetic material that is homologous in all of the enterobacteria.

C. Regulation

Further evidence of genetic similarity could be provided in gene regulation studies. It will be interesting to discover the regulatory processes that might be found in *Erwinia* (Chatterjee *et al.*, 1981). Will the genes be regulated in an operon mechanism with positive and negative control? Is virulence turned on and off? The first such regulatory gene may have been mapped in *E. chrysanthemi* (Chatterjee, 1978; Chatterjee and Starr, 1977). When a fully virulent strain of *E. carotovora* is placed on sodium polypectate, the intracellular levels of PATE remain high. However, when glucose is added the level of PATE is decreased. Exogenously supplied adenosine 3′,5′-cyclic monophosphate (cAMP) reversed the repression and increased activity of PATE (Hubbard *et al.*, 1978). This system is analogous to that of carbon-catabolite repression in *E. coli* (Ide, 1971). Two classes of mutants with a pleiotrophic negative phenotype have been isolated in *E. chrysanthemi* that were found to be unable to utilize many sugars including galacturonate, polygalacturonate, and polygalacturonic acid (Chatterjee and Starr, 1977, 1978, 1980; Mount *et al.*, 1979). Levels of PATE were reduced in both mutants. PATE levels were increased when cAMP was exogenously supplied to one class of mutant, but the other class, labeled *mcu*, still could not utilize polygalacturonic acid after the addition of cAMP. The mutant has been mapped on the *E. chrysanthemi* chromosome and is separate from *pat*. Its function and gene location are similar to the cAMP-receptor protein

(CRP) found in *E. coli* (Ide, 1971; Mount *et al.*, 1978). Therefore, both pat^+ and mcu^+ are required for PATE synthesis. This establishes a cAMP–CRP system in the expression and regulation of the virulence locus in *E. chrysanthemi* (Chatterjee and Starr, 1980).

Acknowledgments

We wish to thank A. Karu for assistance and for providing the *rec* A protein and the monoclonal antibodies, Ms. E. Allingham for technical assistance in the unpublished research and for assistance in the preparation of the manuscript, and Mrs. BettyAnn Merrill for her excellent clerical assistance.

References

Bachman, B. J., and Low, K. B. (1980). *Microbiol. Rev.* **44,** 1–56.
Boistard, P., and Boucher, C. (1978). *Proc. Int. Conf. Plant Pathog. Bact., 4th, Angers* pp. 17–30.
Boucher, C., Message, B., Debieu, D., and Zischek, C. (1981). *Phytopathology* **71,** 639–642.
Brenner, D. J., Fanning, G. R., and Steigerwalt, A. G. (1972). *J. Bacteriol.* **110,** 12–17.
Catchside, D. G. (1977). *In* "The Genetics of Recombination" (K. R. Lewis and B. John, eds.), pp. 103–158. University Park Press, Baltimore.
Cerda-Olmedo, E., Hanawalt, P. C., and Guerola, N. (1968). *J. Mol. Biol.* **33,** 705–719.
Chatterjee, A. K. (1978). *Proc. Int. Conf. Plant Pathog. Bact., 4th, Angers* pp. 3–16.
Chatterjee, A. K. (1980). *J. Bacteriol.* **142,** 111–119.
Chatterjee, A. K., and Brown, M. A. (1980). *J. Bacteriol.* **143,** 1444–1449.
Chatterjee, A. K., and Brown, M. A. (1981). *Curr. Microbiol.* **6** (in press).
Chatterjee, A. K., and Starr, M. P. (1972a). *J. Bacteriol.* **111,** 169–176.
Chatterjee, A. K., and Starr, M. P. (1972b). *J. Bacteriol.* **112,** 576–583.
Chatterjee, A. K., and Starr, M. P. (1973). *J. Bacteriol.* **116,** 1100–1106.
Chatterjee, A. K., and Starr, M. P. (1977). *J. Bacteriol.* **132,** 862–869.
Chatterjee, A. K., and Starr, M. P. (1978a). *Proc. Int. Conf. Plant Pathog. Bact., 4th, Angers* pp. 81–88.
Chatterjee, A. K., and Starr, M. P. (1978b). *Proc. Int. Conf. Plant Pathog. Bact., 4th, Angers* pp. 89–94.
Chatterjee, A. K., and Starr, M. P. (1980). *Annu. Rev. Microbiol.* **34,** 645–676.
Chatterjee, A. K., Thurn, K. K., and Tyrell, D. J. (1981a). *Proc. Int. Conf. Plant Pathog. Bact., 5th, Cali, Colombia* pp. 252–262.
Chatterjee, A. K., Brown, M. A., Ziegle, J. S., and Thurn, K. K. (1981b). *Proc. Int. Conf. Plant Pathog. Bact., 5th, Cali, Colombia* pp. 389–402.
Cho, J. J., Panopoulos, N. J., and Schroth, M. N. (1975). *J. Bacteriol.* **80,** 362–368.
Currier, T. C., and Morgan, M. K. (1981). *Phytopathology* **71,** 869 (Abstr.).
Dixon, R., and Cannon, F. (1976). *Nature (London)* **260,** 268–271.
Dixon, R., and Postgate, J. R. (1971). *Nature (London)* **234,** 47–48.
Dye, M. H. (1958). *N. Z. J. Agric. Res.* **1,** 44.
Dye, D. W. (1968). *N. Z. J. Sci.* **11,** 509–607.
Dye, D. W. (1969a). *N. Z. J. Sci.* **12,** 81–97.
Dye, D. W. (1969b). *N. Z. J. Sci.* **12,** 223–236.
Dye, D. W. (1969c). *N. Z. J. Sci.* **12,** 833–839.

Eisenstark, A. (1977). *Annu. Rev. Genet.* **11,** 369–396.
Ercolani, G. L. (1970). *Phytopathol. Mediterr.* **9,** 145–150.
Errington, J., and Vivian, A. (1981). *J. Gen. Microbiol.* **124,** 439–442.
Fulbright, D. W., and Leary, J. V. (1978). *J. Bacteriol.* **136,** 497–500.
Fulton, R. W. (1950). *Phytopathology* **40,** 936–949.
Gantotti, B. V., Patil, S. S., and Mandel, M. (1979). *Mol. Gen. Genet.* **174,** 101–103.
Garber, E. D. (1956). *Am. Nat.* **90,** 183–194.
Garber, E. D. (1959). *Bot. Gaz.* **120,** 157–161.
Gardner, J. M., and Kado, C. I. (1972). *Int. J. Syst. Bacteriol.* **22,** 201–209.
Gross, D. C., and Vidaver, A. K. (1981). *Phytopathology* **71,** 221 (Abstr.).
Guerola, N. J., Ingraham, L., and Cerda-Olmedo, E. (1971). *Nature (London) New Biol.* **230,** 122–125.
Guimaraes, W. V. (1976). Ph.D. thesis, University of California, Berkeley.
Guimaraes, W. V., Panopoulos, N. J., and Schroth, M. N. (1978). *Proc. Int. Conf. Plant Pathog. Bact., 4th, Angers* pp. 53–65.
Holloway, B. W. (1978). *J. Bacteriol.* **133,** 1078–1082.
Holloway, B. W. (1979). *Plasmid* **2,** 1–19.
Holloway, B. W., and Fargie, B. (1960). *J. Bacteriol.* **80,** 362–368.
Hubbard, J. P., Williams, J. D., Niles, R. N., and Mount, M. S. (1978). *Phytopathology* **69,** 95–99.
Ide, M. (1971). *Arch. Biochem. Biophys.* **144,** 262–268.
Kleckner, N., Roth, J., and Botstein, D. (1977). *J. Mol. Biol.* **116,** 125–159.
Kopecko, D. J. (1980). *In* "Progress in Molecular and Subcellular Biology" (F. E. Hahn, H. Kersten, W. Kersten, and W. Szybalski, eds.), Vol. 7, pp. 135–234. Springer-Verlag, Berlin and New York.
Lacy, G. H. (1978). *Phytopathology* **68,** 1323–1330.
Lacy, G. H., and Leary, J. V. (1975). *J. Gen. Microbiol.* **88,** 49–57.
Lacy, G. H., and Leary, J. V. (1976). *Genet. Res.* **27,** 363–368.
Lacy, G. H., and Leary, J. V. (1979). *Annu. Rev. Phytopathol.* **17,** 181–202.
Lederberg, J., Cavalli, L. L., and Lederberg, E. M. (1952). *Genetics* **37,** 720.
Matsumoto, H., and Tazaki, T. (1971). *Jpn. J. Microbiol.* **15,** 11–20.
Mergeay, M., and Gertis, J. (1978). *J. Bacteriol.* **135,** 18–28.
Mount, M. S., Begman, P. M., Mortlock, R. P., and Hubbard, J. P. (1979). *Phytopathology* **69,** 117–120.
Murata, N., and Starr, M. P. (1974). *Can. J. Microbiol.* **20,** 1545–1565.
Muskavitch, K. M. T., and Linn, S. (1981). *Enzymes* **14,** 233–250.
Panopoulos, N. J., Grumaraes, W. V., Cho, J. J., and Schroth, M. N. (1975). *Phytopathology* **65,** 380–388.
Pérombelon, M. C. M., and Boucher, C. (1978). *Proc. Int. Conf. Plant Pathog. Bact., 4th, Angers* pp. 47–52.
Pugashetti, B. K., and Starr, M. P. (1975). *J. Bacteriol.* **122,** 485–491.
Pugashetti, B. K., Chatterjee, A. K., and Starr, M. P. (1978). *Can. J. Microbiol.* **24,** 448–454.
Radding, C. M. (1973). *Annu. Rev. Genet.* **7,** 87–111.
Riker, A. J. (1940). *In* "The Genetics of Pathogenic Organisms" (F. R. Moulton, ed.), pp. 46–56. Science Press, Princeton, New Jersey.
Russell, P. E. (1975). *J. Appl. Bacteriol.* **39,** 175–180.
Sanderson, K. E. (1976). *Annu. Rev. Microbiol.* **30,** 327–349.
Sato, M. (1978). *Ann. Phytopathol. Soc. Jpn.* **44,** 255–261.
Sato, M., Staskawicz, B., Panopoulos, N. J., Peters, S., and Hanna, M. (1981). *Plasmid* **6,** 325–331.

Schwesinger, M. (1977). *Microbiol. Rev.* **41,** 872–902.
Stall, R. E., and Thayer, P. L. (1962). *Plant Dis. Rep.* **46,** 389.
Starr, M. P., and Chatterjee, A. K. (1972). *Annu. Rev. Microbiol.* **26,** 389–426.
Thayer, P. L., and Stall, R. E. (1961). *Phytopathology* **51,** 568.
Thomas, M. D., and Leary, J. V. (1980a). *J. Gen. Microbiol.* **121,** 349–355.
Thomas, M. D., and Leary, J. V. (1980b). *Phytopathology* **70,** 310–312.
Twiddy, W., and Liu, S. C. Y. (1972). *Phytopathology* **62,** 794 (Abstr.).

Chapter **12**

Plasmids in Plant Pathogenic Bacteria

DAVID L. COPLIN

I. INTRODUCTION

The genetic information of a bacterium is contained in a large circular DNA molecule, termed the chromosome, and a variable number of accessory genetic elements comprised of plasmids, bacteriophages, and transposable elements. In general, accessory elements as defined by Campbell (1981) have two characteristics. First, they do not contain genes which are unconditionally required for the viability of their host cell, and second, they either replicate autonomously or can overreplicate their DNA with respect to the chromosome. Plasmids are a class of accessory elements which are capable of stable autonomous replication, i.e., they are maintained as physically separate entities from the

Phytopathogenic Prokaryotes, Vol. 2

Copyright © 1982 by Academic Press, Inc.
All rights of reproduction in any form reserved.
ISBN 0-12-509002-1

chromosome. Another class of accessory DNA, the transposable elements, are DNA sequences which are able to move from one location to another within the bacterial genome and are not capable of autonomous replication. They consist of insertion sequences (IS), which are short and have no known phenotype other than their effect on the genes that they are inserted into, and transposons, which are larger and carry genes which affect cellular phenotype. An important property of transposable elements is their ability to mediate many kinds of genetic rearrangements.

The distinction between different types of accessory elements is not always clear. Plasmids and lysogenic phages can insert themselves into the chromosome by additive recombination so they do not always replicate autonomously. Some phages, such as P1, can exist in the lysogenic state as plasmids while others, such as Mu, behave as transposons. Transposable elements have become part of both the chromosome and the genomes of plasmids and phages. The flow of information between chromosomal and accessory DNA, accompanied by dissemination of accessory elements to other strains, species, and genera, forms the basis for much of the variability which is characteristic of bacteria.

This chapter will focus on the occurrence of plasmids in plant pathogenic bacteria and the roles that they might serve as determinants of pathogenicity and survival and as agents of accelerated evolution.

A. The Nature of Plasmids

Bacterial plasmids are supercoiled, covalently closed-circular (CCC) DNA molecules. They range in size from small 0.7 megadalton (md) plasmids whose only function appears to be self-replication to giant 500 md "megaplasmids" which could be thought of as minichromosomes. Most bacteria harbor from one to three plasmids, but plasmidless strains are also common. At the other extreme, some bacteria contain as many as 13 plasmids comprising 25% of their genome.

Plasmid genes fall in two groups—those controlling plasmid replication and dissemination and those conferring a new phenotype on their host. The former group will be mentioned only briefly here because they have been discussed by Mills and Gonzalez (Vol. 1, Chapter 5). All plasmids contain sites for initiation of DNA synthesis and generally depend on host enzymes to carry out this process. The number of plasmid copies per chromosome is characteristic of a particular plasmid and is strictly regulated. Conjugation is also a plasmid-specified process which requires genes for synthesis of sex pili and replicative transfer of DNA. To prevent wasteful synthesis of transfer gene products, these genes are usually repressed. Unproductive plasmid transfer is also reduced by mechanisms which block mating pair formation between cells carrying the same plasmid (surface exclusion) and establishment of a plasmid in a cell which already contains a closely related plasmid (incompatibility). Some nonconjugative plasmids lack genes for synthesis of pili but still contain sites for DNA transfer. They can be mobilized by conjugative plasmids present in the same cell.

B. Role of Plasmids in Adaptation and Evolution

Reanny (1976) suggests that the role of plasmids in nature is to distribute the gene pool available to a species among a number of individuals. This enables bacteria to enjoy a rapid multiplication rate because no individual strain is required to replicate the entire genetic load of the species. Adaptation to changes in the environment could therefore come about by selection for strains containing an advantageous plasmid or by spread of the plasmid through an existing population, just as well as by selection of strains with different chromosomal properties.

Most plasmids described in the literature have a readily identifiable phenotype such as drug resistance. These plasmids undoubtedly do give a selective advantage to their host under certain conditions. However, under other conditions they must constitute a bionomic load. Furthermore, many plasmids lack obvious phenotypes and are genetically cryptic. Why then are plasmids maintained in the apparent absence of phenotypic selection? Campbell (1981) argues that overreplication of plasmid DNA with respect to chromosomal DNA, either through high copy number or conjugal transfer, is sufficient to maintain a plasmid in a population for a fairly long time but eventually it must provide an advantage to its host or be lost by dilution.

In many bacteria, especially plant pathogens, we simply do not have enough knowledge to say what functions their plasmids might possess or whether or not they might be advantageous. The nearly unrestricted flow of genes between chromosomal and accessory DNA means that almost any gene in a bacterium could become part of a plasmid. Since most studies on plasmid phenotypes usually focus on what effect eliminating a particular plasmid has on its host, it is quite possible that the presence of indispensable functions on plasmids has gone unnoticed since cured strains would not be viable. However, Campbell feels that this does not occur too frequently. The observation that within taxonomic groups the organization of genes on the chromosome is highly conserved, has led him to conclude that the bacterial chromosome represents a balanced and highly coadapted collection of genes which are not likely to be improved upon by reorganization. Plasmids, on the other hand, appear to be genetic nomads which contain genes that are adapted to function in a wide range of hosts. Thus, whereas the flow of genes between plasmid and chromosomal DNA occurs regularly, over time these may really represent two distinct classes of genes, one of which is specialized, the other of which functions in diverse genetic backgrounds.

The genetic complexity of plasmids indicates that they are products of long and successful evolution. Thus, the ability of plasmids to replicate, interact with chromosomal genes, and disseminate themselves may in itself be of value to their host by accelerating its evolution. Plasmids can do this in their role as vectors of transposable elements which, in addition to inactivating the gene they are inserted into can cause deletions, inversions, and transpositions of adjacent chromosomal DNA. As part of the transposition process they also create replicon fusions. When this results in the integration of a conjugative plasmid into the chromosome, the plasmid can then mobilize chromosomal markers either by Hfr transfer followed by substitutive recombination or through the formation of prime plasmids containing chromosomal DNA. The merodiploidy brought about by prime plasmids allows gene amplification and genetic drift to occur.

C. Phenotypic Functions of Plasmids

Plasmids were first discovered in human clinical strains of bacteria exhibiting infectious multiple drug resistance. Acquisition of these plasmids, called R plasmids, endowed their hosts with resistance to many antibiotics at once. Because of the health consequences, methods were developed for the physical and genetic characterization of R plasmids. In the process, microbiologists soon discovered that plasmids were a general phenomenon in bacteria and could confer many new traits on their hosts. In addition to antibiotic resistance, plasmids can specify (1) resistance to heavy metals and pesticides, (2) production of bacteriocins, (3) sensitivity or resistance to phages and bacteriocins, (4) catabolic pathways such as those for degradation of sugars, organic acids, and hydrocarbons, (5) synthesis of restriction enzymes, (6) symbiotic nitrogen fixation, and (7) pathogenicity to animals and plants.

In many cases the phenotype of a plasmid has been discovered when it was noticed that a particular trait was variable or unstable and then the trait was correlated with the presence of a particular plasmid. This is a valuable preliminary observation, but more lines of evidence are usually needed to prove that the genes of interest are, in fact, located on a plasmid. A good first step in proving this is to treat the culture with agents known to eliminate or "cure" plasmids and look for concomitant loss of both the trait and the plasmid. Effective curing agents are intercalating dyes, such as acridine orange or mitomycin C, high temperatures, detergents, rifamycin, coumeromycin, and pilus-dependent phages. It should be noted, however, that many of the chemicals used for this purpose are mutagens and may lead one to false conclusions. The best approach, but not always the easiest, is to transfer the plasmid to a plasmidless strain by conjugation or transformation and demonstrate linkage between the trait and other plasmid markers or plasmid DNA. In the absence of selectable markers on the plasmid, its transfer may be detected if it can mobilize a nonconjugative plasmid or it it can be mobilized by an R plasmid. By curing a strain and then transferring the plasmid back into it, one can essentially complete Koch's postulates with the plasmid and in the process obtain homogenic strains for physiological comparison. If transposons can be introduced into the strain, they can be used to provide selectable markers on the plasmid so that its transfer or curing can be detected. Furthermore, transposon insertions in the plasmid may inactivate the genes of interest and provide a means of mapping them on the plasmid. Special "suicide plasmids" can be used to create transposon insertions. These are plasmids which can transfer into a species but subsequently fail to replicate or else are very unstable. Selection for transfer of a transposable marker on the plasmid usually yields low frequency transconjugants with transposon-induced mutations. Several suicide plasmids are available which work in plant pathogens. Beringer *et al.* (1978) have constructed an incompatibility group P1 plasmid, pJB4JI, which contains a Mu prophage and Tn5. This plasmid works well in the Rhizobiaceae and some enterics. Sato *et al.* (1981) have combined a ColE1 plasmid with a replication deficient RK2 plasmid which contains Tn7. This plasmid can transfer to *Pseudomonas* from *Escherichia coli* (Migula) Castellani & Challmers but cannot replicate in *Pseudomonas.* An *Erwinia stewartii* (Smith) Dye plasmid containing Tn10 and Mu *cts62 kan* insertions is unstable after transfer from *E. coli* to *E. stewartii* and has been used to isolate Mu-induced avirulent mutants (McCammon and Coplin, 1981). Brown *et al.* (1981) isolated a temperature-sensitive mutant of the broad host range plasmid pUT13 which they used to obtain Tn406-induced auxotrophic mutants in *Erwinia chrysanthemi* Burkholder *et al.*

In order to appreciate the possible significance of plasmids in plant pathogenic bacteria, we need to examine the important role that they play in determining the pathogenic potential of many animal pathogens. Major virulence factors such as toxins, adherence antigens, and iron sequestering compounds are frequently encoded by plasmids. This subject has recently been reviewed by Elwell and Shipley (1980) and the reader is referred to their excellent article for references to the following work on plasmids in *E. coli* and *Staphylococcus aureus* Rosenbach.

Escherichia coli is probably the best studied system in which plasmids control pathogenicity. Certain enteropathogenic strains of *E. coli* cause diarrheal illnesses in man and animals. These strains produce one or both of two types of enterotoxins: a heat-labile toxin (LT) which is a high-molecular-weight antigenic protein and a heat-stable toxin (ST) which is a low-molecular-weight nonantigenic polypeptide. In order to proliferate and be retained in the intestines, these strains must be able to adhere to epithelium cells. Colonization is associated with the presence of certain pilus-like surface antigens. In porcine strains these are the K88 antigens and in human strains they are the CFAI and CFAII antigens.

Plasmids have been shown to carry determinants for either or both the ST and LT enterotoxins and are grouped according to which toxins they encode. Plasmids carrying both ST and LT range from 55 to 61 md. Genetic and physical analysis has shown that they are highly related to each other and to plasmids of the F incompatibility complex. ST plasmids, on the other hand, are quite diverse. This is probably because ST genes, unlike LT genes, are transposable and have located themselves on a number of different plasmids. Not as much is known about the genetics of plasmids which specify only LT toxin. It appears that they may also be heterogeneous. It is also possible for the ST and LT genes to occur on separate plasmids in the same strain. Enteropathogenic strains routinely harbor five or more plasmids including some R plasmids. It is not surprising, therefore, that strains have been found in which toxin production and antibiotic resistance have become linked. Colonization antigens are also found on plasmids. Genes for the porcine K88 antigens and raffinose utilization are often linked on the same plasmid and in a human strain the CFAI genes were located on an ST plasmid.

Another group of *E. coli* strains causes extraintestinal infections in man and animals. Isolates from these infections are usually hemolytic, produce colicin V, hemagglutinate red blood cells in the presence of D-mannose, and kill 13-day-old chick embryos. Invasiveness is associated with carriage of the Col V plasmid. This plasmid makes the bacterium more resistant to host defenses, primarily those dependent on antibody and complement. It also specifies production of a novel iron uptake system mediated by the hydroxamate siderophore aerobactin. This compound allows bacteria to grow in the presence of transferrin, an iron binding protein found in serum.

A few invasive strains of *E. coli* produce a toxin which is lethal for rabbits, mice, and chickens. Genes for its production are located on Vir plasmids which also specify a surface antigen. Two Vir plasmids have been characterized. They are both 92 md in size, conjugative, and appear to be related to each other but not identical. Fortunately, Vir plasmids are rare at present and it is not known what, if any, role they play in human disease.

Other Gram-negative bacteria which contain virulence plasmids are *Shigella sonnei* (Levine) Weldin (Sansonetti *et al.*, 1981), *Yersinia pestis* (Lehmann & Neumann) Loghem (Ben-Gurion and Shafferman, 1981), *Y. enterocolitica* (Schleifstein & Coleman) Frederikun (Portnoy *et al.*, 1981), *Y. pseudotuberculosis* (Pfeiffer) Smith & Thal (Ben-Gurion and Shafferman, 1981), and *Vibrio anguillarum* Bergeman (Crosa *et al.*, 1977). In *V. cholerae* Pacini, however, the situation is reversed and certain plasmids are associated with attenuated strains (Sinha and Scrivastava, 1978).

Plasmids are determinants of toxin production in Gram-positive bacteria too. *Staphylococcus aureus* has a small, 0.75 md plasmid that apparantly regulates expression of chromosomal genes for synthesis of enterotoxin B, the toxin involved in food poisoning. Other strains of *S. aureus*, which cause epidermal infections, produce an extracellular toxin called exfoliative toxin. Structural genes for this toxin are situated on either or both a 3.3 md plasmid and the chromosome. It is interesting that the toxins produced by plasmid and chromosomal genes differ in molecular weight and antigenic specificity.

II. OCCURRENCE OF PLASMIDS IN PLANT PATHOGENIC BACTERIA

A. Isolation Techniques

Small plasmids are probably the easiest of all macromolecules to isolate because of their CCC form. In any plasmid isolation procedure the basic steps are lysis of the bacteria with lysozyme and detergent followed by separation of CCC DNA from linear and open-circular (OC) plasmid DNA and sheared chromosome fragments. Usually the plasmid preparation is deproteinized with phenol or chloroform-isoamyl alcohol and then concentrated by ethanol or isopropanol precipitation. This produces a "cleared lysate" which can be analyzed directly by agarose gel electrophoresis or rate zonal sucrose density gradient centrifugation. Alternatively, the DNA can be further purified by isopynic centrifugation in CsCl density gradients containing ethidium bromide. This technique is based on the ability of ethidium bromide to bind to DNA and lower its buoyant density. Physical constraints on CCC DNA do not permit it to bind as much ethidium bromide as linear or OC DNA so that it bands at a higher density in the presence of the dye.

Various procedures are used to separate plasmid and chromosomal DNA during extraction. Small plasmids (<70 md) can be separated from chromosomal DNA by selective release from cells treated with nonionic detergents, sedimentation of chromosomal DNA along with cellular debris, or precipitation of large DNA by high polyethylene glycol or salt concentrations. Extremely large plasmids require a different approach to reduce shear and obtain better recovery. Currier and Nester (1976) found that if DNA is denatured by alkali and then rapidly neutralized, CCC DNA, whose strands remain concatenated, can reanneal whereas linear and OC DNA cannot. Remaining single-stranded DNA can then be removed from the preparation by a combination of salt precipitation, phenol extraction, and differential alcohol precipitation. A number of variations of this method have appeared (Birnboim and Doly, 1979; Casse *et al.*, 1979; Hanson and Olsen, 1978) and they are excellent for examination of plasmids in plant pathogens because they give good recovery of plasmids which range in size from 3 to over 200 md. The rapid microscale technique of Birnboim and Doly is especially useful for screening a large number of strains.

Megaplasmids (300–500 md) have been recently discovered in strains previously thought to be plasmid-free using a modification (Gonzalez *et al.*, 1981; Zischek *et al.*, 1982) of the technique of Eckhardt *et al.* (1978). In this procedure cells are gently lysed in the wells of the electrophoresis gel.

B. Distribution

Plasmids have now been reported in all genera of plant pathogenic bacteria. A list of the species shown to contain plasmids is given in Table I. With the exceptions of *Erwinia stewartii* and *Pseudomonas solanacearum* (Smith) Smith, which are discussed below, plant pathogens are not unusual in terms of the size or number of plasmids they harbor. Most studies to date have only reported the presence of plasmid DNAs; very little is known about their genetics.

Giant megaplasmids have been found in *P. solanacearum* by Zischek *et al.* (1982) using a modified Eckhardt (1978) procedure. Accurate sizing of these plasmids is impossible due to the unavailability of appropriate electrophoresis standards and the slow mobility of such large molecules on gels, but they appear to be at least 300 to 500 md in size. Eight of nine strains examined contained these plasmids. Considering their size, which may account for almost 25% of the genome, it is quite possible that these plasmids will be found to specify what are normally considered chromosomal functions.

Erwinia stewartii is unusual because it has a complex plasmid system which also comprises as much as 25% of its genome. In a survey of 39 strains of *E. stewartii*, Coplin *et al.* (1982) found that virulent strains had at least eight plasmids and most strains contained between 11 and 13 plasmids ranging in molecular weight from 2.7 to ca. 210 md (Fig. 1). Eight size classes of "common" plasmids, 210, 68, 49, 43, 29.5, 16.8, 8.8, and 2.8 md, were found in 87% or more of the strains. Other size classes of plasmids were also quite frequent; 23, 33, 34.5, and 51 md plasmids were found in 29 to 65% of the strains. Molecular weights of the plasmids in strains SW2 and SS104 were determined by both electron microscopy and agarose gel electrophoresis (Coplin *et al.*, 1981b). Multiple plasmids were present in all *E. stewartii* strains examined from midwestern, southern, and eastern states. Moreover, strains isolated in 1940

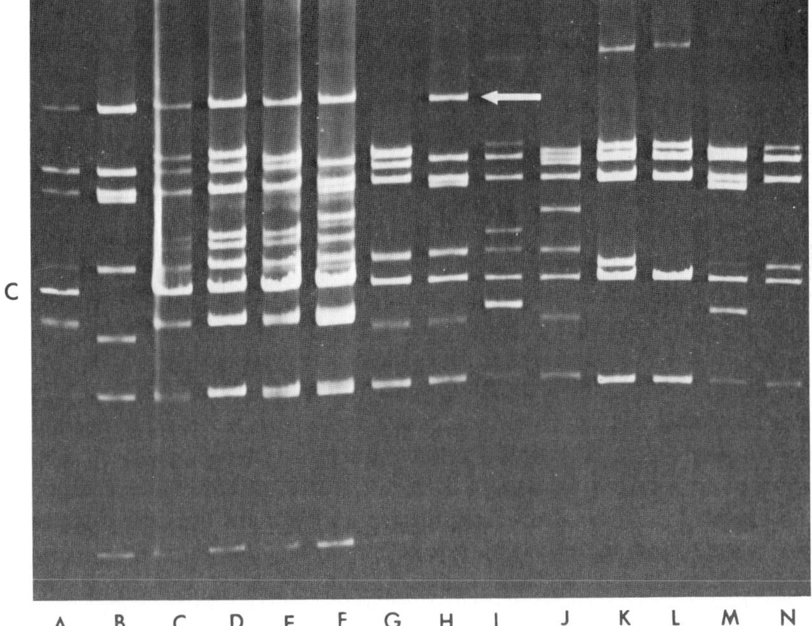

Figure 1. Agarose gel electrophoresis of plasmid DNA from *Erwinia stewartii* strains (A) SW18, (B) SS104, (C) SW2, (D) SW14, (E) SW13, (F) SW3, (G) GC6, (H) LC, (I) DC150, (J) ES-4, (K) SS10, (L) SS12, (M) SS11, and (N) SS13. Strains in lanes A–H are virulent and in lanes I–N are avirulent. The arrow indicates the 68 md plasmids and C denotes chromosomal DNA.

Table I. Plant Pathogenic Bacteria Reported to Contain Indigenous Plasmids[a]

Bacterium	Number of strains with plasmids	Number of plasmids per strain	Range of molecular weights (md)	Reference
Agrobacterium				
radiobacter	19/21	1–3	11–182	Merlo and Nester (1977); Sheikholeslam *et al.* (1978)
rhizogenes	3/3	1–3	107–259	White and Nester (1980)
tumefaciens	26/26	1–4	24–158	Sciaky *et al.* (1978)
Corynebacterium				
flaccumfaciens				
pv. *oortii*	1/1	2	46–48	Gross *et al.* (1979)
fascians	7/7	1–2	77–100	Gross *et al.* (1979); Murai *et al.* (1980)
michiganense				
pv. *insidiosum*	5/5	2–3	23–53	Gross *et al.* (1979)
pv. *michiganense*	7/7	1–2	24–52	Gross *et al.* (1979)
pv. *rathayi*	1/1	1	47	Gross *et al.* (1979)
pv. *sepedonicum*	1/1	1	33	Gross *et al.* (1979)
pv. *tritici*	3/3	1	35	Gross *et al.* (1979)
nebraskense	5/22	1	34	Gross *et al.* (1979)
poinsettiae	2/2	1	35	Gross *et al.* (1979)
Erwinia				
amylovora	3/3	1–3		Panopoulos *et al.* (1978)
chrysanthemi pv. *zeae*	1/1	2	5–50	Sparks and Lacy (1980)
herbicola	3/3	1–3	7–41	Lacy and Sparks (1979)
stewartii	39/39	8–13	3–210	Coplin *et al.* (1980a,b)
Pseudomonas				
solanacearum	8/9	1	>300	Zichek *et al.* (1982)
syringae				
pv. *coronafaciens*	1/1	1	40	Piwowarski and Shaw (1982)
pv. *glycinea*	4/4	1–2	25–87	Curiale and Mills (1978)
pv. *phaseolicola*	39/39	1–3	4–110	Gantotti *et al.* (1979); Panopoulous *et al.* (1979); Jamieson *et al.* (1981); Quant and Mills (1982)

Table I (*continued*)

Bacterium	Number of strains with plasmids	Number of plasmids per strain	Range of molecular weights (md)	Reference
pv. *lachrymans*	1/1	2	58–86	Yano *et al.* (1979)
pv. *savastanoi*	1/1	4	22–38	Comai and Kosuge (1980)
pv. *tabaci*	8/8	1	30–50	Piwowarski and Shaw (1982)
Spiroplasma citri	8/8	2–6	1–26	Ranhand *et al.* (1980)
sp. (corn stunt)	1/1	2	4–9	Ranhand *et al.* (1980)
Xanthomonas campestris				
pv. *manihotis*	?	2	3–17	Lin and Chen (1978)
pv. *vesicatoria*	7/7	2–3	—	Dahlbeck *et al.* (1977)

[a] The bacterial names used are the names suggested by Skerman *et al.* (1980) or Dye *et al.* (1980).

(Fig. 1, lanes K–N) had plasmids typical of contemporary strains indicating that these plasmids are stable both in culture and in nature. Plasmid profiles of *E. stewartii* strains show such remarkable similarities that they can be used as a practical means of identifying this species. We have examined several cultures of the closely related species, *E. milletiae* (Kawakami and Yoshida) Margrow and *E. herbicola* (Löhnis) Dye and they did not contain a large number of plasmids comparable to those of *E. stewartii* (Coplin, unpublished results). Cultures of the later species from corn (*Zea mays* L.) were similar to *E. stewartii* in nutritional capabilities, phage sensitivity, and agglutination by an anti-SW2 serum. Similar results were obtained by Lacy and Sparks (1979) who reported three size classes of plasmids in several strains of *E. herbicola*.

It will be interesting to see if future hybridization studies confirm our notion that similar sized plasmids in different strains of *E. stewartii* are in fact the same plasmids. Preliminary evidence that this is the case comes from comparison of restriction digests of total plasmid DNA from six strains (Coplin *et al.*, 1982). Virulent strains shared 21–23 *Bam*HI fragments even though they contained several different plasmids. This result also suggests the possibility that there is some redundancy among the plasmids of a strain due to the presence of cointegrates.

Although multiple plasmid carriage is known in the Enterobacteriaceae, it is a usually characteristic of individual strains rather than a species. Why *E. stewartii* has evolved such a complex plasmid system is a mystery. Only *Bacillus megaterium* deBary and *B. thuringiensis* Berliner have as many different plasmids in a single strain. We need more knowledge of the phenotypes of these plasmids, especially the common ones, in order to say what advantage there might be in maintaining so many genes as plasmids rather than chromosomal DNA. Certainly the plasmid system of *E. stewartii* must represent a coadapted group of genes. One possible explanation for the stability of this system may be due to the periodic alternation of ecological niches that *E. stewartii* undergoes. This bacterium must be able to colonize the alimentary tract of the corn flea beetle (*Chaetocnema pulicaria* Melsh.) in order to overwinter and it must be able to infect corn plants between generations of beetles. Thus, traits which enable it to grow both in plants and insects must be stable for many generations in the absence of phenotypic selection.

Common plasmids are also present in various pathovars of *P. syringae* van Hall. Quant and Mills (1982) and Mills and Gonzalez (Vol. 1, Chapter 5) compared plasmids in five strains of *P. s.* pv. *phaseolicola* (Burkholder) Young *et al.* for number, size, and relatedness. Comparison of *Bam*HI and *Eco*RI digests of total plasmid DNA from strain PP612, which contains 1.4 and 96 md plasmids, with DNA of the single 108 md plasmid in strain PP622 revealed at least 92% sequence homology between the plasmids in these two strains. Two other strains, PP601 and PP631, shared a 72.5 md plasmid and in addition PP601 contained a 28.5 md plasmid and PP631 had a 26.8 md plasmid. *Eco*RI digests indicated at least 81% homology between the plasmids in these strains. By the same criteria, PP652 had a 70 md plasmid and a 33 md plasmid which shared 70% homology with PP601 and 65% homology with PP631 plasmids. Among all strains there was 46% homology. Solution hybridization also confirmed a high level of homology between these strains. Jamieson *et al.* (1981) also looked at plasmids in *P. s.* pv. *phaseolicola* and reported hybridization between the 22.5 md plasmids present in three strains.

Piwowarski and Shaw (1982) examined the plasmids in five strains of *P. s.* pv. *tabaci* (Wolf & Foster) Young *et al.* and one strain of *P. s.* pv. *coronafaciens* (Elliot) Young *et al.* which produced tabtoxin. They also looked at three tabtoxin minus strains that had previously been identified as *P. angulata* (Fromme & Murray) Holland. All of the strains contained a single plasmid species between 29.5 and 49.8 md. Plasmids were compared by restriction analysis and Southern blot hybridization. Three of the *P. s.* pv. *tabaci* strains had an identical 44.5 md plasmid,

JP1; a fourth *P. s.* pv. *tabaci* strain and the three "angulata" strains shared the same 49.8 md plasmid, JP27. The JP1 group of plasmids had an 8.8 md region of homology with the JP27 group. *P. s.* pv. *coronafaciens* had a 39.7 md plasmid which contained the common 8.8 md region plus additional regions of homology with either JP1 or JP27. In contrast, strain PTBR-2, the only strain of *P. s.* pv. *tabaci* from beans (*Phaseolus vulgaris* L.) rather than tobacco (*Nicotiana tobacum* L.), had a 30.4 md plasmid which lacked detectable homology with any of the other plasmids.

In contrast to these studies, Gonzalez and Vidaver (1980) examined three strains of syringomycin producing *P. s.* pv. *syringae* van Hall from millet (*Eleusine coracana* Gaertn.), almond (*Prunus amygdalus* Batsch), and apricot (*P. americana* Marsh.). Each strain had a 35 md plasmid but their restriction patterns were different.

Strains of *Agrobacterium tumefaciens* (Smith & Townsend) Conn all contain one or more large plasmids ranging in size from 95 to 158 md. One of these, the Ti plasmid, is always necessary for tumor induction. This subject has been reviewed by Kemp (Vol. 1, Chapter 18), Merlo (this volume, Chapter 13), Mills and Gonzalez (Vol. 1, Chapter 5), and Nester and Kosuge (1981) so that *Agrobacterium* plasmids will be discussed only briefly in this chapter and the reader is referred to these reviews for references. Ti plasmids generally fall into three groups according to their ability to code for the degradation of either octopine, nopaline, or agropine. Wide host range octopine plasmids and the few agropine plasmids examined seem to be related on the basis of sequence homology. The narrow host range octopine plasmids and the nopaline plasmids appear to be heterogeneous. Octopine and nopaline plasmids share a highly conserved 5.5 md region of DNA, called "common DNA," which is involved in oncogenicity. Other regions of these plasmids involved in tumorigenesis are also highly conserved. Sequence relationships between Ti plasmids are discussed in detail by Mills and Gonzalez (Vol. 1, Chapter 5).

For most plant pathogens, only the physical descriptions of plasmids have been published and they remain genetically cryptic. It is significant, therefore, that the few studies which have compared sequence homology between plasmids in a species have pointed up instances where whole plasmids or parts of plasmids seem widely distributed in nature. Since plasmids can easily undergo insertions and deletions and form cointegrates with other plasmids, it is possible that wider use of restriction analysis and Southern hybridization techniques will uncover even more instances of relatedness between plasmids of different sizes. While we are still blessed with ignorance, it is tempting to speculate that, as in the case of *A. tumefaciens,* this DNA is somehow involved in determining pathogenicity, since this trait is sometimes all that distinguishes a given pathogen from other pathovars or closely related species. From another viewpoint, the occurrence of common plasmids might be more than just coincidental if we are inadvertantly building bias into our culture collections by using a plasmid-encoded characteristic to identify cultures or by continually isolating them from an environment, i.e., a diseased plant, in which plasmid carriage is advantageous.

III. FUNCTIONS OF PLASMIDS

A. Pathogenicity

The family Rhizobiaceae is comprised of two genera, *Rhizobium* and *Agrobacterium.* Bacteria in both genera are able to cause plant cell proliferation. The presence of large plasmids (>80 md) is a general feature of this family (Casse *et al.,* 1979; Zaenen *et al.,* 1974) and they have been shown to control oncogenicity, nitrogen fixation, nodulation, and host specificity. Although *Rhizobium* is not a plant pathogen, it is of great interest to plant pathologists; studies on recognition of the capsular polysaccharides of *Rhizobium* spp. by plant lectins (Bauer, 1981) have provided the basis for many current theories which invoke host–pathogen recognition phenomena as part of disease resistance.

Species of *Rhizobium* exhibit host specificity; *R. leguminosarum* (Frank) Frank nodulates peas (*Pisum sativum* L.) and vetches (*Vicia* spp.), *R. phaseoli* Dangeard nodulates beans, and *R. trifolii* Dangeard nodulates clover (*Trifolium* spp.). Evidence that genes necessary for symbiosis and host specificity are on a plasmid came from studies on pRL1JI, a transmissible, 130 md, bacteriocinogenic plasmid from *R. leguminosarum.* A Tn5-containing derivative of this plasmid, pJB5JI, was transmissible at high frequency (10^{-2}) to isolates to *R. leguminosarum, R. trifolii,* and *R. phaseoli* that were nodulation deficient (Nod^-) or could not fix nitrogen (Fix^-) (Johnston *et al.,* 1978; Brewin *et al.,* 1980a). This plasmid was able to complement the defects in both nodulation and nitrogen fixation. Moreover, in another set of crosses between *R. leguminosarum* strains, the transconjugants acquired the host range of the donor strain. The ability to nodulate the pea cv. Afganistan and the primitive pea line JI241 was transferred with a 160 md plasmid, pRL5JI (Brewin *et al.,* 1980b). This plasmid is apparently compatible with pRL1JI and it is Nod^+ Fix^+ but nonbacteriocinogenic. In later studies (Beylon *et al.,*

1980), pJB5JI was transferred to *R. phaseoli* strain 1233. Most of the transconjugants carried the pigment marker of *R. phaseoli* and nodulated both peas and beans poorly. These transconjugants contained both plasmids normally found in 1233 plus pJB5JI. However, after reisolation of the bacteria from peas, the transconjugants had lost pigment production and could effectively nodulate peas but not beans. Examination of plasmids in the recovered strains revealed that the smaller of the two 1233 plasmids had been lost. These results suggest that genes for host specificity in *R. leguminosarum* and *R. phaseoli* reside on plasmids of the same incompatibility group and that host passage of the transconjugants was able to select for strains in which the smaller resident plasmid of 1233 had been displaced by pJB5JI.

Another symbiotic plasmid has been reported in *R. trifolii* (Hooykaas *et al.*, 1981). In similar studies, this plasmid was labeled with Tn5, shown to be conjugative at low frequencies, and used to complement Nod^- heat-cured derivatives of the same strain. Transfer of this plasmid to *R. leguminosarum* resulted in strains capable of nodulating not only peas and vetches but clover as well, indicating that host specificity is a function of this plasmid too. In addition, the plasmid was able to complement Fix^- mutants of *R. leguminosarum* showing that it contains part of the *nif* structural genes as well. The transfer of this plasmid to *A. tumefaciens* gave some surprising results. Transconjugants caused small, slow developing, nonfixing nodules on clover. Examination of the infection process revealed that *A. tumefaciens* could carry out most of the steps of nodule formation, i.e., root hair curling, host recognition, infection thread initiation, and release of membrane-enclosed bacteria into the plant cell. This work is dramatic evidence of the close relationship between *Agrobacterium* and *Rhizobium*.

The Ti plasmids of *Agrobacterium* spp. are probably the best known and most extensively studied virulence plasmids of any bacterium. Both *A. tumefaciens* (Watson *et al.*, 1975) and *A. rhizogenes* (Moore *et al.*, 1979; White and Nester, 1980a,b) strains contain large plasmids which enable their host bacteria to cause crown galls and hairy root, respectively. In addition to genes for tumor induction these plasmids also have determinants for (1) tumor morphology, (2) synthesis of indoleacetic acid (IAA) from tryptophan, (3) production of zeatin ribonucleotides, (4) host range, (5) periplasmic proteins, (6) cell wall recognition sites which may function in attachment of bacteria to plant cells, (7) utilization of opines and sometimes arginine, (8) synthesis of opines by tumor cells, and (9) sensitivity to Agrocin 84.

Another pathogen which produces hyperplasias in plants is *P. s.* pv. *savastanoi* (Smith) Young *et al.*, which causes knots and galls in olives

(*Olea europaea* L.) and oleanders (*Nerium oleander* L.). Bacterial synthesis of IAA *in planta* produces galls. IAA production is a major virulence factor in this disease since mutants unable to synthesize IAA fail to cause galls and mutants with an increased level of IAA synthesis incite more severe symptoms (Smidt and Kosuge, 1978). Two enzymes are involved in synthesis of IAA from tryptophan; tryptophan 2-monooxygenase (*iaa*M) converts tryptophan to indoleacetamide and indoleacetamide hydrolase (*iaa*H) catalyzes the hydrolysis of indoleacetamide to IAA and ammonia. The pathway is especially suitable for genetic analysis because IAA^- mutants and IAA overproducers are resistant to α-methyl tryptophan and IAA^+ strains are resistant to 5-methyl tryptophan because this inhibitor is detoxified by tryptophan monooxygenase. This makes selection for IAA genes possible. Comai and Kosuge (1980) isolated four plasmids from strain 2009 of *P. s.* pv. *savastanoi* with molecular weights of 38, 34, 27, and 22 md. IAA^- mutants selected for resistance to α-methyl tryptophan or obtained from acridine orange curing were missing the 34 md plasmid, designated pIAA1. Cured strains lacked both *iaa*M and *iaa*H activities and were avirulent on oleanders. When pIAA1 was transferred back to the cured strains by cotransformation with RSF1010, *iaa*M and *iaa*H activities were restored and the strains became virulent again. To further prove that IAA genes were located on the plasmid and to establish that the IAA genes alone were required for virulence, they cloned a 2.75 kb *Eco*RI fragment from pIAA1 into RSF1010 and then transformed the recombinant plasmid into *E. coli* (Comai and Kosuge, 1982). The cloned fragment contained only the *iaa*M gene and it was transcribed from an RSF1010 promoter in *E. coli*. When the recombinant plasmid was introduced into a pIAA1less strain of *P. s.* pv. *savastanoi*, virulence was restored indicating that only the *iaa*M locus from pIAA1 is necessary for IAA synthesis in this strain of *P. s.* pv. *savastanoi* and suggesting that *iaa*H may be duplicated on its chromosome.

Analysis of additional IAA^- α-methyl tryptophan-resistant mutants revealed that some of these still had pIAA1. However, in these strains, small 0.8 md insertions were detected in or very near the *iaa*M locus on pIAA1. The insertions had polar effects on both *iaa*M and *iaa*H suggesting that they are arranged in an operon.

The work with pIAA plasmids in *P. s.* pv. *savastanoi* is truly significant because it is the first instance where both the plasmid-encoded nature of a plant virulence gene and its product are known. So far only two strains of *P. s.* pv. *savastanoi* have been shown to have pIAA plasmids. It will be interesting to see whether *iaa* genes are located on similar plasmids or the chromosome in other strains, if they are transposable, and what other functions might be linked to them.

There is some evidence that plasmids may affect the virulence of *E. stewartii.* Garibaldi and Gibbins (1975) reported that *E. stewartii* strain SS104 lost virulence and pigment production at high frequencies following growth at 37°C, a finding which suggested loss of a plasmid. Coplin *et al.* (1982) compared plasmids in virulent and avirulent strains of *E. stewartii* using agarose gel electrophoresis. Among the avirulent strains examined were two nonpigmented variants isolated by Garibaldi and Gibbins (1975). These strains were missing the 49, 41.5, 22.5, and 8.8 md plasmids found in their parent strain. This study also showed that avirulent strains tended to have fewer plasmids than virulent strains. The most notable correlation was between virulence and the presence of 68 md plasmids; six of eight avirulent strains were missing this size class whereas only 1 out of 31 virulent strains were missing it (Fig. 1). The apparent exception among the virulent strains (Fig. 1, lane G) was examined further. *Bam*HI digests of total plasmid DNA from this strain contained seven fragment bands that were identical in size to fragments of the 68 md plasmid found in other strains. This suggests that the sequences from the missing plasmid may have been present on one of two smaller unique plasmids found in this strain.

Another series of experiments also suggests that the 68 md plasmid may affect virulence (Coplin, 1982). A derivative of this plasmid from strain SS104 has been constructed that contains Mu *cts*62 pf7701, a kanamycin-resistant derivative of bacteriophage Mu (Thompson and Howe, 1979). Strain SS104 carrying Mu pf7701 was heat shocked to induce Mu replication and then used as a donor in matings with DC350; selection was made for kanamycin resistance. Strain DC350 is a derivative of an avirulent strain isolated by Garibaldi and Gibbins (1975) from SS104 and described above. In this cross, it was expected that one of the plasmids present in SS104 but missing in DC350 would "pick up" a replicating Mu pf7701 prophage and transfer it to DC350. Instead, the only insertion obtained was in the 68 md plasmid, pDC190. To test the ability of this new plasmid to complement avirulent mutants, it was transferred to several strains that were missing 68 md plasmids, but it failed to restore virulence. This negative finding could have been explained by several hypotheses: (1) The avirulence of the recipients was not due solely to loss of the 68 md plasmid; (2) insertion of Mu into pDC190 inactivated the virulence genes carried by it; (3) pDC191 was derived from the resident plasmid in DC350 which may already have been defective; or (4) pDC191 has nothing at all to do with virulence.

Transfer of pDC191 to virulent strains, however, resulted in simultaneous loss of the resident 68 md plasmid and virulence. This result supported either hypothesis 2 or 3 above, but further examination of the transconjugants revealed a more complicated picture. Acquisition of pDC191 was often accompanied by the gain of various smaller plasmids, possibly the result of dissociation of the resident pDC190 plasmid. The transconjugants were either virulent or avirulent depending upon which new plasmids were present. Furthermore, when avirulent pDC191 transconjugants were cured of PDC191, the resulting strains were unstable and reverted to virulence. Reversion was accompanied by appearance of the same new plasmids. At present, these results suggest that pDC190 is a cointegrate plasmid and that incompatibility between it and pDC191 is resolved by dissociation of pDC190 and integration of some of the component plasmids into the chromosome. If integration then occurs at preferred sites, it is possible that the process inactivates either a plasmid or chromosomal gene for virulence. Precise excision of the integrated plasmid would be required to restore virulence. Hybridization studies are needed to test these hypotheses.

Attempts to associate plasmids with other traits of *E. stewartii* have been unproductive. A major virulence factor of this pathogen is extracellular polysaccharide. Mutants which cannot make capsules and slime can cause lesions but not systemic wilting. Analysis of a large number of nonencapsulated mutants did not reveal any consistent differences in plasmid content (Bradshaw-Rouse *et al.*, 1981). Likewise attempts to associate plasmids with antibiotic and heavy metal resistance, nutritional capabilities, and bacteriocin production have been negative. In addition all *E. stewartii* plasmids are compatible with R plasmids from over 13 different incompatibility groups originating in the Enterobacteriaceae (Ashbaugh, 1980).

The pathovars of *P. syringae* form a closely related group of bacteria which are primarily distinguished on the basis of host specificity. Many members of this group produce chlorosis or necrosis inducing toxins. Often the ability to produce a given toxin is found in several pathovars. For example, tabtoxin is produced by both *P. s.* pv. *tabaci* and *P. s.* pv. *coronafaciens.* Related "angulata" strains are identical to pv. *tabaci* except that they cannot produce tabtoxin and consequently form lesions without halos. A lot of effort has logically gone into investigating the possible relationship between plasmids and toxin production in these pathovars. In both *P. s.* pv. *syringae* and *P. s.* pv. *phaseolicola,* an apparent association between plasmid carriage and toxin production has been reported (Gantotti and Patil, 1979; Gonzalez and Vidaver, 1979). Unfortunately in both of these studies the researchers relied on curing data and subsequent work has shown that their results may have been due to mutations caused by UV light and acridine orange which were used to cure the strains. The correlation between phaseotoxin production and the 22.5 md plasmid in pv. *phaseolicola* did not hold up after more strains were examined (Jamieson *et al.*, 1981; Panopoulos *et al.*, 1979). In the case of the putative syringomycin plasmid, Gonzalez and Olsen (1981) completed their studies by labeling it with drug resistance markers and then transferring it to cured strains where it failed to restore toxin production. Lack of correlation between tabtoxin production and plasmids has also been reported in pv. *tabaci* and pv. *coronafaciens* (Piwowarski and Shaw, 1982). Although discouraging, these results are by no means conclusive. To unequivocably determine the location of toxin genes in these pathovars the genes will have to be cloned and used as hybridization probes to see whether they are homologous with plasmid or chromosomal DNA.

Studies on the relationship between pathogenicity and plasmids are really just beginning. The findings with *Agrobacterium, Rhizobium,* and animal pathogens show that a wide range of properties known to affect virulence may be plasmid-borne. Of particular interest in the future will be the role of plasmids in determining the surface properties of phytopathogenic bacteria. Plasmids are well known to affect the outer membrane protein, lipopolysaccharide, and extracellular polysaccharide composition of their hosts. Such effects are usually manifested as changes in phage and bacteriocin sensitivity or antigenicity. These are the same surface properties that have been implicated in virulence (El-Banoby *et al.*, 1980) and host–pathogen recognition phenomena. Host specificity has been shown to be plasmid-borne in agrobacteria and rhizobia and it is possible that future studies on common plasmids in pseudomonads will show that they too determine host range. Other possible roles for plasmids may be in the detoxification of phytoalexins and other inhibitors in plants. Also, plasmid-specified production of siderophores may enable the pathogen to grow better in the presence of hydroxamate compounds in plants which strongly chelate iron.

B. Ecological Fitness

As discussed earlier in this chapter, plasmids are usually advantageous to the survival of their hosts by enabling them to adapt to changing environmental conditions and compete with other microorganisms. While growing in plant tissues, plant pathogens encounter a comparatively constant environment in terms of the kinds of nutrients available to them, the inhibitors they must contend with, and freedom from microbial competition. As a result they have become more fastidious than their saphrophytic cousins. Many of them are also capable of living in soil, water, and plant debris, on the surfaces of leaves and roots, and even in insect intestines. It is clear that many of the traits known to be carried by plasmids, i.e., nutritional capabilities, antibiotic resistance, adherence factors, and production/resistance to bacteriocins, could be useful to plant pathogens in adapting to their environment and competing with other microflora.

All genera of plant pathogenic bacteria are known to produce bacteriocins (Vidaver, 1976) but the genetic basis for this is not well known in this group. A 96 md bacteriocinogenic plasmid in *E. herbicola* is the only one that has been studied (Gantotti and Beer, 1982). Likewise phytopathogenic bacteria exhibit nutritional variability within species but there is only one instance where a plasmid has been implicated. The *Agrobacterium* Ti plasmids encode for the catabolism of either octopine, nopaline, or agropine. Plasmid DNA which has been integrated into the DNA of tumor cells directs synthesis of the same opine that is utilized by the strain that incited the tumor. Since the plants cannot utilize opines, *Agrobacterium* has in effect engineered the plant to produce a nitrogen source for its own use. Of related interest is a transmissible lactose plasmid found in a clinical strain of *E. herbicola* (Chatterjee and Starr, 1973) and a possible relationship between thiamine prototrophy and a 350 md plasmid in plant strains of *E. herbicola* (Gantotti and Beer, 1982).

Given the prevalence of R plasmids in soil bacteria and the exposure of plant pathogenic bacteria to both naturally occurring and commercially applied antibiotics, it is surprising that infectious drug resistance is not more common. Here again only one instance of a possible R plasmid has been reported. Yano *et al.* (1979) found that 13 out of 109 strains of *P. s.* pv. *lachrymans* (Smith & Bryan) Young *et al.* resistant to dihydrostreptomycin from Japan could donate resistance at high frequencies to other strains of pv. *lachrymans,* but not to *E. coli* or *Pseudomonas aeruginosa* (Schroeter) Migula. Two plasmids were present in the one donor strain examined by gel electrophoresis but they did not appear to be present in any of its transconjugants. Although this transfer may be due to conjugation, further study is needed to obtain evidence for plasmid involvement. In a study of streptomycin-resistant mutants of *E. amylovora* (Burrill) Winslow *et al.* from California orchards that had been sprayed with the antibiotic, Schroth *et al.* (1979) felt that resistance was entirely due to chromosomal mutations.

Plant pathogenic erwinias which depend on insects for dispersal and/or overwintering may have developed special properties which enable them to colonize insects. By analogy with work on animal pathogens, adherence antigens, bacteriocin resistance and production, special nutritional capabilities, iron uptake mechanisms, and serum resistance could facilitate colonization of insects. All of these traits can be borne on plasmids, so that studies on plasmids, such as those in *E. stewartii*, may be useful in defining the relationship between phytopathogenic bacteria and their insect vectors.

IV. ROLE OF INDIGENOUS PLASMIDS IN GENETIC EXCHANGE

It is well established that plant pathogenic bacteria can accept R plasmids and sex factors from *E. coli* and *P. aeruginosa* (Chatterjee and Starr, 1980; Lacy and Leary, 1979). For the most part these plasmids behave as they do in their original hosts. They replicate, conjugate, and express phenotypic markers. Plasmids such as F'*lac*$^+$ and R68.45 even mobilize chromosomal genes and are useful for mapping studies. Also, transposable elements borne on these plasmids, such as drug resistance transposons and bacteriophage Mu, can carry out their normal functions. In short, there is no evidence from studies on introduced plasmids to suggest that the potential of naturally occurring plasmids to participate in gene exchange is in any way altered in phytopathogenic bacteria. All that is necessary is that the native plasmids be conjugative and able to interact with the chromosome via accessory elements or regions of homology.

Conjugative plasmids are found in a number of phytopathogenic bacteria. In most cases, these plasmids lack a selectable marker so that in order to demonstrate conjugation they have to be labeled with a drug resistance transposon or used to mobilize a nonconjugative R plasmid. The Ti plasmids of *A. tumefaciens* are the only instance of a conjugative plasmid in a plant pathogen where a selectable marker is already present. Transfer of Ti plasmids can be detected by selecting for opine utilization. *In vitro*, their transfer genes are normally repressed but they can be induced by the same opine that the strain is capable of utilizing and enabling the gall to produce. This explains why transfer of Ti plasmids was detected *in planta* long before it was *in vitro*.

Erwinia amylovora (Panopoulos *et al.*, 1978) and *E. stewartii* (Coplin and Rowan, 1978) contain conjugative plasmids which can mobilize a nonconjugative ColE1 *kan* plasmid, pML2. Plasmids in several strains of *E. stewartii* can mobilize pML2 to *E. coli* and other strains of *E. stewartii*. The best characterized of these is a 33 md plasmid designated pDC250.

This plasmid and a 34.5 md plasmid also present in strain SW2 mobilized pML2 to strains of *E. stewartii* lacking these plasmids at high frequency (10^{-3} to 10^{-2} per donor cell) (Coplin and Rowan, 1978). pDC250 also mobilized pML2 to *E. coli* at low frequencies, but most of the transconjugants from such a mating contained only pML2. A stable *E. coli* transconjugant containing pDC250 which could redonate pML2 was obtained. pDC250 was subsequently transferred from this strain to another strain of *E. coli* which had a copy of Tn10 on its chromosome. pDC250 was then labeled by asking it to transfer Tn10 to a third *E. coli* strain. The resulting plasmid, designated pDC251, contained a Tn10 insertion (Coplin and Rowan, unpublished results). pDC251 transferred at high frequencies (10^{-1} to 1 per donor cell) in intrastrain matings in *E. coli* and *E. stewartii* indicating that its transfer functions are derepressed. The host range of pDC251 included many species of *Salmonella, Shigella, Enterobacter,* and *Erwinia* (Coplin and Emch, unpublished results). A survey of 31 strains (Coplin *et al.*, 1982) revealed 33 md plasmids in over half of the strains. Furthermore, pDC251 was incompatible with the 33 md plasmid in several other strains. This suggests that pDC250 is widely distributed in strains of diverse geographic origin.

Unfortunately the high transfer frequency of pDC250 and the 34.5 md plasmid in SW2 has prevented the detection of other conjugative plasmids in this strain which might be repressed, but a similar set of experiments with SS104, which does not have these plasmids, has shown that it too contains conjugative plasmids. In this case, the plasmids which were obtained after mobilization of pML2 to *E. coli* did not correspond in size to any found in the donor (Coplin and Rowan, 1978). These plasmids may have been part of a large cointegrate plasmid which dissociated after its transfer to *E. coli*.

The only evidence that *E. stewartii* plasmids are capable of integrating into the chromosome comes from the work on pDC190 discussed earlier in this chapter. The appearance of new plasmids in pDC191 transconjugants and their cured derivatives suggests that parts of pDC190 can integrate to avoid incompatibility with pDC191 and then excise when pDC191 is lost from the strain. Interaction of plasmids with the chromosome can also be inferred from their ability to mobilize chromosomal markers, but a native gene transfer system has not been detected in *E. stewartii*. By itself pDC250 does not have chromosome mobilizing ability, although a derivative of it containing Tn1 and Tn10 can transfer auxotrophic markers at low frequency in SS104 (McCammon and Coplin, unpublished results).

Members of the *P. syringae* group also contain conjugative plasmids. Staskawicz *et al.* (1980) have reported that a 30 md plasmid, pBW, from

P. s. pv. *tabaci* can mobilize RSF1010 to *E. coli*. Plasmid pCG133 from *P. s.* pv. *syringae* HS191 is also conjugative. Gonzalez and Olsen (1981) were able to add markers to this plasmid by cloning it into a nonconjugative derivative of RP1. Transfer of the recombinant plasmid between *P. s.* pv. *syringae* strains was then detected at frequencies of 10^{-4} to 10^{-6} per donor cell.

Szabo *et al.* (1982) have investigated the properties of a 98 md plasmid common in *P. s.* pv. *phaseolicola* strains. This plasmid, designated pMC7105, is not conjugative but it can spontaneously integrate into the chromosome. Excision of pMC7105 produces either prime plasmids containing chromosomal DNA or deleted plasmids (Szabo *et al.*, 1982; Mills and Gonzalez, Vol. 1, Chapter 5).

A fertility system has been recently discovered in a Race 1 isolate of *P. s.* pv. *morsprunorum* (Wormald) Young *et al.* (Errington and Vivian, 1981). Crosses between derivatives of strain C28, each carrying two genetic markers, gave recombinants for both selected recipient markers and unselected donor markers. Some mutant strains always acted as donors and others as recipients. Linkage data indicated that fairly large regions of the chromosome were transferred. It is tempting to speculate that the gene transfer is due to conjugation and represents an important means of genetic recombination in nature. However, the researchers have not yet been able to demonstrate the presence of a conjugative plasmid consistently associated with donor strains.

V. AREAS FOR FUTURE RESEARCH

We now know that plasmids are as widely distributed in most plant pathogenic bacteria as they are in other groups of bacteria. Physical and genetic analysis of Ti plasmids represents the state of the art in molecular biology and has already added significantly to our understanding of plasmids in general. Although plasmids in plant pathogens are similar to the more characterized plasmids in *E. coli* and *P. aeruginosa* in many respects, they undoubtedly have diverged at some point in the course of their evolution and now have unique properties which make them worthy of study in their own right.

Answers to a number of important questions are needed. What traits are located on plasmids and why is it advantageous for them to be there? How should the knowledge of plasmid-encoded properties influence our notions of taxonomy and phylogeny? Do plasmids play a role in genetic exchange and the evolution of new races and strains in nature? Is it likely that genes for resistance to new bacteriocides will appear on plasmids? If Ti plasmids can confer pathogenicity upon *A. radiobacter* then is it conceivable that conversion of other epiphytic and rhizosphere bacteria to pathogens could also take place via plasmids? Should epidemiologists consider the spread of virulence plasmids among an indigenous population of "nearly pathogenic" bacteria to be a contributing factor in epidemics?

The finding of pathogenicity genes on plasmids has and will be important to geneticists and physiologists because such genes can be readily isolated and studied. This will lead to understanding the structure and function of these genes and the expression of pathogenicity. Although this chapter concerns the functions of plasmids, it must be emphasized that most pathogenicity genes will be chromosomal. Even *Agrobacterium,* with so much of the information for its pathogenicity on Ti plasmids, is dependent upon chromosomal genes in order to infect plants. Certainly a large part of the genome of a plant pathogen is needed to adapt it to growth in a plant and to survive and spread in nature; there is usually not enough plasmid DNA in a bacterium to account for all of these functions. It is now time that equal emphasis be given to studying the chromosomal genetics of plant pathogenic bacteria. Our knowledge of the behavior of indigenous and introduced plasmids will be valuable in these studies because plasmids will serve as vectors for recombinant DNA and mediators of genetic exchange.

References

Ashbaugh, M. F. (1980). M. S. thesis, Ohio State University.

Bauer, W. D. (1981). *Annu. Rev. Plant Physiol.* **32,** 407–449.

Ben-Gurion, R., and Shafferman, A. (1981). *Plasmid* **5,** 183–187.

Beringer, J. E., Beylon, J. L., Buchanan-Wollaston, A. V., and Johnston, A. W. B. (1978). *Nature (London)* **276,** 633–634.

Beylon, J. L., Beringer, J. E., and Johnston, A. W. B. (1980). *J. Gen. Microbiol.* **120,** 421–429.

Birnboim, H. C., and Doly, J. (1979). *Nucleic Acids Res.* **7,** 1513–1523.

Bradshaw-Rouse, J. J., Whatley, M. H., Coplin, D. L., Woods, A., Sequeira, L., and Kelman, A. (1981). *Appl. Environ. Microbiol.* **43,** 344–350.

Brewin, N. J., Beringer, J. E., Buchanan-Wollaston, A. V., Johnston, A. W. B., and Hirsch, P. R. (1980a). *J. Gen. Microbiol.* **116,** 261–270.

Brewin, N. J., Beringer, J. E., and Johnston, A. W. B. (1980b). *J. Gen. Microbiol.* **120,** 413–420.

Brown, M. A., Ziegle, J. S., and Chatterjee, A. K. (1981). *Phytopathology* **71,** 863 (Abstr.).

Campbell, A. (1981). *Annu. Rev. Microbiol.* **35,** 55–83.

Casse, F., Boucher, C., Juliot, J. S., Michel, M., and Dénarié, J. (1979). *J. Gen. Microbiol.* **113,** 229–242.

Chatterjee, A. K., and Starr, M. P. (1973). *Infect. Immun.* **8,** 563–572.

Chatterjee, A. K., and Starr, M. P. (1980). *Annu. Rev. Microbiol.* **34,** 645–676.

Comai, L., and Kosuge, T. (1980). *J. Bacteriol.* **143,** 950–957.

Comai, L., and Kosuge, T. (1982). *J. Bacteriol.* **149,** 40–46.
Coplin, D. L., and Rowan, R. G. (1978). *Proc. Int. Conf. Plant Pathog. Bact., 4th, Angers.* pp. 67–73.
Coplin, D. L., Rowan, R. G., Chisholm, D. A., and Whitmoyer, R. E. (1981). *Appl. Environ. Microbiol.* **42,** 599–604.
Coplin, D. L., Frederick, R. D., Tindal, M. H., and McCammon, S. L. (1982). *Proc. Int. Conf. Plant Pathog. Bact., 5th, Cali, Colombia* pp. 379–388.
Crosa, J. H., Schiewe, M. H., and Falkow, S. (1977). *Infect. Immun.* **18,** 509–513.
Curiale, M. S., and Mills, D. (1978). *J. Bacteriol.* **131,** 224–228.
Currier, T. C., and Morgan, M. K. (1981). *Phytopathology* **71,** 869 (Abstr.).
Currier, T. C., and Nester, E. W. (1976). *Anal. Biochem.* **76,** 431–441.
Dahlbeck, D., Pring, D. R., and Stall, R. E. (1977). *Proc. Am. Phytopathol. Soc.* **4,** 176 (Abstr.).
Dye, D. W., Bradbury, J. F., Goto, M., Hayward, A., Lettiot, R. A., and Schroth, M. N. (1980). *Rev. Plant Pathol.* **59,** 153–168.
Eckhardt, J. (1978). *Plasmid* **1,** 584–588.
El-Banoby, F. E., Rudolf K., and Mendgen, K. (1981). *Physiol. Plant Pathol.* **18,** 91–98.
Elwell, L. P., and Shipley, P. L. (1980). *Annu. Rev. Microbiol.* **34,** 465–496.
Errington, J., and Vivian, A. (1981). *J. Gen. Microbiol.* **124,** 439–442.
Gantotti, B. V., and Beer, S. V. (1982). *Phytopathology* **72,** 260–261 (Abstr.).
Gantotti, B. V., Patil, S. S., and Mandel, M. (1979). *Appl. Environ. Microbiol.* **3,** 511–516.
Garibaldi, A., and Gibbins, L. N. (1975). *Can. J. Microbiol.* **21,** 1282–1287.
Gonzalez, C. F., and Olsen, R. H. (1981). *Phytopathology* **71,** 220 (Abstr.).
Gonzalez, C. F., and Vidaver, A. K. (1979). *Curr. Microbiol.* **2,** 75–80.
Gonzalez, C. F., and Vidaver, A. K. (1980). *Phytopathology* **70,** 223–225.
Gonzalez, J. M., Dulmage, H. T., and Carlton, B. C. (1981). *Plasmid* **5,** 351–365.
Gross, D. C., Vidaver, A. K., and Keralis, M. B. (1979). *J. Gen. Microbiol.* **115,** 479–489.
Hanson, J. B., and Olsen, R. H. (1978). *J. Bacteriol.* **135,** 222–238.
Hooykaus, P. J. J., van Brussel, A. A. N., Den Dulk-Ras, H., van Slogteren, G. M. S., and Schilperoort, R. A. (1981). *Nature (London)* **291,** 351–353.
Jamieson, A. F., Bieleski, R. L., and Mitchell, R. E. (1981). *J. Gen. Microbiol.* **122,** 161–165.
Johnston, A. W. B., Beynon, J. L., Buchannan-Wollaston, A. V., Setchell, S. M., Hirsch, P. R., and Beringer, J. E. (1978). *Nature (London)* **276,** 635–636.
Lacy, G. H., and Leary, J. V. (1979). *Annu. Rev. Phytopathol.* **17,** 181–202.
Lacy, G. H., and Sparks, R. B. Jr. (1979). *Phytopathology* **69,** 1293–1297.
Lin, B.-C., and Chen, S. J. (1978). *Int. Congr. Plant Pathol., 3rd Munich* (Abstr.).
McCammon, S. L., and Coplin, D. L. (1981). *Phytopathology* **71,** 240 (Abstr.).
Merlo, D. J., and Nester, E. W. (1977). *J. Bacteriol.* **129,** 76–85.
Moore, L. W., Warren, G., and Strobel, G. (1979). *Plasmid* **2,** 617–626.
Murai, N., Skoog, F., Doyle, M. E., and Hanson, R. S. (1980). *Proc. Natl. Acad. Sci. U.S.A.* **77,** 619–623.
Nester, E. W., and Kosuge, T. (1981). *Annu. Rev. Microbiol.* **35,** 531–565.
Panopoulos, N. J., Guimaraes, W. V., Hua, S., Sabersky-Lehman, C., Resnik, S., Lai, M., and Shaffer, S. (1978). *In* "Microbiology 78" (D. Schlesinger, ed.), pp. 238–241. Amer. Soc. Microbiol., Washington, D.C.
Panopoulos, N. J., Staskawicz, B. J., and Sandlin, D. (1979). *In* "Plasmids of Microbial, Environmental and Commercial Importance" (K. W. Timmis and A. Pühler, eds.), pp. 365–372. Elsevier, Amsterdam.
Piwowarski, J. M., and Shaw, P. P. (1982). *Plasmid* **7,** 85–94.
Portnoy, D. A., Moseley, S. L., and Falkow, S. (1981). *Infect. Immun.* **31,** 775–782.

Quant, R., and Mills, D. (1982). *Proc. Int. Conf. Plant Pathog. Bact., 5th, Cali, Colombia* pp. 412–419.

Ranhand, J. M., Mitchell, W. O., Popkins, T. J., and Cole, R. M. (1980). *J. Bacteriol.* **143,** 1194–1199.

Reanney, D. (1976). *Microbiol. Rev.* **40,** 552–596.

Sansonetti, P. J., Kopecko, P. J., and Formal, S. B. (1981). *Infect. Immun.* **34,** 75–83.

Sato, M., Staskawicz, B. J., Panopoulos, N. J., Peters, S., and Honma, M. (1981). *Plasmid* **6,** 325–331.

Schroth, M. N., Moller, W. J., and Thompson, S. V. *Phytopathology* **69,** 565–568.

Sciaky, D., Montoya, A. L., and Chilton, M.-D. (1978). *Plasmid* **1,** 238–251.

Sheikholeslam, S., Okubara, P. A., Lin, B.-C., Dutra, J. C., and Kado, C. I. (1978). *In* "Microbiology 1978" (D. Schlessinger, ed.), pp. 132–134. Amer. Soc. Microbiol., Washington, D.C.

Sinha, V. B., and Scrivastava, B. S. (1978). *J. Gen. Microbiol.* **104,** 251–255.

Skerman, V. B. D., McGowan, V., and Sneath, P. H. A. (1980). *Int. J. Syst. Bacteriol.* **30,** 225–420.

Smidt, M. L., and Kosuge, T. (1978). *Physiol. Plant Pathol.* **13,** 203–214.

Sparks, R. B., and Lacy, G. H. (1980). *Phytopathology* **70,** 369–372.

Staskawicz, B. J., Sato, M., and Panopoulos, N. J. (1981). *Phytopathology* **71,** 257 (Abstr.).

Szabo, L. J., Curiale, M. S., and Mills, D. (1982). *Proc. Int. Conf. Plant Pathog. Bact., 5th Cali, Colombia* pp. 403–411.

Thompson, C. J., and Howe, M. (1979). *Annu. Meet. Am. Soc. Microbiol.* Abstr. No. S44.

Vidaver, A. K. (1976). *Annu. Rev. Plant Pathol.* **74,** 451–465.

Watson, B., Currier, T. C., Gordon, M. P., Chilton, M. D., and Nester, E. W. (1975). *J. Bacteriol.* **123,** 255–264.

White, F. F., and Nester, E. W. (1980a). *J. Bacteriol.* **141,** 1134–1141.

White, F. F., and Nester, E. W. (1980b). *J. Bacteriol.* **144,** 710–720.

Yano, H., Fuji, H., Mukoo, H., Fukuyasu, T., Terakado, N., and Isayama, Y. (1979). *Ann. Phytopathol. Soc. Jpn.* **45,** 201–206.

Zaenen, I., Van Larabeke, N., Teuchy, H., Van Montagu, M., and Schell, J. (1974). *J. Mol. Biol.* **86,** 109–127.

Zischek, C., Boistard, P., Tuyén, L. T. K., and Boucher, C. (1981). *Proc. Int. Conf. Plant Pathog. Bact., 5th, Cali, Colombia* pp. 427–437.

Chapter **13**

Bridging the Gap to Plants: Bacterial DNA in Plant Cells

DONALD J. MERLO

I. INTRODUCTION

This chapter will focus on some of the biological and genetic aspects of the induction of crown gall tumors. These neoplasias, induced on dicotyledenous plants by virulent strains of *Agrobacterium tumefaciens* (Smith & Townsend) Conn (Smith and Townsend, 1907), are the result of a remarkable interaction between the bacterial causal agent and the cells of the host plant. The most unusual feature of the disease is the transfer of genetic information from the bacterium to the plant cell. This results in a persistent perturbation of the control of cell growth and nitrogen

Phytopathogenic Prokaryotes, Vol. 2

Copyright © 1982 by Academic Press, Inc.
All rights of reproduction in any form reserved.
ISBN 0-12-509002-1

metabolism of the tumor cell, and these changes benefit the inducing bacteria.

Rather than presenting a comprehensive review of the many aspects of crown gall disease, I will discuss three topics which deal primarily with the mechanism of DNA transfer from pathogen to host, and the ultimate results of this transfer. Progress in this field is being made at an extremely rapid pace, but I will review some of the pertinent publications available by mid-1981 concerning (1) the process of DNA transfer from bacterial cell to plant cell, (2) the amounts of DNA transferred and the physical organization of bacterial DNA in the plant cell, and (3) the potential use of this transfer system for the genetic modification of higher plants.

For the reader desiring a more comprehensive review there are many selections available (Braun, 1978; Drlica and Kado, 1975; Kado, 1976: Lippincott and Lippincott, 1975; Merlo, 1981; Nester and Kosuge, 1981; Schell and Van Montagu, 1980; Schell *et al.*, 1979; Schilperoort *et al.*, 1980).

II. THE PROCESS OF Ti PLASMID TRANSFER TO PLANT CELLS

Crown gall disease was the first plant disease in which an extrachromosomal DNA element was unequivocally shown to be responsible for pathogenicity of the causal organism (for other examples, see Coplin, this volume, Chapter 12). This extrachromosomal DNA, called Ti ("tumor-inducing") plasmid, exists in the bacterium as a covalently closed circle of double-stranded DNA, and is present in about one copy per each copy of the bacterial genote. Genes borne on the Ti plasmid are essential in conferring to the bacterium the ability to induce crown gall tumors (Van Larebeke *et al.*, 1974; Watson *et al.*, 1975), and during the induction process a portion of the plasmid DNA is transferred to, maintained in, and expressed in, the plant cell (discussed in detail below).

A question which arises therefore concerns the physical mechanism by which this DNA is transferred from prokaryotic cell to eukaryotic cell. As we shall see, however, very little is known about this process.

A. Requirement for Binding of Cells

Work by the Lippincotts and others (Glogowski and Galsky, 1978; Lippincott and Lippincott, 1969; Lippincott *et al.*, 1977) suggests that within the first 10 to 30 min after inoculation, a specific binding of the bacterial cell to the plant cell wall occurs. This binding probably involves the bacterial envelope lipopolysaccharide (LPS) and the plant cell middle lamella (Lippincott and Lippincott, 1977; Whatley *et al.*, 1976). Evidence to support these claims comes primarily from experiments in which avirulent bacteria were shown to inhibit tumor formation when applied to the plant wound site before the addition of virulent bacteria, whereas no effect on tumor formation was seen when the avirulent cells were added sometime after the virulent cells. Also, homogenates of plant cells which were enriched in particular cell wall fractions were inhibitory to tumor formation, when virulent cells were incubated with these fractions before inoculation into the plant wound site. This was taken as evidence that the binding sites on the bacteria were saturated during preincubation, and these cells, which would be unable to bind to plant cell walls in the wound site, would therefore be decreased in overall tumor-inducing capacity. Similarly, bacterial LPS fraction inhibited tumor formation when applied to the wound site before, but not after, the addition of tumorigenic bacteria. This result suggests a saturation of the available binding sites in the wound by the LPS, thereby reducing the susceptibility of the plant cells to transformation.

One might criticize these studies in that the event measured, tumor formation, is temporally far removed from the steps presumed to occur during the first minutes of infection. Matthysse *et al.* (1978) and others (Smith and Hindley, 1978) have employed a more direct assay to measure cell–cell binding. After incubation of tobacco (*Nicotiana tabacum* L.) or carrot (*Daucus carota* L.) cell suspension cultures with bacteria, and filtration to remove nonbound bacterial cells, the plant cells were collected by centrifugation and plated on bacteriological media to assay bacterial cell numbers. The results of these assays suggest that bacterial LPS is involved in binding, and that plasmid-borne genes may control binding, as also suggested by Whatley *et al.* (1978).

In electron microscope studies, *A. tumefaciens* cells were seen adhered to plant cell walls but it is not known whether or not the particular bacteria/plant cell pairs observed were in fact involved in a tumor-inducing event (Schilperoort, 1969; Matthysse *et al.*, 1981). Treatment of bacterial cells in the wound site with ribonuclease or deoxyribonuclease has been shown to decrease tumor formation (reviewed by Drlica and Kado, 1975), suggesting that free (unprotected) nucleic acid may be involved in tumor induction, and perhaps suggesting that intimate contact between bacteria and plant cell is not a necessary feature of the induction process. It is difficult to assess, however, the relative importance of secondary effects of these nucleases on either the bacteria or plant cells, and no firm conclusions can be drawn.

Recent results of Matthysse *et al.* (1981), obtained with the scanning electron microscope, demonstrated that *A. tumefaciens* cells, following initial binding to either dead or alive plant cells, soon became bound to the plant cell wall surface by means of cellulose fibrils synthesized by the bacteria. The multiplication of the bacteria either directly attached or entrapped by these fibrils resulted in multicellular clusters of bacteria which were hypothesized to facilitate transfer of Ti plasmid DNA to the underlying plant cell.

Further evidence pointing to a role of cell–cell binding in tumor induction is found in the observation that plant tissues which are resistant to infection by *A. tumefaciens* possess cell walls that do not bind the bacteria, and cell wall preparations from these tissues are noninhibitory when mixed with virulent cells. Specifically, Lippincott and Lippincott (1978) found that cell wall preparations from monocotyledons and from crown galls grown either on the host plant or in tissue culture were noninhibitory. Treatment of these cell wall preparations with pectinesterase to remove methyl groups rendered the preparations inhibitory. Additionally, cell walls from embryonic (3-day-old) host plant tissues were noninhibitory, although similar preparations from 7-day-old plants were inhibitory. These observations suggest that walls of crown gall tumor cells may be chemically similar to embryonic cell walls, and may partially explain why plants regenerated from crown gall teratoma shoots are resistant to superinfection by *A. tumefaciens* (Turgeon *et al.*, 1976; Wullems *et al.*, 1980). Subsequent work by Wullems *et al.* (1981a), however, suggests that supraoptimal cytokinin levels in the regenerated plants, rather than altered cell walls, may be responsible for the resistance of those plants to crown gall infections.

B. Similarity to Bacterial Conjugation

The observation that the conjugal transfer of Ti plasmids between bacterial cells is sensitive to the same temperature regime that inhibits tumor formation prompted Tempé *et al.* (1977) to suggest that the two phenomena are controlled by a common regulatory pathway. However, no mutations of Ti plasmids have been reported that simultaneously inactivate oncogenicity (onc) and conjugal transfer (tra) functions (Schell *et al.*, 1979; Ooms *et al.*, 1980). This, of course, does not rule out the involvement of an unidentified plasmid or chromosomal gene. It is an open question, therefore, whether a conjugation-like process is responsible for transfer of the Ti plasmid from the bacteria to the plant cell, and probably a similar, but not identical process is involved in bacteria–plant cell transfer as in bacteria–bacteria transfer.

C. Liposome-Mediated Transfer

Besides the actual mechanism of Ti plasmid DNA transfer from bacterium to host cells, there also exists the question of the amount of the total Ti plasmid which is transferred to the initial transformed cell. As we shall see in a later section, different independently derived tumor lines maintain varying amounts of the Ti plasmid DNA (T-DNA, see below) during years of axenic culture, but it is difficult to design experiments which can measure the amount of Ti plasmid sequences present in plant cells during the very early stages of infection. This is due to the continued presence of viable, Ti plasmid-containing bacteria in the plant tissue for extended periods after infection.

At least two possibilities must be considered. In the first case, reactions which take place in the bacterial cell would cleave out from the whole Ti plasmid [perhaps by mechanisms analogous to lambda phage excision in *Escherichia coli* (Migula) Castellani & Chalmers] that portion of the plasmid destined to become T-DNA. This pre-T-DNA would then be transferred to the host cell, and recombine with plant DNA.

In the second case, the whole Ti plasmid would be transferred to the plant cell, and the reactions which ultimately result in the integration of the T-DNA into plant DNA would be catalyzed therein. That these reactions can occur without the intervention of bacterial cells is shown by the results of experiments performed by S. Dellaporte *et al.* (personal communication). Whole Ti plasmid DNA was first encapsulated in artificially produced liposomes, and these DNA-containing liposomes were then fused to tobacco cell protoplasts, resulting in the transfer of the whole Ti plasmid into the tobacco cell cytoplasm. Following subsequent selection and screening procedures, it was found that a very small fraction of the initial protoplasts had maintained and expressed Ti plasmid sequences that were identical to those that are found as T-DNA in tumor lines incited by the parental *A. tumefaciens* strain. Therefore, it is clear that plant cells do possess the ability to catalyze all the reactions involved in T-DNA excision/integration. It is not known, however, if the enzymes which catalyze those reactions are encoded by the plant genome, or rather are produced early in infection through expression of Ti plasmid DNA sequences. It is intriguing to speculate that the latter is the case, as this might provide a rationale for the uniform large size of naturally occurring Ti plasmids. Further experiments involving the introduction into plant cell protoplasts of Ti plasmids that have been mutated in various regions may provide answers to these questions (Ooms *et al.*, 1981). The question also remains, of course, as to the extent that liposome-mediated fusion processes may be relevant to the actual crown gall induction process by virulent bacteria.

III. AMOUNTS OF T-DNA IN TUMOR CELLS

Several experimental approaches are available by means of which one may estimate the amounts of DNA sequences homologous to Ti plasmid sequences which are present in a particular tumor tissue. In any case, those sequences of the tumor DNA which are represented in the Ti plasmid DNA are called the T-DNA (for "tumor" DNA, or "transferred" DNA). Conversely, the region of a Ti plasmid which is homologous to T-DNA is called the T-region. The first type of analysis used to define T-DNA involved monitoring the reassociation kinetics of individual, radiolabeled Ti plasmid DNA restriction fragments in the presence of a large excess of tumor tissue DNA (Chilton *et al.*, 1977; Merlo *et al.*, 1980; Yang *et al.*, 1980a,b). Alternately, the labeled DNA fragments may be hybridized to a Southern blot of restriction enzyme-digested tumor tissue DNA, as illustrated by Thomashow *et al.* (1980a). Another method involves hybridizing radioactively labeled messenger RNA isolated from tumor tissue to a Southern blot of restriction enzyme-digested Ti plasmid DNA (Drummond *et al.*, 1977; Ledeboer, 1978; Yang *et al.*, 1980b,c). Each method has particular advantages and disadvantages which will not be dealt with here; rather I will try to present a compilation of the results garnered by the three approaches.

A. Types of Ti Plasmids

Based on the studies of several independent research groups, it is generally believed that there exist three major types of Ti plasmids. These classifications are based on physical, physiological, and genetic studies, and include the majority of Ti plasmids studied thus far.

1. *Octopine (oct)-Type Plasmids*

These plasmids encode genes (occ) that enable agrobacteria which harbor the plasmid to catabolize octopine as a source of nitrogen or carbon (or both). They also encode genes (*ocs*) which catalyze octopine synthesis by the plant tumor cell (Bomhoff *et al.*, 1976; Montoya *et al.*, 1977). DNA–DNA homology studies (Currier and Nester, 1976; Drummond and Chilton, 1978) and restriction enzyme digest patterns ("fingerprints"; Sciaky *et al.*, 1978) have shown that these plasmids are, for the most part, highly conserved, bearing greater than 90% homology to one another and having almost identical fingerprints. Recently, however, Thomashow *et al.* (1981) have distinguished wide host range (WHR) and limited host range (LHR) types of octopine plasmids, the latter types being primarily isolated from grapevine (*Vitis vinifera* L.)

crown galls. The LHR Ti plasmids bear only 6–15% DNA homology to the standard WHR octopine Ti plasmids, and therefore constitute a new subgroup of the octopine-type plasmids.

As will be discussed in further detail below, the WHR octopine Ti plasmids and most nopaline-type (see below) Ti plasmids share a highly conserved region of DNA base sequences (the "common" DNA) which comprise 5.5 to 6.7 × 10^6 daltons (Chilton *et al.*, 1978; Depicker *et al.*, 1978, 1980). Since the common DNA sequences were a part of the T-DNA of all tumor lines of both octopine and nopaline types which have been examined, it was hypothesized that they were intimately concerned with oncogenicity. Surprisingly, the LHR octopine plasmids, while clearly capable of tumor induction, contain only a very small degree of sequence homology to the common DNA (Thomashow *et al.*, 1981). If the common DNA is indeed involved in oncogenicity in the WHR octopine-type and the nopaline-type Ti plasmids, then either the LHR plasmids induce the tumor growth habit via a different mechanism than that employed by the former plasmid types, or a clearly distinct set of genes is utilized by the LHR plasmids in inducing a common mechanism. It is also possible that the lack of the common DNA sequences is in some way related to the narrow host range of the LHR plasmid-bearing strains. It will be of interest to learn the extent of T-DNA present in tumors induced by the LHR strains, since the T-DNA of several other octopine-producing tumor lines has been found to be quite different from line to line (see below and Fig. 1).

2. *Nopaline (nop)-Type Plasmids*

These plasmids, analogously to the octopine-type plasmids, were classified as those plasmids which encoded nopaline catabolism (*noc*) by the bacteria, and nopaline synthesis (*nos*) in tumors induced by bacteria harboring these plasmids. From the standpoint of DNA homology and restriction enzyme fingerprints, these plasmids were found to be clearly distinct both from octopine-type Ti plasmids and from each other (Currier and Nester, 1976; Sciaky *et al.*, 1978).

Until recently, it was generally held that tumors induced on plants of high regenerative capacity (e.g., *Kalanchöe* sp.) by nopaline *A. tumefaciens* strains were usually of the teratoma type, developing spontaneous abnormal shoots, buds, and other plant structures. Indeed, fertile, normal-appearing plants have been regenerated from teratoma shoots derived from tumor tissues established from a single tumor cell (Braun, 1980; Braun and Wood, 1976; Turgeon *et al.*, 1976; Wood *et al.*, 1978). In contrast, most tumors induced by octopine-type Ti plasmids were of the unorganized type, whether the host plant be of high or low regenerative

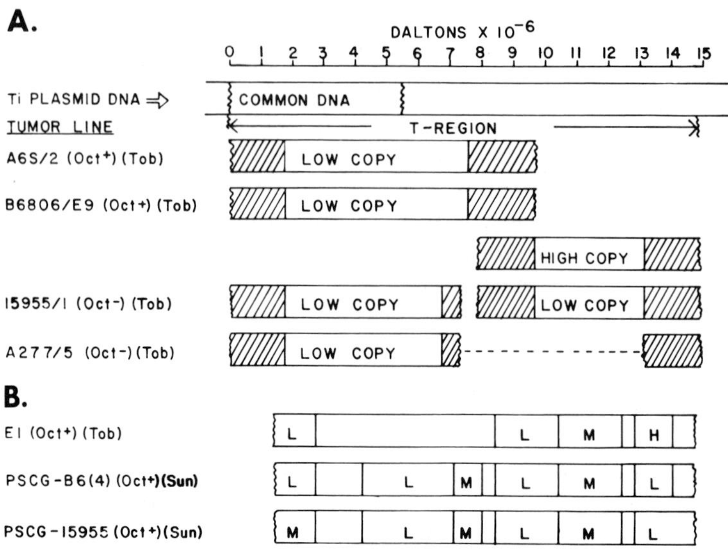

Figure 1. (A) T-DNA of tobacco crown gall tumors incited by *A. tumefaciens* strains harboring octopine-type Ti plasmids. Extents of the T-DNA, as determined by DNA–DNA homology studies, are aligned with the physical map of the Ti plasmid T-region. Boxes with the diagonal markings and ragged ends indicate that the ends of the T-DNA, although not precisely located, are known to occur within the regions depicted. Low- and high-copy refer to the numbers of the respective fragments determined per diploid tumor cell DNA equivalent, and are 1–2, and 18–30, respectively. Oct^+ and Oct^- indicate the octopine synthetic capacities of the respective tumor tissues. Common DNA has been represented to include all of *Sma*I fragments 16a and 17, and *Hpa*I fragment 14 (Chilton *et al.*, 1976). (B) T-DNA of tobacco (E1) and sunflower ("PSCG") crown gall tumors incited by *A. tumefaciens* strains harboring octopine-type Ti plasmids. Extents of the T-DNA were determined by hybridizing radiolabeled tumor RNA to restriction fragments of the plasmid T-region. L, M, and H refer respectively to light, moderate, and heavy transcription levels of the indicated regions. Regions showing no transcriptional activity are therefore only presumed to be present in the tumor DNA by analogy with the T-DNA's of the tumor lines shown in A.

capacity. However, there are now several reports of octopine-producing tobacco tumor tissues which have spontaneously organized shoots (Einset and Cheng, 1979; L. Owens, personal communication; Wullems *et al.*, 1981a,b). Therefore, it seems that while tumors induced by nopaline-type plasmids possess an inherently greater propensity for structural organization, the tumor cells induced by octopine-type plasmids are also able to suppress the expression of the unorganized tumor trait. The consequences of this regenerative capacity of tumor cells will be discussed in a later section.

3. *Null-Type, or Agropine-Type Plasmids*

This class of Ti plasmids was originally termed the "null" type by Sciaky *et al.* (1978) since neither octopine, nopaline, nor any of several other tumor-specific compounds (Kemp, 1978; Nester and Kosuge, 1981) were detected in the tumors induced by *A. tumefaciens* harboring these plasmids. Moreover, this group of plasmids did not confer to the host bacteria any catabolic capabilities for the known opines. [Opines is the generic term applied to compounds such as octopine and nopaline. Generally, opines are defined (Schell *et al.*, 1979) as compounds whose biosynthesis in crown gall cells is directed by the T-DNA, and which can be catabolized by *A. tumefaciens* via Ti plasmid-encoded pathways to supply carbon and nitrogen to the bacteria. In some cases, opines also induce conjugal transfer of Ti plasmids between bacterial cells.] Agropine was first isolated from octopine-producing tobacco crown gall tissues, and was found to comprise as much as 7% of the tissue dry weight (Firmin and Fenwick, 1978). Subsequently, agropine was isolated from "null-type" tumors; hence the more correct classification of these tissues and Ti plasmids should be "agropine-type" (Guyon *et al.*, 1980).

Agropine differs markedly in its chemical composition from the earlier described opines. Octopine, and the other commonly detected opines found in octopine-producing tumors (histopine, lysopine, and octopinic acid), are condensation products of basic amino acids (arginine, histidine, lysine, and ornithine, respectively) with pyruvate. Nopaline, and the sister compound ornaline (nopalinic acid), are the condensates of arginine and ornithine, respectively, with glutamate (Kemp, 1978). Agropine, on the other hand, appears to be a bicyclic derivative of glutamic acid and a hexitol sugar (Coxon *et al.*, 1980). On the basis of these physiological differences the agropine plasmids appear to be distinct from the other groups. However, the significant homology of one agropine plasmid with an octopine-type plasmid (Drummond and Chilton, 1978), and the observation that octopine-producing tumor tissues often also contain agropine, may point to a common evolutionary ancestry for the agropine and the octopine plasmids (Firmin and Fenwick, 1978).

Four new opines have recently been reported (Ellis and Murphy, 1981). These opines, collectively called agrocinopines, were found in nopaline-producing tumors or in agropine-producing tumors. The chemical composition of the agrocinopines, which includes sugars such as glucose, fructose, and arabinose, as well as phosphorus, clearly marks them as a different class of opines from all those previously reported.

B. T-Region of Octopine-Type Ti Plasmids

1. *Amounts of T-DNA in Tumors*

The work of Chilton *et al.* (1977) provided the first definitive proof for the existence, in axenic crown gall tumor tissue, of DNA sequences that are homologous to Ti plasmid DNA sequences. Subsequent work has investigated both the extent of the T-DNA sequences in the tumor line examined in the previous work, and the T-DNA contents of tumor lines of independent origin which were incited by octopine-type *A. tumefaciens* strains. The results of some of these experiments are summarized in Fig. 1. For purposes of clarity, I have omitted the names and numbers of the individual restriction enzymes and DNA fragments; these may be found in the original publications (Gurley *et al.*, 1979; Merlo *et al.*, 1980; Thomashow *et al.*, 1980a).

Several conclusions may be drawn from these data. First, it is clear that a particular *A. tumefaciens* Ti plasmid can induce tumors which maintain different organizations of T-DNA. For example, the tumor lines B6806/E9 and A277/5 were both induced on Xanthi nc tobacco by *A. tumefaciens* strains harboring the Ti plasmid of strain B6806, yet the extent and amounts of T-DNA found in the two tumor lines differ greatly.

Second, it appears that DNA sequences that are found in the general region of the common DNA of the Ti plasmid are able to be rearranged and fused or separated as they are incorporated as the T-DNA of the tumor cell. For example, the tumor lines B6806/E9, 15955/1, and A277/5 have T-DNA which is represented as left- and right-hand portions of the T-region. As shown in Fig. 1 for tumor line A277/5, these two portions are not contiguous in the Ti plasmid T-regions. However, in the DNA of tumor line A277/5, it appears that a deletion/fusion event has occurred, such that these two sets of DNA sequences are contiguous in the tumor DNA (as shown by the dotted line in Fig. 1). Similar, but apparently more complex types of fusion were seen in tumor DNA from lines 15955/1 (Thomashow *et al.*, 1980a) and A6S/2 (Thomashow *et al.*, 1980b). It may be noted, however, that no rearrangements of the T-region in the left-hand portions of the T-DNAs have been detected, and this "core" T-DNA (which includes, but apparently is not limited to, the common DNA) is colinear in the tumor and the Ti plasmid.

Also, it appears that the right-hand T-DNA portion, while quite variable in size, is also variable in copy number. In tumor line B6806/E9 for example, only one or two copies of the left-hand portion were found per tumor cell, whereas 18–30 copies of the right-hand portion have been detected. In the tumor line 15955/1, however, which contains approximately the same extent of T-DNA as B6806/E9, the left- and right-hand portions of the T-DNA were present in apparently equal (low) copy numbers. The significance of these variations, and the mechanisms by which they arise, are intriguing but unanswered questions.

Another feature raised by examination of the results shown in Fig. 1 is the ubiquitous presence of the common DNA sequences in all four tumor lines. (It is pertinent to remind the reader at this point that the common DNA comprises those sequences that are most highly conserved between octopine-, nopaline-, and agropine-type Ti plasmids.) This shared feature of the tumors incited by octopine-type Ti plasmids (and which is also a feature of tumors of the nopaline type, see Fig. 2B) suggests that these sequences may be involved in tumor induction, tumor maintenance, or both phenomena. That this is indeed the case with octopine-type Ti plasmids is shown by the works of Koekman *et al.* (1979), Garfinkel and Nester (1980), and Ooms *et al.* (1980, 1981) in which insertions or deletions of the common DNA sequences were found to affect virulence on some plant hosts or tumor morphology on other hosts. It is apparent, however, that not all insertions into the common DNA lead to avirulence on all plants.

The relatively small amount of T-DNA found in tumor line A6S/2 provides a clue as to the location of the octopine-synthesis genes of these Ti plasmids; since this tumor line produces octopine, the *ocs* gene(s) must lie somewhere within the T-DNA region depicted. Probably, those genes lie somewhere at the right-hand end of the A6S/2 T-DNA, since neither of the two tumor lines 15955/1 and A277/5, which have suffered rearrangements immediately within the right end of the A6S/2 T-DNA equivalent, is an octopine producer (Thomashow *et al.*, 1980a).

Finally, one must raise the question of the extent of T-DNA to be found in tumors incited by the limited host range, octopine-type Ti plasmids (see Section III,A). Since these plasmids apparently lack the common DNA sequences, the composition of the T-DNA of those tumor lines is an exciting question yet to be answered.

2. *Physical Status of T-DNA*

Faced with the evidence that crown gall tumor cells contain DNA sequences homologous to, and therefore derived from, a bacterial plasmid, it was of interest to determine, first, the physical location of those DNA sequences within the tumor cells, and, second, whether or not the bacterially derived DNA was covalently attached to plant DNA or rather existed as a free replicon. Both questions have recently been answered. Thomashow *et al.* (1980a,b) concluded that most, if not all, of the T-DNA

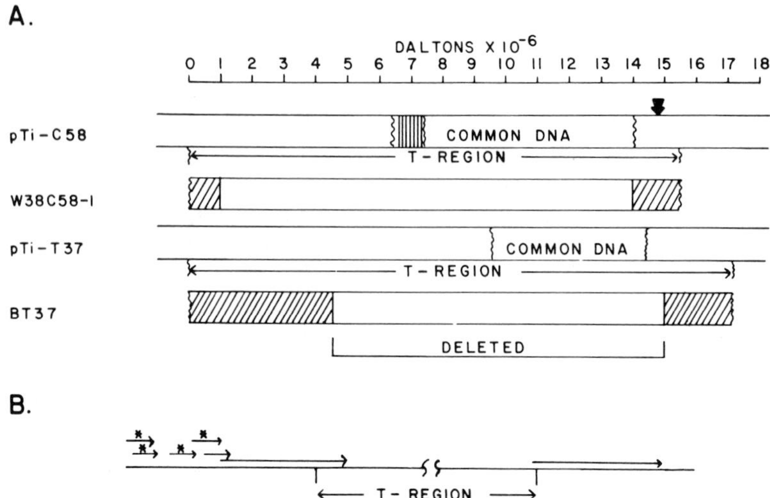

Figure 2. (A) T-DNA of tobacco crown gall tumors incited by *A. tumefaciens* strains harboring nopaline-type Ti plasmids (pTi-C58 or pTi-T37). Extent of T-DNA as determined by DNA–DNA homology studies is aligned under the physical map of the plasmids present in the inducing strain. Markings have same meanings as in Fig. 1. Common DNA region of pTi-C58 (comprising ca. 6.6×10^6 daltons) taken from Depicker *et al.* (1980); that of pTi-T37 (ca. 4.8×10^6 daltons) is from Yang and Simpson (1981). The size difference of the T-DNAs, as well as a discrepancy in size estimates of the BT37 T-DNA (14.5×10^6, Lemmers *et al.*, 1980; vs 17.2×10^6, Yang and Simpson, 1981) probably reflect different estimates of the positions of the T-DNA ends. Lemmers *et al.* (1980) found the extents of T-DNA in W38C58-1 and BT37 to be identical, except for the absence of 1×10^6 daltons of DNA in BT37 tumor DNA, which is also deleted in pTi-T37 (vertically barred region to left of common DNA in map of pTi-C58). Bracket under T-DNA of BT37 indicates region that is deleted in T-DNA of teratoma-derived plants regenerated from BT37 tumor cells (Yang and Simpson, 1981). Arrow above pTi-C58 map indicates position at which transposon insertion destroys nopaline synthesis activity (Hernalsteens *et al.*, 1980). (B) Positions of directly repeated DNA sequences at the ends of the T-region of pTi-T37, and of Chi (short arrows; GCTGGTGG) or Chi-like sequences (different from Chi by one or two bases, indicated by asterisk above arrow). The long directly repeated sequences which overlap the ends of the T-region comprise 25 bases, and are not perfect repeats, differing by a total of 6 bases. Data provided by Yadav and Chilton (personal communication).

of octopine-type tumors was covalently attached to highly repetitive plant nuclear DNA, and found no evidence that the T-DNA was linked to chloroplast or mitochondrial DNA. They point out, however, that there is as yet no formal evidence to prove that the T-DNA is physically integrated into a tobacco chromosome.

Willmitzer *et al.* (1980) found that the T-DNA of another octopine-type tumor line also resided in the cell nucleus, and further showed that the nucleus was responsible for synthesis of RNA homologous to the T-DNA sequences.

3. *Transcription of the T-DNA*

The results of Gurley *et al.* (1979) have confirmed and extended the earlier results of Drummond *et al.* (1977) and Ledeboer (1978) concerning transcription of the T-DNA. As shown in Fig. 1B, not all regions of the T-DNA are transcribed with equal frequency, and some regions apparently are not represented at all in the total RNA. Also, the transcription patterns of tobacco and sunflower (*Helianthus annuus* L.) tumor tissues appear to be substantially different from each other.

C. T-Region of Nopaline-Type Ti Plasmids

1. *Amounts of T-DNA in Tumors*

The propensity of tobacco teratoma tumors to organize shoots and other plant structures has enabled not only the determination of the extent of T-DNA in the original, cloned tobacco teratoma tissues, but also the examination of the fate of the T-DNA during regeneration of whole plants from the teratoma shoots. In Fig. 2A are presented results summarized from several sources (Lemmers *et al.*, 1980; Yang *et al.*, 1980a,b,c; Yang and Simpson, 1981; Zambryski *et al.*, 1980). In order that the extents of the T-regions of octopine- and nopaline-type Ti plasmids may be directly compared, the common DNA sequences are indicated.

Generally speaking, tumor tissues established from primary crown galls (i.e., those which form on an inoculated host plant) have been found to contain the T-DNA regions indicated in Fig. 2A (Lemmers *et al.*, 1980; Yang and Simpson, 1981). Some important exceptions have been found, however. Braun and Wood (1976), Turgeon *et al.* (1976), and Wood *et al.* (1978) have described the regeneration of tobacco shoots and entire plants from single-cell clones of a tobacco teratoma (BT37) induced by *A. tumefaciens* harboring pTi-T37, and the differential expression of tumor traits in the regenerated plants. Although initial studies involving only one of the regenerated plants (and its progeny) showed that the T-DNA was not maintained through meiotic cell divisions (Yang *et al.*, 1980a,b), subsequent studies (Wullems *et al.*, 1981a,b; Yang and Simpson, 1981) have shown that portions of the T-DNA (see Fig. 2A) can be retained during meiosis, and are expressed in F_1 progeny of teratoma-derived, regenerated plants. While some plants had normal-appearing morphology, others were quite abnormal; yet each retained the same portions (the ends) of the T-DNA. These results give renewed hope to the prospect of utilizing the Ti plasmid as a plant genetic engineering vector (see below).

2. *Physical Status of T-DNA*

As in the case of the T-DNA of octopine-producing tumors, the T-DNA of nopaline-type tumors has been found to be covalently linked to plant nuclear DNA (Chilton *et al.*, 1980; Yadav *et al.*, 1980; Zambryski *et al.*, 1980). The precise physical nature of this linkage is as yet undetermined. Zambryski *et al.* (1980) and Yadav *et al.* (1980) found that at least one end of the T-DNA is attached to repeated-sequence plant DNA, but the attachment does not result in the simple insertion of the T-DNA into a particular segment of plant DNA. Rather, the right-hand and left-hand ends of the T-DNA appear to be covalently joined in some tumor DNA fragments, yielding a structure that suggests either the tandem duplication of T-DNA units, or the formation of circular, free replicons (Lemmers *et al.*, 1980; Zambryski *et al.*, 1980). There is, however, no evidence of extrachromosomal elements the size of the T-DNA being present in tumor DNA preparations, so the former interpretation is regarded as the more likely (Lemmers *et al.*, 1980; Zambryski *et al.*, 1980). There have been no reports of the presence of nopaline-type T-DNA in copy numbers equivalent to the high values (20–30) seen in some octopine-type tumors. In addition, except for the shortened T-DNA formed in regenerated plants from the teratomas discussed earlier, there is no evidence for gross rearrangements of the T-DNA in the nopaline-type tumors. The arrangement of the T-DNA is probably one of a few tandemly repeated units of T-DNA that are colinear to the T-region of the inducing plasmid (Lemmers *et al.*, 1980).

3. *Transcription of T-DNA*

Studies on the transcription of T-DNA in nopaline-type tumors have not been reported in detail equal to that summarized in Fig. 1 for octopine-type tumors. Although Yang *et al.* (1980b) originally reported the finding of transcripts only of the T-DNA ends, subsequent work (Yang *et al.*, 1980c) has shown that apparently all the T-DNA sequences present in BT37 tumor cells are represented in the polyadenylated RNA isolated from that tissue. Furthermore, the right-hand end of the T-DNA, which has been shown to control oncogenicity and nopaline synthesis (Depicker *et al.*, 1980), was found to be the most heavily transcribed region.

4. *DNA Sequence Analysis*

Transposable DNA sequences (transposons) are capable of movement from a particular position in a replicon to a different position in the same or a different replicon (for review, see Calos and Miller, 1980). A general feature of a transposon, whether present in prokaryotic or eukaryotic cells, is the occurrence of similar or identical DNA sequences at the ends of the transposon in either direct or inverted repeat orientations (see Calos and Miller, 1980). Since the T-region DNA generally falls into the category of a transposon (i.e., capable of movement from the Ti plasmid and insertion into plant DNA), it was of interest to examine the DNA base sequences of the ends of the T-region. Yadav and Chilton (personal communication) determined the base sequences of the ends of the T-region of pTi-T37 (Fig. 2B), and found several surprising features that are summarized as follows: (1) a sequence of about 25 base pairs is imperfectly directly repeated at the ends of the T-region, but the majority of the bases in the repeats lie *outside* the DNA segment that is incorporated into the plant genome. This result is in direct contrast to the results of transposon movement, wherein the repeated sequences at the transposon ends are an integral part of the transposon, and therefore move with the transposon. In general, the direct or inverted repeats of transposons are much larger than 25 base pairs (although transposon Tn3 has only a 38 base pair terminal inverted repeat; Ohtsubo *et al.*, 1979), and therefore the analogies of T-region movement and transposon movement, and the involvement of these short direct repeats, may not be biologically relevant considerations. Further support of this conclusion is found in the observation that the T-DNA of octopine-type tumors (Fig. 1) is extremely variable in size, and therefore apparently contradicts the transposon model. (However, as transposons have in many cases been shown to be responsible for the formation of DNA inversions or deletions, one might hypothesize that such events are responsible for the variations seen in the size of the octopine-type T-DNA.) (2) Chi sequences are found in the *E. coli* bacteriophage lambda, and serve as recombinational hotspots promoted by the RecBC pathway of *E. coli* (Stahl, 1979). An examination of the Ti plasmid base sequence to the left of the T-region (Fig. 2B) reveals the presence of five sets of sequences which are identical to Chi, or differ from it by only one or two bases. While the function of these Chi-like sequences is not known, it is certainly tempting to speculate that they are involved in some way in the excision (via recombination with plant DNA; Thomashow *et al.*, 1980b) of the T-region DNA from the plasmid. No Chi-like elements have been found in the sequences which have so far been determined to the right of the T-region. However, since Chi sequences are thought to be involved in the resolution of recombinant structures, rather than in the formation of Holliday or Aviemore structures proposed to initiate recombination (Stahl, 1979), it is possible that the Chi sites adjacent to the left end of the T-region are involved in determining precisely the left end of the T-DNA, through termination of a recombination event initiated by sequences at the right-hand end of the T-region.

Lemmers *et al.* (1980) provided evidence both supporting and refuting the idea that sequences at the right end of the T-region play a role in determining the size of the T-DNA. Specifically, they observed that the left end of the T-DNA (i.e., T-region) was very closely conserved in all tumor lines examined, but there was a slight amount of variation in the position of the right boundary when different tumor lines incited by wild-type Ti plasmid were examined. In addition, when transposon Tn7 was inserted into the right-hand end of the T-region of pTi-T37 (at a position equivalent to that of the arrow above the pTi-C58 map in Fig. 2A; Hernalsteens *et al.*, 1980), it was found that all of the Tn7 sequences, as well as the "normal" T-DNA complement, were transferred to, and maintained in, tumor tissue which resulted from inoculation of tobacco by bacteria carrying the altered Ti plasmid. The right-hand boundary of the T-DNA (which was increased in size by the size of Tn7) of these tumors was found to lie in almost the same position as found for nonaltered plasmids, suggesting that DNA sequences at the right-hand end (or possibly just outside) of the T-region are important in specifying the exact end of the T-DNA.

Another set of experiments (Lemmers *et al.*, 1980) examined the T-DNA of a tumor line incited by bacteria harboring pTi-C58 plasmid into which transposon Tn1 had been inserted. The nature of this insertion was such that a deletion of a large portion of pTi-C58 occurred, resulting in a fusion of the T-region (at a point approximately at the right-hand end of the common DNA) to the Tn1 DNA. The sequences which normally comprise the T-region right-hand boundary were therefore deleted. The right-hand end of the T-DNA of the resultant tumor tissue was found to lie within the Tn1 sequences. This result shows that wild-type plasmid sequences are not essential for delimiting the right-hand boundary of T-DNA; other sequences can apparently substitute. One might speculate however, that the Tn1 DNA bases that constitute the new right-hand terminus bear a sequence or structural resemblance to the wild-type terminus, and therefore were chosen in the integration event. DNA base sequence analysis of the appropriate regions will surely answer this question.

A final question which arises when considering recombinational mechanisms of integration of the T-DNA into plant DNA sequences is the presence of DNA sequence homology between the target plant DNA and Ti plasmid DNA. Thomashow *et al.* (1980a) and Yang and Simpson (1981) have reported that Ti plasmid DNA hybridizes to normal tobacco DNA. At present the physical location of these homologous sequences in the Ti plasmid is not known. If, in fact, they are found to lie nearby to the right of the right-hand end of the T-region, then one might imagine that the integration of T-DNA into plant DNA occurs in three steps (see Stahl, 1979). First, an Aviemore structure is formed involving strand switching of a plant DNA strand and a plasmid DNA strand. This event is presumed to be catalyzed at the homology region assumed to lie to the right of the T-region. Second, DNA synthesis and branch migration occur, resulting in a copy of one T-DNA strand becoming covalently attached at the right-hand end to the plant DNA strand involved in formation of the Aviemore structure. Finally, an event catalyzed by Chi sequences to the left of the T-region results in joining of the left end of the T-DNA single strand to plant DNA. Synthesis and ligation of the T-DNA complementary strand would complete the integration process.

IV. PROSPECTS FOR GENETIC ENGINEERING

Of the several host-vector systems proposed for exploitation in plant genetic engineering (reviewed by Kado, 1979; Kado and Lurquin, this volume, Chapter 14), *A. tumefaciens* and the Ti plasmid comprise the only system whose successful use has been unequivocally proven (Hernalsteens *et al.*, 1980). The utility of any vehicle of genetic engineering will ultimately be limited by the ease with which *in vitro* and *in vivo* manipulations may be performed with the vehicle. (In this discussion, I will use the term vehicle to refer to the nucleic acid to which the engineering gene is attached to facilitate its entrance into the plant cell. The term vector, although sometimes used interchangeably with vehicle, seems more appropriately employed in this context to refer to the *A. tumefaciens* cell, liposome, etc. that is used to introduce the vehicle into the host cell.) Because the normal host for the Ti plasmid is a bacterium, genetic manipulation of the plasmid is feasible using the techniques of microbial genetics which have been so successfully employed in modern molecular biology. Indeed, techniques such as transposon mutagenesis and deletion analyses have already enabled the elucidation of many traits controlled by Ti plasmid genes (reviewed by Nester and Kosuge, 1981). The use of the Ti plasmid is further facilitated by the ability to culture large quantities of bacterial cells and subsequently prepare large amounts of Ti plasmid for physical or genetic analysis.

The best defined systems available today for the cloning, characterization, and amplification of genes employ *E. coli* cells and various plasmids or phages. It is therefore extremely fortunate that there exist efficient means of transfer of genetic information between *E. coli* and *A.*

tumefaciens. The availability of these systems (see below) allows one to perform all the initial cloning and modification steps for the gene of choice in a system (*E. coli*) that is comparatively well defined and easily manipulated. When deemed appropriate, the cloned gene may then be moved into *A. tumefaciens* cells, and inserted into specific sites of the Ti plasmid for eventual transfer to the host plant.

That foreign genes inserted into the Ti plasmid can indeed be transferred to plant cells was first shown by Hernalsteens *et al.* (1980). The drug-resistance transposon Tn7 was first inserted randomly into the pTi-T37 plasmid, and the mutated plasmids were then screened for their ability to induce tumors which did not synthesize nopaline. One such plasmid was found, and subsequent analysis revealed that Tn7 had been integrated into the T-region (at a position equivalent to that of the arrow above the pTi-C58 map in Fig. 2A). Hybridization analysis of the T-DNA of the nopaline-minus tumor tissue revealed the presence of Tn7 DNA sequences, in the same relative position of the T-DNA as it had occurred in the plasmid T-region. Lemmers *et al.* (1980) have also reported the transfer of Tn1 sequences to tobacco plant cells.

The insertion of the foreign DNA into the Ti plasmid in the above experiments depended on the transpositional ability of the foreign DNA itself, and the eventual site of integration was not under the experimenter's control. Another method, which we may call marker-exchange, has recently been developed and exploited to move DNA fragments (which do not necessarily have to be self-transposable) into selected sites of the Ti plasmid. The marker-exchange system was originally exploited by Ruvkun and Ausubel (1981) to specifically insert Tn5 into the *Rhizobium meliloti* Dangeard genome. Specifically, an *R. meliloti* (Rm) DNA fragment which had been cloned in *E. coli* was mutagenized by Tn5 insertion. A plasmid containing the mutagenized Rm DNA was then transferred to *R. meliloti,* wherein homologous recombination catalyzed by the flanking Rm DNA enabled the replacement of the wild-type Rm DNA with the mutagenized version. In this way, site-directed mutagenesis of any cloned fragment of Rm DNA would theoretically be possible.

The general applicability of the method to site-directed insertion into the Ti plasmid has recently been shown (Garfinkel *et al.,* 1981; Matzke and Chilton, 1981; J. Kemp, personal communication). Basically, the technique requires first the cloning in *E. coli* of the wild-type Ti plasmid sequences into which the ultimate insertion of the foreign DNA is to take place (e.g., a restriction fragment of T-DNA). The foreign DNA of choice is then inserted by recombinant DNA techniques into the Ti plasmid fragment such that Ti plasmid DNA sequences extend on each end of the foreign DNA. The plasmid bearing the altered Ti plasmid fragment is then introduced into *A. tumefaciens* by transformation, and by means of various genetic selection techniques one is able to eventually isolate Ti plasmids in which the wild-type sequences have been replaced with the altered sequences, the result being the integration of the foreign DNA into the Ti plasmid. Infection of plants with bacteria harboring these altered plasmids then results in the mobilization of the foreign genes into the plant cell, wherein they are stably maintained as part of the T-DNA.

There are several real and potential problems which must be overcome before the Ti plasmid system can be generally useful in plant genetic engineering. First, it may be important to derive a vehicle capable of DNA transfer but incapable of tumor induction. However, should this prove not to be feasible, the recent findings of Wullems *et al.* (1981a,b) and Yang and Simpson (1981), that normal-appearing tobacco plants may be obtained from regenerated teratomas, and that T-DNA remnants are present in these plants and in their sexual progeny, give us reason to hope that the present system will prove generally useful for many species of plants.

Second, it is not clear that proper expression of the foreign genes in the engineered plant will occur. There are several facets to this consideration, and the relative importance of each depends in part upon the ultimate goal of the engineering venture. Questions such as the requirement for eukaryotic-type promoters, termination signals, and intervening sequences may limit the expression of prokaryotic genes in the plant cell. Other considerations such as the degree and timing of various control mechanisms may limit the usefulness of eukaryotic genes cloned into the plant. The effects of the cloned genes on such important aspects of plant metabolism as disease resistance and agronomic yield are impossible to estimate *in vitro,* but clearly are not important considerations if the goal of the research is to design plant tissue cultures which overproduce important secondary metabolites such as drugs or insecticides. There is obviously much research still needed to address these questions, and one may feel confident that the next decade will provide many new exciting perspectives in plant biology.

Acknowledgments

Sincere thanks are extended to A. Fitzpatrick for artwork and help with the literature compilation, to R. Dalke for typing the manuscript, and to M. Zarowitz for critical reading of the manuscript. I acknowledge the research support extended by the United States Department of Agriculture during the preparation of this chapter.

References

Bomhoff, G., Klapwijk, P. M., Kester, C. M., and Schilperoort, R. A. (1976). *Mol. Gen. Genet.* **145**, 177–181.

Braun, A. C. (1978). *Biochim. Biophys. Acta* **516**, 167–181.

Braun, A. C. (1980). *In Vitro* **16**, 38–48.

Braun, A. C., and Wood, H. N. (1976). *Proc. Natl. Acad. Sci. U.S.A.* **73**, 496–500.

Calos, M. P., and Miller, J. H. (1980). *Cell* **20**, 579–595.

Chilton, M.-D., Drummond, M. H., Merlo, D. J., Sciaky, D., Montoya, A. L., Gordon, M. P., and Nester, E. W. (1977). *Cell* **11**, 263–271.

Chilton, M.-D., Drummond, M. H., Merlo, D. J., and Sciaky, D. (1978). *Nature (London)* **275**, 147–149.

Chilton, M.-D., Saiki, R. K., Yadav, N., and Gordon, M. P. (1980). *Proc. Natl. Acad. Sci. U.S.A.* **77**, 4060–4064.

Coxon, D. T., Davies, A. M. C., Fenwick, G. R., and Self, R. (1980). *Tetrahedron Lett.* **21**, 495–498.

Currier, T. C., and Nester, E. W. (1976). *J. Bacteriol.* **126**, 157–165.

Depicker, A., Van Montagu, M., and Schell, J. (1978). *Nature (London)* **275**, 150–153.

Depicker, A., DeWilde, M., DeVos, G., DeVos, R., Van Montagu, M., and Schell, J. (1980). *Plasmid* **3**, 193–211.

Drlica, K. A., and Kado, C. I. (1975). *Bacteriol. Rev.* **39**, 186–196.

Drummond, M., and Chilton, M.-D. (1978). *J. Bacteriol.* **136**, 1178–1183.

Drummond, M. H., Gordon, M. P., Nester, E. W., and Chilton, M.-D. (1977). *Nature (London)* **269**, 535–536.

Einset, J. W., and Cheng, A. (1979). *In Vitro* **15**, 703–708.

Ellis, J. G., and Murphy, P. J. (1981). *Mol. Gen. Genet.* **181**, 36–43.

Firmin, J. L., and Fenwick, G. R. (1978). *Nature (London)* **276**, 842–844.

Garfinkel, D. J., and Nester, E. W. (1980). *J. Bacteriol.* **144**, 732–743.

Garfinkel, D. J., Simpson, R. B., Ream, L. W., White, F. F., Gordon, M. P., and Nester, E. W. (1981). *Cell* **27**, 143–153.

Glogowski, W., and Galsky, A. G. (1978). *Plant Physiol.* **61**, 1031–1033.

Gurley, W. B., Kemp, J. D., Albert, M. J., Sutton, D. W., and Callis, J. (1979). *Proc. Natl. Acad. Sci. U.S.A.* **76**, 2828–2832.

Guyon, P., Chilton, M.-D., Petit, A., and Tempé, J. (1980). *Proc. Natl. Acad. Sci. U.S.A.* **77**, 2693–2697.

Hernalsteens, J. P., Van Vliet, F., De Beuckeleer, M., Depicker, A., Engler, G., Lemmers, M., Holsters, M., Van Montague, M., and Schell, J. (1980). *Nature (London)* **287**, 654–656.

Kado, C. I. (1976). *Annu. Rev. Phytopathol.* **14**, 265–308.

Kado, C. I. (1979). *In* "Genetic Engineering" (J. K. Setlow and A. Hollaender, eds.), Vol. 1, pp. 223–239. Plenum, New York.

Kemp, J. D. (1978). *Plant Physiol.* **62**, 26–30.

Koekman, B. P., Ooms, G., Klapwijk, P. M., and Schilperoort, R. A. (1979). *Plasmid* **2**, 347–357.

Ledeboer, A. M. (1978). Ph.D. dissertation, (University of Leiden).

Lemmers, M., DeBeuckeleer, M., Holsters, M., Zambryski, P., Depicker, A., Hernalsteens, J. P., Van Montagu, M., and Schell, J. (1980). *J. Mol. Biol.* **144**, 353–376.

Lippincott, B. B., and Lippincott, J. A. (1969). *J. Bacteriol* **97**, 620–628.

Lippincott, B. B., Whatley, M. H., and Lippincott, J. A. (1977). *Plant Physiol.* **59**, 388–390.

Lippincott, J. A., and Lippincott, B. B. (1975). *Annu. Rev. Microbiol.* **29**, 377–405.

Lippincott, J. A., and Lippincott, B. B. (1977). *In* "Cell Wall Chemistry Related to Specificity in Host-Plant Pathogen Interactions" (B. Solheim and J. Raa, Eds.), pp. 439–451. Scandinavian University Books, Oslo.

Lippincott, J. A., and Lippincott, B. B. (1978). *Science* **199,** 1075–1078.

Matthysse, A. G., Wyman, P. M., and Homes, K. V. (1978). *Infect. Immun.* **22,** 516–522.

Matthysse, A. G., Holmes, K. V., and Gurlitz, R. H. G. (1981). *J. Bacteriol.* **145,** 583–595.

Matzke, A. J. M., and Chilton, M.-D. (1981). *J. Mol. Appl. Genet.* **1,** 39–49.

Merlo, D. J. (1981). *In* "Advances in Plant Pathology" (P. Williams and D. Ingram, eds.), Vol. 1, pp. 139–178. Academic Press, New York.

Merlo, D. J., Nutter, R. C., Montoya, A. L., Garfinkel, D. J., Drummond, M. H., Chilton, M.-D., Gordon, M. P., and Nester, E. W. (1980). *Mol. Gen. Genet.* **177,** 637–643.

Montoya, A. L., Chilton, M.-D., Gordon, M. P., Sciaky, D., and Nester, E. W. (1977). *J. Bacteriol.* **129,** 101–107.

Nester, E. W., and Kosuge, T. (1981). *Annu. Rev. Microbiol.* **35,** 531–565.

Ohtsubo, H., Ohmori, H., and Ohtsubo, E. (1979). *Cold Spring Harbor Symp. Quant. Biol.* **43,** 1269–1277.

Ooms, G., Klapwijk, P. M., Poulis, J. A., and Schilperoort, R. A. (1980). *J. Bacteriol.* **144,** 82–91.

Ooms, G., Hooykaas, P. J. J., Moolenaar, G., and Schilperoort, R. A. (1981). *Gene* **14,** 33–50.

Ruvkun, G. B., and Ausubel, F. M. (1981). *Nature (London)* **289,** 85–88.

Schell, J., and Van Montagu, M. (1980). *In* "Genome Organization and Expression in Plants" (C. J. Leaver, ed.), pp. 453–470. Plenum, New York.

Schell, J., Van Montagu, M., DeBeuckeleer, M., DeBlock, M., Depicker, A., De Wilde, M., Engler, G., Genetello, C., Hernalsteens, J. P., Holsters, M., Seurinck, J., Silva, B., Van Vliet, F., and Villarroel, R. (1979). *Proc. R. Soc. London Ser. B* **204,** 251–266.

Schilperoort, R. A. (1969). Ph.D. dissertation, University of Leiden.

Schilperoort, R. A., Klapwijk, P. M., Ooms, G., and Wullems, G. J. (1980). *In* "New Perspectives on the Genetic Origin of Tumor Cells" (F. J. Cleton and J. W. I. M. Simons, eds.), pp. 87–108. Nijhoff, The Hague.

Sciaky, D., Montoya, A. L., and Chilton, M.-D. (1978). *Plasmid* **1,** 238–253.

Smith, E. F., and Townsend, C. O. (1907). *Science* **25,** 671–673.

Smith, V. A., and Hindley, J. (1978). *Nature (London)* **276,** 498–500.

Stahl, F. W. (1979). *Annu. Rev. Genet.* **13,** 7–24.

Tempé, J., Petit, A., Holsters, M., Van Montagu, M., and Schell, J. (1977). *Proc. Natl. Acad. Sci. U.S.A.* **74,** 2848–2849.

Thomashow, M. F., Nutter, R., Montoya, A. L., Gordon, M. P., and Nester, E. W. (1980a). *Cell* **19,** 729–739.

Thomashow, M. F., Nutter, R., Postle, K., Chilton, M.-D., Blattner, F. R., Powell, A., Gordon, M. P., and Nester, E. W. (1980b). *Proc. Natl. Acad. Sci. U.S.A.* **77,** 6448–6452.

Thomashow, M. F., Knauf, V. C., and Nester, E. W. (1981). *J. Bacteriol.* **146,** 484–493.

Turgeon, R., Wood, H. N., and Braun, A. C. (1976). *Proc. Natl. Acad. Sci. U.S.A.* **73,** 3562–3564.

Van Larebeke, N., Engler, G., Holsters, M., Van den Elsacker, S., Zaenen, I., Schilperoort, R. A., and Schell, J. (1974). *Nature (London)* **252,** 169–170.

Watson, B., Currier, C., Gordon, M. P., Chilton, M.-D., and Nester, E. W. (1975). *J. Bacteriol.* **123,** 255–264.

Whatley, M. H., Bodwin, J. S., Lippincott, B. B., and Lippincott, J. A. (1976). *Infect. Immun.* **13,** 1080–1083.

Whatley, M. H., Margot, J. B., Schell, J., Lippincott, B. B., and Lippincott, J. A. (1978). *J. Gen. Microbiol.* **107,** 395–398.

Willmitzer, L., DeBeuckeleer, M., Lemmers, M., Van Montagu, M., and Schell, J. (1980). *Nature (London)* **287,** 359–361.

Wood, H. N., Binns, A. N., and Braun, A. C. (1978). *Differentiation* **11,** 175–180.

Wullems, G. J., Molendijk, L., and Schilperoort, R. A. (1980). *Theor. Appl. Genet.* **56,** 203–208.

Wullems, G. J., Molendijk, L., Ooms, G., and Schilperoort, R. A. (1981a). *Cell* **24,** 719–727.

Wullems, G. J., Molendijk, L., Ooms, G., and Schilperoort, R. A. (1981b). *Proc. Natl. Acad. Sci. U.S.A.* **78,** 4344–4348.

Yadav, N. S., Postle, K., Saiki, R. K., Thomashow, M. F., and Chilton, M.-D. (1980). *Nature (London)* **287,** 458–461.

Yang, F., and Simpson, R. B. (1981). *Proc. Natl. Acad. Sci. U.S.A.* **78,** 4151–4155.

Yang, F.-M., Montoya, A. L., Nester, E. W., and Gordon, M. P. (1980a). *In Vitro* **16,** 87–92.

Yang, F.-M., Montoya, A. L., Merlo, D. J., Drummond, M. H., Chilton, M.-D., Nester, E. W., and Gordon, M. P. (1980b). *Mol. Gen. Genet.* **177,** 707–714.

Yang, F.-M., McPherson, J. C., Gordon, M. P., and Nester, E. W. (1980c). *Biochem. Biophys. Res. Commun.* **92,** 1273–1277.

Zambryski, P., Holsters, M., Kruger, K., Depicker, A., Schell, J., Van Montagu, M., and Goodman, H. (1980). *Science* **209,** 1385–1391.

Chapter **14**

Prospectus for Genetic Engineering in Agriculture

CLARENCE I. KADO *and* PAUL F. LURQUIN

I. INTRODUCTION

Novel approaches in the direct genetic modification of plants for food, fiber, and aesthetic purposes have been horizons long sought by plant and animal breeders. After the gradual acceptance that DNA was the nature of genes (for historical review, see Hotchkiss, 1979), direct manipulation of this genetic material became the center of intensive attention, particularly when the structural details became known and could be related to function. Biochemical tools for the precise dissection and rejoining of the DNA molecule made it feasible to easily rearrange genes

Copyright © 1982 by Academic Press, Inc.
All rights of reproduction in any form reserved.
ISBN 0-12-509002-1

from one source to that of another (Timmis *et al.*, 1978; Helling and Lomax, 1978). The technologies for the insertion of reassembled genes into various recipient cells were developed in parallel to these biochemical endeavors. Therefore, it is not surprising that applications of these technologies are being put to use. With crop plants, knowledge that they can be regenerated from a single cell is of primary importance and provides the added advantage that is presently lacking in animal systems. The totipotent nature of plant cells therefore provides the immediate potential for direct foreign gene insertions into the cell system with the culmination of a utilitarian crop plant.

The overall scheme of these technologies is coined under an umbrella term "genetic engineering." Thus, the genetic engineering of crop plants usually involves the reconstruction of sets of genes that will be stably incorporated in the plant genome and successfully express the traits that were initially selected *in vitro*.

We describe herein the means of assembling genes for genetically modifying bacteria and crop plants. The main concerns have been (1) a means to introduce foreign genes into recipient plant cells; (2) stable maintenance and inheritance of those genes; (3) expression of the genes into the suitable phenotype selected; (4) phenotypic stability under environmental and biological stress; and (5) economic suitability and importance.

The genetic concerns are discussed in the forthcoming section of this chapter. Various model systems portraying the current approaches are described.

II. COMPLEXITY OF THE PROBLEM

Foreign genes can be supplied to plant cells as (1) purified DNA in association with compounds destined to protect it from nuclease degradation or (2) as chromosomal DNA present in whole bacteria or bacterial spheroplasts. In the first case, gene-size DNA molecules must face both mechanical (cell wall, plasmalemma) and biochemical (integration, transcription, translation, and enzymatic function) barriers which may all prevent its expression in the recipient cells. The nature of these barriers has been extensively reviewed elsewhere (Lurquin, 1977; Kleinhofs and Behki, 1977; Kado and Kleinhofs, 1980). Recent progress made in the field of yeast and mammalian cell transformation has indicated that molecular barriers may be easier to surmount than originally thought, provided that the foreign genes (eukaryotic and prokaryotic) are coupled to suitable promoters and/or included in a suitable replicon (Yoder and Ganesan, 1981; Cocking *et al.*, 1981; Smith and Danner,

1981). Thus, properly engineered prokaryotic genes have been shown to be expressed in eukaryotic cells (Jiminez and Davies, 1980; Mulligan and Berg, 1980). Even though convenient plant vectors still have to be developed, it can be anticipated that molecular barriers present in plants may not be more difficult to avoid than those presented by yeast and mammalian cells.

Plant cell walls can be removed by a variety of cellulolytic enzymes. The process releases single protoplasts with plasmalemma that display interesting properties such as their capability to fuse with the plasmalemma of other protoplasts, microorganisms, and even lipid vesicles (for review, see Cocking *et al.*, 1981). Therefore, higher plant protoplasts may very well be recipients of choice in DNA uptake experiments. Unfortunately, so far only a few plant species produce totipotent protoplasts.

A further complication resides in the fact that conditional lethal plant auxotrophs are extremely rare. Among those, the best candidates for transformation experiments seem to be the tobacco nitrate reductase mutants isolated by Muller and Grafe (1978). Indeed, genetic engineering experiments must rely on the possibility to screen for transformants. The latter can be detected only if auxotrophs can be reversed to a prototrophic condition after DNA uptake. Another possibility, however, is to select transformants on the basis of a novel trait which does not normally exist in these cells. Hormone independence conferred by *Agrobacterium tumefaciens* T-DNA insertion into plant nuclear DNA or antibiotic resistance acquired through prokaryotic transposon expression are two examples of this approach (see Section V,B).

It is clear that biochemical analysis on the fate of donor genes does not prove that transformation has or will occur. Nevertheless, those studies have indicated in what directions efforts should be made and in three cases, such studies (Lurquin and Kado, 1977; Lurquin, 1979; Rollo *et al.*, 1981) have paved the way to the demonstration that optimized nucleic acid uptake conditions lead to their biological expression in plant protoplasts (Davey *et al.*, 1980; Dellaporta and Fraley, 1981; Fukunaga *et al.*, 1981; Watanabe *et al.*, 1982).

III. GENE VECTOR SYSTEMS

A. Construction of Gene Vectors

Potential plant host vectors have already been extensively discussed (Kado, 1979). Plant replicons and promoters are not yet available. However, it is conceivable that mammalian cell promoters such as those from

SV40 and from the Herpes thymidine kinase genes may be recognized by plant cell RNA polymerase II. Therefore, a recombinant DNA molecule consisting of a selected eukaryotic or prokaryotic gene flanked by such a promoter may very well be transcribed in plant cells. This composite molecule might in turn be introduced into the yeast 2-μm nuclear plasmid in order to possibly allow replication of the chimeric molecule. However, it must be pointed out that it is not known whether the yeast plasmid is able to replicate independently in other eukaryotic cells.

Other independent replicons such as DNA of plant viruses of the caulimo- and genimi-virus groups could also be considered as potential gene vectors. Here, some progress has been made toward the utilization of those circular DNA molecules as potential plant host vectors. The genome of cauliflower mosaic virus (CaMV) is a relaxed circular DNA molecule about 8 kb in length that harbors three naturally occurring nicks (Franck *et al.*, 1980). This DNA possess unique sites for restriction endonucleases *Sal*I and *Xho*I. These sites can be used to open the CaMV DNA into a linear molecule which then can be ligated to a suitable *E. coli* plasmid vector such as pBR322 or pBR325 (Bolivar, 1978), resulting in the formation of a hybrid plasmid molecule. The CaMV DNA thus can be cloned and amplified in *E. coli*. The resulting cloned CaMV DNA is infectious when excised from the hybrid plasmid (S. Daubert, personal communication).

Cloned CaMV DNA from *E. coli* no longer possesses the three nicks; however, these nicks reappear when CaMV DNA is isolated from cauliflower plants that were inoculated with the cloned-exised CaMV DNA. The virus also appears capable of either gene conversion or genetic recombination, since coinoculation with two different insertion mutants yields CaMV DNA like the wild-type strain, the genome of which carries again the three nicks (S. Daubert, personal communication). Analogous types of experiments seem to support this hypothesis (Howell *et al.*, 1981). Two basic problems as a vector are obvious: (1) the inability to package foreign DNA greater than about 800 base pairs in the CaMV genome and still retain virulence. (2) The host range of CaMV is narrow, although the barriers might be either at the cell wall level or at the level of intercellular transport in nonhosts.

The maintenance of foreign genes in plant cells may not be required if the genes were cloned within plant DNA sequences homologous to that of the host cells. Such regions of homology could lead to foreign gene integration through recombination. This phenomenon is well-documented in yeast (Hinnen *et al.*, 1978) and in mammalian cells (Pellicer *et al.*, 1980).

Integration in the absence of homology could even occur if the cloning vector consisted of maize transposable elements. However, those transposable elements have not yet been cloned and it is not known whether or not they will be functional in other plant species.

The last and so far most promising plant host vector is the *A. tumefaciens* pTi plasmid whose T-DNA region is integrated in crown gall nuclear DNA (for review, see Nester and Kosuge, 1981). The fate of this T-DNA in plants regenerated from crown gall tumors is presently unclear. However, it seems that at least a portion of this T-DNA can go through meiosis (Yang and Simpson, 1981). Therefore, it may be possible to engineer this pTi plasmid, i.e., by marker exchange in such a way that desirable genes may accompany residual T-DNA fragments in progeny plants (Matzke and Chilton, 1981). Such experiments are technically feasible since border fragments resisting meiosis have been identified. Moreover, many T-DNA restriction endonuclease fragments have been cloned in amplifiable *E. coli* plasmids.

B. Packaging and Maintenance of Vectors

It has long been recognized that plant protoplasts are refractory to DNA uptake and degrade DNA in the medium. Polycations such as poly-L-orinthine, polyethylene glycol, or a combination of both have been shown to increase the donor DNA half-life and its uptake (Lurquin and Kado, 1977; Fernandez *et al.*, 1978; Lurquin and Marton, 1979). It has been found recently that lipid vesicles (liposomes) composed of a variety of lipids have the capability to sequester recombinant plasmids and to strongly interact with a variety of plant protoplasts (Lurquin, 1979, 1981, Rollo *et al.*, 1981; Lurquin *et al.*, 1981; Lurquin and Sheehy, 1982). Biochemical experiments indicate that DNA transferred by liposomes suffers minimal damage. One report strongly suggests that liposome-mediated transformation of plant protoplasts may be a reality (Dellaporta and Fraley, 1981). Liposome-mediated transformation of mammalian cells has been demonstrated (Fraley *et al.*, 1981).

Alternatively, *Agrobacterium tumefaciens* cells (Smith and Hindley, 1978; Marton *et al.*, 1979) and spheroplasts (Hasezawa *et al.*, 1981) have been shown to induce crown gall transformation of tobacco cells and protoplasts. This technique efficiently bypasses uptake and maintenance problems presented by isolated DNA molecules since it relies on a purely natural phenomenon. However, for the time being, it is limited to the case of pTi DNA transfer to plant cells.

IV. SUITABLE GENES AND STRATEGIES FOR PLANT DISEASE CONTROL

Strategies to prevent or curb plant diseases have resulted from data gathered over long periods from empirical tests, from shotgun approaches, and from field observations, many of which were subjective. Absolute disease control is difficult to achieve and often too costly to attempt. By far the most effective means of disease control have been the development of resistant, immune, or tolerant cultivars. Disease control by genetic manipulations has been limited by several parameters. First, the precise mechanism by which a pathogen causes disease remains either uncertain, unestablished, or totally unknown. Without complete knowledge of disease mechanisms, even classical genetic approaches remain limiting and yield to emperical approaches, which nonetheless have resulted in some degree of success because of continued costly, persistent, and tasking work by plant breeders and pathologists. It is therefore obvious that most logical approaches are to examine the nature of the pathogen and determine its inherent weaknesses.

Tremendous impetus regarding a given plant disease comes about when the pathogenic organism is carefully and thoroughly studied rather than host–parasite interactions or the host itself (Kado, 1976a). A great deal of energy has been expended on examining host responses. Such studies unfortunately have been rewarded with small gains. Molecular biological approaches aimed at the pathogenic organism generate answers to a number of disease control problems. Knowing that genes of the pathogen code for products, which in turn directly or indirectly cause the disease response in the plant host, is the primary point of focus. Such knowledge contributes toward large gains in understanding the cause of disease and toward its control.

There are a number of genes that confer virulence and pathogenicity on the pathogen. We define virulence as the degree of aggressive ability of the pathogen to colonize the host, and in turn we define pathogenicity as the ability of the pathogen to perturb higher cells, the result of which collectively is recognized as a disease response. Thus, the genes for virulence are there for the pathogen to grow and colonize the host and the genes for pathogenicity code products that alter cell function. Hence, a thorough understanding of gene functions in virulence and pathogenicity is imperative in the determination of the weaknesses of the pathogen. Knowledge of these factors permits the development of suitable control strategies. It is obvious that compounds affecting virulence (i.e., the degree of aggressive ability of the pathogen to grow in the host) or pathogenicity (i.e., elaboration of a perturbant or cell killing agent by the pathogen) of the pathogen may potentially be candidates for use in disease control.

A. Genes That Code for Fungicidal Products

In nature, microorganisms effectively compete among each other to retain or gain access to a given ecological niche. In environments such as soil where various organisms compete for space and food, those organisms that effectively compete against fungi possess mechanisms that either prohibit fungal growth or kill the competing fungus directly. Fungi that persist in such soils probably are equipped with protective mechanisms. On the other hand soil-borne plant pathogenic fungi are probably less well equipped and seek the plant as the sheltered environment, in which to colonize and ultimately to become the final niche of the pathogen. Soil bacteria are probably the best candidates from which genes that code for fungicidal compounds can be easily isolated. This is not to say that other fungi and Actinomycetes are not good candidates. Some examples of such compounds will be discussed here, emphasizing the fact that these are examples of compounds that can alter the physiology of a given fungus culminating in cessation of growth or in their death.

1. Chitinase

Alterations of fungal cell wall synthesis may lead to fungicidal action. Fungal cell walls are mainly composed of chitin microfibrils, polysaccharides, and their chemical complexes with proteins (Farkas, 1979). β-Glucans and crystalline polysaccharides support cell wall structure (Bartnicki-Garcia, 1970; Farkas, 1979). Compounds affecting the synthesis of chitin should prove effective in retarding or inhibiting fungal growth. With the knowledge that synthesis of chitinous cell wall occurs during spore germination (Selitrennikoff *et al.*, 1976), and during septum formation during cell division and during mating (Schekman and Brawley, 1979), chitin synthase (UDP-2-acetamido-2-deoxy-D- glucose : chitin 4-β-acetamidodeoxy-D-glucosyltransferase, EC 2.4.1.16) inhibiting compounds may prove effective biofungicides. Fungal inhibitating bacteria can be readily isolated from soil by simple screening procedures. These bacteria can be examined for inhibitory activity on chitin synthase. The gene(s) that code for this activity may be cloned in an appropriate plasmid vehicle in an appropriate recipient bacterium. The recipient bacterium was derived from its normal niche in which the pathogenic fungi invades to initiate infection. The presence of this bacterium now endowed with the chitin synthase inhibitor makes this niche a very unsuitable environment for the fungus, thereby protecting the plant host from potential infection.

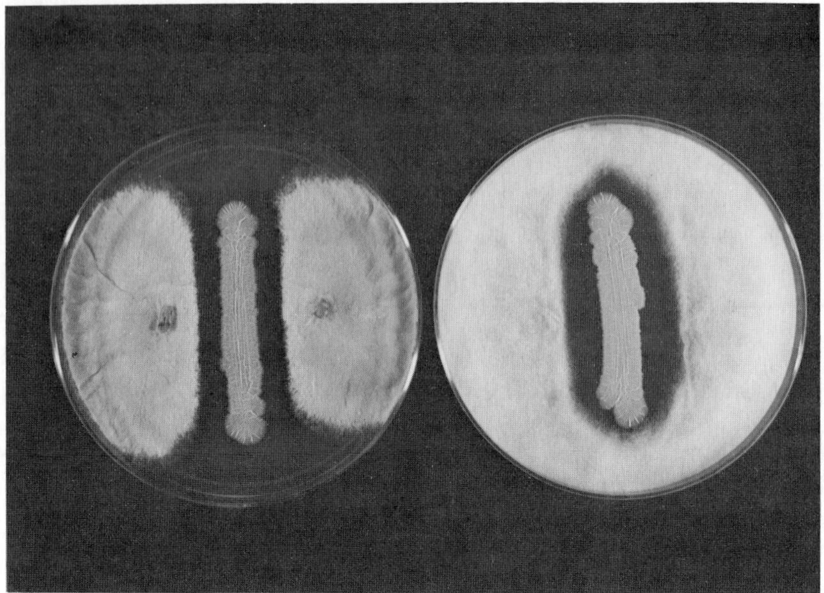

Figure 1. Production of a mycocidal compound by a Gram-negative soil bacterium that was grown on a rich agar medium. Left petri plate shows zone of inhibition of a cotton (*Gossypium hirsutum* L.) strain of *Rhizoctonia solani* Kuehn. Right petri plate shows zone of inhibition of a cotton strain of *Pythium ultimum* Trow. (Data from C. I. Kado, W. C. Schnathorst, H. R. Azad, and J. Davis.)

2. *Mycocidal Compounds*

There are numerous microorganisms that elaborate compounds besides the chitin synthase inhibitor that prevent fungal growth. These microorganisms can be specifically selected for activity against a given plant pathogenic fungus. Of these organisms, bacteria are the most suitable candidates because of their smaller genomic size and less genetic complexity than lower eukaryotes. The mycocides elaborated by these bacteria can be characterized and those that show high degree of stability and ability to penetrate fungi are selected. Furthermore, if such mycocides are coded by genes on plasmids, the effort expended in isolating those genes is enormously reduced. Thus, it is important to obtain bacteria that show mycocidal activities and harbor cryptic plasmids. A mycocide-producing bacterium such as the one shown in Fig. 1 may not possess the potentials to serve as a protecting biocide because it may not survive successfully in the potential sites of infection (i.e., the infection court). It would be necessary then to look for one of these bacterium that naturally occupies the infection court. This bacterium can be tailored to be the recipient of the mycocidal genes derived from the first bacterium.

B. Genes That Code for Bacteriocidal Products

Similar to the approaches in selecting mycocidal organisms harboring the genes coding for bacteriocidal compounds, namely bacteriocins, can be obtained from soil and plant inhabiting bacteria and Actinomycetes. Bacteriocins elaborated by bacteria are generally coded by plasmids (Tagg *et al.*, 1976). They are high-molecular-weight extracellular antibiotics that are active against closely related species of bacteria, in contrast to antibiotics of relatively low molecular weight, which have wider activity spectrum. Bacteriocins that are polypeptides have the best potentials for being coded directly by plasmid genes. When this is the case, like the mycocide genes, the bacteriocin coding genes can be isolated with relative ease and cloned in an appropriate plasmid vehicle.

Several bacteriocins showing activity against plant pathogenic bacteria have been studied and those that have been tested show little promise in prevention or for therapeutic use on systemic diseases (Vidaver, 1976). Nevertheless, bacteriocins have excellent potential if there are means to prevent the development of resistance to the bacteriocin. One means is to employ more than one type of bacteriocin. Superficially, the easiest approach would be to use two different bacteria, each producing a different bacteriocin. However, there are several limitations that surface when this concept is put to application. These are listed in Table I. To avoid these limitations, it is best to design a bacteriocinogenic bacterium. Such bacteria are selected from the ecosystem

Table I. Limiting Factors on the Use of Bacteriocinogenic Bacteria for Plant Disease Control

Observation	Probable cause	Solution
A. Gradual steady decrease in effective control	Mutation to resistance by the pathogen	Employ more than one bacteriocin (see text)
B. Decrease in control and rapid spread of the ineffectiveness	Transfer of bacteriocin genes to the pathogen	Employ bacteriocinogenic bacteria with transfer deficient plasmids
C. Rapid ineffective control	Transfer of bacteriocin-resistance genes to the pathogen	Employ more than one bacteriocin coded by transfer-deficient plasmid
D. Control effective only in certain regions or on certain crop plants	Presence of naturally occurring bacteriocin inhibitors and/or antagonists are present. Low survival of bacteriocinogenic bacteria	Eliminated by using proper recipient strains

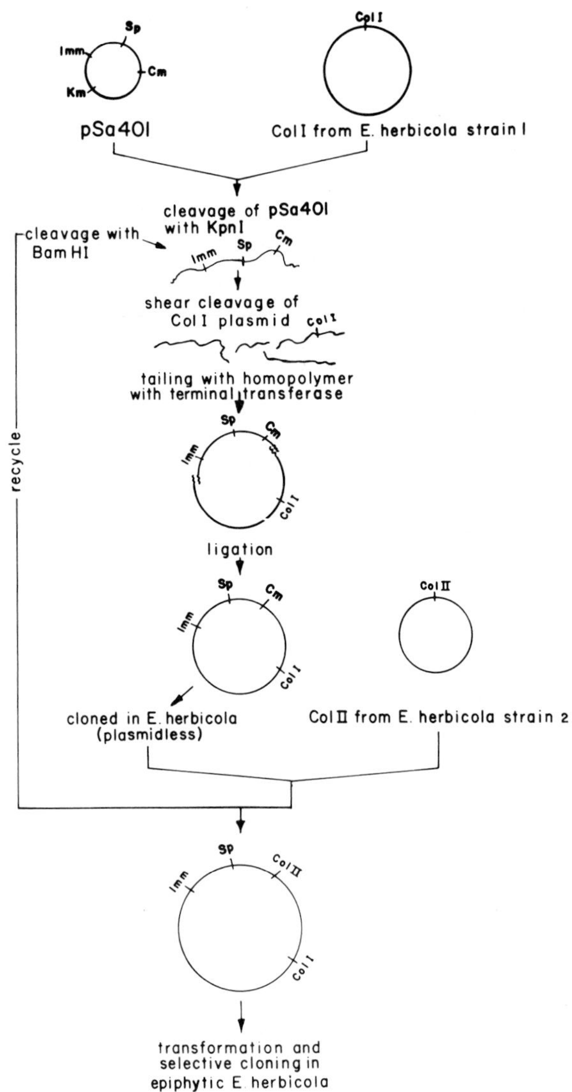

Figure 2. Strategy on the construction of a biological control bacterium by recombinant DNA methodologies. The cloning vector pSa401 carries a unique *Kpn*I site in the kanamycin resistance gene (Km) into which the *Col*I gene of *Erwinia herbicola* is inserted and ligated by first cleaving the *E. herbicola* DNA by mechanical shearing, alligning the ends with exonuclease III and tailing the termini with a homopolymer such as poly(dT). Alternatively, the ends are blunted and then ligated without tailing. Following ligation of the DNA pieces to pSa401, clones carrying the *Col*I gene is scored for the bacteriocin activity on *E. amylovora*. Subsequently, a second different *Col*II gene can be inserted in the unique *Bam*HI site of pSa401 by the same procedure. Clones now harboring both *Col*I and *Col*II

in which the plant pathogen must survive. Take for example the fireblight disease of pear. It is well established that the pear blossom is the primary site of infection owing to the transfer of *Erwinia amylovora* by the insect vectors and natural elements such as wind blown rain, etc. The pear blossom harbors a natural population of *Erwinia herbicola* and yeasts. These organisms should be considered prime candidates as recipients of bacteriocin genes. We have reported previously a strategy on the use of *E. herbicola* as a recipient of a hybrid plasmid composed of two or more bacteriocin genes for control of fireblight (Kado, 1976b). The same version of this strategy is presented in Fig. 2. Many strains of *Erwinia* including *E. amylovora*, are sensitive to colicins and bacteriocins (Azad, 1979; Beer and Rundle, 1980). A plasmid vector system such as pSa401 may be used in the cloning of bacteriocin genes. Colicinogenic strains of *Erwinia herbicola* are easily isolated for pear buds and blossoms. These strains harbor plasmids, one of which apparently codes for *Col*I (Gantotti *et al.*, 1981) as shown in Fig. 3. The colicin coding gene (designated *Col*I, II, III etc.) can be easily cloned into the unique *Kpn*I site of the kanamycin resistance gene of pSa401. A second colicin gene from a distinct *E. herbicola* strain can be spliced into the unique *Bam*HI site of the vector plasmid.

The result of this cloning strategy (Kado, 1976b), as shown in Fig. 2, is a composite plasmid harboring two or more genes that code for distinct bacteriocins (colicins) directed against *E. amylovora*. Because the recipient bacterium *E. herbicola* was a natural resident of the pear bud and blossom, the problem of survivability of a biocontrolling agent is avoided. The recipient *E. herbicola* strains tested in our laboratory are generally resistant to their own colicin but certain strains have been sensitive to bacteriocins from other strains, e.g., as in Fig. 2, *E. herbicola* strain I. When such strains are chosen as the recipient it would be necessary to initially construct a *Col*II-resistant mutant that is not a *Col*II permease mutant.

C. Genes That Code for Nematocidal Products

Interactions between plant nematodes and parasitic bacteria have been reported (Mankau, 1975; Sayre and Wergin, 1977; Sayre, 1980). The

---

yield a recombinant DNA molecule that produces all two bacteriocins. The existing chloramphenicol resistance gene (Cm) aborts in the absence of selective pressure (Farrand *et al.*, 1981). The recipient *E. herbicola*, resistant to each of the bacteriocins, is able to inhibit growth of *E. amylovora*. Since, this particular strain of *E. herbicola* was isolated from pear blossoms, it is effective in protecting the blossoms from infection by *E. amylovora*. (This strategy was based on that of Kado, 1976b.)

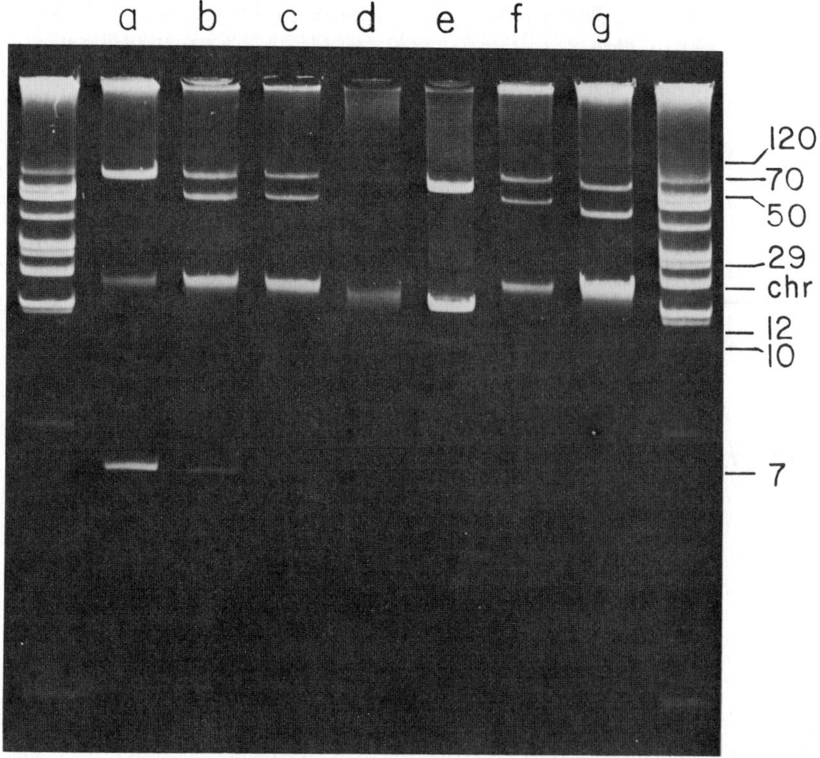

Figure 3. Plasmids of *Erwinia herbicola* strains resolved in a agarose gel by electrophoresis using plasmids isolated by a miniscreen procedure of Kado and Liu (1981). Lanes a through g are respectively *E. herbicola* strains 25D3, 25D31, 25D32, 25D33, 25D34, 25D35, and 25D36. The lanes that flank lanes a–g show plasmids of *E. stewartii* (Smith) Dye strain SW2 used as molecular weight standards. (Data from C. I. Kado and T. J. Quayle).

bacteria in these cases were parasitic, in that their spores penetrate the nematode's body during germination. Such mechanisms are mainly mechanical followed by parasitism and therefore not amenable to gene-cloning technologies. Bacteria that elaborate nematocidal compounds have not been reported. This does not imply that such bacteria do not exist in nature. The strategies used to obtain such bacteria are essentially the same as that used for those organisms discussed above. However, because plant parasitic nematodes are obligate parasites, single member culture technologies have not been described. Nematocidal bacteria are usually associated in soil harboring large populations of a parasitic nematode. These bacteria can be screened for by directly testing them for effects on the viability of the nematode. This can be accomplished as follows. Test bacteria are streaked in a straight line down the center of agar plates and allowed to grow for 24–48 hr at 30°C on minimal agar medium. After the bacteria have grown, wells are made with a 5-mm-diameter cork borer in a diagonal to the streaked bacteria using a template. Two such lines of well are placed in the petri plate (Fig. 4). Aliquots of about 20 nematodes are dispensed in to each well. The dish is covered and incubated at 16°C for several hours, the length of time being standardized to make the assay reproducible. After a given time, the nematodes are viewed directly in each well by using an inverted microscope and individual nematodes tested by pricking them with a needle. Nematodes in wells nearest the streaks are first tested. This

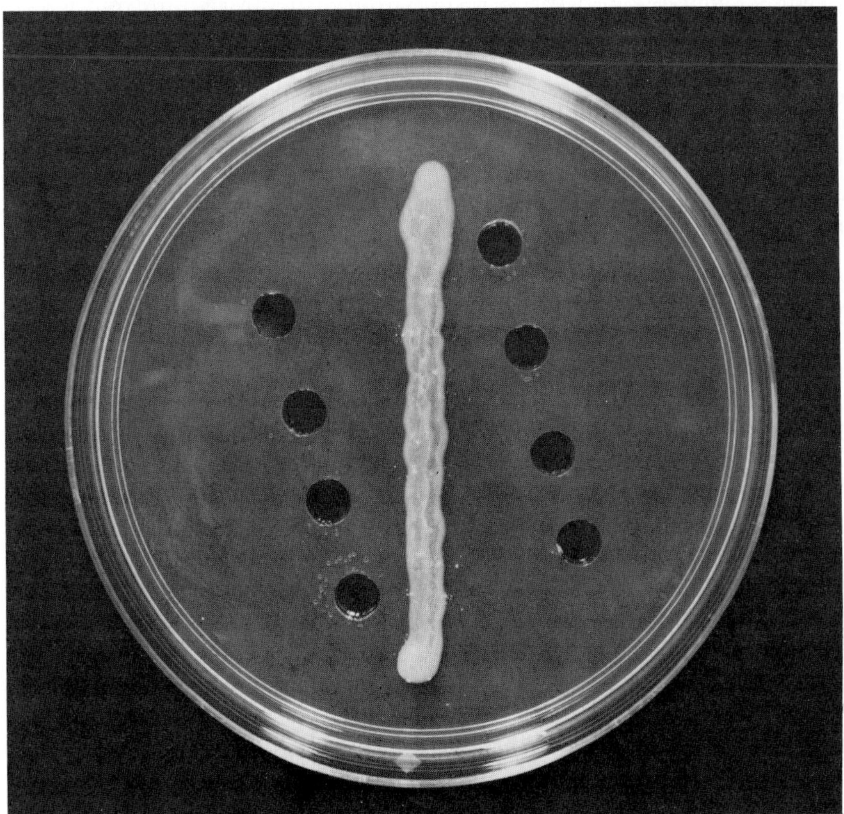

Figure 4. A Gram-negative soil bacterium, with activity against the root-knot nematode (*Meloidogyne* sp.), was streaked on agar medium, diagonally to the parallel wells in the agar. After a set time of growth, an equal number of live nematodes are dispensed into each well and their survival scored by motility.

facilitates the assay since effective nematocidal compounds would have permeated the closest wells first. Those compounds showing no activity will generally have live nematodes in the first wells and therefore the plates can be discarded without further assessments. Bacteria with high nematocide activity can then be rescreened and their nematocidal compound characterized.

V. TRANSFORMATION OF HIGHER CELLS

Insertion of extrachromosomal DNA molecules by transformation has been well established for various bacteria. A number of techniques have become available for the transformation of various eukaryotic organisms. These procedures are essential for achieving success in genetic modification of higher cells. There are two means by which extrachromosomal DNA can be maintained in transformed cells. First the introduced DNA is allowed to integrate in the genomic DNA of the recipient cell by designing a suitable vector that is known to possess integration functions. The second means is to introduce DNA that replicate as an independent replicon.

A. Fungi

The successful transformation of yeast (*Saccharomyces cerevisiae*) has been reported by Hinnen *et al.* (1978) and Beggs (1978). In this case, spheroplasts were first prepared by exposure of actively growing yeast cells to Glusulase (Endo Laboratories) or Helicase (Industrie Biologigue Francaise) in 1–1.2 *M* sorbitol. The spheroplasts were then treated with 10 m*M* $CaCl_2$ in 1 *M* sorbitol, 0.01 *M* Tris–HCl, pH 7.5, before exposure to plasmid DNA (10–60 μg/ml). The spheroplasts were allowed to fuse in the presence of 40% polyethylene glycol 4000, sedimented by centrifugation, and aliquots of the resuspended spheroplasts were plated on regeneration medium and minimal medium. After 2–4 days incubation of 29°C, transformants can be seen on the minimal plates.

An efficient transformation system has also been developed for *Neurospora crassa* (Case *et al.*, 1979). The general procedures for transformation of yeasts were adapted for *N. crassa* with slight modifications. Freshly germinated conidia were subjected to Glusulase to generate spheroplasts. The spheroplasts washed with 1 *M* sorbitol and then treated with 0.05 *M* $CaCl_2$ in 1 *M* sorbitol, 0.01 *M* 4-morpholinepropane sulfonic acid, pH 6.3, followed by a 30-sec 37°C shock treatment and placed on ice. Plasmid DNA (60 μg/ml) was then added and the mixture was subjected to a 30-sec 45°C shock treatment. The spheroplasts were fused in 40% polyethylene glycol 4000 in buffered $CaCl_2$ solution. The washed spheroplasts were plated on minimal regeneration medium and the resulting transformants collected.

These techniques are applicable to other fungi. For example, there is much interest in mycorrizae. These are fungi that establish symbiotic associations with roots and are viewed as important in sustaining increased availability of nutrients to its host plants. Mycorrhizal fungi are found in most agronomic species and are widespread in the two major crop families, Leguminosae and Graminae. Unfortunately, these fungi have not been cultured as pure fungal cultures and therefore they are not easily amenable to recombinant DNA technologies for the construction of new beneficial endosymbionts. It is obvious that efforts made in the pure culture of mycorrhizal fungi can yield tremendous benefits.

Much of the recombinant DNA work has concentrated on the yeast *Saccharomyces cerevisiae* because it is the only eukaryote where the propagation of extrachromosomal DNAs (plasmids) can be ensured by selecting for the expression of a linked marker such as a gene capable of complementing a host lesion. Several yeast genes have been isolated as hybrid plasmid molecules that were capable of complementing *E. coli* auxotrophs (Struhl *et al.*, 1976; Ratzkin and Carbon, 1977; Bach *et al.*, 1979). Conversely, a chimeric plasmid carrying the yeast marker *leu* 2 was able to complement auxotrophic yeast mutants (Hinnen *et al.*, 1978). In this case, the transforming DNA was found integrated into the host chromosome in several different places. Hinnen *et al.* (1978) used the plasmid pYe*leu* 10,.which is a hybrid DNA molecule composed of the *Escherichia coli* plasmid ColE1 and a segment of yeast DNA from chromosome III. This plasmid complements *leu* B mutants of *E. coli* and contains the yeast *leu* 2^+ gene which encodes the leucine biosynthetic enzyme β-isopropylmalate dehydrogenase. Although the mechanism of insertion of the pYe*leu* 10 plasmid into yeast DNA is presently unknown, Hinnen *et al.* (1978) demonstrated that ColE1 DNA sequences were integrated in yeast chromosomal DNA. Since ColE1 and its derivatives are well established as cloning vectors (Hershfield *et al.*, 1974), pYe*leu* 10 may be used as a vector to shuttle eukaryotic genes between *E. coli* and *S. cerevisiae*. However, eukaryotic genes on such shuttle vectors that integrate the genes into the yeast chromosome yield a low frequency of transformation and in its integrated form may not function appropriately. To circumvent these difficulties, it would be desirable to design a vector that replicates autonomously in the absence of recombination with the yeast genome. Struhl *et al.* (1979) have designed yeast transformation vectors with the following properties: the ability to replicate in yeast and *E. coli* cells; genetic characteristics selectable in yeast or *E. coli* after DNA transformation into either of these organisms; sites of cleavage into which essentially any fragment of DNA can be inserted; and capability to isolate hybrid DNAs as covalently closed circles in at least one of these organisms. These vectors were derivatives of pBR322 carrying yeast chromosomal DNA and/or yeast plasmid Scp1 DNA. They therefore combine *E. coli* and yeast genetics into a single system, making it possible for cloning foreign genes directly into yeast cells. The vectors, showing high frequency of transformation, harbored a yeast chromosomal sequence and replicated autonomously. Such vectors have proved valuable as a general means for the cloning of any eukaryotic gene. Stinchcomb *et al.* (1979) reported vectors carrying the *ars* 1 (autonomously replicating sequence) sequence are capable of autonomous replication in the absence of recombination with the yeast genome. Thus, when transformed into yeast, a chimeric molecule carrying an *ars* sequences or its equivalent origin of replication has a readily selectable property of high-frequency transformation. Hence, DNA sequences from *Neurospora crassa, Dictyostelium discoideum, Caenorhabditis elegans, Drosophila melanogaster,* and *Zea mays* were cloned and replicated in yeast cells (Stinchcomb *et al.,* 1980). It would be interesting to test whether such eukaryotic DNA sequences are stably maintained in various eukaryotic systems besides yeast.

Recently, expression of the *E. coli* plasmid chloramphenicol acetyltransferase gene has been shown to occur in yeast cells (*Saccharomyces cerevisiae*) (Cohen *et al.,* 1980). In this experiment a composite vector was used consisting of the *E. coli* plasmid pBR325 (Bolivar, 1978), the yeast 2-μm DNA plasmid (Hollenberg *et al.,* 1976), and a fragment of DNA containing the yeast *leu* 2 structural gene derived from plasmid pYe*leu*1 (Ratzkin and Carbon, 1977). When a leucine-require yeast strain, 21D, carrying a double mutation in the *leu* 2 gene, was transformed to leucine prototrophy with this composite plasmid, the LEU^+ transformants showed resistance to chloramphenicol at 500 μg/ml in agar medium containing the nonfermentable energy sources glycerol and ethanol. Cellular metabolism and growth on these carbon sources require functional mitochondria which, in yeast, is the cellular target of chloramphenicol. Therefore, only cells that are resistant to chloramphenicol will grow on the medium. These transformants were shown to contain the detoxification enzyme, chloramphenicol acetyltransferase. It remains uncertain at this time whether or not bacterial or yeast DNA sequences are controlling the expression of this gene.

B. Plants

Transformation of plants by the application of exogenous DNA has been reported from time to time but the experimental results were never clearly verified. These past experiments have been viewed as early attempts to qualitatively modify plants (Kleinhofs and Bekhi, 1977; Lurquin, 1977; Lurquin and Kado, 1979; Kado and Kleinhofs, 1980). The early approaches were clearly deficient in addressing a number of fundamental questions, of which the genetic and biochemical barriers (Kado, 1979) confronting a foreign genetic element were poorly understood (see Section II). It is now clear that foreign DNA molecules, for example, hybrid DNA molecules generated and amplified as independent replicons in bacteria such as *E. coli*, will survive in the protoplasts of carrot, cowpea, and turnip (Lurquin and Kado, 1979; Fernandez *et al.*, 1978), and barley (Hughes *et al.*, 1979), potato, and lettuce (C. I. Kado, unpublished results). The Ti plasmid of *Agrobacterium tumefaciens* was shown to survive as relatively intact linear molecules in cowpea protoplast nuclei (Lurquin and Kado, 1979).

To incorporate exogenous DNA (usually as a hybrid plasmid) into protoplasts, various additives such as poly-L-ornithine (Lurquin and Kado, 1977; Fernandez *et al.*, 1978; Hughes *et al.*, 1979), high pH and Ca^{2+} (Sarkar *et al.*, 1974), polyethylene glycol (Cassells and Barless, 1978; G. J. Wullems, personal communication), and lyposomes (Lurquin, 1980) have been used successfully (see Section III,B). Similarly, for gene transfer to mammalian cells, the method of Graham and van der Eb (1973), in which DNA is coprecipitated with calcium phosphate and the precipitate is added directly to a cell monolayer, has been used successfully. Although the mechanism by which plasmid DNA is taken up by protoplast is not well understood, all of the above constituents promote DNA incorporation. The degree of promoting transfer by each of these reagents is about the same once each of the systems is optimized. From these data it is clear that plasmid DNA can be directly inserted into plant protoplasts.

One of the limiting factors has been the lack of selectable markers that are useful in directly screening for transformants. Generally, antibiotic markers that confer resistance to prokaryotic antibiotics do not confer the same resistance in plant cells. It has been reported that plantlets obtained from tobacco protoplasts treated with ColE1 plasmid DNA carrying a gene conferring resistance to kanamycin, failed to express expected levels of resistance to kanamycin (Owens, 1979).

Certain antibiotics such as chloramphenicol may prove useful as was shown with yeast as discussed in the preceding section. Antibiotics that inhibit prokaryotic transcription and translation might be effective in inhibiting these processes is chloroplasts and mitochondria. However, it has been shown that antibiotics such as rifampicin (or its derivatives) did not inhibit chloroplasts RNA polymerases of wheat (Bottomley *et al.*, 1971) or maize (Polya and Jagendorf, 1971). Hernalsteens *et al.* (1980) have shown that Tn7, the transposon which encodes streptomycin, spectinomycin, and trimethoprim resistance, can be inserted into tobacco DNA by means of *A. tumefaciens* mediated transfer of the T-DNA carrying Tn7 to the tobacco plant. In this case, crown gall tumors were obtained from infection by an *A. tumefaciens* harboring a Ti plasmid, in which Tn7 had inserted in the right-hand region of the T-DNA of the plasmid. This region, which encodes nopaline synthase, was observed to be unessential for crown gall tumor production and did not obstruct integration of the T-DNA into tobacco DNA. Resistance to streptomycin, spectinomycin, or trimethoprim by the transformed tobacco calli was not reported by Hernalsteens *et al.* (1980). Apparently, in this case, the Tn7-encoded dihydrofolate reductase was not expressed. On the other hand, it has been shown that mammalian cells can be rendered resistant to low levels of methotrexate (amethopterin), a specific inhibitor of dehydrofolate reductases like trimethoprim (Lewis *et al.*, 1980; Wigler *et al.*, 1980), using total genomic DNA from a methotrexate-resistant mutants of a Chinese hamster cell line.

Besides antibiotics, certain sugars, sugar alcohols, or organic acid might serve as a means to select transformants. Certain sugars either limit growth or are toxic to plants (Stenlid, 1959; Malca *et al.*, 1967; Faludi *et al.*, 1963; Hoffman *et al.*, 1971; Goring *et al.*, 1968; Roberts *et al.*, 1971; Hoffmannowa, 1964). Therefore transformants carrying genes coding for an enzyme catalyzing the breakdown of one of these sugars (as for example, the gene coding for β-galactosidase) might be selected on medium containing lactose. A strategy like this was used in early studies attempting plant cell transformation with heterologous DNA (Doy *et al.*, 1973; Johnson *et al.*, 1973).

Other selectable markers are those that are already recognized as normal plant functions which seemed to shut-off when plant cells are maintained in tissue culture. Generally tissue cultures require exogenous supply of auxin and cytokinin to grow properly and indefinitely. The strategy of inserting genes that either permit the switching-on of existing phytohormone genes or code for the phytohormone itself may prove successful. Phytohormone prototrophy has been long known as a means for selection of cells that have been converted to crown gall tumor cells through infection of host plants with *Agrobacterium tumefaciens* (White and Braun, 1941; Braun and White, 1943). Thus, transformants have been successfully obtained either by exposing cells in suspension culture to the bacterium (Smith and Hindley, 1978; Marton *et al.*, 1979) or protoplasts to the bacterial Ti plasmid DNA (Dellaporta and Fraley, 1981; G. J. Wullems, personal communication).

A second limiting factor is the expression of the inserted genes in a foreign biochemical and genetic environment of the plant cell. However it has been clearly demonstrated that specific genes can be introduced into cultured mammalian cells by chromosome-mediated gene transfer (McBride and Ozer, 1973; Willecke and Ruddle, 1975; Willecke *et al.*, 1979) and by purified DNA-mediated gene transfer (Baccheti and Graham, 1977; Maitland and McDougall, 1977; Wigler *et al.*, 1977; Robins *et al.*, 1981). Furthermore, expression of various cloned genes in the mammalian cell systems has been demonstrated (Bacchetti and Graham, 1977; Maitland and McDougall, 1977; Wigler *et al.*, 1977, 1979; Capecchi, 1980; Hanahan *et al.*, 1980). Knowledge of efficient promoter sequences in the plant host used as the recipient of the foreign gene will certainly obviate some concerns about adequate expression of the gene (Meagher and McKnight, 1980). Encouragement comes from the fact that functional expression of a number of bacterial genes in yeast (*Saccharomyces cerevisiae*) has been reported (Hollenberg, 1979; Cohen *et al.*, 1980; Panthier *et al.*, 1980; Jiminez and Davies, 1980; Rose *et al.*, 1981; Roggenkamp *et al.*, 1981). In these experiments, a 2-μm DNA vector of the yeast was cloned into a widely used *E. coli* plasmid vector pBR322 or pBR325 and carried the promoter. Likewise, mouse fibroblasts have been transformed to methotrexate resistance by using plasmids consisting of SV40 early gene promoter and cap sites, sequences coding for methotrexate-resistant dihydrofolate reductases of bacterial origin, with donor and acceptor splice sites and a polyadenylation site from a rabbit β-globin gene (O'Hare *et al.*, 1981). Therefore, it is without doubt that vectors currently being designed will be able to carry genes that are fully expressed in plant cells. Thus, expression of various genes, even with intervening sequences, introduced into plant cells may not be as limiting as it currently appears. One of the primary limitations already discussed has been the finding of means to directly select for bona fide transformants. The lack of adequate plant cell mutants hinders this progress.

A third limiting factor is in the ability of the transferred gene to be maintained stably in the plant cell. Both mitotic and meiotic processes may quickly result in the loss of either all or part of the gene, rendering the loss of expression. The question arises whether or not such genes could only be stabilized by maintaining mutant cell lines under a selective pressure. The question also arises whether it is best to maintain genes on an independent replicon in the nucleus or in a form integrated with one of the chromosomes. Genes that do not survive or become altered through meiosis may be maintained stably only by subculture of plant cells or plants regenerated from such transformed cells.

VI. FUTURE PROSPECTS

In the near future, technological advances will be achieved in the plant sciences. The methodologies are now available for introducing foreign genes into plant cells, protoplasts, and even intact plants. Active studies are currently being made to design gene vectors that will be able to replicate, carry one or more selectable markers, carry DNA sequences for integration or maintenance as an independent replicon, and carry a plant promoter sequence. The genes being surveyed are those that make plant crops refractory to: infection by pathogens, invasion by pests, drought stress, high salt concentrations, temperatures that induce cold and frost injury, shock due to replanting, and to a variety of other stress-inducing factors. Also included are genes that make the crop plants more nourishing, enhance productivity, and provide year round production and/or enjoyment.

As emphasized in this chapter, models were proposed for tailoring bacteria for use in the biological control of pathogens and parasites. These models may be adapted in the design of bacteria to protect crop plants from other stress-related injuries. That bacteria and yeasts can be modified to produce desired products is already established, making the above goals easily attainable. On the other hand, modification of plants by introducing foreign DNA from genetically unrelated sources will require exquisite vector designs, might lead to unanticipated problems and surely will require great deal of effort and time. It remains to be seen if foreign genes can confer the desired traits on a given crop plant and, if so, will the modification result in unexpected traits? Nevertheless, efforts being made in this area are logical (although perhaps simplistic) and should eventually yield successful results. Active efforts by many laboratories will help pave the way for this success by providing valuable information on gene function in plants.

Acknowledgments

The authors thank Tom Quayle, Diana Fogle, and Jeff Hall for technical assistance. This work was supported, in part, by grants from the NIH and USDA SEA Competitive Research Grants Program (to C. I. Kado) and USDA SEA Competitive Grants Program grant 59-2531-0-1-465-0 and by funds provided to Washington State University through the NIH Biomedical Research Support Grant (to P. F. Lurquin).

References

Azad, H. R. (1979). Ph.D. thesis, University of California, Davis.

Azad, H. R., and Kado, C. I. (1980). *J. Gen. Microbiol.* **120,** 117–129.

Bacchetti, S., and Graham, F. L. (1977). *Proc. Natl. Acad. Sci. U.S.A.* **74,** 1590–1594.

Bach, M. L., Lacronte, F., and Botstein, D. (1979). *Proc. Natl. Acad. Sci. U.S.A.* **76,** 386–390.

Bartnicki-Garcia, S. (1970). *In* "Phytochemical Phylogeny" (J. B. Hasborne, ed.), pp. 81–103. Academic Press, New York.

Beer, S. V., and Rundle, J. R. (1980). *Phytopathology* **70,** 459 (Abstr.).

Beggs, J. D. (1978). *Nature (London)* **275,** 104–109.

Bolivar, F. (1978). *Gene* **4,** 121–136.

Bottomley, W., Smith, H. J., and Bogorad, L. (1971). *Proc. Natl. Acad. Sci. U.S.A.* **68,** 2412–2416.

Braun, A. C., and White, P. R. (1943). *Phytopathology* **33,** 85–100.

Capecchi, M. R. (1980). *Cell* **22,** 479–488.

Case, M. E., Schweizer, M., Kushner, S. R., and Giles, N. H. (1979). *Proc. Natl. Acad. Sci. U.S.A.* **76,** 5259–5263.

Cassells, A. C., and Barless, M. (1978). *Virology* **87,** 459–462.

Cocking, E. C., Davey, M. R., Pental, D., and Power, J. B. (1981). *Nature (London)* **293,** 265–270.

Cohen, J. D., Eccleshall, T. R., Needleman, R. B., Federoff, H., Buchferer, B. A., and Marmur, J. (1980). *Proc. Natl. Acad. Sci. U.S.A.* **77,** 1078–1082.

Davey, M. R., Cocking, E. C., Freeman, J., Pearce, N., and Tudor, I. (1981). *Plant Sci. Lett.* **18,** 307–313.

Dellaporta, S. L., and Fraley, R. T. (1981). *Plant Mol. Biol. Assoc. Newslett.* **2,** 59–66.

Doy, C. H., Gresshoff, P. M., and Rolfe, B. G. (1973). *Proc. Natl. Acad. Sci. U.S.A.* **70,** 723–727.

Faludi, B., Daniel, A. F., Gyurjan, I., and Anda, S. (1963). *Acta Biol. Acad. Sci. Hung.* **14,** 183–190.

Farkas, V. (1979). *Microbiol. Rev.* **43,** 117–144.

Farrand, S. K., Kado, C. I., and Ireland, C. R. (1981). *Mol. Gen. Genet.* **181,** 44–51.

Fernandez, S. M., Lurquin, P. F., and Kado, C. I. (1978). *FEBS Lett.* **87,** 277–282.

Fraley, R., Subramanian, S., Berg, P., and Paphadjopoulos, D. (1981). *J. Biol. Chem.* **21,** 10431–10435.

Franck, A., Guilley, H., Jonard, G., Richards, K., and Hirth, L. (1980). *Cell* **21,** 285–294.

Fukunaga, Y., Nagata, T., and Takebe, I. (1981). *Virology* **113,** 752–760.

Gantotti, B. V., Kindle, K. L., and Beer, S. V. (1981). *Curr. Microbiol.* **6,** 377–381.

Goring, V. H., Reckin, E., and Kaiser, M. V. R. (1968). *Physiol. Biochem.* **159,** 82–103.

Graham, F. L., and van der Eb, A. J. (1973). *Virology* **52,** 456–467.

Hanahan, D., Lane, D., Lipsich, L., Wigler, M., and Botchan, M. (1980). *Cell* **21,** 127–139.

Hasezawa, S., Nagata, T., and Syono, K. (1981). *Mol. Gen. Genet.* **182,** 206–210.

Helling, R. B., and Lomax, M. I. (1978). *In* "Genetic Engineering" (A. M. Chakrabarty, ed.), pp. 1–30. CRC, West Palm Beach, Florida.

Hernalsteens, J.-P., DeBeuckeleer, M., Depicker, A., Engler, G., Lemmers, M., Holsters, M., Van Montagu, M., and Schell, J. (1980). *Nature (London)* **287,** 654–656.

Hershfield, V., Boyer, H. W., Yanofsky, C., Lovett, M. A., and Helinski, D. R. (1974). *Proc. Natl. Acad. Sci. U.S.A.* **71,** 3455–3459.

Hinnen, A., Hicks, J. B., and Fink, G. R. (1979). *Proc. Natl. Acad. Sci. U.S.A.* **75,** 1929–1933.

Hoffmann, F., Kull, U., and Jeremias, K. (1971). *Z. Pflanzenphysiol.* **64,** 223–231.

Hoffmannowa, A. (1964). *Acta Soc. Botan. Pol.* **33,** 193–210.
Hollenberg, C. P. (1979). *In* "Plasmids of Medical, Environmental and Commercial Importance" (K. N. Timmis and A. Puhler, eds.), pp. 481–494. Elsevier, Amsterdam.
Hollenberg, C. P., Degelman, A., Kustermann-Kuhn, B., and Royer, H. D. (1976). *Proc. Natl. Acad. Sci. U.S.A.* **73,** 2072–2076.
Hotchkiss, R. D. (1979). *Ann. N.Y. Acad. Sci.* **325,** 321–342.
Howell, S. H., Walker, L. L., and Walden, R. M. (1981). *Nature (London)* **293,** 483–486.
Hughes, B. G., White, F. G., and Smith, M. A. (1977). *FEBS Lett.* **79,** 80–84.
Jiminez, A., and Davies, J. (1980). *Nature (London)* **287,** 869–871.
Johnson, C. B., Grierson, D., and Smith, H. (1973). *Nature (London) New Biol.* **244,** 105–107.
Kado, C. I. (1967a). *Ann. Rev. Phytopathol.* **14,** 265–308.
Kado, C. I. (1976b). *In* "Beltsville Symposium in Agricultural Research, Vol. 1, Virology in Agriculture" (J. A. Romberger, ed.), pp. 249–266.
Allanheld, Osmun, Monteclair, New Jersey.
Kado, C. I. (1979). *In* "Genetic Engineering" (J. K. Setlow and A. Hollaender, eds.), Vol. 1, pp. 223–239. Plenum, New York.
Kado, C. I., and Kleinhofs, A. (1980). *Int. Rev. Cytol. Suppl.* **11B,** 47–80.
Kado, C. I., and Liu, S.-T. (1981). *J. Bacteriol.* **145,** 1365–1373.
Kleinhofs, A., and Behki, R. (1977). *Annu. Rev. Genet.* **11,** 79–101.
Lewis, W. H., Srinivasan, P. R., Stokoe, N., and Siminovitch, L. (1980). *Somatic Cell Genet.* **6,** 333–347.
Lurquin, P. F. (1977a). *Prog. Nucleic Acid Res. Mol. Biol.* **20,** 161–207.
Lurquin, P. F. (1977b). *Mol. Gen. Genet.* **154,** 113–121.
Lurquin, P. F. (1979). *Nucleic Acids Res.* **6,** 3773–3784.
Lurquin, P. F. (1981). *Plant Sci. Lett.* **21,**.31–40.
Lurquin, P. F., and Kado, C. I. (1979). *Plant Cell Environ.* **2,** 199–203.
Lurquin, P. F., and Marton, L. (1980). "Advances in Protoplast Research," pp. 389–405. Pergamon, Oxford.
Lurquin, P. F., and Sheehy, R. E. (1982). *Plant Sci. Lett.* **25,** 133–146.
Lurquin, P. F., Sheehy, R. E., and Rao, N. A. (1981). *FEBS Lett.* **125,** 183–187.
McBride, D. W., and Ozer, H. C. (1973). *Proc. Natl. Acad. Sci. U.S.A.* **70,** 1258–1262.
Maitland, N. J., and McDougall, J. K. (1977). *Cell* **11,** 233–241.
Malca, I., Endo, R. M., and Long, M. R. (1977). *Phytopathology* **57,** 272–281.
Mankau, R. J. (1975). *Invertebr. Pathol.* **26,** 333–339.
Marton, L., Wullems, G. J., Molendijk, L., and Schilperoort, R. A. (1979). *Nature (London)* **277,** 129–131.
Matzke, A. J. M., and Chilton, M.-D. (1981). *Mol. Appl. Genet.* **1,** 39–49.
Meagher, R. B., and McKnight, T. K. (1980). *In* "Genomic Organization and Expression in Plants" (C. J. Leaver, ed.), pp. 63–75. Plenum, New York.
Muller, A. J., and Grafe, R. (1978). *Mol. Gen. Genet.* **161,** 67–76.
Mulligan, R., and Berg, P. (1980). *Science* **209,** 1422–1429.
Nester, E. W., and Kosuge, T. (1981). *Annu. Rev. Microbiol.* **35,** 531–565.
O'Hare, K., Benoist, C., and Breathnach, R. (1981). *Proc. Natl. Acad. Sci. U.S.A.* **78,** 1527–1531.
Owens, L. D. (1979). *Plant Physiol.* **63,** 683–686.
Panthier, J. J., Fournier, P., Heslot, H., and Rambach, A. (1980). *Curr. Genet.* **2,** 109–113.
Pellicer, A., Robins, D., Wold, B., Sweet, R., Jackson, J., Lowy, I., Roberts, J. M., Sim, G. K., Silverstein, S., and Axel, R. (1980). *Science* **209,** 1414–1422.
Polya, G. M., and Jagendorf, A. T. (1971). *Arch. Biochem. Biophys.* **146,** 649–657.

Ratzkin, E., and Carbon, J. (1977). *Proc. Natl. Acad. Sci. U.S.A.* **74,** 487–491.

Roberts, R. M., Heishman, A., and Wicklin, C. (1971). *Plant Physiol.* **48,** 36–42.

Robins, D. M., Ripley, S., Henderson, A. S., and Axel, R. (1981). *Cell* **23,** 29–39.

Roggenkamp, R., Kusterman-Kuhn, B., and Hollenberg, C. P. (1981). *Proc. Natl. Acad. Sci. U.S.A.* **78,** 4466–4470.

Rollo, R., Galli, M. G., and Parisi, B. (1981). *Plant Sci. Lett.* **20,** 347–354.

Rose, M., Casadaban, M. J., and Botstein, D. (1981). *Proc. Natl. Acad. Sci. U.S.A.* **78,** 2460–2464.

Sarkar, S., Upadhya, M. D., and Melchers, G. (1974). *Mol. Gen. Genet.* **135,** 1–9.

Sayre, R. M. (1980). *J. Nematol.* **12,** 260–270.

Sayre, R. M., and Wergin, W. P. (1977). *J. Bacteriol.* **129,** 1091–1101.

Schekman, R., and Brawley, V. (1979). *Proc. Natl. Acad. Sci. U.S.A.* **76,** 645–649.

Selitrennikoff, C. P., Allin, D., and Sonneborn, D. R. (1976). *Proc. Natl. Acad. Sci. U.S.A.* **73,** 534–538.

Smith, H. O., and Danner, D. B. (1981). *Annu. Rev. Biochem.* **50,** 41–68.

Smith, V. A., and Hindley, J. (1978). *Nature (London)* **276,** 498–500.

Stinchcomb, D. T., Struhl, K., and Davis, R. W. (1979). *Nature (London)* **282,** 39–43.

Stinchcomb, D. T., Thomas, M., Kelley, J., Selker, E., and Davis, R. W. (1980). *Proc. Natl. Acad. Sci. U.S.A.* **77,** 4559–4563.

Struhl, K., Cameron, J. R., and Davis, R. W. (1976). *Proc. Natl. Acad. Sci. U.S.A.* **73,** 1471–1475.

Struhl, K., Stinchcomb, D. T., Scherer, S., and Davis, R. W. (1979). *Proc. Natl. Acad. Sci. U.S.A.* **76,** 1035–1039.

Tagg, J. R., Dajani, A. S., and Wannamaker, L. W. (1976). *Bacteriol. Rev.* **40,** 722–756.

Timmis, K. N., Cohen, S. N., and Cabello, F. C. (1978). *In* "Progress in Molecular and Subcellular Biology" (F. E. Hahn, H. Kersten, W. Kersten, and W. Szybalski, eds.), pp. 1–58. Springer-Verlag, Berlin and New York.

Vidaver, A. K. (1976). *Annu. Rev. Phytopathol.* **14,** 451–465.

Watanabe, Y., Ohno, T., and Okada, Y. (1982). *Virology* **120,** 478–480.

White, P. R., and Braun, A. C. (1941). *Science* **94,** 239–241.

Wigler, M., Silverstein, S., Lee, L., Pellicer, A., Cheng, Y., and Axel, R. (1977). *Cell* **11,** 223–232.

Wigler, M., Pellicer, A., Silverstein, S., Axel, R., Urlaub, G., and Chasin, L. (1979). *Proc. Natl. Acad. Sci. U.S:A.* **76,** 1373–1376.

Wigler, M., Perucho, M., Kurtz, K., Dana, S., Pellicer, A., Axel, R., and Silverstein, S. (1980). *Proc. Natl. Acad. Sci. U.S.A.* **77,** 3567–3571.

Willecke, K., and Ruddle, F. H. (1975). *Proc. Natl. Acad. Sci. U.S.A.* **72,** 1792–1796.

Willecke, K., Klomfass, M., Mierau, R., and Dohmer, J. (1979). *Mol. Gen. Genet.* **170,** 179–185.

Yang, F., and Simpson, R. B. (1981). *Proc. Natl. Acad. Sci. U.S.A.* **78,** 4151–4155.

Yoder, J. I., and Ganesan, A. T. (1981). *Mol. Gen. Genet.* **181,** 525–531.

Part **IV**

Strategies for Control

The ultimate goal of phytopathology is to provide information useful for control of plant–prokaryote interactions for the benefit of mankind. A. W. Saettler and M. S. Mount (Chapter 15) emphasize the importance of understanding the biology of phytopathogenic prokaryotes, the biology of their host plants, and the effects of agronomic practices in designing disease control measures. In the following chapters, E. L. Civerolo (Chapter 16) discusses cultural practices for disease management, D. J. Hagedorn (Chapter 17) describes the importance of host breeding for disease resistance, A. K. Vidaver (Chapter 18) presents concepts for biological control of diseases with prokaryotes, and A. L. Jones (Chapter 19) reviews the state of chemical control for prokaryote-incited diseases.

Chapter **15**

Manipulation of Plant–Prokaryote Interaction

ALFRED W. SAETTLER *and* MARK S. MOUNT

I. INTRODUCTION

Prokaryotic phytopathogens have coexisted for long periods with various plant species, during which time they both have undoubtedly evolved unique ways in which to interact successfully with the "life style" of their partners (Sands *et al.*, Vol. 1, Chapter 4). Pathogens have developed different methods to survive when their hosts are not present, to spread from host to host, to avoid host defenses, and to secure nutrients from their hosts. Knowledge about the manner in which

Copyright © 1982 by Academic Press, Inc.
All rights of reproduction in any form reserved.
ISBN 0-12-509002-1

specific pathogenic prokaryotes accomplish these parts of their life cycles provides the starting point for designing disease control systems.

Plants also possess adaptive mechanisms which are manifested in their interactions with phytopathogenic prokaryotes. The process of recognition between host and parasite is believed to involve specific glycoprotein-like compounds, lectins, which immobilize incompatible bacteria by envelopment, thereby inhibiting their successful multiplication and establishment (Sequeira, 1978). Another class of host-elaborated materials, phytoalexins, are elicited in response to the presence of numerous biological, chemical, and physical stimuli (Kuć, 1972). These materials are inhibitory to a number of microorganisms, and their production may constitute a mechanism whereby the host plant can recognize and eliminate potential pathogens. Further, the life cycles of cultivated host plants affect the degree of their interactions with pathogens. For instance, the developmental stage of the host, the tissue present, the length of the growing season, and the genetics of the host all may affect disease development.

Finally, both hosts and pathogens interact in an environment in which the temperature, moisture, light, and presence or absence of supplementary pathogen hosts or pathogen vectors may vary widely during a single growing season, or even from year to year. The factorial nature of the possible interactions among pathogens, their hosts, and the environment (the disease triangle) should clearly indicate that disease control is a complex matter with variable success from season to season.

Progress has been made in reducing crop loss due to prokaryote-caused diseases. In most cases, control measures such as breeding resistant cultivars, applying biocidal chemicals, or using disease-free planting stock have afforded useful levels of crop protection. However, in several cases where successful measures were developed, control was not of long-term duration. For example, crop cultivars or lines developed for tolerance to specific bacterial pathogens have been shown to harbor the pathogen in the absence of disease symptoms. While no obvious economic loss is incurred in plantings of such cultivars, neighboring fields of susceptible cultivars are exposed to possible infection due to secondary spread. Several studies also suggest that the pathogen may acquire altered virulence patterns upon exposure to tolerant cultivars (Brinkerhoff, 1970). New strains of pathogens may be selected by disease control measures as occurred with the emergence of streptomycin-resistant strains of *Erwinia amylovora* (Burrill) Winslow *et al.* in streptomycin-sprayed California fruit orchards (Moller *et al.*, 1981). Thus, the ability of the pathogen to acquire altered virulence (Schnathorst, 1970), or tolerance to a biocide, or the ability of a tolerant host to support the pathogen in the absence of disease symptoms, suggests that traditional control measures may only be of short-term value in disease control programs. We suggest that vast improvements in management of prokaryote-induced plant diseases will become possible only as our understanding of basic host and pathogen life cycles and their interactions is extended. The purpose of this chapter is to explore certain aspects of the life cycles of both pathogen and host that may give us basic insights into more useful means for control of disease interactions and to introduce the disease control topics pursued in the following chapters by E. L. Civerolo, D. J. Hagedorn, A. K. Vidaver, and A. L. Jones.

II. THE PATHOGEN

The well-known disease triangle concept involves pathogen, host, and environment. Disease in the context of this chapter is considered a condition of abnormal structure or function of a host plant, characterized by reduced economic yield and/or quality. For purposes of organization, and brevity, this discussion will examine the disease concept initially from the point of view of the pathogen's life cycle relative to its host. Of particular importance is a basic understanding of the various stages in the life cycle of the pathogen.

A. Survival Stage

This stage represents, in most instances, the primary inoculum source. Therefore, it constitutes the single most important factor for the successful survival and subsequent establishment of the prokaryotes on or in plants. The ability to survive from one host crop to the next may involve association with the planting/propagation material of the particular host or association with other plants, plant residues, vectors, or soil. Many pathogens have more than one such association for survival "between" hosts, suggesting that control strategies may have to be directed toward several targets. Since this subject is carefully reviewed by J. R. Venette (this volume, Chapter 1), we will only briefly examine some potential sources of primary inoculum.

1. Plant-Propagation Material

Association of pathogens with planting stock of their host is responsible for both short- and long-distance dissemination. Contamination of true botanical seed may be both surface and internal (Cafati and Saettler, 1980b, Elango and Lozano, 1980; Katherman *et al.*, 1980), but, in most cases, the former is amenable to simple eradication by biocidal treatments. With internal contamination, the pathogen may be associated with cotyledons, embryos, or parts of the seed coat. In any case, one must know the precise location of the pathogen to consider control measures.

Pathogen contamination of vegetative planting stock (Lozano and Sequeira, 1974), such as "seed" potatoes (*Solanum tuberosum* L.), and cuttings of ornamental and fruit crops, are effective sources of primary inoculum, and often lead to serious epiphytotics. With some vegetables, planting stock in the form of transplants may become infected in the transplant bed, either from planting infected seed or from secondary disease spread.

2. *Supplementary Host Plants*

In temperate climates, few plant diseases caused by prokaryotes develop from primary inoculum associated with weed, other crop, or noncrop host plants. This is because freezing temperatures kill most herbaceous plants, thus eliminating tissue harboring the pathogens. One exception is the brown spot disease of bean (*Phaseolus vulgaris* L.) caused by *Pseudomonas syringae* pv. *syringae* van Hall in which the pathogen may survive the winter on leaves of a perennial weed, hairy vetch (*Vicia villosa* Roth) (Ercolani *et al.*, 1974). In tropical and semitropical climates, it is probable that numerous pathogens may move among crop or weed plants to natural hosts. Such movement might be of considerable importance where crops are grown in associated or mixed culture (Cafati and Saettler, 1980a). In these cases, it is practically impossible to distinguish primary from secondary disease spread.

As techniques for the detection and enumeration of prokaryotes are improved and refined, more and more pathogens will be detected on supplementary hosts (Hopkins, 1981; Moller *et al.*, 1981; Mulrean and Schroth, 1981). For example, the black rot pathogen, *Xanthomonas campestris* pv. *campestris* (Pammel) Dowson, was found to be associated with symptom-free cruciferous weeds in, and/or near, cabbage (*Brassica oleracea* var. *capitata* L.) fields in Georgia and California (Schaad and Dianese, 1981). Rifampin-resistant isolates of *X. c.* pv. *phaseoli* (Smith) Dye, causing bacterial blight of bean, were utilized to demonstrate that common weed species and nonhost crop plants may be important inoculum sources under certain conditions (Cafati and Saettler, 1980a).

3. *Plant Residues*

Many prokaryotes are associated with various residues of their hosts after harvest of the economic part or organ. Leaves, stems, branches, fruits, and seeds may be contaminated with the pathogen when such parts are returned to the soil. In general, prokaryotes survive relatively short periods in and on the soil in temperate climates with alternating periods of freezing and thawing. Seldom does the survival period exceed 1 year, which emphasizes the value of rotation and plowing for encouraging destruction of plant debris.

4. *Vectors*

Some prokaryotes survive from year to year in their insect vectors (A. J. Purcell, Vol. 1, Chapter 6). For example, *Erwinia stewartii* (Smith) Dye principally overwinters in the bodies of the corn flea beetle (*Chaetocnema pulicaria* Melsh.). The survival of the Stewart's wilt pathogen is directly related to the survival of the corn flea beetle. Severe winters reduce the numbers of beetles and consequently the number of primary infections during the following spring. The causal agent of bacterial wilt of cucurbits, *Erwinia tracheiphila* (Smith) Bergey *et al.*, does not overwinter in infected plant debris, but is totally dependent on insect vectors for its survival. The organism overwinters within the intestine of the striped cucumber beetle (*Acalymma vittata* Fabricius) and the spotted cucumber beetle (*Diabrotica undecimpunctata* Barber).

5. *Soil*

Several prokaryotes possess survival phases in the soil—notably *P. solanacearum* and *Agrobacterium* spp., and possibly *Erwinia* spp. (Buddenhagen, 1965; DeBoer, Vol. 1, Chapter 12; Jackson and Gonzalez, 1981; Leben, 1974; Pérombelon and Kelman, 1980; Schuster and Coyne, 1975; Stanghellini, Vol. 1, Chapter 10). Most other prokaryotes are quite poor competitors away from their living hosts, even in plant residues.

6. *Physiological State*

The physiological condition or state of the pathogen is important relative to devising control strategies involving primary inoculum. Certain phytobacterial pathogens are believed to survive in a reduced metabolic or hypobiotic state. Since uptake of chemical compounds is restricted in this state, biocidal chemicals or physical treatments may be less effective in killing such dormant cells compared to actively metabolizing cells.

B. Pathogenic State

1. *Primary Infection*

Pathogenesis involves the successful establishment, growth, and production of disease by the pathogen in a susceptible host. The initial site of primary infection is often determined by location and type of the primary inoculum. In many seed-borne diseases of vegetables and grain legumes, pathogenic bacteria are lodged under the seed coat and on cotyledon surfaces and infection of the host tissues occurs through rifts in the cotyledon during seed germination. From these initial infection sites, bacteria rapidly colonize other host tissues. Primary inoculum in diseases caused by mycoplasmalike organisms and fastidious walled bacteria is situated primarily in diseased tissues (Hopkins, 1981), and initial disease develops upward and outward from such tissues in stems and branches. In general, primary inoculum is localized within a certain host tissue or tissues, and spreads from such sites only as the host begins active growth. In cases where primary inoculum may be physically separated from the host plant (in plant debris, supplementary hosts, or soil), the pathogen must be transported to the host tissue surface for infection to develop. Such movement may be mediated by agents like insects, rain, hail, aerosols, machinery, and/or wind-blown soil particles (Venette, this volume, Chapter 1).

Dispersal of pathogens to susceptible hosts may result in colonization, but not pathogenesis (Pérombelon, this volume, Chapter 3). The list of prokaryotic plant pathogens which exhibit a peaceful coexistence phase of growth or resident phase on plants (Leben, 1981) continues to grow (Cafati and Saettler, 1980c; Crosse, 1966; Daub and Hagedorn, 1981; Ercolani *et al.*, 1974; Mew and Kennedy, 1971; Schnathorst, 1970; Surico *et al.*, 1981). In most cases, plants harboring significant pathogen numbers show no evident disease (Hayward, 1974). Recognition of these widespread resident phases for pathogenic bacteria would require modification of some existing disease control concepts.

Phytopathogenic bacteria possess no independent means to penetrate intact host tissues and therefore require some means of ingress into the host. Infection courts for plants vary depending on plant part or organ, but can generally be divided into natural openings (stomata, hydathodes, lenticels) and artificial openings (wounds caused by insects, wind-blown soil particles, wind, hail, and machinery) (Goodman, Vol. 1, Chapter 3). In the latter class could be included "pseudowounds" such as those sites where secondary lateral roots erupt. Root invasion is a common means for primary infection by *P. solanacearum* and *Agrobacterium* spp. Certain plant pathogenic bacteria are motile by means of flagella (Kelman and Hruschka, 1973), which allow limited chemotactic movement toward infection courts (Chet *et al.*, 1973). In the case of *P. s.* pv. *phaseolicola* (Burkholder) Young *et al.*, motility appears to be essential for the optimum expression of virulence (Panopoulos and Schroth, 1974).

2. *Growth*

Numerous studies, especially with leaf spotting *Pseudomonas* and *Xanthomonas* spp., have revealed rather typical bacterial growth curves *in planta* in susceptible reactions (Cafati and Saettler, 1980c; Daub and Hagedorn, 1980; Laurence and Kennedy, 1974; Mew and Kennedy, 1971; Surico *et al.*, 1981; Weller and Saettler, 1980). However, temperature and other environmental variables may alter the duration and associated populations of the individual growth stages.

3. *Symptom Production*

Development of disease symptoms in infected tissues is believed to be dependent upon the pathogenic population reaching a critical level (Weller and Saettler, 1980). Below this population, symtoms are minimal or absent. Regardless, most population studies have shown that pathogenic inocula for secondary spread are available before visible symptoms appear.

4. *Production of Disease*

It is not within the scope of this chapter to discuss in detail the specific mechanisms whereby prokaryotes inflict damage on their hosts. Since potential control strategies could be directed at them, it is important to briefly mention them here and the reader is referred to selected chapters discussing these mechanisms. Such mechanisms may involved phytotoxins (Patil, 1977; Durbin, Vol. 1, Chapter 17), macerating enzymes (Collmer *et al.*, Vol. 1, Chapter 16), extracellular polysaccharides (Bradshaw-Rouse *et al.*, 1981; Van Alfen, Vol. 1, Chapter 19), and growth regulators (Kosuge and Kimpel, Vol. 1, Chapter 15).

5. *Secondary Infection*

Successful primary infection usually leads to the production of pathogen cells available for further dissemination. Secondary spread may occur over relatively short, intra- or interplant, or long distances to widely spaced plants within a field, or field to field. Dissemination of secondary inoculum occurs by the same methods as those described for primary spread.

Epiphytic growth and development and colonization of growing points are believed responsible for systemic, secondary infection of bean and soybean (*Glycine max* (L.) Merr.) plants by *X. c.* pv. *phaseoli* (Smith) Dye and *P. s.* pv. *glycinea* (Coerper) Young *et al.*, respectively. Resident phases have been reported for *P. s.* pv. *syringae* on wheat (*Triticum aestivum* L.) and *X. c.* pv. *vesicatoria* on tomato (*Lycopersicon esculentum* Mill.) (Leben, 1974). The significance of the resident phase lies in the fact that sufficient inoculum may be present on tissue surfaces for secondary dissemination prior to symptom development (Blakeman, Vol. 1, Chapter 13). Most of the economic damage to a crop is due to repeating cycles of secondary disease spread and development. Environmental factors, especially temperature and moisture, are important in determining the number of cycles.

At some point in the disease cycle, the host is either killed or matures, and the economic part of the plant is harvested. The pathogen then enters the survival stage again until such time that another host is available and environmental conditions are favorable for new primary infections.

III. THE HOST

A. Crop Production Practice

Plant pathologists are primarily interested in disease control, and often give less than adequate attention to understanding the life cycle of the host. Even though disease is defined in terms of physiological or morphological variation from the healthy or normal condition, we commonly have more difficulty in defining what is normal than abnormal. A plant and its parts can respond to a pathogen in totally different ways during different stages of plant development. Certainly one must understand unique aspects for production of a particular crop, and be aware how these characters can affect the disease initiation and development processes. Specifically these may include, but are not limited to, the various parameters listed below.

1. *Length of Growing Season*

The growing season extends from the date of planting to harvest for most annual or biennial crops. For perennial crops, it is the annual period including active growth and/or fruiting, and harvest. The growing season is usually dictated by a narrow range of temperature, moisture, and light regimes to which the particular host is acclimated. Pathogenic prokaryotes must also be adapted to these same regimes to be successful pathogens on that host.

2. *Nutrient Status*

Nutrients are required for crop production, but the host nutrient status affects pathogen establishment, growth, and pathogenesis. For instance, nitrogen fertilization may increase the incidence and severity of fire blight (Civerolo, this volume, Chapter 16).

3. *Tillage*

Any practice during the growing season which disturbs the soil has the potential of uncovering inoculum, either in the form of true soil-borne pathogenic bacteria, or pathogen-infested plant residue. Plowing infested refuse down after crop harvest is, of course, a practice which encourages destruction of the pathogen. Tillage may also result in injury to host plant tissues, thereby increasing the number of available infection sites. Various farm implements and machinery may also transmit pathogens from infection points to healthy plants in the field (Civerolo, this volume, Chapter 16; Venette, this volume, Chapter 1).

4. *Pest Control*

Pest control procedures for weeds, insects, and diseases may also affect disease control. Weed control is a sound agronomic practice for many crops because it eliminates not only plants which compete for moisture and nutrients, but also eliminates other plants which could serve as reservoir hosts of the pathogen (Venette, this volume, Chapter 1). Moreover, at least with row crops, weed control permits a more rapid drying of excess moisture on crop plants and on the soil surface, thereby decreasing the period of leaf wetness during which bacterial infection could occur. Spraying host plants for insect and disease control could lead to limited spread of the pathogen by dispersion by spray droplets or aerosols during treatment. Various insecticides, fungicides, and bactericides may affect the pathogen directly in an inhibitory or stimulatory manner, or indirectly by altering the normal microflora of the host and its environment.

5. *Associated Culture or Mixed Cropping*

Associated culture or mixed cropping of plants is a common practice of crop production in numerous countries. Such systems alter the physical environment of the host plant in terms of light, temperature, and moisture levels. The biological environment, including microflora, associated with both crops is also affected. This may affect either the pathogen, or disease progression. For example, the use of systemic and contact insecticides to control the flea beetle (*Chaetocnema pulicaria*) vector of *Erwinia stewartii* confers *in vivo* resistance to the pathogen in artificially inoculated seedlings of susceptible cultivars (Sands *et al.*, 1979).

B. Host Anatomy and Development

Additional morphological or physiological characteristics of the host plant are important relative to disease development (Anderson, this volume, Chapter 6; Goodman, Vol. 1, Chapter 3). These include (1) the types of natural infection courts, such as stomata, lenticels, and hydathodes, that are present and functional throughout the growing season. For instance, since stomatal density varies in different cultivars of the same crop (Butler and Tibbitts, 1979), it might therefore be possible to breed cultivars possessing fewer infection courts. (2) Susceptibility of plant tissues, parts, and organs may be affected by the stage of plant development and the relative susceptibilities of plant parts during vegetative and reproductive growth of the host. One example of such an interaction is xanthomonas bacterial blight of bean, in which plants in the reproductive stage of development are generally more susceptible to the pathogen than plants in the vegetative stage (Saettler, 1977).

IV. STRATEGIES FOR MANIPULATING PLANT–PROKARYOTE INTERACTIONS

A. Economic Threshold

Certain practical aspects relating to disease and its management should be considered before discussing specific strategies in depth. Perhaps the most important aspect is whether or not control is necessary. The term "economic threshold" suggests that plants can tolerate a certain minimum level of damage before control costs are justified economically. Once that threshold is reached, the costs involved in applying pest control procedures will be regained through the economic benefit gained from the increased yield or reduced disease losses. This concept can be applied to plant diseases caused by prokaryotes. However, application of economic threshold is most useful in those instances where control strategies involve an immediate, identifiable cost liability, e.g., spray applications, planting disease-free stock, chemical treatment of seed or other plant propagative part. In cases where the strategy involves the development of technology or materials, e.g., breeding host cultivars, it is almost impossible to apply the threshold concept.

B. Strategies

While there are several ways in which to discuss the development and application of disease management strategies, we chose to approach the subject in terms of the target in the disease triangle concept to which a strategy is directed—environment, host, and pathogen.

1. *Environment*

Because physical environmental parameters such as temperature and moisture are cardinal determinants for the ecological niche of phytopathogenic prokaryotes, it may be possible to restrict or even prevent their activity on a particular host by either of the following: (1) altering the date of planting, or (2) altering the location of host planting. One example of such a strategy is the development of the vegetable seed industry in semiarid or arid areas of the western United States, where devastating seed-borne bacterial pathogens are unable to spread by rain splash. This is an example of the value of producing initial planting stock of the host under environmental conditions unfavorable for pathogen activity. Little is known of the subtle effects on phytopathogenic prokaryotes of other environmental parameters such as light intensity quality or duration, soil physical properties, etc.

2. *Host*

The most obvious strategy for control of prokaryote-caused disease through host manipulation is the breeding and use of pathogen-tolerant cultivars (Hagedorn, this volume, Chapter 17). A thorough understanding of the physiological–morphological bases for development of incompatible host–pathogen reactions would be useful, but is not prerequisite to such an effort. Breeding programs for resistance to phytopathogenic prokaryotes have traditionally been based on selection of genotypes exhibiting no, or reduced amounts of visible disease symptoms after exposure to the pathogen under artificial or natural conditions of infection. Critical parameters for effective selection procedures include recognizing pathogenic variation, possible differential disease reactions of various tissues and organs of the host, and environmental influences on disease development and progression. Recently, there have been reports that tolerant genotypes of several crop species support relatively large populations of pathogenic bacteria in the absence of disease symptoms. In several cases, systemic colonization of the tolerant plants may serve as a source of inoculum for disease spread. However, at least one bean genotype showed resistance to systemic epiphytic colonization by *X. c.* pv. *phaseoli* [var. *fuscans sensu* (Burkholder) Starr & Burkholder] (Cafati and Saettler, 1980a), and is being utilized in a breeding program.

One could theorize several additional novel criteria for breeders and pathologists to consider in efforts to develop disease-tolerant crop varieties. For example, breeders could select genotypes (1) in which no or limited growth and colonization of prokaryotes occur on or in vegetative and reproductive tissues; (2) in which the pathogen is incapable of, or has a reduced ability for contaminating the developing seed or other propagative material; (3) in which a reduced number of infection courts is conferred; (4) in which water congestion occurs with difficulty or to a reduced degree (Panopoulos and Schroth, 1974), thereby reducing the number of infections in leaves; (5) in whose tissues the pathogen possesses reduced survivability; and (6) which possess a plant canopy more receptive to the deposition of sprays, but less favorable for systemic colonization by the pathogen and reducing leaf wetness periods conducive to infection.

3. *Pathogens*

The quantity and the quality of the pathogenic inoculum are very important in disease control. The pathogen is generally at its lowest population density and distribution when it exists as primary inoculum. Thus, treatments should be devised to eradicate or decrease the populations of the pathogen at this point. Unfortunately, in many cases, the sources of primary inoculum are not well known. Even when the sources are known, the pathogen may be in such a physiological or physical state that treatments are not effective. For example, in common bean blight, *X. c.* pv. *phaseoli* infects developing seed during the reproductive stage of plant development. As the maturing seed loses moisture, the bacteria also become more resistant to desiccation. Viable *X. c.* pv. *phaseoli* has been recovered from 30-year-old infected seed stored at room temperature. Treatments to eradicate *X. c.* pv. *phaseoli* from bean seed must have the ability to kill such dormant bacteria, or else the bacteria must be induced to enter an active physiological condition to become susceptible to the treatments.

Sbragia (1975) and others suggested several tactics useful for possible chemical control of pathogens: (1) Compounds that adversely affect bacterial motility (Panopoulos and Schroth, 1974) and/or chemotactic activity (Chet *et al.*, 1973) could be designed to interfere with these processes and, therefore, reduce primary or secondary infections. (2) Chemicals that alter or interfere with the production of extracellular polysaccharides (EPS) by phytopathogenic bacteria may allow the host to recognize the altered EPS of the pathogen and lead to pathogen immobilization. Enzymes, known to degrade EPS, might be used in this manner. (3) Broad spectrum antiprokaryotic chemicals should be developed to supplement those used in traditional chemical spray control programs (Jones, this volume, Chapter 19). (4) New methods of chemical application, such as using organic solvents as carriers for antibiotics into plant materials such as seeds and tubers, may be developed. (5) Chemical treatments which could directly modify the host susceptibility to a pathogen. (6) Compounds such as lectins which would specifically immobilize the pathogen, or induce the elaboration of phytoalexin-type chemicals with inhibitory activity toward prokaryotes (Gnanamanickam and Smith, 1980).

Biological control of prokaryotic plant pathogens is still in the early stages of development. The only notable commercial success is the control of *A. tumefaciens* by *A. radiobacter* (Beijerinck & van Delden) Conn strain 84. However, reports of isolation of antagonistic bacteria from soil, seed, leaves and other plant parts are abundant, and additional research in this area is warranted (Blakeman, Vol. 1, Chapter 13, Blakeman and Brodie, 1976; Foster and Bowen, Vol. 1, Chapter 7; Godfrey, 1976). Biological control with antagonists represents a relatively simple, economical, and ecologically sound strategy of disease management (Vidaver, 1976, and this volume, Chapter 18).

Physical methods of treatment, such as UV irradiation, high temperature, and microwaves, might also be useful in eradicating pathogens from plant materials not damaged excessively by such treatments.

In the following chapters in this section, other authors will consider in more detail certain strategies for manipulating prokaryotic–plant interactions for disease control. Specifically, E. L. Civerolo (Chapter 16) will discuss management by cultural practices and environmental control, D. J. Hagedorn (Chapter 17) will consider breeding resistant host plants, A. K. Vidaver (Chapter 18) will provide perspectives for biological control, and A. L. Jones (Chapter 19) will review chemical controls.

References

Blakeman, J. P., and Brodie, I. D. S. (1976). *In* "Microbiology of Aerial Plant Surfaces" (C. H. Dickinson and T. F. Preece, eds.), pp. 529–557. Academic Press, New York.

Bradshaw-Rouse, J. J., Whatley, M. H., Coplin, D. L., Woods, A., Sequeira, L., and Kelman, A. (1981). *Appl. Environ. Microbiol.* **42,** 344–350.

Brinkerhoff, L. A. (1970). *Annu. Rev. Phytopathol.* **8,** 85–110.

Buddenhagen, I. W. (1965). *In* "Ecology of Soil-borne Plant Pathogens" (K. F. Baker and W. C. Snyder, eds.), pp. 269–284. Univ. of California Press, Berkeley.

Butler, L. K., and Tibbitts, T. W. (1979). *J. Am. Soc. Hortic. Sci.* **104,** 213–216.

Cafati, C. R., and Saettler, A. W. (1980a). *Plant Dis.* **64,** 194–196.

Cafati, C. R., and Saettler, A. W. (1980b). *Phytopathology* **70,** 638–640.

Cafati, C. R., and Saettler, A. W. (1980c). *Phytopathology* **70,** 675–679.

Chet, I., Zilberstein, Y., and Henis, Y. (1973). *Physiol. Plant Pathol.* **3,** 473–479.

Crosse, J. E. (1966). *Phytopathology* **56,** 291–310.

Daub, M. E., and Hagedorn, D. J. (1980). *Phytopathology* **70,** 429–436.

Daub, M. E., and Hagedorn, D. J. (1981). *Phytopathology* **71,** 547–550.

Elango, F., and Lozano, J. C. (1980). *Plant Dis.* **64,** 784–786.

Ercolani, G. L., Hagedorn, D. J., Kelman, A., and Rand, R. E. (1974). *Phytopathology* **64,** 1330–1339.
Gnanamanickam, S. S., and Smith, D. A. (1980). *Phytopathology* **70,** 894–896.
Godfrey, B. E. S. (1976). *In* "Microbiology of Aerial Plant Surfaces" (C. H. Dickinson and T. F. Preece, eds.), pp. 433–439. Academic Press, New York.
Hayward, A. C. (1974). *Annu. Rev. Phytopathol.* **12,** 87–97.
Hopkins, D. L. (1981). *Phytopathology* **71,** 415–418.
Jackson, M. T., and Gonzalez, L. C. (1981). *Phytopathology* **71,** 690–693.
Katherman, M. J., Wilkinson, R. E., and Beer, S. V. (1980). *Plant Dis.* **64,** 857–859.
Kelman, A., and Hruschka, J. (1973). *J. Gen. Microbiol.* **76,** 177–188.
Kuć, J. (1972). *Annu. Rev. Phytopathol.* **10,** 207–232.
Laurence, J. A., and Kennedy, B. W. (1974). *Phytopathology* **64,** 1470–1471.
Leben, C. (1974). *Spec. Circ. Ohio Agric. Dev. Center, Wooster, Bull.* 100.
Leben, C. (1981). *Plant Dis.* **65,** 633–637.
Lozano, J. C., and Sequeira, L. (1974). *Phytopathology* **64,** 83–88.
Mew, T. W., and Kennedy, B. W. (1971). *Phytopathology* **61,** 715–716.
Moller, W. J., Schroth, M. N., and Thompson, S. V. (1981). *Plant Dis.* **65,** 563–568.
Mulrean, E. N., and Schroth, M. N. (1981). *Phytopathology* **71,** 336–339.
Panopoulos, N. J., and Schroth, M. N. (1974). *Phytopathology* **64,** 1389–1397.
Patil, S. S. (1974). *Annu. Rev. Phytopathol.* **12,** 259–279.
Pérombelon, M. C. M., and Kelman, A. (1980). *Annu. Rev. Phytopathol.* **18,** 361–387.
Saettler, A. W. (1977). *Fitopatol. Brasil.* **2,** 179–186.
Sands, D. C., Heithel, G. H., and Krung, J. B. (1979). *Plant Dis. Rep.* **63,** 631–633.
Sbragia, R. J. (1975). *Annu. Rev. Phytopathol.* **13,** 257–269.
Schaad, N., and Dianese, J. C. (1981). *Phytopathology* **71,** 902.
Schnathorst, W. C. (1970). *Phytopathology* **60,** 258–260.
Schuster, M. L., and Coyne, D. P. (1975). *Agric. Exp. Sta., Univ. Neb. Res. Bull.* 268.
Sequeira, L. (1978). *Annu. Rev. Phytopathol.* **16,** 453–481.
Surico, G., Kennedy, B. W., and Ercolani, G. L. (1981). *Phytopathology* **71,** 532–536.
Vidaver, A. K. (1976). *Annu. Rev. Phytopathol.* **14,** 451–465.
Weller, D. M., and Saettler, A. W. (1980). *Phytopathology* **70,** 500–506.

Chapter **16**

Disease Management by Cultural Practices and Environmental Control

E. L. CIVEROLO

Copyright © 1982 by Academic Press, Inc.
All rights of reproduction in any form reserved.
ISBN 0-12-509002-1

I. INTRODUCTION

All plant diseases are affected by variations in the pathogen, host, and environment, and by the interactions of these factors. Most phytopathogenic prokaryotes replicate very rapidly, require free water for survival and for growth, and may be protected from prophylactic bacteriocide treatments in or on plant tissue. Thus, the diseases caused by them often develop extremely rapidly during damp or rainy periods when bactericides or other control measures are most difficult to apply and least effective. Consequently, these diseases are generally difficult to manage. These diseases are most effectively managed, before environmental conditions are suitable for epiphytotic development, by integrated systems of compatible practices whereby use of resistant varieties is supplemented with appropriate cultural practices and chemical or antibiotic treatments (Apple, 1977; Zadoks and Shein, 1979). Reliable systems for forecasting disease occurrence based on various environmental conditions and epidemiological factors are also useful for management of these diseases.

Several basic strategies underlie the integrated systems designed to manage plant diseases caused by prokaryotes. Specifically, these methods avoid, exclude, or eradicate the pathogen to reduce the amount of inoculum available for infection, to reduce spread of the pathogen, to increase the resistance of plants to infection at critical infection periods, and to create an environment or conditions unfavorable to the pathogen, infection, and/or disease development. The following discussion will review some of the tactics used to implement these strategies.

II. PATHOGEN-FREE PLANTING AND PROPAGATING MATERIAL

A. Production

Several phytopathogenic prokaryotes survive and are disseminated in association with seeds or vegetative propagating material of their plant host. Latent or subclinical infections by some phytopathogenic prokaryotes in propagating material produced in a specific environment may result in disease occurrence in the subsequent crop when environmental conditions in the same or another environment are conducive to disease development. Therefore, production, inspection, certification, and use of pathogen-free or nearly pathogen-free seed or propagating material are essential for the management of several diseases caused by phytopathogenic prokaryotes. Cucumber (*Cucumis sativus* L.), bean (*Phaseolus vulgaris* L.), and pea (*Pisum sativum* L.) seed production in arid or semiarid areas is based on the low frequency of infections in such areas of *Corynebacterium flaccumfaciens* pv. *flaccumfaciens* (Hedges) Dowson, *C. f.* pv. *flaccumfaciens* var. *aurantiacum* Schuster & Christianson, *C. f.* pv. *flaccumfaciens* var. *violaceum* Schuster, Vidaver & Mandel, *Pseudomonas syringae lachrymans* (Smith & Bryan) Young *et al.*, *P. s.* pv. *phaseolicola* (Burkholder) Young *et al.*, *P. s.* pv. *syringae* van Hall, *Xanthomonas campestris* pv. *phaseoli* (Erw. Smith) Dye, and *X. c.* pv. *phaseoli* var. *fuscans* (Burkholder) Starr & Burkholder (Grogan, 1971; Deshodt and Strijdom, 1979; Wallen and Galway, 1979; Schuster and Coyne, 1981), and/or environmental conditions that do not favor infection and disease development.

Large scale production of *Erwinia* spp.-free potato (*Solanum tuberosum* L.) planting stocks by stem cuttings (Perombelon, 1979) and by tissue culture techniques (Perombelon and Kelman, 1980; Roca *et al.*, 1978) avoids contamination from the mother tuber, the primary source of pathogen. Clonal selection and multiplication by stem cutting and tissue culture techniques are effective for reducing occurrence of bacterial potato ring rot disease caused by *C. michiganense* pv. *sepodonicum* (Spieckermann & Kothoff) Dye & Kemp (Velupillai, 1979).

A bud-rooting method to obtain cassava (*Manihot esculenta* Crantz) planting stock free of the cassava bacterial blight disease (CBBD) pathogen, *X. c.* pv. *manihotis* (Berthet & Bondar) Dye, is based on the absence of the bacterium in mature woody tissues of most cassava cultivars (Lozano and Sequeira, 1974). Stem pieces with two or three axillary buds, or individual buds from leaf axils, are selected from mature woody, but symptomless, branches and stems of infected plants are rooted individually. More than 90% of the plants from the stem cuttings and all of the plants from pathogen-free seeds may be obtained from disease-free plants.

Production of *P. solanacearum* (Smith) Smith-free potato seed at high elevations is based on the important role of temperature in the development and epidemiology of bacterial wilt disease of potato (French, 1979; Kelman, 1979a). Precautions must be taken, however, to avoid contaminating potato seed production fields with latently infected tubers. Alternatively, the use of true seed in potato production instead of tuber seed may effectively eliminate pathogens carried in tubers and reduce infection associated with cut tuber seed pieces (Thurston, 1980). *P. s.* pv. *syringae* associated with gummosis and bacterial canker disease of deciduous fruit trees, as well as other graft-transmitted, fastidious prokaryotes can be avoided by use of pathogen-free scion and rootstock material for propagation.

B. Treatment

Various treatments of seed and vegetative propagating material are part of many overall sanitation programs. Reliable seed treatment methods that are consistently effective and ecologically safe are not always available (Schaad *et al.*, 1980). *X. c.* pv. *campestris* (Pammel) Dowson may be reduced in or eradicated from naturally infected crucifer seeds by soaking seeds in hot acidic cupric acetate (Schaad *et al.*, 1980). Although the rate of germination of seed treated with the cupric acetate was generally reduced, the amount of reduction depended upon the treatment temperature, species, and cultivar (Schaad *et al.*, 1980). Soaking *Brassica* spp. seeds in streptomycin followed by a water rinse and soak in sodium hypochlorite (NaOCl) may be useful for eradicating seedborne *X. c.* pv. *campestris* without causing seed damage or phytotoxicity to seedlings (Humaydan *et al.*, 1980). Soaking zinnia (*Zinnia elegans* Jacq.) seed in NaOCl reportedly eradicated *X. c.* pv. *zinniae* Hopkins & Dowson without significant reduction in germination rate (Strider, 1979). The seedling phase of angular leafspot disease (ALSD) of cucumbers, caused by *P. s.* pv. *lachrymans*, was reduced in the field by treating seeds at 50°C and 75% relative humidity for 3 days and then drying (Leben, 1981).

Soaking infested cassava seed in hot water to eradicate *X. c.* pv. *manihotis* without affecting seed germination (Persley, 1979) and use of aerated steam to eradicate *C. michiganense* pv. *michiganense* (Smith) Jensen from tomato (*Lycopersicon esculentum* Mill.) seed and *X. c.* pv. *campestris* from cauliflower (*Brassica oleracea* var. *botrytis* L.) seeds but not *X. c.* pv. *malvacearum* (Erw. Smith) Dye from cotton (*Gossypium hirsutum* L.) seed (Navaratnam, 1980) have been reported. However, the detection methods used may not have been sensitive enough to detect low levels of these pathogens (Elango and Lozano, 1980). Nevertheless, significant reductions in occurrence of these diseases resulted from treating infested seed.

III. PLANTING SITE SELECTION

Planting site selection as a plant disease management practice is based on soil type, adequate drainage, absence of pathogens, presence of antagonistic soil microorganisms, and history of previous crops. Drainage may be improved by tilling and the soil can be amended or treated. For tree crops, new infections may be prevented by not planting young trees next to older trees that are severely infected with canker bacteria or insect-transmitted fastidious prokaryotes such as mycoplasmlike organisms (MLO).

Increased occurrence and severity of fireblight disease (FBD) of pome fruits, caused by *Erwinia amylovora* (Burrill) Winslow *et al.* on heavy, poorly drained, or highly acid soils is related to poor biological nitrification (Aldwinckle and Beer, 1979). On moderately acid, well-drained soils, soil temperature and aeration increase early in the season. As a result, biological nitrification is favored and nitrate nitrogen is available for proper tree growth when it is needed most (Aldwinckle and Beer, 1979). Delay of nitrification and late supply of nitrate nitrogen results in development of late tree growth highly susceptible to fireblight development with high foliar nitrogen (Aldwinckle and Beer, 1979).

Prunus bacterial spot disease (PBSD) caused by *X. c.* pv. *pruni* (Erw. Smith) Dye occurs where stone fruit trees are grown in soil types ranging from coarse sand to fine sandy loam (Matthee and Daines, 1968; Moffett, 1973). Infection by *X. c.* pv. *pruni* is favored by large stomatal openings and increased water congestion associated with increasing oxygen concentrations in light, well-aerated soils (Matthee and Daines, 1968, 1969).

Reduced incidence of black rot disease (BRD) of cabbage (*Brassica oleracea* var. *capitata* L.) in Hawaii was associated with soils at high elevations and with high organic matter content, high water holding capacity, high clay content, high calcium content, and high pH (Alvarez and Cho, 1978). These factors may affect host susceptibility and/or survival of the pathogen *X. c.* pv. *campestris.*

Planting site may be selected on the basis of the presence of disease-suppressive soils. Soils in coastal Peru may be antagonistic to *P. solanacearum* race 3 (French, 1979). These sites can be identified by planting indicator plants in potted field soil. However, attention must be given to appropriate indicator plants depending upon the climatic conditions and the possible presence of pathotypes, biotypes, or races of specific pathogens.

Occurrence of common potato scab disease is reduced in soils continuously cropped to potatoes than in soils in which potatoes are grown intermittently or in rotation with a variety of other crops (Cook and Baker, 1974). Since actinomycetes are generally more active in the dry, neutral-alkaline soils, common potato scab [*Streptomyces scabies* (Thaxter) Waksman & Henrici *incertae sedis*] and sweet potato soil rot [*S. ipomea* (Person & Martin) Waksman & Henrici] diseases are managed, in part, by maintaining soil pH below 5.2–5.5 (Baker and Cook, 1974). Growth of the bacteria may be directly affected by low pH.

IV. HOST NUTRITION

Various elements essential for plant development influence the occurrence and severity of plant diseases. In nature, plant resistance to infection by specific phytopathogenic prokaryotes may be determined not only by the presence or absence of nutrients, but also by the relative proportion, forms, and specific availability of nutrients (Huber, 1980; Huber and Watson, 1974; Sharvelle, 1979). The environment within the host may affect pathogen growth directly or inhibit mechanisms of pathogenesis (Huber, 1980). *In planta* growth of *E. stewartii* in tracheal sap is limited in nitrogen-deficient sweet corn [*Zea mays* L. var. *saccharata* (Sturte.) Bailey] seedlings. Conversely, increased levels of available nitrogen in soil or potassium deficiency increase the severity of the bacterial wilt disease (Huber, 1980). Similarly, *in planta* growth of *C. m.* pv. *michiganense* in tomato phloem is enhanced by nitrate nitrogen (Huber, 1980). High nitrogen and low potassium levels favor stomatal opening and water congestion in peach [*Prunus persica* (L.) Batsch] leaves resulting in increased susceptibility to infection by *X. c.* pv. *pruni* (Matthee and Daines, 1969). Therefore, improper fertilization with excessive nitrogen and inadequate potassium may increase the incidence of PBSD. In glasshouse tests, lesion lengths on rice (*Oryza sativa* L.) leaves of cultivars with specific resistance to *X. c.* pv. *oryzae* (Ishiyama) Dye were not affected by high nitrogen levels (Mew *et al.*, 1979). However, on leaves of cultivars susceptible to *X. c.* pv. *oryzae*, lesion length increased with increased levels of nitrogen (Ho and Lim, 1978; Mew *et al.*, 1979). Addition of potassium and phosphorus may reduce the severity of bacterial blight disease of rice grown on lateritic soils (Dath *et al.*, 1978). On the other hand, susceptibility of cotton to bacterial blight disease associated with nitrogen deficiency can be reduced by providing an adequate supply of nitrogen (Sharvelle, 1979).

In management of FBD of pome fruits, the proper nitrogen, phosphorus, and potassium balance to minimize tree susceptibility is maintained by nutrient applications based on soil and leaf analyses (Aldwinckle and Beer, 1977). Incidence and severity of bacterial vascular necrosis and rot disease (BVNRD) of sugar beets (*Beta vulgaris* L.) infected by *E. carotovora* subsp. *betavasculorum* Thomson *et al.* was directly related to wider in-row spacing of plants (Thomson *et al.*, 1981). This was attributed in part to increased nitrogen availability and larger beets with more growth cracks and split petioles in widely spaced compared to closely spaced plants.

Plant disease management may be achieved in part by manipulating the specific forms of nitrogen available to plants that affect host resistance, pathogen growth or virulence, microbial interactions, or any combination of these factors (Huber and Watson, 1974). Thus, while infection of peaches and plums (*Prunus domestica* L.) by *X. c.* pv. *pruni* may not be prevented by application of ammonium- or nitrate-nitrogen, rapid periderm development on plums supplied with ammonium-nitrogen causes cankers to heal promptly and reduced defoliation of peaches and plums supplied with nitrate-nitrogen minimizes the severity of PBSD (Huber and Watson, 1974). Lesions on rice leaves infected by *X. c.* pv. *oryzae* and *X. c.* pv. *translucens* (Jones *et al.*) Dye were longer on plants fertilized with ammonium sulfate or urea than on control plants or plants fertilized with calcium ammonium nitrate (Rao *et al.*, 1978; Naidu *et al.*, 1979). This was attributed to increased concentrations of phenolic compounds and sugar and reduced concentrations of nitrogen in the leaves of calcium ammonium nitrate-treated leaves.

V. SANITATION

A. Disinfestation

The basis for disinfesting all tools, equipment, stores, and personnel, as well as seeds, propagating material, and fruit or other products before distribution, is to reduce the spread of phytopathogenic prokaryotes. Copper-containing compounds, sodium or calcium hypochlorite, mercuric chloride, formaldehyde, and quaternary ammonium are readily available, inexpensive chemical disinfestants that are generally effective against many phytopathogenic bacteria. Environmental and toxic hazards, and corrosiveness limit the usefulness of some effective disinfestants. Methods to overcome some of these problems without reducing the effectiveness of useful disinfestants need to be developed. Other disinfestation treatments include hot air, aerated steam, and chemical fumigation.

B. Eradication

A plant pathogen may be introduced into areas other than those in which the disease it causes is endemic. This may occur despite efforts to preclude such introduction. A plant disease epidemic may occur if the pathogen becomes established. In order to prevent a plant disease epidemic or to reduce further losses resulting from spread of the pathogen, the pathogen may be effectively eliminated by eradication of host plants. Citrus bacterial canker disease (CBCD) was controlled by host eradication in some *Citrus*-growing areas in the United States (Florida and Gulf states), Australia, Mozambique, New Zealand, and South Africa (Garnsey, 1979). In Florida, more than 257,000 citrus grove trees and three million nursery trees were destroyed over 18 years in order to achieve successful eradication of CBCD (Garnsey *et al.*, 1979).

Eradication of host plants of insect vectors is potentially effective in the management of certain plant diseases caused by prokaryotic phytopathogens (McClure *et al.*, 1982). The rate of occurrence of peach trees with X-disease symptoms was directly related to the number of leafhoppers on the trees and that are known to transmit the causal agent of X-disease from wild hosts (McClure *et al.*, 1982). In addition, the number of leafhoppers on peach trees depended upon the species of plants growing under the trees in the orchard (McClure *et al.*, 1982). Thus, it is possible that populations of insect vectors of phytopathogenic fastidious prokaryotes may be reduced by eradication of preferred food and oviposition hosts, thereby reducing the incidence of plant diseases caused by these pathogens.

C. Roguing

Removing and destroying diseased plants, perennial or biennial nonhosts, and infested debris reduce or eliminate many phytopathogens. Many phytopathogenic bacteria survive epiphytically in a resident phase associated with various host and nonhost plants either internally, externally, or in the rhizosphere (Leben, 1974). However, the epidemiological significance of nonhost plants with respect to the ecology and survival of many phytopathogenic prokaryotes, as sources of inoculum for host plants under natural conditions, is not completely understood. Nevertheless, reciprocal spread of *X. c.* pv. *phaseoli* was detected between bean cultivars susceptible to bean common bacterial blight disease (CBBD) and nonhost plants (*Chenopodium album* L. and *Amaranthus retroflexus* L.) with which the pathogen was associated epiphytically (Cafati and Saettler, 1980). Thus, in some cases nonhost weeds and associated crops may be sources from which phytopathogenic bacteria are disseminated primarily or secondarily to host plants. The incidence of X-disease in *Prunus* species is reduced when infected chokecherry (*Prunus virginiana* L.) plants near stone fruit orchards are eradicated (Jones, 1981; Yadava and Doud, 1980). *P. solanacearum* affects a large number of important economic, as well as ornamental and weed, solanaceous and nonsolanaceous plants (Martin, 1979). Development of bacterial wilt disease of potatoes was reduced when weeds were controlled by spraying with a contact herbicide (Jackson and Gonzalez, 1979; Martin, 1979).

D. Pruning

Cankers are primary sources of inocula of many phytopathogenic bacteria of fruit trees in the spring, as well as sources of inocula for secondary spread of these pathogens during the growing season. Removal of overwintering cankers and other infected plant tissues or organs during the year is an important practice in managing FBD of pome fruits (Aldwinckle and Beer, 1979) and CBCD of citrus (Kuhara, 1978). Removal of spring and summer cankers from infected stone fruit trees is helpful in reducing incidence of PBSD under some conditions. Satisfactory management of CBBD was achieved by pruning back heavily infected cassava plants to 20–30 cm in the dry season (Lozano and Sequeira, 1974). The effectiveness of pruning for eliminating sources of inocula of phytopathogenic bacteria may depend on timing and extent of pruning (Yadava and Doud, 1980).

E. Defoliation

Defoliation of citrus trees affected by CBCD with contact herbicides is being evaluated as a CBCD management practice to reduce the amount of *X. c.* pv. *citri* (Hasse) Dye inoculum available for further infections (DuCharme, 1981). This practice is a potential alternative to eradication of entire trees where CBCD may appear. Presumably only 1 or 2 years of fruit production on defoliated trees would be lost instead of several years of lost fruit production which would result from eradication of diseased and surrounding trees, and replanting young trees.

In Argentina, citrus trees were defoliated completely or partially by spraying with Diquat (1,1-ethylene-2-2-bipyridylium ion present in formulation as dibromide monohydrate salt). Within 6 days, defoliation is nearly complete and young branches are killed back about 38–45 cm. New growth begins within 30 days in properly maintained groves. The defoliated leaves must be destroyed by burning or burying as viable *X. c.* pv. *citri* have been detected in or on dead leaves up to about 1 month after defoliation. Additional protection of the new growth with protective sprays of copper-containing compounds will enhance the effectiveness of defoliation in CBCD management. The following year, CBCD reoccurred on about 12% of completely defoliated and 5% of partially defoliated trees.

VI. OTHER CULTURAL PRACTICES

A. Crop Rotation

Some phytopathogenic bacteria survive in residue and debris of infected plants. Elimination of some phytopathogenic bacteria can be achieved by crop rotation with nonhost plants. Crop rotation may be supplemented by fallow periods of various lengths. This practice is generally most effective in the management of diseases caused by those bacteria with limited host range and that do not survive for long periods of time in the soil.

Rotation with nonhost crops is variably effective for managing BRD of crucifers, CBBD of cassava, halo blight disease of beans, bacterial blight disease of soybeans [*Glycine max* (L.) Merr.], bacterial pustule disease of soybeans, ALSD of cucurbits, bacterial blight of cereals and grasses, bacterial soft rot diseases of vegetables, bacterial wilt disease of poatoes, crown gall disease, and common scab disease of potato.

Long-term survival of *P. solanacearum* in the rhizosphere on soil may depend on infection of a wide variety of presumed nonhost plants (Granada and Sequeira, 1981). Thus, corn, sorghum (*Sorghum vulgare* Pers.), bean, peas, and soybean grown in *P. solanacearum*-infested soil were apparently systemically infected by the bacterium. If infection of presumed nonhost plants is essential for long-term survival of phytopathogenic bacteria, management by crop rotation of plant diseases caused by these bacteria may need to be reevaluated.

B. Irrigation

Judicious irrigation as part of plant disease management programs is based on maintaining soil moisture conditions that are optimum for host growth and adverse for phytopathogens. Excess moisture, surface irrigation, overhead irrigation, and flooding are primary means by which some phytopathogenic bacteria are disseminated from plant to plant, and from field to field. Prolonged flooding, especially when used where paddy rice is grown in rotation with potatoes, reduces *P. solanacearum* survival in the soil, but probably does not eradicate the pathogen (French, 1979). Potato blackleg disease tends to occur more often in waterlogged soil (Perombelon, 1979). The incidence of rice bacterial blight disease, caused by *X. c.* pv. *oryzae*, was higher in submerged transplants than in rainfed transplants and transplants in saturated soil (Sharma *et al.*, 1979). Maintaining soil water near field capacity during tuber formation is important in the management of common potato scab disease (Baker and Cook, 1974). Suppression of *S. scabies* in wet soil may be related to an increase in the bacteria antagonistic to *S. scabies* or to the increased competitive advantage of other bacteria over actinonycetes (Baker and Cook, 1974).

C. Cultivation

Cultivation late in the growing season encourages highly FBD-susceptible late growth of pome fruit trees with high foliar nitrogen as a result of reduced cover crop competition for available nitrogen (Aldwinckle and Beer, 1979). Similarly, the cover crop, well mowed early in the season, is allowed to grow after mid-summer to reduce vigorous tree growth and development of tissue highly susceptible to infection by *E. amylovora* (Aldwinckle and Beer, 1979).

C. f. pv. *flaccumfaciens*, *C. f.* pv. *flaccumfaciens* var. *aurantiacum*, *P. s.* pv. *syringae*, *X. c.* pv. *phaseoli*, and *X. c.* pv. *phaseoli* var. *fuscans*, which can overwinter in bean straw on the soil surface, may be eliminated by turning in the straw below the soil surface (Schuster and Coyne, 1981). Diseases caused by some strains of *P. solanacearum*, like Moko disease or bacterial wilt of banana [*Musa paradisiaca* subsp. *sapientum* (L.) Kuntze], may be effectively managed by discing several centimeters of soil frequently during the dry season, followed by about a 1 year fallow (Sequeira, 1958).

The incidence of peach X-disease may be reduced by discouraging leafhopper vectors of the causal agent from invading peach orchards (McClure *et al.*, 1982). Based on recent work this might be effectively accomplished by keeping the orchard floor free of weeds and grasses, or maintaining a ground cover free of naturally occurring, wild plant species that are preferred hosts of insect vectors of phytopathogenic prokaryotes. Thus, significantly fewer leafhopper vectors of the causal organism of peach X-disease occurred on peach trees when the orchard floor was kept free of plants by weekly tilling, or when a ground cover of orchard grass (*Dactylis glomerata* L.) was maintained (McClure *et al.*, 1982).

D. Rootstock–Scion Combinations

The susceptibility of apple (*Malus sylvestris* Mill.) scion cultivars to FBD is influenced by the rootstock (Aldwinckle and Beer, 1979; Bonn,

1978; Boyce, 1970; Cummins and Norton, 1974; Keil and van der Zwet, 1975; Mowry, 1969; Thompson, 1971). Thus, strong induction of scion susceptibility has been reported for rootstocks MM106, M26 (Bonn, 1979; Boyce, 1970; Keil and van der Zwet, 1975; Mowry, 1969; Thompson, 1971), and M9 (Aldwinckle *et al.*, 1979), and M9/MM111 interstem (Aldwinckle *et al.*, 1979). It is not possible, however, to predict the susceptibility of the scion cultivar based on the rootstock alone. In addition, FBD susceptibility of scion cultivars is affected by climatic factors, soil conditions, and tree nutrition. Nevertheless, the possibility that certain size-controlling rootstock sensitize some apple scion cultivars to infection by *E. amylovora* should be considered in planning new apple orchards where FBD is a potential problem.

Fewer plum trees on peach rootstocks are affected by bacterial canker disease (*P. s.* pv. *syringae*) than those on various clonal plum rootstocks (Cameron, 1971; Westwood *et al.*, 1973). Cherry (*Prunus avium* L. and *P. cerasus* L.) trees on *P. avium* cv. Mazzard rootstock are generally less affected by X-disease than trees on *P. mahaleb* L. rootstock (Jones, 1981; Yadava and Doud, 1980). The incidence and severity of pear decline in pear (*Pyrus communis* L.) scions are also affected by specific rootstocks and interstocks (Yadava and Doud, 1980). Generally, pear decline is less severe ("slow decline" form) in pear scions on *P. communis* L. cvs. Bartlett, Anjou, Winter Nelis and Bosc, nondwarfing *P. betulaefolia* Bunge, and *P. calleryana* Decne. than on *P. serotina* Rehd. or *P. ussuriensis* Maxim. ("quick decline" form) (Woodbridge *et al.*, 1957; Yadava and Doud, 1980).

E. Bacterization

Bacterization is the process of inoculating seed, seed pieces, and roots with specific root-colonizing bacteria or rhizobacteria (Brown, 1974). Some strains of these bacteria are known as plant growth-promoting rhizobacteria (PGPR) (Kloepper *et al.*, 1980). Enhanced growth and increased yields of sugar beets, potatoes, and radishes (*Rhaphanus sativus* L.) have resulted from bacterization with PGPR (Kloepper and Schroth, 1979; Kloepper *et al.*, 1980). High concentrations of PGPR are applied directly to seed or seed pieces and bacterization effects are greatest in crops with short cropping periods (Kloepper and Schroth, 1979).

Selection for PGPR is based on their ability to inhibit fungal and bacterial pathogens, as well as miscellaneous rhizosphere bacteria and fungi. They may act, at least in part, as biological control agents. Additionally, however, PGPR may displace harmful microorganisms that commonly colonize roots or inhibit toxigenic nonparasitic or slightly parasitic microorganisms (Brown, 1974; Kloepper and Schroth, 1979; Kloepper *et al.*, 1980). Direct suppression of phytopathogenic bacteria may also result from bacterization (Brown, 1974; Kloepper and Schroth, 1979).

Other naturally occurring antagonistic bacteria, as well as PGPR, may function in reducing the occurrence and severity of diseases caused by phytopathogenic bacteria. Such microorganisms need to be identified and developed further for increased effectiveness against phytopathogenic bacteria by genetic engineering techniques. Specific microorganisms could be designed and developed for specific plant disease management purposes.

F. Cross Protection, Interference, Immunization

Crown gall disease on stone fruits and rose (*Rosa* spp.), associated with *Agrobacterium tumefaciens* (Smith & Townsend) Conn., has been successfully managed by preplanting treatment of seeds, roots, or young plants or cuttings with suspensions of a nonpathogenic strain of *A. radiobacter* (Beijerinck & van Delden) Conn (Kerr, 1980). Limited success has been achieved using strains of *E. herbicola* (Löhnis) Dye and other bacteria antagonists to *E. amylovora* to reduce FBD of pome fruits (Aldwinckle and Beer, 1979). Generally, however, *E. amylovora* may be suppressed by *E. herbicola* strains introduced into apple blossoms before or shortly after inoculation with *E. amylovora*. Localized infections of tobacco mosaic virus (TMV) and tobacco necrosis virus (TNV) induced systemic and long-lived resistance in tobacco (*Nicotiana tabacum* L.) against *P. s.* pv. *tabaci* (Wolf & Foster) Young *et al.* (Lovrekovich *et al.*, 1968; McIntyre *et al.*, 1981). However, plant immunization to activate mechanisms of resistance (Kuc, 1977), cross protection, and interference are undeveloped as practices to manage diseases caused by phytopathogenic prokaryotes.

VII. ENVIRONMENTAL CONTROLS

A. Growing Conditions

Effective management of brown blotch disease of mushrooms [*Agaricus campestris* v. *bisporus* (Lang.) Singer caused by *P. tolaasi* (Paine)] in houses with high relative humidity depends on adequate ventilation and precise temperature regulation within 0.1°C (Baker and Cook, 1974). In addition, mushroom mummy disease (*Pseudomonas* sp.)

incidence is reduced by proper thermal manipulations and adequate ventilation during composting and casing soil treatment (Baker and Cook, 1974).

B. Storage Conditions

The temperature at which potato tubers are stored after harvest may affect the incidence of soft rot caused by *E. chrysanthemi* Burkholder *et al.* (Hidalgo and Echandi, 1981). At 4°C, soft rot increased in *S. tuberosum* L. ssp. *tuberosum* and *S. tuberosum* L. ssp. *andigena* clones following tuber inoculation with *E. chrysanthemi*. In contrast, soft rot incidence did not increase in tubers of the same cultivars and clones stored at 23°C. Reducing sugar content was lower and less soft rot developed in *E. carotovora* subsp. *atroseptica* (van Hall) Dye-inoculated tubers stored at 21–26°C than in tubers stored at 3–6°C (Otazu and Secor, 1981). However, the relationship(s) between reducing sugar content and potato soft rot is not clear.

In controlled or modified atmospheres, O_2 concentration is reduced and/or CO_2 concentration is increased (El-Goorani and Sommer, 1981). Generally, respiration and ethylene production rates are reduced, and ripening or senescence is delayed under these conditions. Postharvest diseases may be suppressed in controlled or modified atmospheres as a result of maintenance of host resistance and altered pathogen growth (El-Goorani and Sommer, 1981).

Generally, the soft rot *Erwinia* species are facultative anaerobes. While *in vitro* growth of soft rot bacteria is generally inhibited or reduced at low O_2 (3%) and high CO_2 (0–30%) concentrations at 21°C (El-Goorani and Sommer, 1981; Perombelon and Kelman, 1980; Wells, 1974) reducing O_2 concentration from about 21 to 0.25–1% generally has little effect on suppressing bacterial soft rot diseases of stored asparagus (*Asparagus officinalus* L.) spears at 6°C, potatoes at 15 and 20°C, radishes at 10°C, and lettuce (*Lactuca sativa* L.) (El-Goorani and Sommer, 1981). In atmospheres with less than 1% O_2, stored fruit and vegetables may be susceptible to other injuries (El-Goorani and Sommer, 1981). Bacterial soft rots of stored potato tubers are generally most extensive when the O_2 concentration exceeds 30% (Nielsen, 1968) or when the tubers are maintained under anacrobic conditions (Lund and Nichools, 1970; Lund and Wyatt, 1972; Perombelon and Kelman, 1980). On the other hand, soft rot susceptibility of potato tubers increases with lower O_2 concentrations in environments with high relative humidity (De Boer and Kelman, 1978). Higher incidence of soft rot of stored potatoes under anaerobic rather than aerobic conditions may be due to inhibition by low O_2 concentration on the resistant response of the tuber (Perombelon and Kelman, 1980). Tomatoes inoculated with *E. carotovora* (Jones) Bergey *et al.* and held for 6 days at 12.5°C developed less soft rot in a controlled atmosphere of 3% O_2 and 5% CO_2 than in air (Parsons and Spalding, 1972).

C. Storage Design and Management

Effective design and management of crop storage systems is essential for minimizing losses in storage due to a wide range of soft-rotting erwinia (*E. carotovora* subsp. *atroseptica*, *E. carotovora* subsp. *carotovora* (Jones) Bergey *et al.*, and *E. chrysanthemi*) and pectolytic bacteria (*Bacillus* spp., *Pseudomonas* spp., *Aerobacter* spp., *Flavobacterium* spp., and *Clostridium* spp.) (Booth, 1979; Kelman, 1979; Nielsen, 1968; Perombelon, 1979). In managing bacterial decay of stored tubers resulting from field infections, the tubers are not cured and the temperature of the tubers is reduced as soon as possible (Booth, 1979). In other cases, however, management of bacterial decay resulting from infection of tubers in storage is based on carefully selecting tubers for storage, and curing them at 15°C and 95% RH to permit healing of wounds that might occur during harvesting and handling (Booth, 1979). During storage, adequate ventilation and insulation are necessary to prevent moisture condensation and development of anaerobic conditions. Wet tubers placed into storage must also be dried rapidly by high levels of ventilation (Booth, 1979). Rapid depletion of O_2 within the tuber occurs at 22°C when there is a continuous film of water on the tuber surface. Inadequate ventilation during storage may result in increased temperature, humidity, and CO_2 concentration, and decreased O_2 concentration (Booth, 1979).

D. Windbreak Systems

Plant-to-plant spread of the pathogen in the direction of prevailing winds and correlation of disease incidence with amount of rainfall are characteristic of many diseases caused by phytopathogenic bacteria. Rainfall, and especially wind-driven rain, provides the necessary conditions for mobilization, distribution, and penetration of inoculum.

Use of windbreak systems is a basic component of the integrated system used in Japan to manage CBCD (Kuhara, 1978). Windbreak trees or nets are placed at 20–50 m intervals (10–20 m intervals for plantings on steep slopes) to reduce wounding caused by shoots being severely whipped in strong winds. In addition, dissemination of the *X. c.* pv. *citri* to potential infections sites during strong wind-driven rains is also reduced. The incidence of pear decline in pome fruit trees was also reduced when the trees were protected with windbreaks of *Poplar* spp. (Yadava and Doud, 1980).

VIII. CONCLUSIONS

Clearly the most effective management of plant diseases caused by phytopathogenic prokaryotes is by the development and implementation of specific integrated systems of compatible cultural practices and environmental control methods. Design of integrated plant disease management systems requires precise knowledge about the biology and ecology of phytopathogenic prokaryotes and about the epidemiology of the diseases they cause. Specifically, more information about phytopathogenic prokaryotes is needed regarding recognition, detection, and identification of races, biotypes, and pathotypes; location and mechanism of survival; epidemiologically significant sources of inocula; the epidemiological significance of nonhost plants; the nature and mechanisms of pathogenesis; and the nature and mechanism(s) of host resistance. Such information would also aid in development of reliable disease forecasting systems as part of the management of diseases caused by phytopathogenic prokaryotes.

Increasing the resistance of plant hosts to infection by phytopathogenic prokaryotes and/or creating conditions unfavorable for infection and disease development can be achieved by manipulation of temperature, soil moisture, soil fertility, plant nutrition, and storage conditions. Many plants can be protected against infection by sanitary and cultural practices. More attention, however, needs to be given to the effects of specific scion–rootstock combinations, immunization with plant viruses, and cross-protection or interference by other microorganisms on development of diseases caused by phytopathogenic prokaryotes.

References

Aldwinckle, H. S., and Beer, S. V. (1979). *Hortic. Rev.* **1**, 423–474.

Aldwinckle, H. S., Preczewski, J. L., and Beer, S. V. (1979). *Proc. Int. Conf. Plant Pathog. Bact. 4th, Angers 1978* **2**, 505–512.

Alvarez, A. M., and Cho, J. J. (1978). *Phytopathology* **68**, 1456–1459.

Apple, J. L. (1977). *In* "Plant Disease: An Advanced Treatise" (J. G. Horsfell and E. B. Cowling, eds.), Vol I, pp. 79–102. Academic Press, New York.

Baker, K. F., and Cook, R. J. (1974). "Biological Control of Plant Pathogens." Freeman, San Francisco, California.

Bonn, W. G. (1979). *Proc. Int. Conf. Plant Pathog. Bact., 4th, Angers 1978* **2,** 493–497.
Booth, R. H. (1979). *Report Plan. Conf. Dev. Control Bact. Dis. Potatoes, Lima* pp. 120–124.
Boyce, B. R. (1970). *Plant Dis. Rep.* **54,** 638–640.
Brown, M. E. (1974). *Annu. Rev. Phytopathol.* **12,** 181–197.
Cafati, C. R., and Saettler, A. W. (1980). *Plant Dis.* **64,** 194–196.
Cameron, H. R. (1971). *Plant Dis. Rep.* **55,** 421–423.
Cummins, J. N., and Norton, R. L. (1974). *N. Y. Food Life Sci. Bull.* **41,** 1–15.
Dath, A. P., Padmanabhan, S. Y., and Devadath, S. (1978). *Sci. Cult.* **44,** 417–418.
DeBoer, S. H., and Kelman, A. (1978). *Potato Res.* **21,** 65–80.
Deshodt, C. C., and Strijdom, B. W. (1979). *Phytophylactica* **11,** 187–189.
DuCharme, E. P. (1981). *Citrus Canker Coord. Comm. Meet. Workshop, Winter Haven* pp. 45–48.
Elango, F., and Lozano, J. C. (1980). *Plant Dis.* **64,** 784–786.
El-Goorani, M. A., and Sommer, N. F. (1981). *Hortic. Rev.* **3,** 412–461.
French, E. R. (1979). *Rep. Plan. Conf. Dev. Control Bact. Dis. Potatoes, Lima* pp. 72–81.
Garnsey, S. M., DuCharme, E. P., Lightfied, J. W., Seymour, C. P., and Griffiths, J. T. (1979). *Citrus Ind.* **60,** 5–6, 8, 10, 13.
Granada, G. A., and Sequeira, L. (1981). *Abstracts Int. Conf. Plant Pathog. Bact., 5th, Cali, Colombia* pp. 23–24 (Abstr.).
Grogan, R. G., Lucas, L. T., and Kimble, K. A. (1971). *Plant Dis. Rep.* **55,** 3–6.
Hidalgo, O., and Echandi, E. (1981). *Phytopathology* **71,** 224–225.
Ho, B. L., and Lim, W. C. (1978). *Mardi Res. Bull.* **6,** 29–35.
Huber, D. M. (1980). *In* "Plant Disease: An Advanced Treatise" (J. G. Horsfall and E. B. Cowling, eds.), Vol. 5, pp. 381–405. Academic Press, New York.
Huber, D. M., and Watson, R. D. (1974). *Annu. Rev. Phytopathol.* **12,** 139–165.
Humaydan, H. S., Harmon, G. E., Nedrow, B. L., and DiNitto, L. V. (1980). *Phytopathology* **70,** 127–131.
Jackson, M. T., and Gonzalez, L. C. (1979). *Rep. Plan. Conf. Dev. Control Bact. Dis. Potatoes, Lima* pp. 66–71.
Jones, A. L. (1981). *Am. Fruit Grower* **101,** 16, 20.
Kaiser, W. J., and Teemka, L. R. (1979). *Plant Dis. Rep.* **63,** 780–784.
Keil, H. L., and van der Zwet, T. (1975). *Fruit Var. J.* **29,** 30–33.
Kelman, A. (1979a). *Rep. Plan. Conf. Dev. Control Bact. Dis. Potatoes, Lima* pp. 20–27.
Kelman, A. (1979b). *Rep. Plan. Conf. Dev. Control Bact. Dis. Potatoes, Lima* pp. 125–130.
Kerr, A. (1980). *Plant Dis.* **64,** 25–30.
Kloepper, J. W., and Schroth, M. N. (1979). *Proc. Int. Conf. Plant Pathog. Bact., 4th, Angers 1978* **2,** 879–882.
Kloepper, J. W., Schroth, M. N., and Miller, T. D. (1980). *Phytopathology* **70,** 1078–1082.
Kuc, J. (1977). *Neth. J. Plant. Pathol.* **83** (Suppl. 1), 463–471.
Kuhara, S. (1978). *Rev. Plant Protect. Res.* **11,** 132–142.
Laurence, J. A. (1981). *Z. Pflanzenkr. Pflanzenschutz* **87,** 156–172.
Leben, C. (1974). *Ohio Agric. Res. Dev. Ctr. Spec. Circ.* 100.
Leben, C. (1981). *Phytopathology* **71,** 235.
Lovrekovich, L., Lovrekovich, H., and Stahmann, M. A. (1968). *Phytopathology* **58,** 1034–1035.
Lozano, J. C., and Sequeira, L. (1974). *Phytopathology* **64,** 83–88.
Lukens, R. J., Miller, P. M., Walton, G. S., and Hitchcock, S. W. (1971). *Plant Dis. Rep.* **55,** 645–647.
Lund, B. M., and Nichols, J. C. (1970). *Potato Res.* **13,** 210–214.
Lund, B. M., and Wyatt, G. M. (1972). *Potato Res.* **15,** 174–179.

McClure, M. S., Andreadis, T. G., and Lacy, G. H. (1982). *J. Econ. Entomol.* **75,** 64–68.
McIntyre, J. L., Schneider, H., Lacy, G. L., Dodds, J. A., and Walton, G. S. (1979). *Phytopathology* **69,** 955–958.
McIntyre, J. L., Dodd, J. A., and Hare, J. D. (1981). *Phytopathology* **71,** 297–301.
Martin, C. (1979). *Rep. Plan. Conf. Dev. Control Bact. Dis. Potatoes, Lima* pp. 63–65.
Matthee, F. N., and Daines, R. H. (1968). *Phytopathology* **58,** 1298–1301.
Matthee, F. N., and Daines, R. H. (1969). *Phytopathology* **59,** 285–287.
Mew, T. W., Cruz, C. M. V., and Reyes, R. C. (1979). *Int. Rice Res. Newslett.* **4,** 12–13.
Moffett, M. (1973). *Aust. J. Biol. Sci.* **26,** 171–179.
Mowry, J. B. (1969). *J. Hort. Sci.* **4,** 128–130.
Naidu, V. D., Rao, B. S., and Rao, C. S. (1979). *Phytopathol. Z.* **96,** 83–86.
Navaratnam, S. J., Shuttleworth, D., and Wallace, D. (1980). *Aust. J. Exp. Agric. Animal Husb.* **20,** 97–101.
Nielsen, L. W. (1968). *Am. Potato J.* **45,** 174–181.
Otazu, V., and Secor, G. A. (1981). *Phytopathology* **71,** 290–295.
Parsons, C. S., and Spalding, D. H. (1972). *J. Am. Soc. Hortic. Sci.* **97,** 297–299.
Perombelon, M. C. M. (1979). *Rep. Plan. Conf. Dev. Control Bact. Dis. Potatoes, Lima* pp. 94–119.
Perombelon, M. C. M., and Kelman, A. (1980). *Annu. Rev. Phytopathol.* **18,** 361–387.
Persley, G. J. (1979). *Ann. Appl. Biol.* **93,** 159–160.
Rao, C. S., Rao, B. S., and Naidu, V. D. (1978). *Indian J. Phytopathol.* **31,** 547–548.
Roca, W. M., Espinoza, N. O., Roca, M. R., and Bryan, J. E. (1978). *Am. Potato J.* **55,** 691–701.
Schaad, N. W., Gabrielson, R. L., and Mulanax, M. W. (1980). *Appl. Environ. Microbiol.* **39,** 803–807.
Schuster, M. L., and Coyne, D. P. (1981). *Hortic. Rev.* **3,** 28–58.
Sequeira, L. (1958). *Phytopathology* **48,** 64–69.
Sharma, G. L., Modgal, S. C., and Gautum, R. C. (1979). *Int. Rice Res. Newslett.* **4,** 12–13.
Sharvelle, E. G. (1979). "Plant Disease Control." AVI Publ., Westport, Connecticut.
Strider, D. L. (1979). *Plant Dis. Rep.* **63,** 873–876.
Thompson, J. M. (1971). *Hort. Sci.* **6,** 167.
Thomson, S. V., Hills, F. J., Whitney, E. D., and Schroth, M. N. (1981). *Phytopathology* **71,** 605–608.
Thurston, H. D. (1980). *Plant Dis.* **64,** 252–257.
Velupillai, M. (1979). *Rep. Plan. Conf. Dev. Control Bact. Dis. Potatoes, Lima* pp. 131–137.
Wallen, V. R., and Galway, D. A. (1979). *Can. J. Plant Pathol.* **1,** 42–46.
Wells, J. M. (1974). *Phytopathology* **64,** 1012–1015.
Westwood, M. N., Chaplin, M. H., and Roberts, A. N. (1973). *J. Am. Soc. Hortic. Sci.* **98,** 352–357.
Woodbridge, C. G., Blodgett, E. C., and Diener, T. O. (1957). *Plant Dis. Rep.* **41,** 569–572.
Yadava, U. L., and Doud, S. L. (1980). *Hortic. Rev.* **2,** 1–116.
Zadoks, J. C., and Schein, R. D. (1979). "Epidemiology and Plant Disease Management." Oxford Univ. Press, London and New York.

Chapter 17

Control of Prokaryotes by Host Breeding

D. J. HAGEDORN

I. INTRODUCTION

Breeding host plants for disease resistance is without doubt the most important method for controlling plant diseases. Nelson (1973) considered it "likely that more than 75 percent of the current agricultural acreage in the United States is planted with varieties resistant to one or more plant diseases." Twenty years previous to that Coons (1953) estimated that up to $750,000,000 per year was saved by growers using resistant crop cultivars on 50% of the United States cropland. Beitz (1954) estimated that the value of breeding United States wheat (*Triticum vulgare* L.) for disease resistance, writing that "the increased income from wheat alone at $2 per bushel would return four-fold the annual cost of all tax-supported agricultural research." If one considers

Phytopathogenic Prokaryotes, Vol. 2

Copyright © 1982 by Academic Press, Inc.
All rights of reproduction in any form reserved.
ISBN 0-12-509002-1

the use of disease resistant cultivars all around the world, the financial and social benefits may be viewed as monumental.

The breeding of host plants for resistance to prokaryotes is also a very important way to control these plant pathogens. Perhaps one of the most important examples of breeding for resistance to these organisms involved the breeding of alfalfa (*Medicago sativa* L.) for resistance to bacterial wilt caused by *Corynebacterium michiganense* pv. *insidiosum* (McCulloch) Dye & Kemp. This classic research and other examples will be discussed later, but it is valuable to here be advised that this research has been considered by Hanson (1972) as one of the two greatest contributions to alfalfa improvement ever achieved. (The other was the development of winter hardiness.) Kehr *et al.* (1972) wrote that "Bacterial wilt-resistant varieties alone are saving farmers more than $100 million annually."

II. EARLY RESEARCH ON BREEDING FOR RESISTANCE

Even though there are numerous references to early research on breeding plants for disease resistance (starting in the mid-1800s), very few, if any, mention researching resistance to diseases incited by prokaryotes. Perhaps one of the first references to research on resistance to bacterial diseases was made by Orton in 1902, wherein he indicated that he was studying resistance to bacterial wilt of potato, (*Solanum tuberosum* L.) incited by *Pseudomonas solanacearum* (Smith) Smith, and angular leaf spot of cotton (*Gossypium hirsutum* L.) (now called bacterial blight) incited by *Xanthomonas campestris* pv. *malvacearum* (Smith) Dye.

One of the early researches concerning host resistance "control" of the fireblight disease, incited by *Erwinia amylovora* (Burr.) Winslow *et al.*, was by Reimer (1925) who studied the reaction of various strains of pears (*Pyrus communis* L.) to the pathogen. He and other scientists found that even though some cultivars of apples (*Malus sylvestris* Mill.) and pears possess helpful levels of tolerance, none was immune and very few highly resistant. High levels of disease resistance to fireblight in commercial cultivars are still being sought since this disease remains a very important malady.

As early as 1895 Stewart (1897) observed a bacterial wilt of sweet corn [(*Zea mays* var. *saccharata* (Sturtev.) Bailey] on Long Island which caused very serious losses—up to 100%. Inoculation studies with the pathogen, *Erwinia stewartii* (E. F. Smith) Dye, indicated that although sweet corn was susceptible, dent corn, popcorn [*Z. mays* var. *everta* (Sturtev.) Bailey] and teosinte (*Euchlaena mexicana* Schrad.) were resistant. Rand and Cash (1921) and Thomas (1924) reported that early sweet corn cultivars were more seriously affected than late cultivars.

III. BREEDING CROP PLANTS FOR RESISTANCE TO PROKARYOTES

Many crop plants are attacked by pathogenic prokaryotes and there is substantial literature reporting research on breeding for resistance to the diseases involved. Due to space limitations only selected researches can be summarized in the following paragraphs and in Table I.

A. Field Crops

1. Alfalfa

Jones (1925) first reported alfalfa bacterial wilt incited by *C. m.* pv. *insidiosum* in the upper midwestern states of Illinois and Wisconsin. The disease spread widely and became a very serious problem in practically all of the major alfalfa producing areas of the United States.

This disease caused striking reductions in stand and forage yield, however, resistance was reported by Weimer and Madson (1936) in the cultivars Ladak, Turkestan, and Hardistan. These cultivars served as sources of resistance in intensive alfalfa breeding programs which were extremely successful. They were the first researches on breeding for disease resistance in alfalfa. As a result Ranger and Buffalo, the first wilt-resistant cultivars, were released by the Agricultural Experiment Stations in Nebraska and Kansas in cooperation with the USDA. Many alfalfa cultivars with various percentages of wilt-resistant plants have subsequently been developed. For many years cultivar (cv.) Vernal, with about 46% resistant plants was a very popular and widely grown cultivar in the mid-United States. It served as a standard for comparing bacterial wilt resistance of new alfalfa breeding lines and cultivars.

A number of inoculation methods involving one or more techniques for introducing the pathogen into the host have been used successfully to determine the reaction of alfalfa populations to *C. m.* pv. *insidiosum.* Jones (1930) scrapped roots under a bacterial suspension; bacterial inoculum was injected into roots or crowns (Cormack *et al.,* 1957) or cotyledons were wounded (Kreitlow, 1963) or petioles punctured (Graham, 1960). Perhaps the most effective method is to soak the roots of dug and washed 8- to 10-week-old plants in a bacterial suspension from

Table 1. Examples of Prokaryote-Incited Plant Disease Control through Host Resistance

Crop name					
Common	Scientific	Disease	Pathogen	Resistant cultivar(s)	Reference(s)
Alfalfa	*Medicago sativa*	Bacterial wilt	*Corynebacterium insidiosum*	Ladak, Turkestan	Weimer and Madson (1936)
Corn	*Zea mays*	Stewart's wilt	*Erwinia stewartii*	Golden Bantam	Ivanoff and Riker (1936)
Cotton	*Gossypium* spp.	Bacterial blight	*Xanthomonas malvacearum*	Kufra, Oasis, Wagad 8	Knight (1956)
Rice	*Oryza sativa*	Bacterial blight	*Xanthomonas oryzae*	Lead; TKM 6	Sakaguchi *et al.* (1968)
Soybean	*Glycine max*	Bacterial blight	*Pseudomonas glycinea*	P.I. 68708	Dunleavy *et al.* (1960)
Soybean	*Glycine max*	Bacterial pustule	*Xanthomonas phaseoli* var. *sojensis*	CNS Wayne, Clark 63	Chamberlain (1962) Dunleavy (1973)
Sugarcane	*Saccharum*	Leaf scald	*Xanthomonas albilineans*	Ebenè 1-37, Pinder	Martin (1965)
Tobacco	*Nicotiana tabacum*	Bacterial wilt	*Pseudomonas solanacearum*	Oxford 26	Smith and Clayton (1948)
Pear	*Pyrus communis*	Fireblight	*Erwina amylovora*		Layne (1968)
Poplar	*Populus* spp.	Canker	*Aplanobacter populi*	Blom, Rap, Barn	Koster (1973)
Bean	*Phaseolus vulgaris*	Common blight	*Xanthomonas phaseoli*	Jules, Tara	Coyne and Schuster (1969a)
Bean	*Phaseolus vulgaris*	Halo blight	*Pseudomonas phaseolicola*	Wisconsin HBR-40	Hagedorn *et al.* (1974)
Bean	*Phaseolus vulgaris*	Bacterial brown spot	*P. syringae*	Wisconsin (BBSR) 130	Hagedorn and Rand (1980)
Cucumber	*Cucumis sativum*	Angular leaf spot	*P. lachrymans*	P.I. 197087	Barnes (1961)
Potatoes	*Solanum tuberosum*	Bacterial wilt	*P. solanacearum*		Sequeira (1979)
Pepper	*Capsicum fructescens*	Bacterial spot	*Xanthomonas vesicatoria*	G-2 Deva	Greenleaf (1960)

comminuted fresh or frozen infected roots for 20–30 min before transplanting. After 12–16 weeks in the field they are dug to determine disease severity by the extent of internal discoloration in root cross-section. Barnes *et al.* (1971) and Frosheiser (1966) have successfully used a combination of the cotyledon wounding and the root soak methods of inoculation to test large populations of young alfalfa plants.

Even though pure cultures of the pathogen may be used for inoculum, they are less virulent than inoculum from diseased host tissue (Kernhamp and Hemerick, 1952). Cormack (1961) and Cormack *et al.* (1957) found that infected plant material was easily stored and may provide a mixture of strains of the pathogen.

Several methods of plant breeding have been used successfully for incorporating bacterial wilt resistance into new alfalfa cultivars. They include recurrent phenotype selection, a modified backcross program, and recombination of selected alfalfa clones. Although many researchers have attempted to elucidate the nature of inheritance and resistance in alfalfa, these phenomena have not been conclusively explained (Brink *et al.*, 1934; Donnelly, 1952; Haun and LeBeau, 1962; Jones, 1934; Pearson and Elling, 1960; Pettier and Tysdal, 1934; Theurer and Elling, 1963). However, several investigators (Donnelly, 1952; Fulkerson, 1960; Pearson and Elling, 1960; Tysdal and Crandall, 1948) have found that resistance of parents and progeny is correlated positively, making possible excellent progress in the development of resistant cultivars.

2. *Corn*

Stewart's bacterial wilt of corn, incited by *Erwinia stewartii*, was a very important problem, especially on sweet corn, until resistant cultivars were developed and adopted. Valleau (1934) noted that corn cultivars with large plants were generally more resistant; and Thomas (1924) and Rand and Cash (1921) reported that late maturing cultivars showed lower infection percentages, thus were less seriously affected. Reddy and Holbert (1928) found that all progenies of certain inbreds of like maturity showed a high level of bacterial wilt resistance, while those of other lines were all susceptible. This key study demonstrated the feasibility of breeding wilt resistance into early, commercially acceptable sweet corn.

Ivanoff and associates, especially Riker (1936), studied some important phenomena concerning resistance in inbreds of cv. Golden Bantam sweet corn. Three types of resistance were recognized: (1) resistance correlated with increased height, (2) late maturity, and (3) "true" resistance. Ivanoff (1936) found that dent corn cultivars of a given maturity and height were no more resistant than sweet corn and flint corn (also Z.

mays L.) cultivars of the same maturity and height. He concluded that the resistance of open-pollinated dent corn was similar in type and degree to that in open-pollinated flint and sweet corn.

The genetics of resistance to Stewart's bacterial wilt was studied by Wellhausen (1935) and associates and by Ivanoff and Riker (1936). Wellhausen found that all gradations of disease reaction (highly susceptible to highly resistant) occurred in 56 inbred lines of dent, flint, and sweet corn and 14 crosses from these lines. Most of the field corn inbreds were resistant, the cv. Evergreen group intermediate, and the early sweet corns susceptible. The F_1 generations were resistant and two major dominant genes, and a modifying gene were involved. Other researchers found that resistance in corn hybrids was generally dominant, tall and late hybrids appeared to be more resistant, and hybrid sweet corn developed from highly resistant inbreds showed high resistance regardless of maturity. However, Elliott (1941) reported that some inbred dent corns, resistant to the leaf blight phase of the disease, were susceptible in later growth stages. She urged test inoculations later in the growth cycle of the plants to obtain accurate determination of "true" resistance. Koehler (1955) reported that resistance to *E. stewartii* and *Helminthosporium turcicum* Pass. was well correlated.

The resistant hybrid sweet corn cv., Golden Cross Bantam, was released for use in 1932 and 1933, both epidemic Stewart's wilt seasons. This new cultivar was readily accepted, and it provided great impetus for the rapid development of more yellow, early maturing sweet corn hybrids with the result that the threat of crop losses due to Stewart's bacterial wilt had practically disappeared by 1954.

A modified hypodermic syringe technique for rapidly inoculating large numbers of plants was described by Ivanoff (1934). Lockwood and Williams (1957) studied inoculation and disease rating methods, and developed a rapid, very effective, new method for inoculating seedling plants. The coleoptile tips of seedlings (7–9 days after planting, 1–2 leaf stage) were clipped and either wiped with absorbent cotton contaminated with a suspension of the bacterium or sprayed with the suspension. Symptoms in plants inoculated by either wiping or spraying were similar to those in plants inoculated with hypodermic syringes.

The disease rating system used by Lockwood and Williams (1957) involved the assignment of a disease rating of 0 to 5 to individual leaves, based on amount of wilting and severity and area of lesions. These researchers found that the disease severity was reduced when the time interval between clipping and inoculation was increased, and that disease severity was not significantly influenced by moisture conditions.

3. Cotton

During the past 30 years very good progress has been made in breeding cotton (*Gossypium* spp.) for resistance to bacterial blight incited by *X. c.* pv. *malvacearum*. Key contributions to this effect were made by Knight (1957) and Innes (1965) who identified 13 independent genes with measurable effects on resistance and assigned symbols to them. Other researchers (Blank and Hunter, 1955; Brinkerhoff, 1970) reported additional important sources of resistance and genes governing such resistance. The use of minor and modifying genes, in combination with major genes, has been well established as a proper scientific approach to the development of highly resistant or immune cottons. Bird and Blank (1951) published an excellent bulletin describing the methods used to successfully breed cotton for resistance to bacterial blight, and Brinkerhoff (1970) prepared a very helpful review on variation in the pathogen in relation to control.

Several techniques have been used successfully for determining the reaction of cotton plants to *X. c.* pv. *malvacearum*. Bird and Blank (1951) grew the pathogen on potato–carrot–dextrose agar for 5–7 days at 24–28°C. The bacteria from one Petri plate were added to 9.5 liters of water for field inoculations, or to 1 liter of water for greenhouse inoculation. Pressure spraying the inoculum onto the lower surfaces of leaves was the preferred method of inoculation. This forced the bacteria through the open stomata. In the field a wheelbarrow sprayer was used which maintained 8.8 to 10.6 kg/cm^2 pressure through the nozzle held 30.5 cm from the leaves. In the greenhouse a hand sprayer was used at 7.0 kg/cm^2 pressure and the nozzle was held 15 cm from the leaves. An abrasion method of inoculation developed by Brinkerhoff (1949) has also been used.

Bird and Blank (1951) also developed a disease severity rating system which they believed was very satisfactory for Texas conditions. They used the numbers 1 through 7, wherein 1 represented immunity and 7 complete susceptibility. Useful illustrations and written descriptions of the leaf symptoms used in the disease severity determinations were presented.

There are a number of races of the pathogen and the list of races had expanded as more differential hosts are studied (Hunter *et al.*, 1968). Although the presence of races earlier caused real problems in cotton breeding for resistance to bacterial blight, more recent research has been very successful because (1) several important races of *X. c.* pv. *malvacearum* have been used and (2) more breeding material containing the

"B" genes (genes for resistance to bacterial blight), especially B2, B3, B4, and B6 has been incorporated into the breeding effort. Bird (1973) considers that concepts and procedures for developing bacterial blight-resistant cotton lines should be used as a model for obtaining disease control through host resistance.

4. *Rice*

Bacterial blight incited by *Xanthomonas campestris* pv. *oryzae* (Ishiyama) Dye of rice (*Oryza sativa* L.) is one of the three most serious diseases of this very important food crop. This disease has become particularly serious in Asia since the widespread planting of the new high-yielding rice cultivar "IR8" which is very susceptible. Symptoms in temperate zones are white, blighted leaves; but in the tropics leaves yellow and the plant is stunted or seedlings wilt and die. Seedling death is known as the "Kresek" symptom. Generally, bacterial blight is more serious in the tropics because of higher temperature and rainfall and the presence of more virulent strains of the pathogen. Under such conditions whole fields are lost from kresek, while in Japan a serious loss would be a 30% reduction in yield (Ou, 1973).

Rice plants are generally inoculated with *X. c.* pv. *oryzae* by (1) spraying leaves with a bacterial suspension, (2) needle-pricking the leaves, or (3) dipping seedlings into inoculum. The first method is very useful for identifying resistant and susceptible plants, but is not always satisfactory for determining intermediate levels of disease reaction. Needle-pricking is good for determining intermediate reactions, and this inoculation technique compares well with natural infection. Ou (1973) found that resistance in the seedling and flowering stages was generally correlated positively.

The search for resistance and breeding for disease resistance have been undertaken in Japan and at the International Rice Research Institute (IRRI) in the Philippines. In Japan a series of new rice cultivars have been developed through the years but many are no longer resistant to the current virulent strains of *X. c.* pv. *oryzae*. Sakagushi *et al.* (1968) tested 863 lines of rice for reaction to the pathogen. Two lines of wild rice, plus the cvs. Nigeria 5, Lead, and TKM-6 were resistant. At IRRI more than 8000 rice cultivars and lines have been inoculated in the field with *X. c.* pv. *oryzae*. Resistant selections were tested and retested with the result that 30 resistant cultivars were developed. In India many of these rice lines were somewhat susceptible, however, giving added evidence of differing virulence in strains of the pathogen. Such cultivars as "BJ1" and "TKM-6" have a wider genetic base for resistance, thus offer more promise as germplasms for breeding programs designed to control the disease via host resistance. By combining the genes for resistance from several different genetic backgrounds better control should be realized eventually (Ou, 1973).

The most serious deterrent to the achievement of this goal is the wide variability in *X. c.* pv. *oryzae*, especially with regard to virulence of strains and isolates. Ou (1973) reported that 50 strains of the pathogen were studied on 24 rice cultivars and four pathogenic patterns were distinguished. Bacterial strains in Pattern I were highly virulent and caused an intermediate disease reaction on resistant cultivars, a susceptible reaction on intermediate cultivars, and death in susceptible cultivars. On the other end of the pattern scale, the strains in Pattern II were weakly virulent, showing an immune reaction on resistant cultivars and a moderate reaction on susceptible rices. Other combinations of disease reaction were displayed in Patterns III and IV. Weakly virulent bacterial strains never caused severe damage to resistant cultivars, but a few virulent strains caused damage to cultivars resistant to most virulent strains. In general, bacterial strains from tropical countries were more virulent than those from temperate areas, some from India and Indonesia being the most virulent.

5. *Soybeans*

Bacterial blight of soybeans [*Glycine max* (L.) Merr.] is incited by *Pseudomonas syringae* pv. *glycinea* (Coerper) Young *et al.* This bacterium is widespread throughout the soybean production areas of the world. Severe losses due to bacterial blight occur occasionally but not commonly, although yield reductions of up to 22% have been reported. The seed-borne nature of the bacterium adds to its potential as a troublesome pathogen.

Dunleavy *et al.* (1960) were the first to discover resistance to *P. s.* pv. *glycinea* in soybean cv. P.I. 68708. Seven races of the pathogen were described by Cross *et al.* (1966) after determining the disease reaction on leaves of seven soybean cultivars. The most resistant cultivar was Chippewa which was intermediate in reaction to race 4, but resistant to the other six races. Inoculation of soybean plants may be accomplished by gently rubbing carborundum-dusted leaves with a cloth pad saturated with inoculum containing 10^7 cells/ml in sterile water. However, Kennedy and Cross (1966) preferred the use of an artist's airbrush for the precise inoculations needed for differentiating races of the pathogen. Dunleavy *et al.* (1960) researched a motor-driven sprayer at 5.6 kg/cm^2 for inoculation of soybeans in the field; Dunleavy (1973) later described a similar but improved inoculation method which involved the use of a motor-driven compressed air paint sprayer, with 600 mesh carborundum added to the inoculum at 2 g/liter. Inoculum can be grown on PDA or trypticase soy agar at pH 7.0 for 48–72 hr or in trypticase soy broth at 28°C on a shaker for 24 hr (Dunleavy, 1973). The same researcher and associates described a rating system for disease reactions on inoculated plants (Dunleavy *et al.*, 1960).

Soybean bacterial pustule is incited by *X. c.* pv. *phaseoli* (Smith) Dye var. *sojensis* (Hedges) Starr & Burkh. Jones (1961) reported the southern United States weed, red vine (*Brunnichia cirrhosa* Gaertn.), as a natural host of the pathogen and implicated this plant as a primary source of inoculum. According to Elliott (1951), lima bean (*Phaseolus limensis* Macf.) and common bean (*P. vulgaris* L.) are also alternate hosts. Although the disease occurs in most of the soybean-growing areas of the world, severe economic losses due to its presence are not common.

Inoculum preparation and inoculation methods similar to those indicated above for *P. s.* pv. *glycinea* are generally appropriate, although it is important to incubate cultures and inoculated plants at 30°C. A unique technique for preparing inoculum was reported by Jones and Hartwig (1959). Infected leaves were sealed in glass jars, frozen, and stored in that state for use the next season. Thawed leaves were macerated in a food chopper with 10 chopped leaves added to 300 ml of water. After 2 hr the preparation was filtered through two thicknesses of cheesecloth and the volume increased to 3.8 liters. This inoculum was pressure-sprayed on field-grown plants. It is often difficult to accurately identify resistant plants in a segregating progeny in the greenhouse unless temperature and inoculum concentration are well controlled. However, Chamberlain (1962) was able to successfully separate plants of the resistant cv. CNS from those of the susceptible Lincoln.

The soybean cultivar CNS has been the source of resistance used by United States soybean breeders in their researches to develop cultivars resistant to *X. c.* pv. *phaseoli* var. *sojensis*. Resistance is governed by a recessive single gene *rpx*, but modifying genes influence levels of susceptibility. Resistance is commonly more strongly expressed in the field than in the greenhouse. Most soybean cultivars grown in the southern United States are resistant to bacterial-pustule, while very few, i.e., Wayne and Clark 63, northern United States cultivars are resistant (Dunleavy, 1973).

6. Sugarcane

Sugarcane (*Saccharum officinarum* L.) leaf scald is caused by the bacterium *Xanthomonas albilineans* (Ashby) Dowson. This disease is widespread in the world's sugarcane production areas where it may cause severe epiphytotics. In its chronic phase the disease appears as narrow white strips on leaves or as blanched leaves on stunted stalks with many shoots. The acute phase is manifested by rapid wilting and death of shoots (Martin and Robinson, 1961). These same authors indicate that Wilbrink's agar is appropriate for isolation of the pathogen and maintenance of stock cultures. The fact that cultivar reaction to the pathogen is different in different countries suggests that there are strains of the bacterium.

Cultivars and sugarcane lines are tested for reaction to *X. albilineans* by using the aluminum cap method of artificial inoculation devised by Koike (1965). Inoculum, consisting of a water suspension of 7- to 10-day-old culture of the bacteria, was sprayed on the cut surfaces of primary cane shoots 20–30 cm tall. The cuts were made a few centimeters above the shoot apex. Inoculated shoots were capped with aluminum foil. Egan (1969) agreed that this method of inoculation provided a rapid and efficient way of identifying the most resistant and most susceptible plants, but intermediate reactions were not determined reliably.

Stevenson (1965) reported that there are resistant cultivars within the genera *S. officinarum* and *S. spontaneum* L., but those classified as *S. robustum* (Brandes and Jesw.) Grassl. were susceptible. Martin (1965) listed 15 resistant hybrids from 5 different countries.

7. *Tobacco*

Granville or bacterial wilt of tobacco (*Nicotiana tabacum* L.) is incited by *Pseudomonas solanacearum*, a pathogen with a very wide host range, especially in the Solanaceae. This tobacco disease is found in most warm tobacco-growing areas of the world. For many years before 1940 it caused annual 40–100% crop losses valued at up to 40 million dollars in Granville County, North Carolina. Lucas (1975) reviewed the literature concerning this and other tobacco diseases, including the research on breeding for disease resistance.

Resistance in *N. tabacum* was discovered by Clayton and Foster (1940) in T.I. 448A. It was the only tobacco line which was resistant among 1100 lines tested. Oxford 26, released in 1945 by Smith and Clayton (1948), was the first resistant cultivar and it was an all-important parent in the subsequent development of many flue-cured tobaccos. Resistance was inherited from T.I. 448A in a recessive and polygenic manner. Resistance to bacterial wilt and to the black shank disease incited by *Phytophthora parasitica* var. *nicotianae* (Breda de Haan) Tucker appeared to be linked genetically.

An important problem encountered in researching the pathogen in the laboratory was that in culture it was genetically variable, often losing virulence (Kelman, 1953). He developed a method for isolating and maintaining virulent cultures using differential media. Other researchers (Okobe and Goto, 1963) used host specificity to identify races of *P. solanacearum*. In studying tobacco plants for reaction to bacterial wilt it is common to use naturally infested field nurseries. Although the pathogen often persists well in such testing sites the inoculum level can be raised by the addition of infested soil and/or diseased plant debris, and Moore *et al.* (1963) reported that the use of 8×10^6 virulent bacterial cells per ml in 50 ml/plant of the transplant water was a very effective field inoculation technique.

B. Trees

1. *Apple and Pear*

The important bacterial disease of apple and pear is fireblight incited by *Erwinia amylovora*. Although it is a very troublesome disease of apple, it is a devastating malady of pear and is often the limiting factor in pear production.

There is no immunity in *Malus* sp. but there some apples lines show considerable resistance to the spread of the bacteria within infected shoots. The disease reaction is commonly assessed by inoculation at the tip of actively growing terminal shoots and subsequently measuring the distance the pathogen has invaded the shoots to determine the percentage of the shoot infected. Moore (1946) considered that resistance is polygenically controlled. Nonnecke (1948) reported that different biological races of the pathogen exist, a fact that apple breeders and pathologists must take into account.

Because of the great importance of fireblight to pear production the breeding for host resistance has received substantial attention by scientists for many years. Layne and Quamme (1975) have prepared a publication which includes a very good treatment of this subject. These authors wrote that the pioneer work of Reimer (1925) set the stage for an intensive effort at breeding for fire blight resistance. Sources of resistance were identified among the Oriental pear lines introduced by Reimer (Reimer 1925; Lamb, 1960; Thompson *et al.*, 1962). This provided screening methods, resistant germplasm, and a rational approach to blight resistance breeding.

The inoculation technique used for many years was similar to the one mentioned above and used by apple scientists. However, van der Zwet and Oitto (1973) developed a new method to efficiently inoculate large numbers of small pear plants. Tips of succulent seedling shoots were injured with a group of metal pins in a clamp which simultaneously released the bacterial inoculum through a sponge on the clamp opposite the metal pins. The sponge was connected to a plastic bottle containing the inoculum that was suspended above a backpack. The inoculated seedlings were incubated on the enclosed bench at 85–100% RH and 21–27°C for 6–8 weeks.

Layne (1968) and Layne *et al.* (1968) have intensively researched the breeding of fireblight-resistant pears for 18 years and have tested many different resistance sources and breeding techniques. *Pyrus ussuriensis* Maxim. resistance sources were slightly more efficient than *P. pyrifolia* (Burm.) Nakai which were slightly better than *P. communis.* But there were always important exceptions so there was a tendency to show continued interest in the best *P. communis* sources because of their superior fruit size, appearance, and quality. They considered it important to continue the breeding program only with the most advanced backcross selections with the best fruit quality.

Van der Zwet *et al.* (1970) developed an efficient and accurate disease rating system for determining blight resistance in the field following natural infection. Its widespread adoption was recommended by Layne and Quamme (1975). These authors wrote that "the inheritance of resistance to fire blight in *Pyrus* is not yet established." There is some evidence that resistance is polygenically inherited, and in some cases major gene inheritance is indicated; in others monogenic resistance is thought to exist.

An important complication in breeding pear for fireblight resistance was the discovery of van der Zwet and Oitto (1972) that some cultivars are shoot resistant and trunk susceptible, others are shoot susceptible and trunk resistant, and others show both shoot and trunk to be either susceptible or resistant. This may well necessitate the field testing of greenhouse shoot resistant seedlings for trunk reaction to *E. amylovora.*

2. *Poplar*

One of the major bacterial diseases of forest trees is found on poplar (*Populus* spp.) in Europe and is known as poplar canker incited by *Aplanobacter populi.* Gremmen and Koster (1972) made an extensive study of more than 1100 clones and hybrids of several poplar species. Clones were vegetatively propagated from softwood cuttings and 10 1-year-old plants of each clone were planted in early spring and shortly thereafter shoots were cut back to ground level. Fresh leaf scars were inoculated in September of the following year when the clone's 2-year-old roots were bearing a 1⅓-year-old shoot.

Inoculum was grown on a yeast–peptone–glucose medium at neutral pH. To obtain quantities of inocula the pathogen was stimulated by subculturing *Aplanobacter* isolates 1 month prior to inoculation, and 4–5 days before inoculation the isolates were mixed together and plated onto medium in Petri dishes. "Small amounts of slime" were delivered to the fresh leaf scars presumably via a hypodermic syringe at two sites per plant at heights of 50 and 75% of the total shoot length. Disease severity data during and at the end of 2 years following inoculation were rated using 5 severity scores, descriptive photographs, and text for the scores are available. The most resistant poplar species was *Populus nigra* L. which showed that 92.3% of the 196 clones tested were resistant. These researchers, Gremmer and Koster (1972), suggested two changes in their technique: (1) inoculate in August in the Netherlands, and (2) use two tests instead of one, the second under different "circumstances." Koster (1973) reported that the new clones Blom, Rap, Barn, and Donk can be regarded as completely resistant. Nowadays all poplar selection being released in Europe are screened for reaction to bacterial canker.

C. Vegetables

1. Beans

It is very likely that the common blight disease incited by *Xanthomonas campestris* pv. *phaseoli* Smith (Dye) is the most serious malady of beans (*Phaseolus vulgaris* L.). The disease occurs in practically every country where beans are grown, and is serious because (1) the pathogen is seed-borne, (2) highly resistant cultivars are not commonly available and (3) the pathogen is variable with the sudden occurrence of highly virulent strains. These factors combine to slow disease resistance breeding. Bean improvement programs at CIAT in Colombia, South America, the University of Nebraska, Cornell University, and at Michigan State University are emphasizing the breeding of resistance to common blight and to its "sister" disease, fuscans blight incited by *X. phaseoli* var. *fuscans* (Burkholder) Starr & Burkholder. One of the most significant contributions in this effort was made by Coyne and Schuster (1969a) by the development of the cultivar "Jules," which has high tolerance to both common blight and fuscans blight.

The bean disease halo blight incited by *Pseudomonas syringae* pv. *phaseolicola* (Burkholder) Young *et al.* has caused very troublesome epiphytotics, especially in snap bean production fields. In more recent times (the last 15–20 years) these disease outbreaks have been occasional instead of usual, and were highly and positively correlated with infected seed supplies. The University of Wisconsin has been very active in breeding for resistance to this disease; Hagedorn *et al.* released the first resistant snap beans in 1974.

Inoculum of *Xanthomonas* or *Pseudomonas* pathogens can be grown on nutrient dextrose agar or in nutrient broth. It is advisable to use inoculum which has been growing on/in these media for 24–48 hr. Inoculum concentration should be standardized at a moderately high level depending upon several factors including the virulence of the bacterial isolate, plant age, and incubation environment. Usually 10^{4-6} cells/ml is satisfactory.

Bean plants can be successfully inoculated in several ways. Andrus (1948) described the multiple needle puncture technique whereby a metal flower stem holder with 15–25 needles is dipped into inoculum just prior to being pressed against the surface of half-expanded bean leaves. The use of a pressurized atomizer to forcibly watersoak bean leaves with inoculum was described as an inoculation method in 1955 by Schuster. Goth in 1965 reported that needle-pricking leaves or pods through drops of inoculum was effective. More recently Antonius and Hagedorn (1981) have developed a technique for efficiently and reliably inoculating large numbers of bean seedlings using a hypodermic needle to introduce *P. syringae* pv. *syringae* van Hall.

The reaction of inoculated plants can be evaluated and recorded in several ways, and it may be important to do so using a system which can be quantified. Coyne *et al.* (1973) used a disease rating system where numbers indicated bean common blight disease severity on individual plants as follows: 1 = no visible symptoms; 2 = slight, small lesions on about 1–5% of leaves; 3 = moderate lesions of various sizes, some leaves chloratic; 4 = severe, many large lesions on most leaves, pronounced chlorosis and necrosis; 5 = very severe, plants chlorotic, necrotic, and largely defoliated. This system could be transformed into a disease index (D.I.) by changing the numerical disease severity ratings to 0 through 4 and then calculating a D.I. according to the method of Sherwood and Hagedorn (1958).

During the past 20 years, very significant progress has been made in the breeding of beans for resistance to bacterial diseases. A good number of field beans with resistance to common blight have been released from the breeding programs mentioned above, and we have developed new processing-type bean lines with resistance to halo blight. An interesting phenomenon noted in both the common blight and halo blight breeding activities is that different genes govern foliage and pod resistance. Coyne and Schuster (1980) have summarized the sources of resistance to the bacterial diseases of beans and also listed the cultivars and lines developed for resistance.

The most important disease of snap beans grown for processing in the United States midwest is bacterial brown-spot incited by *P. s.* pv. *syringae*. Bean crops grown there are often sprayed two to four times each season with a copper "bactericide" as a control practice. Although the pathogen may not commonly be seed-borne to any significant extent, it is regularly present as an epiphyte on weed hosts, especially hairy vetch (*Vicia villosa* Roth L.) (Ercolani *et al.*, 1974), from which it easily spreads into the bean crop via blowing dust or water.

Tolerance to *P. s.* pv. *syringae* in beans was reported by Coyne and Schuster (1969) and Hagedorn *et al.* (1972), and high level resistance was discovered by Hagedorn and Rand (1975) after exhaustive field and greenhouse tests involving over 1000 bean lines and cultivars. The resistant plants in P.I. 313537 from Mexico were crossed with Slimgreen to develop the first highly resistant bush bean, Wis. (BBSR) 130 released in 1976 (Hagedorn and Rand, 1977). This bean also carried resistance to six other bean pathogens, including *X. c.* pv. *phaseoli* and *P. s.* pv. *phaseolicola*. After further bean breeding efforts to improve plant and pod characteristics, the same two researchers released Wis. (BBSR) 17 and Wis. (BBSR) 28 (Hagedorn and Rand, 1980).

The field testing of hundreds of bean lines for reaction to bacterial brown spot provided a real challenge especially with regard to proper inoculation of the plants. Inoculum was obtained by gathering diseased leaves the previous season, rapidly air-drying them at about 20°C, grinding the dry leaves into a powder, and storing at 4°C. At planting time only seed of the susceptible "spreader" cultivar planted in alternate rows was inoculated. The powdered inoculum was mixed thoroughly with the bean seed at about 340 g inoculum to 100 kg seed. The inoculated seed was planted with a commercial type bean planter. Alternate rows were hand-planted with uninoculated seed of the bean lines to be tested. It was important to plant into moist soil and to apply overhead irrigation regularly to keep the very sandy soil from drying. As disease development progressed in plants in the spreader rows the pathogen gradually moved into the test bean lines aided at times by early morning horizontal spraying with water using a commercial air-blast sprayer.

Greenhouse grown plants were spray inoculated when the first trifoliolate leaves one-quarter to one-third expanded. The undersides of these leaves were thoroughly wetted with a fine mist of inoculum which consisted of a water suspension of 10^7 cells/ml prepared from a 48 hr culture of *P. s.* pv. *syringae* growing on tube slants of nutrient dextrose agar. It was not necessary to cover inoculated plants or incubate them in a moist chamber if the RH in the greenhouse was above 60%. Under such conditions small water-soaked lesions could be observed on susceptible plants in 5 days (Hagedorn and Rand, 1975). In more recent studies concerned with new sources of disease resistance, Antonius and Hagedorn, (1978) have used the pressure sprayer described by Ercolani *et al.* (1974) to watersoak the tissue.

2. *Cucumbers*

The angular leaf spot disease incited by (*Pseudomonas syringae* pv. *lachrymans* (Smith and Bryan) Young *et al.* of cucumbers (*Cucumis sativus* L.) is an important problem in many cucumber production areas. It is an especially troublesome problem in pickling cucumbers because the extent of the infection and tissue discoloration beneath the fruit rind is impossible to discern from the outside. The inciting bacteria are spread by windblown and splashing rain and disease development is optimum at 24–28°C.

Sitterly (1973) maintained this pathogen on nutrient-dextrose agar, and prepared inoculum by growing the pathogen in slant bottles of this medium for 48 hr. Another method of inoculum preparation is to dry and store (up to 1 year) infected leaves in a cardboard box at 15–21°C. When needed, the leaves may be crushed, soaked in water for 1 hr, strained, and diluted to proper concentration. Greenhouse grown plants are inoculated at the fifth leaf stage by spraying the undersides of leaves until watersoaking is visible. The plants are incubated in a moist chamber for 2 days at 21°C and 98% RH. In the field plants are sprayed in the evening at 2.1 to 4.2 kg/cm with a carborundum-amended inoculum (4 cm^3 carborundum/liter).

Chand and Walker (1964) considered that the cucumber PI 169400 possessed a helpful level of resistance to *P. s.* pv. *lachrymans* so they crossed it with Wisconsin SMR 15 and 18. Resistance levels could be increased by repeated selection of resistant plants. These same researchers (1964a) found that older leaves of susceptible plants supported much fewer bacteria than young leaves, and bacterial multiplication was relatively low in resistant plants, high in susceptible, and intermediate in the hybrid between the two. Barnes (1961) found that PI 197087 showed more resistance than PI 169400 and thus could be considered highly resistant.

3. *Potatoes*

Bacterial wilt incited by *Pseudomonas solanacearum* is a major disease of potato (*Solanum tuberosum*), when this crop is grown in the subtropics and tropics. No practical levels of host resistance were found in *S. tuberosum*, but Thurston and Lozano (1968) detected very good resistance in certain Colombian diploids of cultivated *S. phureja* Juzepezuk and Bukasov. This important discovery gave impetus to intensive research at the International Potato Center, Lima, Peru, the University of Wisconsin, and elsewhere. Sequeira (1979) reported on the progress of research to develop resistant hybrid potato clones from the bacterial wilt resistance found in *S. phureja*.

He found that procedures for adequate and reproducible screening for disease resistance were developed, but that the stem inoculation technique proved too cumbersome for testing large populations. Gonzalez *et al.* (1973) developed a rapid and efficient root inoculation technique, but some resistant seedlings carried latent bacterial infections. The most successful procedure involved growing seedlings inoculated and uninoculated from a single clone until they could be vegetatively propagated. If the inoculated tuber survived, tubers from the uninoculated plants were retained.

Resistant clones of *S. phureja* and hybrid clones of *S. tuberosum* reportedly resistant in the tropics were crossed with 24- and 48-chromosome clones of *S. tuberosum*. Sequeira and Rowe (1969) showed that resistance was dependent on multiple, dominant genes.

Differences were found in the proportion of resistant to susceptible plants when progenies were tested at different times of the year in the greenhouse (Sequeira and Rowe, 1969). Constant temperatures above 30°C or light intensities at or below 1300 ft-c eliminated resistance in growth rooms. Thus, recommendations for use of resistant potato clones had to take into account sensitivity to low light intensities and high temperatures.

When the wilt-resistant clones were field-tested in the tropics, other disease problems, late blight, incited by *Phytophthora infestans* (Mont.) DB, and potato viruses (X, Y, A, and S, and the leaf roll virus), caused problems. So late blight-resistant potatoes from Mexico and virus-resistant potatoes from Germany were added to the crossing program. The result was the development of potato clones with resistance to all three disease problems.

4. Pepper

Bacterial spot of pepper (*Capsicum frutescens* L.) is incited by *Xanthomonas campestris* pv. *vesicatoria* (Doidge) Dye. This disease is a troublesome problem in production and marketing of peppers, especially in the important southeastern areas of the United States. One of the first studies on host resistance was conducted by Horsfall and McDonnell (1940) who noted that several commercial cultivars were disease free and showed very few leaf spots. Among these were Bullrose, Harris Earliest,

Harris Early Giant, Sweet Yellow, Waltham Beauty, and Yellow Oshkosh. However, resistance was not evident in Bullrose or Early Giant in Florida (Weber, 1932).

Martin (1948) tested a good number and range of pepper cultivars and types for disease reaction. Plants 12 weeks were old inoculated with a suspension of *X. c.* pv. *vesicatoria* from one Petri dish (7-day-old PDA culture; 10^7 cells/ml), forcibly sprayed on the ventral leaf surfaces at noon when the stomata were open. Inoculated plants were kept in a moist chamber at near 100% RH at 27°C during the day and 18°C at night. Differences in disease reaction were apparent after 5 days and final readings were made 11 days after inoculation. Two hot pepper cultivars that were rated as highly resistant were the Santanka (4a-2-1) and Cayenne (4566).

Other studies by Krupka (1956) involved about 40 commercial pepper cultivars and showed Long Red Cayenne and Calcom to be resistant. Greenleaf (1960) found a Ceylonese pepper, G-2-Deva (P.I. 246331), with a higher level of resistance than any previously tested pepper. This pepper, plus 14 other P.I.s, were reported by Sowell (1960) as possessing sufficient disease resistance to bacterial spot to be of value as sources of resistance for plant breeding purposes. He spray-inoculated 659 pepper lines in the greenhouse when they were 30 days after seeding in flats, and incubated them 40 hr in a moist chamber and recorded data 7–10 days after inoculation. Disease incidence and severity readings were made after the method of Krupka (1956) where incidence was recorded and severity was rated on a scale of 0–3: 0 = 0 spot/leaf; 1 = 1–2 spots/leaf; 2 = 3–14 spots/leaf; 3 = 15 or more spots/leaf.

The inheritance of resistance in pepper to bacterial spot has been studied by Cook and Stall (1963). They listed P.I. 163184, 163189, 183922, 246331, 244670, and 163192 as resistant to the disease in Florida, and they crossed representative plants of each of these P.I.s with susceptible, large fruited "bell" peppers. All F_1 plants (except those derived from P.I. 163192) were intermediate in disease reaction response, indicating multigenic inheritance. There was evidence of dominant resistance in P.I. 163192; but heterogeneity was also found in this pepper. These researchers also cautioned that environmental conditions and pathogen strain differences can cause variability.

IV. TISSUE–CELL CULTURE AND HOST RESISTANCE

One of the classic systems for studying a bacterial plant pathogen in tissue culture concerns the crown gall disease incitant, *Agrobacterium tumefaciens* (Smith and Tounsend) Conn. This research was built upon the knowledge generated by the pioneer tissue scientists Morel (1944, 1948) and White (1934).

The report by Braun (1959) that a whole plant could be grown from a single cell gave great impetus to research on plant cell culture techniques, and excellent progress has been made since that time. Hundreds of publications report this progress; the following useful reviews and books deal with the subject at hand: Brettell and Ingram (1979), Ingram (1977), Ingram and Helgeson (1980), Nickell and Heinz (1973), and Thomas *et al.* (1979). Several of these references include at least summaries and/or discussions of the present and future application to tissue–cell culture in the development of new disease-resistant crop plants.

Even though there are some useful advantages of using this approach to the development of disease-resistant cultivars, plant breeders and plant pathologists have not sufficiently exploited the new technology; and there is only one instance known to the author which indicates that a prokaryote-incited plant disease could be controlled by host resistance obtained through cell–tissue culture. Carlson (1970) studied the reaction of methionone sulfoxime (MSO)-resistant tobacco plants, derived from protoplasts, to the tobacco wildfire pathogen *Pseudomonas syringae* pv. *tabaci* (Wolf and Foster) Young *et al* His studies were built on the discovery by Braun (1955) that the toxin produced by *P. s.* pv. *tabaci* is a structural analog of methionine. He treated tobacco cv Havana Wisconsin 38 cells with the mutagen 0.25% ethyl methanesulfonate, plated them, and 2 weeks later overlaid them with 10 m*M* MSO. The calluses which were resistant to the MSO exposure were grown to whole tobacco plants. The apical region of each test leaf was inoculated twice with 0.1 ml of a 3- to 4-day-old culture of *P. s.* pv. *tabaci* in nutrient broth. The left side of the basal portion of each leaf was treated with methionine sulfoximine. Large chlorotic halos developed only on the control leaf, the reaction of mutant leaves A and B were similar to Burley 21 tobacco which carries a natural resistance to *P. s.* pv. *tabaci*.

As indicated above an important aspect of parasitism by a number of bacteria is the production of toxins which inhibit host metabolism. Bajiaja and Saettler (1970) reported that the culture filtrates of the bacterial bean pathogens *P. s.* pv. *phaseolicola* and *P. s.* pv. *syringae*, and the closely related *P. s.* pv. *morsprunorum* (Wormald) Young *et al.*, could inhibit the growth of *Phaseolus vulgaris* callus tissue. Also, there were interesting similarities in the physiological effects of the toxin-containing filtrates of *P. s.* pv. *phaseolicola* on green-leaf tissue and bean callus. The researchers suggested that callus tissue might be used to investigate the mode of action of the bacterial toxin.

A possible model for studying the inheritance of resistance to bacterial disease can be studied in the work of Helgeson *et al.* (1976). They used a tissue culture system to study the inheritance of resistance in tobacco to black shank disease incited by *Phytophthora parasitica* var. *nicotianae* (Breda de Haan) Tucker. They found that the single dominant genetic factor which conferred disease resistance to intact tobacco plants was also expressed in tobacco pith callus cultures. This was considered the first report of the successful use of tissue culture for such genetic studies.

V. MULTILINES AND RESISTANCE

Nelson (1973) defined multilines as "blends of different genotypes, each of which, in the simplest case, contains a different gene for VR (vertical resistance)." The use of multilines for disease control has been recommended by several researchers (Borlaug, 1965; Browning and Frey, 1969). Frey and Browning stated that advantages of multilines may include (1) a mechanism to synthesize horizontally resistant cultivars, (2) a mechanism to extend the useful life of a single resistance gene, (3) a mechanism to stabilize the cultivars used and enable optimizal production, and (4) a mechanism to distribute cultivars without risk of reducing the germplasm pool on a global scale. Nelson (1973) indicated that multilines, by reducing the amount of initial inoculum available for infection and by curbing subsequent increase of disease, exhibit both VR and horizontal resistance, respectively. Fleming and Person (1978) have developed a mathematical model to theorize disease control through use of multilines. A multiline cultivar program has been successful for the control of crown rust, *Puccinia coronata* Cda. var. *avenae* Fraser and Led., of oats (*Avena sativa* L.) (Frey *et al.*, 1971).

Even though such a program has not been described for the control of diseases incited by prokaryotes, there is good reason to believe that multilines offer promise, especially for the control of such diseases as bacterial blight of rice and other diseases where new strains of the pathogen occur quite readily.

VI. PROSPECTS FOR THE FUTURE

The future should hold real promise for steady, and sometimes perhaps spectacular improvement in host resistance for the control of plant diseases incited by prokaryotes. Our technology should continue to advance, and younger, more highly trained scientists will take over more and more of the research programs which concentrate on developing disease resistance. If indeed this "hope" materializes excellent progress should be made with conventional plant breeding and such promising new researches as those described by Shepard *et al.* (1980) and others on the use of plant protoplasts to increase disease resistance. Excellent scientific knowledge has already been gained on the nature of resistance to bacteria (Kelman and Sequeira, 1972). There may also be some helpful breakthroughs provided by the new and rapidly expanding genetic engineering technology. However, there is a trend on the part of some to deemphasize research programs which concentrate directly on disease control. Such actions will quite likely greatly impede the development of more host resistance to prokaryotic plant pathogens. We need both basic and applied research to solve the problems.

References

Andrus, C. F. (1948). *Phytopathology* **38,** 757–759.

Antonius, S. H., and Hagedorn, D. J. (1978). *Meet. Am. Phytopathol. Soc., 70th* p. 134 (Abstr.).

Baggett, J. R., and Frazier, W. A. (1967). *Plant Dis. Rep.* **54,** 963–905.

Bajiaja, V., and Saettler, A. W. (1970). *Phytopathology* **60,** 1065–1067.

Barnes, D. K., Hanson, C. H., Frosheiser, F. I., and Elling, L. J. (1971). *Crop. Sci.* **11,** 545–546.

Barnes, W. C. (1961). *Proc. Am. Soc. Hortic. Sci.* **77,** 417–423.

Bird, L. S. (1973). *In* "Breeding Plants for Disease Resistance" (R. R. Nelson, ed.), p. 184–185. Penn. State Univ. Press, University Park, Pennsylvania.

Bird, L. S., and Blank, L. M. (1951). *Tex. Agric. Exp. Sta. Bull.* **736.**

Blank, L. M., and Hunter, R. E. (1955). *Proc. Cotton Dis. Council* **16,** 18–19.

Borlaug, N. E. (1965). *Phytopathology* **55,** 1088–1098.

Braun, A. C. (1955). *Phytopathology* **45,** 659–667.

Braun, A. C. (1959). *Proc. Natl. Acad. Sci. U.S.A.* **45,** 932–938.

Brettell, R. I. S., and Ingram, D. S. (1979). *Biol. Rev.* **54,** 329–345.

Brink, R. A., Jones, F. R., and Albrecht, H. R. (1934). *J. Agric. Res.* **49,** 635–642.

Brinkerhoff, L. A. (1949). Personal communication with L. M. Blank.

Brinkerhoff, L. A. (1970). *Annu. Rev. Phytopathol.* **8,** 85–109.

Browning, J. A., and Frey, K. J. (1969). *Annu. Rev. Phytopathol.* **7,** 355–382.

Carlson, P. S. (1970). *Science* **180,** 1366–1358.

Chamberlain, D. W. (1962). *Plant Dis. Rep.* **46,** 707–709.

Chand, J. M., and Walker, J. C. (1964a). *Phytopathology* **54,** 49–51.

Chand, J. M., and Walker, J. C. (1964b). *Phytopathology* **54,** 51–54.

Clayton, E. E., and Foster, H. H. (1940). *Phytopathology* **30,** 4.

Cook, A. A., and Stall, R. E. (1963). *Phytopathology* **53,** 1060–1062.

Coons, G. H. (1953). *In* "Plant Disease, the Yearbook of Agriculture," pp. 174–192. US Govt. Printing Office., Washington, D.C.

Cormack, M. W. (1971). *Phytopathology* **5,** 260–261.

Cormack, M. W., Peake, R. W., and Downey, R. K. (1957). *Can. J. Plant Sci.* **37,** 1–11.

Coyne, D. P., Schuster, M. L., and Fast, R. (1967). *Plant Dis. Rep.* **51,** 20–24.

Coyne, D. P., and Schuster, M. L. (1969a). *Univ. Neb. Agric. Exp. Sta. Bull.* **506,** 1–10.

Coyne, D. P., and Schuster, M. L. (1969b). *Plant Dis. Rep.* **53**, 677–680.

Coyne, D. P., and Schuster, M. L. (1980). *In* "Advances in Legume Science" (Summerfield and Buntings, eds.), pp. 225–233. Royal Botanic Gardens, Kew.

Coyne, D. P., Schuster, M. L., and K. Hill. (1973). *J. Am. Soc. Hortic. Sci.* **98**, 94–99.

Cross, J. E., Kennedy, B. W., Lambert, J. W., and Cooper, R. L. (1966). *Plant Dis. Rep.* **50**, 557–560.

Donnelly, E. D. (1952). *Agron. J.* **44**, 562–568.

Dunleavy, J. (1973). *In* "Breeding Plant Disease Resistance" (R. R. Nelson, ed.), pp. 274–275. Penn State Univ. Press, University Park, Pennsylvania.

Dunleavy, J., Weber, C. R., and Chamberlain, D. W. (1960). *Proc. Iowa Acad. Sci.* **67**, 102–125.

Egan, B. T. (1969). *Int. Soc. Sugar Cane Tech. Proc.* **13**, 1153–1158.

Elliott, C. (1941). *Phytopathology* **31**, 7–8.

Elliott, C. (1951). "Manual of Bacterial Plant Pathogens." Chronica Botanica, Waltham, Massachusetts.

Ercolani, G. L., Hagedorn, D. J., Kelman, A., and Rand, R. E. (1974). *Phytopathology* **64**, 1330–1339.

Fleming, R. A., and Person, C. O. (1978). *Phytopathology* **68**, 1230–1233.

Frazier, W. A. (1970). *Bean Improve. Coop. Rep.* **13**, 12–19.

Frey, K. J., Browning, J. A., and Grindeland, R. L. (1971). Int. Atomic Energy Agency, Vienna. IAEA STI/PUB/271.

Frosheiser, F. I. (1966). *Phytopathology* **56**, 566–567.

Fulkerson, J. F. (1960). *Phytopathology* **50**, 377–380.

Gonzalez, L. C., Sequeira, L., and Rowe, P. R. (1973). *Am. Potato J.* **50**, 96–104.

Goth, R. W. (1965). *Phytopathology* **55**, 930–931.

Graham, J. H. (1960). *Phytopathology* **50**, 637.

Greenleaf, W. H. (1960). *Proc. Assoc. South. Agric. Work.* **57**, 238–239.

Gremmer, J., and Koster, R. (1972). *Eur. J. For. Pathol.* **2**, 116–124.

Hagedorn, D. J., and Rand, R. E. (1975). *Proc. Am. Phytopathol. Soc.* **2**, 49–50.

Hagedorn, D. J., and Rand, R. E. (1977). *Proc. Am. Phytopathol. Soc.* **4**, 133.

Hagedorn, D. J., and Rand, R. E. (1980). *HortScience* **15**, 208–209.

Hagedorn, D. J., Rand, R. E., and Saad, S. M. (1972). *Plant Dis. Rep.* **56**, 325–327.

Hagedorn, D. J., Walker, J. C., and Rand, R. E. (1974). *HortScience* **9**, 402.

Hanson, C. H. (1972). "Alfalfa Science and Technology." Am. Soc. Agric., Madison, Wisconsin.

Hawn, E. J., and Lebean, J. B. (1962). *Phytopathology* **52**, 266–268.

Helgeson, J. P., Haberlach, G. T., and Upper, C. D. (1976). *Phytopathology* **66**, 91–96.

Horsfall, J. G., and McDonnell, A. D. (1940). *Plant Dis. Rep.* **24**, 34–36.

Hunter, R. E., Brinkerhoff, L. A., and Bird, L. S. (1968). *Phytopathology* **58**, 830–832.

Ingram, D. S. (1977). *In* "Plant Tissue and Cell Culture" (H. E. Street, ed.), pp. 463–500. Blackwell, Oxford.

Ingram, D. S., and Helgeson, J. P. (1980). *In* "Tissue Culture Methods for Plant Pathologists," pp. 223–255. Blackwell, Oxford.

Innes, N. L. (1965). *Exp. Agric.* **1**, 189–191.

Ivanoff, S. S. (1934). *Phytopathology* **24**, 74–76.

Ivanoff, S. S. (1935). *Phytopathology* **25**, 992–1002.

Ivanoff, S. S., and Riker, A. J. (1936). *J. Agric. Res.* **53**, 927–954.

Jones, F. R. (1925). *Phytopathology* **15**, 243–244.

Jones, F. R. (1934). *J. Agric. Res.* **48**, 1085–1098.

Jones, J. P. (1961). *Phytopathology* **51**, 206.

Jones, J. P., and Hartwig, E. E. (1959). *Plant Dis. Rep.* **43,** 946.
Kehr, W. R., Frosheiser, F. I., Wilcoxson, R. D., and Barnes, D. K. (1972). *In* "Alfalfa Science and Technology" (C. H. Hanson, ed.), Ch. 15. Am. Soc. Agronomy, Madison, Wisconsin.
Kelman, A., and Sequeira, L. (1972). *Proc. R. Soc. London Ser. B* **181,** 247–266.
Kennedy, B. W., and Cross, J. E. (1966). *Plant Dis. Rep.* **50,** 560–565.
Kernkamp, M. F., and Hemerick, G. (1952). *Phytopathology* **42,** 13.
Knight, R. L. (1957). *Proc. Int. Plant Protect. Conf., 2nd* pp. 53–59.
Kochler, B. (1955). *Plant Dis. Rep.* **39,** 164–165.
Koike, H. (1965). *Phytopathology* **55,** 317–319.
Koster, R. (1973). *Populier* **10,** 5–7.
Kreitlow, K. W. (1963). *Phytopathology* **53,** 800–803.
Krupka, L. R. (1956). M.S. thesis, University of Delaware.
Lamb, R. C. (1960). *Am. Soc. Hortic. Sci. Proc.* **75,** 85–88.
Layne, R. E. C. (1968). *Can. Agric.* **13,** 28–29.
Layne, R. E. C., and Quamme, H. A. (1975). *In* "Advances in Fruit Breeding" (Janick and Moore, eds.), pp. 38–70. Purdue Univ. Press.
Layne, R. E. C., Bailey, C. H., and Hough, L. F. (1968). *Can. J. Plant Sci.* **48,** 231–243.
Lockwood, J. L., and Williams, L. E. (1957). *Phytopathology* **47,** 83–87.
Lucas, G. B. (1975). "Diseases of Tobacco" 3rd ed. Raleigh, North Carolina.
Martin, J. A. (1948). *Proc. Am. Soc. Hortic. Sci.* **52,** 336–340.
Martin, J. P. (1965). *Int. Soc. Sugar Cane Technol. Proc.* **12,** 1213–1225.
Martin, J. P., and P. E. Robinson. (1961). *In* "Sugarcane Diseases of the World," Vol. I, pp. 78–107. Elseview, Amsterdam.
Moore, E. L., Lucas, E. B., Jones, G. L., and Gwynn, G. R. (1962). *North Carolina Agric. Exp. Sta. Bull.* 419.
Moore, E. L., Kelman, A., Powell, N. T., and Bunn, B. H. (1963). *Tobacco Sci.* **7,** 17–20.
Moore, R. C. (1946). *Proc. Am. Soc. Hortic. Sci.* **47,** 49–57.
Morel, G. (1944). *C.R. Bulg. Acad. Sci.* **218,** 50–52.
Morel, G. (1948). *Ann. Epiphyt.* **14,** 137–234.
Nelson, R. R. (1973). "Breed Crop Plants." Penn State Univ. Press, University Park, Pennsylvania.
Nickell, L. G., and Heinz, D. J. (1973). *In* "Genes, Enzymes and Populations" (A. M. Srb, ed.), pp. 109–128. Plenum, New York.
Nonnecke, I. (1948). *Proc. Meet. West. Can. Soc. Hortic. Sci., 4th* pp. 31–32.
Orton, W. A. (1902). *Proc. Meet. Ga. State Hortic. Soc., 26th* pp. 45–46.
Ou, S. H. (1973). *In* "Breeding Plants for Disease Resistance" (R. R. Nelson, ed.), pp. 101–105. Penn State Univ. Press, University Park, Pennsylvania.
Pearson, L. C., and Elling, L. J. (1960). *Agron. J.* **52,** 291–294.
Pettier, G. L., and Tysdal, H. M. (1934). *Neb. Agric. Exp. Sta. Res. Bull.* **76.**
Rand, F. V., and Cash, L. C. (1921). *J. Agric. Res.* **21,** 263–264.
Reddy, C. S., and Holbert, J. R. (1928). *J. Agric. Res.* **36,** 905–910.
Reimer, F. C. (1925). *Oreg. Agric. Exp. Sta. Bull. 214.*
Reitz, L. P. (1954). *Econ. Bot.* **8,** 251–268.
Sakaguchi, S., Suwa, T., and Murta, N. (1968). *Bull. Natl. Inst. Agric. Sci., Tokyo* **18,** 1–29.
Schuster, M. L. (1955). *Phytopathology* **45,** 519–520.
Sequeira, L. (1979). *Int. Potato Ctr. Rep.* pp. 55–62.
Sequeira, L., and Rowe, P. R. (1969). *Am. Pot. J.* **46,** 451–462.
Shepard, J. F., Bidney, D., and Shakim, E. (1980a). *Science* **60,** 313–316.
Shepard, J. F., Bidney, D., and Shakim, E. (1980b). *Science* **208,** 17–24.

Sherwood, R. T., and Hagedorn, D. J. (1958). *Wis. Agric. Exp. Sta. Bull.* 531.

Sitterly, W. R. (1973). *In* "Breeding for Plant Disease Resistance" (R. R. Nelson, ed.), pp. 297–299. Penn State Univ. Press, University Park, Pennsylvania.

Smith, T. E., and Clayton, E. E. (1948). *Phytopathology* **38,** 227–229.

Sowell, G., Jr. (1960). *Plant Dis. Rep.* **44,** 587–590.

Stevenson, G. C. (1965). "Genetics and Breeding of Sugarcane." Longmans, London.

Stewart, F. C. (1897). *N.Y. Agric. Exp. Sta. Bull.* **130,** 422–439.

Theurer, J. D., and Elling, L. J. (1963). *Crop. Sci.* **3,** 50–53.

Thomas, E., King, P. J., and Potryhus, I. (1979). *Z. Pflazenzuecht.* **82,** 1–30.

Thomas, R. C. (1924). *Ohio Agric. Exp. Sta. Mon. Bull.* **9,** 81–84.

Thompson, S. S., Janick, J., and Williams, E. B. (1962). *Am. Soc. Hortic. Sci. Proc.* **80,** 105–113.

Thurston, H. D., and Lozano, J. C. (1968). *Am. Potato J.* **45,** 51–55.

Tysdal, H. M., and Crandall, B. H. (1948). *J. Am. Soc. Agron.* **40,** 293–306.

Valleau, W. D. (1934). *Plant Dis. Rep.* **18,** 106.

van der Zwet, T., and Oitto, W. A. (1973). *Plant Dis. Rep.* **57,** 20–25.

van der Zwet, T., Oitto, W. A., and Brooks, H. J. (1970). *Plant Dis. Rep.* **54,** 835–839.

Weber, G. F. (1932). *Fla. Agric. Exp. Sta. Bull.* **244,** 6–9.

Weimer, J. L., and Malson, B. A. (1936). *J. Agric. Res.* **52,** 547–555.

Wellhausen, E. J. (1935). *Iowa State Coll. J. Sci.* **9,** 539–547.

White, P. R. (1934). *Plant Physiol.* **9,** 585–600.

Zalewski, J. C., and Sequeira, L. (1973). *Phytopathology* **63,** 942–944.

Chapter **18**

Biological Control of Plant Pathogens with Prokaryotes

ANNE K. VIDAVER

I. INTRODUCTION

Microbial interactions of various types occur both in the laboratory and field. It is always a challenge for microbiologists to determine whether interactions *in vitro* have any bearing on microbial interactions in nature. Plant pathologists are interested in the manipulation of such interactions in efforts to minimize plant diseases caused by bacteria and other microorganisms. Biological control as discussed here will include both experimental and commercial examples. Recent general discussions of biological control involving phytopathogenic bacteria are in Anonymous (1978), Baker (1980), Baker and Cook (1974), and Cook (1977). There are scattered reports of bacteria causing diseases of undesirable plants (Klement and Lovrekovich, 1960; Stewart and Brown,

Phytopathogenic Prokaryotes, Vol. 2

Copyright © 1982 by Academic Press, Inc.
All rights of reproduction in any form reserved.
ISBN 0-12-509002-1

1969; Wilson, 1969); biological control of weeds by plant pathogens is not considered here. Hence this chapter deals solely with the protection of agricultural and horticultural crops by controlling plant pathogens.

II. DEFINITIONS AND TERMS

The deliberate use of one species of organism to control or eliminate another is biological control (Singleton and Sainsbury, 1978). This definition incorporates the concept of management or manipulation of interacting microorganisms (Cook, 1977), and for plant pathologists implies that the pathogen is the direct target, with the ultimate aim of reducing disease. This definition also implies an active form of interaction, rather than a passive one of inherent plant resistance or cultural practices.

Biological control is a variation of antagonism. The mechanisms of antagonism are (1) competition for nutrients, physical, and biological sites, or oxygen (it is not known whether other gases are significant), (2) antibiosis by production of metabolites such as antibiotics, (3) predation or parasitism by other microorganisms, and (4) modification of host resistance (Baker, 1980; Cook, 1977). Such mechanisms can be used to explain the multiple types of interactions that may occur between microorganisms and range from stimulation to inhibition and death (Baker, 1980).

III. CONTROL OF PHYTOPATHOGENIC BACTERIA WITH BACTERIA

The control of the crown gall bacterium *Agrobacterium tumefaciens* (Smith & Townsend) Conn by a strain of its nonpathogenic relative, *A. radiobacter* (Beijerinck & van Delden) Conn strain 84, is the most dramatic and economically successful example of biological control of a bacterial plant pathogen (Kerr, 1980; Moore and Warren, 1979; Vidaver, 1981). The recent reviews on this topic cover the physical conditions, concentrations, recommendations, precautions, and occasional failures of its use. In summary, the recommendations are (1) use high concentration of cells, 10^8–10^9 colony-forming units (CFU)/ml, i.e., a "turbid" suspension, (2) treat seed, bare roots, cuttings, or aerial grafts before presumptive exposure to the crown gall bacterium, since only preventive treatment is effective, (3) dip or spray plant parts with strain 84 (spraying is recommended if plant stock is contaminated with pathogenic fungi) (Moore and Warren, 1979), and (4) keep treated plants away from sunlight and from drying out to protect the live cells. Moore and Warren (1979) emphasize that the use of strain 84 will not stop latent infections, presumably because the pathogen is already in a protected site, nor will use of the bacterium substitute for proper sanitation and nursery management.

The failure of strain 84 to control crown gall in some instances is due at least in part to the prevalence of certain strains of *A. tumefaciens*. Biotype (biovar) 2 strains are most susceptible, but insensitive biotype 1 (or 3) strains are prevalent in some geographic areas; such strains appear associated with certain crops (Moore and Warren, 1979). On the other hand, strain 84 has been apparently successful in the field, even when inoculated strains are resistant to the specific antibiotic it produces, agrocin 84. The success of strain 84 is remarkable in view of its being used in so many different environments; no other strain has been found as effective among over 20,000 tested (Kerr, personal communication; Moore and Warren, 1979). Other antagonists isolated from plant roots, namely, species of the fungi *Penicillium, Aspergillus, Trichoderma*, and the bacterium *Bacillus* were not as effective as strain 84, even though they produced potent inhibitors *in vitro* (Cooksey and Moore, 1980).

Bacteriocin (agrocin) production has been postulated as the mechanism by which strain 84 controls *A. tumefaciens* strains. Based on the evidence to date, the probability is low that the bacteriocin itself accounts for the success of crown gall control, either by its elaboration at the plant surface or in concentrations high enough to be effective. Although use of the bacteriocin itself can prevent crown gall (Moore, cited in Moore and Warren, 1979), transfer of the plasmid coding for bacteriocin from strain 84 to a nonproducer gave less satisfactory control by the bacteriocin-producing transconjugants than did the parent (Ellis *et al.*, 1979). Thus, an additional factor(s) besides bacteriocin production was suggested as being necessary for achieving control. This additional factor may explain why, in some cases, bacteriocin-resistant strains can nevertheless be controlled by strain 84 (Moore and Warren, 1979). Moore further suggests that the host plant also may play a role in whether control is achieved or not (Moore and Warren, 1979).

Erwinia herbicola (Löhnis) Dye has often been associated with antagonism to *E. amylovora* (Burrill) Winslow *et al.*, causal agent of fireblight. *Erwinia herbicola* and other bacteria antagonistic to the bacterium *in vitro* are readily isolated from infected plants (see reviews cited above). Beer (1981) found that a bacteriocin-producing strain of *E. herbicola* was equally as effective as a nonproducing strain in controlling fireblight in apple (*Malus sylvestris* Mill.) orchards. Both strains at 10^8

CFU/ml were as effective as 100 μg/ml streptomycin in one field trial and nearly as effective in another. In addition, Beer (1981) found that a nonproducing mutant of a producing *E. herbicola* strain was as effective as streptomycin. Such a strain thus shows promise in control despite the lack of correlation with bacteriocin production *in vitro;* however, as bacteriocin detection is dependent on nutrient and physical conditions, a biologically active compound(s) could be produced *in planta* which is not detected *in vitro*.

Erwinia herbicola has also been implicated in control of citrus (*Citrus* spp.) blight caused by *Xanthomonas campestris* pv. *citri* (Hasse) Dye (Goto *et al.*, 1979). High temperature (30°C) enabled *E. herbicola* to inhibit the growth of *X. c.* pv. *citri in vitro*, but intercellular fluid collected from citrus in summer suppressed *E. herbicola* growth. This observation coincided with severe disease expression of citrus blight, whereas intercellular fluid collected in the fall or early spring was not inhibitory to *E. herbicola*. Injection or spray applications of *E. herbicola* to external parts of plants have not been evaluated for biocontrol activity.

In the studies with *E. herbicola*, none of the investigators has used the same strain, making it difficult to compare evaluations of control effectiveness. Such comparisons may not be appropriate, however, because different *E. herbicola* biotypes may be associated with different plant species. This needs to be determined.

It is not always possible to correlate *in vitro* with *in planta* antagonism. For example, all the phylloplane bacteria effective in disease suppression were not antagonistic to *Xanthomonas campestris* pv. *malvacearum* (Smith) Dye *in vitro* on a peptone–sucrose medium (Verma *et al.*, 1978). They showed that a Gram-negative bacterium identified as a *Flavobacterium* sp. (data not presented) was the most effective of the bacteria tested in suppressing disease, but only when inoculated 8 hr before challenge with strains of *X. c.* pv. *malvacearum*. Simultaneous inoculations or preinoculation at 24 or 48 hr were not effective. Equal concentrations of about 10^7 CFU/spot of both pathogen and antagonists were used in leaf infiltration assays. Other studies (see above) have shown that high antagonist to pathogen ratios provide the most effective biological control. It is unclear whether an inhibitory substance is produced by the protecting bacteria, whether the bacteria induce the host plant to produce a protection factor, or if attachment or competition for sites limits disease development.

Nonspecific control of *Pseudomonas tolaasii* Paine, causal agent of brown blotch of the cultivated mushroom, *Agaricus bisporus* Lange (Imbach), can be achieved commercially by using a mixture of at least 10 : 1 of a strain of either *P. cepacia* (ex Burkholder) nom. rev. Palleroni &

Holmes (syn. *P. multivorans* Stanier *et al.*), *P. fluorescens* Migula, or *Enterobacter aerogenes* Hormaeche & Edwards to the pathogen (Nair and Fahy, 1976). As in the above case, no antibiosis was observed *in vitro*.

Actinomycetes are well known as producers of antibiotics effective against both bacteria and fungi, but their biological control potential against bacterial plant pathogens has not been explored. An actinomycete plant pathogen, the so-called *Streptomyces scabies* (Thaxter) Waksman & Henrici (species *incertae sedis*), causal agent of common potato (*Solanum tuberosum* L.) scab, can be controlled in some environments either by a strain of *Bacillus subtilis* (Ehrenburg) Conn or unidentified antagonists (see Baker, 1980).

Competition between or among pathogenic strains inoculated simultaneously or in some sequence can lead to a variety of effects that range from no effect on disease development, but with predominance of one strain over another (Togashi, 1979) to suppression of disease symptoms (Bantarri and Zeyen, 1979; Marchoux and Giannotti, 1971). The mechanism of such competition might be bacteriocins (Smidt and Vidaver, 1981) or other antimetabolites, differences in growth rate, or surface properties. From a practical point of view, such interactions are not useful for biological control efforts, but should be of interest to plant breeders who use a mixture of strains in inocula.

Protection from pathogens can be achieved with the use of mild or avirulent strains of both walled and wall-less bacteria. Either can suppress multiplication of virulent strains inoculated later (Lawson and Smith, 1981; Sequeira and Hill, 1974). Such cross-protection is of interest in efforts to understand the mechanism of induced resistance. Because of the requirement of prior inoculation, it is of little value in biological control, with the possible exception of high value ornamental plants. There is, however, the prospect of isolating a specific compound or cell component which might be used in protection against some diseases. The cost and manner of production, application, concentration, and stability of such compounds may be limiting factors in use.

IV. CONTROL OF PHYTOPATHOGENIC FUNGI WITH BACTERIA

Among Gram-positive bacteria, streptomyces have shown promise in reducing populations of fungi both *in vitro* and in the field (Baker and Cook, 1974; Dixit and Gupta, 1980; Turhan, 1981). Similarly, there are several reports of *Bacillus* species (Doherty and Preece, 1978; Fravel and Spurr, 1974), particularly *B. subtilis* (Baker and Cook, 1974), controlling soil-borne or seed-associated fungi (Thirumalachar and O'Brien, 1977), as well as pathogens of aerial parts (Swinburne, 1978). However, *B. subtilis* also may be deleterious, at least at high temperatures (30°C or above), as it is implicated in soybean [*Glycine max* (L.) Merr.] seed decay, with attendant poor germination and stand inhibition (Schiller *et al.*, 1977).

Gram-negative bacteria, particularly pseudomonads, are implicated in control of several soil-associated pathogens or quasipathogens. For example, pseudomonads (otherwise unidentified) can be isolated from potato periderm or roots and inoculated on seeds to suppress pathogens and increase growth (Kloepper *et al.*, 1980). These investigators found that potato, sugar beet (*Beta vulgaris* L.), and radish (*Raphanus sativus* L.) inoculation increased growth which was correlated with siderophore production. The production of such iron-chelating compounds apparently is absent or weak in the pathogens tested, but present in the controlling bacteria. It is not clear whether the inhibited microorganisms are pathogens per se or opportunists that cause weakened root growth associated with their external occurrence (see also Suslow, Vol. 1, Chapter 8).

Another *Pseudomonas, P. fluorescens* Migula, has been reported effective in suppression of *Pythium ultimum* Trow induced damping-off of cotton (*Gossypium hirsutum* L.) seedlings (Howell and Stipanovic, 1980). Seedling survival was markedly increased by use of the bacterium alone or with an antibiotic it produces, pyoluteorin, suggesting that this may be its mechanism of action.

Pseudomonads are the most effective bacteria in biological control of take-all of wheat (*Triticum aestivum* L.), caused by *Gaeumannomyces graminis* (Sacc.) Von Arx & Olivier var. *tritici* Walker. Some of the pseudomonad strains effective in biological control produced a hypersensitive reaction in tobacco (*Nicotiana tabacum* L.); this property normally is associated with plant pathogenic pseudomonads (Weller and Cook, 1981), thus raising the question of their relationship to these bacteria. Whether other strains of effective pseudomonads, isolated elsewhere, also produce such a reaction, is not known (Smiley, 1979; Sivasithamparam *et al.*, 1979). In greenhouse experiments, Vrany *et al.* (1981) found strain K11 of *P. putida* (Trevisan) Migula more effective against take-all than other *P. putida* strains or other *Pseudomonas* or *Agrobacterium* strains (otherwise unidentified). However, some of these bacteria, particularly pseudomonads, also can stimulate colonization of the rhizosphere with *G. graminis* (see Stanek, 1979). *Bacillus mycoides* (Flügge) has also been shown effective against this fungus (Campbell and Faull, 1979). In the majority of reports of bacteria antagonistic to fungi, (e.g., Giha, 1976) the bacteria are so poorly identified that evaluation of effectiveness related to other studies is not possible. Thus, this complex problem clearly needs more study in the identification and manipulation of effective bacteria.

V. PHYTOPATHOGENIC BACTERIA AS CONTROL AGENTS

Although phytopathogenic bacteria have shown promise for biological control against some fungi, it is difficult to justify such use. No report shows inactivation of pathogenic properties and the concentrations applied are so high that dissemination to nontarget plants is likely. There is also the possibility of genetic transfer of pathogenic determinants to saprophytes. Much needs to be learned about the genetics of effective control strains so that they can be rendered not only avirulent, but also resistant to transfer of pathogenic determinants from pathogenic strains.

The use of plant pathogenic bacteria in biological control is primarily in early stages of investigation. In greenhouse tests, *Pseudomonas syringae* pv. *phaseolicola* (Burkholder) Young *et al.*, causal agent of halo blight of bean (*Phaseolus vulgaris* L.), can protect a nonhost plant, pea *Pisum sativum* L., against the fungus *Mycosphaerella pinodes* (Berk & Blox) Vest. (Platero Sanz and Fuchs, 1980) without evidence of increased pisatin production. This suggested that this phytoalexin was not involved in this phenomenon. There are preliminary reports of *P. marginata* (McCulloch) Stapp and *P. cichorii* (Swingle) Stapp antagonistic to rusts of iris (*Iris* spp.) and wheat, respectively (Durgapal and Trivedi, 1977), while *Xanthomonas campestris* pv. *translucens* (Jones *et al.*) Dye and *P. cepacia* have been reported antagonistic to *Septoria nodorum* Berk., the causal agent of glume blotch of wheat (Jones and Roane, 1981). *Pseudomonas cepacia* also controlled damping-off of onion (*Allium cepa* L.) seedlings by *Fusarium oxysporum* f. sp. *cepae* (Hanz) Snyd. & Hans. when applied to onion seed prior to planting (Kawamoto and Lorbeer, 1976) and has been implicated in control of fungal brown spot of tobacco (Spurr, 1978, 1981). In the former study, control in greenhouse tests correlated with production of an inhibitor *in vitro*. Not all of the *P. cepacia* strains in these studies were onion pathogens, but the marked similarity of biotypes (Gonzalez and Vidaver, 1979) raises the question of potential genetic transfer of pathogenic properties.

The potential use of *P. syringae* pv. *syringae* van Hall in Dutch elm (*Ulmus americana* L.) disease control is the most interesting and controversial use of a bacterial plant pathogen to control a fungal pathogen. In a patent claim (Strobel, 1981), a strain of *P. s.* pv. *syringae,* DC27+(NRRLB-12050) is described as being used both prophylactically and therapeutically in the control of Dutch elm disease in the field. The mechanism is believed to be due to a high molecular weight antibiotic, a 14 amino acid polypeptide clearly differentiable from syringomycin. Interestingly, the claim is made that injection of purified antibiotic is effective also, but that repeated application is required, compared to a single injection with 10^8 to 10^{11} total cells. The *P. s.* pv. *syringae* lives in the outer bark for at least one season and can be reisolated from it. Since 22 trees were treated on different dates and in different locations, evaluation of effectiveness is difficult to assess, aside from the relatively short treatment time of 2 years. Interestingly, the patent also claims to include the use of any other *P. s.* pv. *syringae* that could produce this unidentified antibiotic, as well as any genetically engineered bacterium that might produce it.

Unfortunately, except for the patent, there are as yet only preliminary publications documenting the use of *P. s.* pv. *syringae* strains or their antibiotics (Myers and Strobel, 1981; Strobel and Myers, 1981) so that it is difficult to assess the validity of the claims made in Dutch elm disease control. More importantly, there is no mention in the patent or elsewhere that *P. s.* pv. *syringae* is a pathogen. At least one strain used apparently produces syringomycin in addition to its unique antibiotic. To date, all syringomycin-producing *P. s.* pv. *syringae* have been pathogens. Thus, it is reasonable to question the use of a probable pathogen in this case. Although the bacterium is contained within a tree, dissemination by insects or breaking branches could occur. Either inactivation of its pathogenic potential or transfer of its antifungal activity to a nonpathogen would be prudent.

VI. BACTERIOPHAGES AND PARASITIC BACTERIA

Bacterial viruses are reasonably specific and relatively easy to propagate and produce. All efforts to use bacterial viruses as biological control agents have been disappointing since they have only delayed symptom expression or reduced the amount of infection. Any success in control has required preventive treatment (see Vidaver, 1976). However, for *E. amylovora*, a bacteriophage has been isolated that codes for a polysaccharide depolymerizing enzyme. This enzyme strips the capsule of virulent strains *in vitro* and resistant colonies are avirulent. The majority of tested *E. amylovora* strains were sensitive to this virus (Ritchie and Klos,

1979). Thus, even if the virus itself is not particularly effective, the depolymerizing enzyme has the potential of being used alone.

Wild-type strains of the minute bacterium *Bdellobvibrio bacteriovorus* Stolp & Starr and associated species are intracellular parasites of other bacteria (Stolp, 1973). The host range of these bacteria is often very broad, however, and this restricts their potential as a control agent. For example, a strain isolated for *X. campestris* pv. *oryzae* (Ishiyama) Dye was equally effective *in vitro* against a strain of *E. carotovora* (Jones) Bergey *et al.* (Uematsu and Ohata, 1979). Other strains were discovered parasitic for many other phytopathogenic strains of *Pseudomonas, Xanthomonas, Erwinia,* and *Agrobacterium* (Scherff, 1973; Stolp, 1973). Further, any limitation on the host bacterium affects growth of the parasite, parasitic strains do not survive well without a host and reproduction is slow with relatively few progeny being produced (Stolp, 1973) compared to the other class of intracellular parasites, bacterial viruses. Although these cases are of interest, in view of the above considerations, their practical application appears quite limited.

VII. PROSPECTS FOR BIOLOGICAL CONTROL AND RECOMMENDATIONS

Bacteria may be present in apparently healthy internal tissues of plants (e.g., Matta, 1971), probably gaining entry through minute injuries or natural openings. Thus, Baker and Cook (1974) suggest the possibility of dipping the base of cuttings or cut seed pieces into suspensions of bacteria found antagonistic to vascular pathogens. Such a suggestion may alleviate problems with bacterial diseases of potatoes, for example, in which cut seed pieces are often used in planting.

The probability of successful biological control may be increased with a mixture of compatible antagonists, but for bacteria, the published work is so fragmentary (e.g., Taylor and Guy, 1981) that it is only possible to suggest the usefulness of such a method. As computer use increases and knowledge accumulates, the interactions of microorganisms should be easier to predict and hence, to control.

Biological control agents should have certain desirable attributes, discussed previously (Vidaver, 1976). These are reasonable persistence, safety, aesthetic acceptability, cost effectiveness, predictable control, and a reasonably broad killing spectrum among target strains. In addition, they should be easy to produce, store, and apply.

While it is improbable that biological control will be the sole method of controlling pathogens within this century, the rapidly developing knowledge in this area and the recognized need for targeting control efforts will increase its use. The need for biological control will be intensified with changes in availability of other control agents, changes in microbial problems associated with plant breeding (including new methods of genetic engineering), as well as changes in cultivation practices. The difficulty of the task (see Schroth and Hancock, 1981) must be surmounted if the world is to have food and fiber at reasonable cost and without further deterioration of the environment.

References

Anonymous. (1978). "Biological Agents for Pest Control, Status and Prospects." USDA Special Report, Washington, D.C.

Baker, K. F. (1980). *In* "Contemporary Microbial Ecology" (D. C. Elwood, M. J. Lathan, J. N. Hedger, J. M. Lynch, and J. H. Slater, eds.), pp. 327–347. Academic Press, New York.

Baker, K. F., and Cook, R. J. (1974). "Biological Control of Plant Pathogens." Freeman, San Francisco, California.

Banttari, E. E., and Zeyen, R. J. (1979). *In* "Leafhopper Vectors and Plant Disease Agents" (K. Maramorosch and K. F. Harris, eds.), pp. 327–348. Academic Press, New York.

Beer, S. V. (1981). *Acta Hortic.* **117,** 123.

Campbell, R., and Faull, J. L. (1979). *In* "Soil-borne Plant Pathogens" (B. Schippers and W. Gams, eds.), pp. 603–610. Academic Press, New York.

Cook, R. J. (1977). *In* "Plant Disease—An Advanced Treatise" (J. G. Horsfall and E. B. Cowling, eds.), Vol. 1, pp. 145–166. Academic Press, New York.

Cooksey, D. A., and Moore, L. W. (1980). *Phytopathology* **70,** 506–509.

Dixit, R. B., and Gupta, J. S. (1980). *Acta Bot. Indica* **8,** 190–192.

Doherty, M. S., and Preece, T. F. (1978). *Physiol. Plant. Pathol.* **12,** 123–132.

Durgapal, J. C., and Trivedi, B. M. (1977). *Curr. Sci.* **46,** 200.

Ellis, J. G., Kerr, A., Van Montagu, M., and Schell, J. (1979). *Physiol. Plant. Pathol.* **15,** 311–319.

Fravel, D. R., and Spurr, H. W., Jr., (1977). *Phytopathology* **67,** 930–932.

Freeman, T. C. (1977). *Aquat. Bot.* **3,** 175–184.

Giha, O. H. (1976). *Plant Dis. Rep.* **60,** 985–987.

Gonzalez, C. F., and Vidaver, A. K. (1979). *J. Gen. Microbiol.* **110,** 161–170.

Goto, M., Tadauchi, Y., and Okabe, N. (1979). *Ann. Phytopathol. Soc. Jpn.* **45,** 618–624.

Howell, C. R., and Stipanovic, R. D. (1980). *Phytopathology* **70,** 712–715.

Jones, J. B., and Roane, C. W. (1981). *Phytopathology* **71,** 229.

Kawamoto, S. O., and Lorbeer, J. W. (1976). *Plant Dis. Rep.* **60,** 189–191.

Kerr, A. (1980). *Plant Dis.* **64,** 24–30.

Klement, Z., and Lovrekovich, L. (1960). *Acta Microbiol.* **7,** 113–119.

Kloepper, J. W., Loeng, J., Teintze, M., and Schroth, M. N. (1980). *Nature (London)* **286,** 885–886.

Lawson, R. H., and Smith, F. F. (1981). *Phytopathology* **71,** 234.

Marchoux, G., and Giannotti, J. (1971). *Physiol. Veg.* **9,** 595–610.

Matta, A. (1971). *Annu. Rev. Phytopathol.* **9,** 387–410.

Moore, L. W., and Warren, G. (1979). *Annu. Rev. Phytopathol.* **17,** 163–179.

Myers, D. R., and Strobel, G. A. (1981). *Phytopathology* **71,** 1006.

Nair, N. G., and Fahy, P. C. (1976). *Aust. J. Agric. Res.* **27,** 415–422.

Platero Sanz, M., and Fuchs, A. (1980). *Neth J. Plant Pathol.* **86,** 181–190.

Ritchie, D. R., and Klos, E. J. (1979). *Phytopathology* **69,** 1078–1083.

Scherf, R. H. (1973). *Phytopathology* **63,** 400–402.

Schiller, C. T., Ellis, M. A., Tenne, F. D., and Sinclair, J. B. (1977). *Plant Dis. Rep.* **61,** 213–316.

Schroth, M. N., and Hancock, J. G. (1981). *Annu. Rev. Microbiol.* **35,** 453–476.

Sequeira, L., and Hill, L. M. (1974). *Physiol. Plant Pathol.* **4,** 447–455.

Singleton, P., and Sainsbury, D. (1978). "Dictionary of Microbiology." Wiley, New York.

Sivasithamparam, K., Parker, C. A., and Edwards, C. S. (1979). *Soil Biol. Biochem.* **11,** 161–165.

Smidt, M., and Vidaver, A. K. (1981). *Phytopathology* **71,** 904.

Smiley, R. W. (1979). *Soil Biol. Biochem.* **11,** 371–376.

Spurr, H. W., Jr. (1978). *Phytopathol. News* **12,** 74.

Spurr, H. W., Jr. (1981). *Phytopathology* **71,** 905.

Stanek, M. (1979). *In* "Soil-borne Plant Pathogens" (B. Schippers and W. Gams, eds.), pp. 247–252. Academic Press, New York.

Stewart, J. R., and Brown, J. M. (1969). *Science* **164,** 1523.

Stolp, H. (1973). *Annu. Rev. Phytopathol.* **11,** 52–76.

Strobel, G. (1981). "Method for Treating Dutch Elm Disease." U.S. Patent No. 4, 277, 462.

Strobel, G. A., and Myers, D. R. (1981). *Phytopathology* **71,** 1007.

Swinburne, T. R. (1978). *Ann. Appl. Biol.* **89,** 94–96.

Taylor, J. B., and Guy, E. M. (1981). *New Phytol.* **87,** 729–732.

Thirumalachar, M. J., and O'Brien, M. J. (1977). *Plant Dis. Rep.* **61,** 543–545.

Togashi, J. (1979). *Ann. Phytopathol. Soc. Jpn.* **45,** 591–595.

Turhan, G. (1981). *Z. Pflanzenkr. Pflanzenschutz* **88,** 422–434.

Uematsu, T., and Ohata, K. (1979). *Ann. Phytopathol. Soc. Jpn.* **45,** 147–155.

Verma, J. P., Chowdhury, H. D., and Singh, R. P. (1978). *Proc. Int. Conf. Plant Pathog. Bact., 4th, Angers* pp. 795–802.

Vidaver, A. K. (1976). *Annu. Rev. Phytopathol.* **14,** 451–465.

Vidaver, A. K. (1981). *In* "Handbook Series in Agriculture, Section D. Pest Management" (D. Pimentel, ed.), pp. 329–334. CRC Press, Cleveland, Ohio.

Vrany, J., Vancura, V., and Stanek, M. (1981). *Folia Microbiol.* **26,** 45–51.

Weller, D. M., and Cook, R. J. (1981). *Phytopathology* **71,** 262.

Wilson, C. L. (1969). *Annu. Rev. Phytopathol.* **7,** 411–434.

Zettler, F. W., and Freeman, T. C. (1972). *Annu. Rev. Phytopathol.* **10,** 455–470.

Chapter 19

Chemical Control of Phytopathogenic Prokaryotes

A. L. JONES

I. INTRODUCTION

For farmers and plant pathologists, controlling bacterial incited diseases of fruit, vegetable, and field crops and of ornamental plants has

Phytopathogenic Prokaryotes, Vol. 2

Copyright © 1982 by Academic Press, Inc.
All rights of reproduction in any form reserved.
ISBN 0-12-509002-1

been a difficult proposition. Compared to fungicides, few bactericides have been developed for the control of bacterial incited diseases of plants, and no new compounds have been developed since the era of the antibiotics. Furthermore, our understanding of the epidemiology of many bacterial diseases is incomplete, making it difficult to properly time chemical control treatments. However, some bacterial diseases are controlled better today than they were before bactericides were developed. Chemical control of diseases caused by mycoplasmal- and rickettsial-like organisms is in its infancy. Following the discovery of mycoplasma as plant disease agents by Doi *et al.* (1969), there has been a resurgence in research on antibiotics, particularly the tetracyclines. In this chapter, I review the development of chemical control strategies for phytopathogenic prokaryotes and discuss possible future directions for chemical control research.

II. CHEMICALS USED FOR CONTROL

Two groups of compounds, coppers and antibiotics, are used most in agriculture to control diseases caused by phytopathogenic prokaryotes.

A. Copper Compounds

The value of copper sulfate as a fungicide dates back to the observation by Millardet in 1882 that Bordeaux mixture controlled downy mildew of grape. Bordeaux mixture was soon adapted for the control of fungal pathogens on fruit and vegetable crops, and led to observations that bacterial incited diseases caused less problems in fields where Bordeaux mixture had been applied. In the late 1920s and early 1930s, Bordeaux mixture was tested extensively for the control of fire blight during the bloom period (van der Zwet and Keil, 1979).

The demonstration that Bordeaux mixture helped to control bacterial incited diseases led to the testing of numerous other copper-containing compounds. Today, both inorganic and organic copper compounds are used in the control of a wide range of bacterial incited diseases. Although these compounds, commonly known as "fixed coppers," are less phytotoxic than Bordeaux mixture, phytotoxicity continues to limit their use. Copper ions replace cofactors of vital bacterial enzymes or complex disruptively with carbohydrates and proteins.

B. Antibiotics

1. *Uses*

Streptomycin and oxytetracycline are the only antibiotics used to control plant diseases used by prokaryotes. The principal usage of streptomycin is for control of fire blight on apple (*Malus sylvestris* Mill.) and pears (*Pyrus communis* L.) caused by *Erwinia amylovora* (Burrill) Winslow *et al.* It is also used in some states under special local need registrations for the control of a few other bacterial incited diseases of local importance.

Commercial use of oxytetracycline has increased during the past decade following its experimental use for the remission of symptoms from diseases of suspected mycoplasma etiology. Currently, oxytetracycline is used in the control of lethal yellowing of coconut (*Cocus nucifera* L.) and Pritchardia (*Pritchardia* spp.) palms, pear decline, and peach X-disease. Oxytetracycline is also used in several peach [*Prunus persica* (L.) Batsch.]-growing states for the control of bacterial spot, caused by *Xanthomonas campestris* pv. *pruni* (Smith) Dye, and in California for the control of fire blight.

2. *Mechanisms of Action*

The mechanisms of action of streptomycin and tetracyclines, including oxytetracycline, in phytopathogenic prokaryotes are probably similar to those described for other bacteria and involve inhibition of bacterial protein synthesis.

a. Streptomycin. Despite much research, the exact mechanism of inhibition of streptomycin and other aminoglycoside antibiotics remains in question. The action of streptomycin is dependent on its ability to bind a particular protein or proteins of the 30 S ribosomal subunit. This probably causes protein conformational changes. On polyribosomes, polypeptide chain elongation is inhibited and free ribosomes are prevented from initiating the translational complex. How either process causes rapid death upon exposure of bacterial cells to streptomycin is unclear (Wallace *et al.*, 1979).

b. Tetracycline. Tetracyclines also inhibit bacterial protein synthesis, bind to the 30 S ribosomal subunits, and inhibit polypeptide chain elongation. However, the mechanism is different since tetracyclines block aminoacyl-tRNA binding to the subunit (Kaji and Ryoji, 1979).

C. Others

Many reports can be found in the literature of tests with miscellaneous compounds for the control of phytopathogenic prokaryotes. Only a few of these will be mentioned here.

1. *Disinfesting Agents*

Disinfestation of tools with alcohol (ethanol or isopropanol, 70%) or sodium hypochlorite (liquid bleach, 0.5%) is effective in preventing the spread of fire blight on apple or pear through pruning wounds. Hypochlorite is also useful for disinfecting potato (*Solanum tuberosum* L.) seed piece cutters to prevent bacterial soft rot, caused by *Erwinia carotovora* subsp. *carotovora* (Jones) Bergey *et al.* and preparing cuttings of ornamental plants to prevent spread of crown gall [caused by *Agrobacterium tumefaciens* (Smith and Townsend) Conn.], and has been used in water used for fluming potatoes and washing tomatoes (*Lycopersicon esculentum* Mill).

2. *Other Fungicides*

Some metal-containing fungicides other than fixed coppers have shown sporatic antibacterial activity, but none approach copper or the antibiotics in effectiveness. Zinc sulfate and lime was used to control bacterial spot of peach until its use was discontinued in the 1960s. The zinc-containing fungicide zineb and the mercury-containing fungicide Puratized Agricultural Spray seemed to have antibacterial activity (Thomas and Henderson, 1952), but control with these compounds was too erratic to be of practical significance. Zinc and mercury, like copper, are generalized biocides and have several possible and probably coordinated modes of action against bacteria.

Captan is another fungicide that is considered to have antibacterial activity, although here again data are conflicting. Generally, captan is either not effective or too weak to give a practical level of control for most bacterial diseases. When captan is mixed with dodine and applied in protective spray programs, the mixture reduces the incidence of bacterial spot on peach fruits (Diener and Carlton, 1960). Dodine appears to contribute most of the control activity in this mixture (Daines, 1960). However, bacterial spot control with this mixture is inferior to control with oxytetracycline (Powell, 1967).

3. *Fumigants*

For soil-borne pathogens such as those causing Granville wilt of tobacco (*Nicotiana tobaccum* L.) caused by *Pseudomonas solanacearaum*

(Smith) Smith or crown gall, fumigation of soil with methyl bromide-chloropicin may be effective. Again, these bromine- and chlorine-containing compounds are general biocides, and act as alkylating agents. However, soil fumigation and other types of chemical soil treatments must be approached with caution because certain treatments cause an increase in the incidence of disease, especially crown gall (Deep and Young, 1965; Deep *et al.*, 1968).

4. *Insecticides*

Several diseases incited by bacteria and by mycoplasma- and rickettsial-like organisms are disseminated by insect vectors. Control of these diseases is often based on control of the vector rather than direct control of the pathogen. An example is Stewart's wilt of corn (*Zea mays* L.) caused by *Erwinia stewartii* (Smith) Dye. Its control is based on using the insecticide carbaryl to control the flea beetles (*Chaetocnema pulicaria* Melsh.) that carry the pathogen from plant to plant. Another example is the reduction in spread of Pierce's disease on moderately susceptible grape varieties with dilute sprays of dimethoate timed to reduce populations of the vector, *Graphocephala atropunctata* (Signoret) (Purcell, 1979).

5. *Acidic Sprays*

In a novel approach to the control of phytopathogenic prokaryotes, Sands and McIntyre (1977a,b) used organic acid sprays to reduce epiphytic bacterial populations by lowering the pH on leaf surfaces of host plants. In greenhouse trials, populations of *E. amylovora* developed slower on pear leaves sprayed with citrate or tartrate then on unsprayed leaves, and lesions from *Pseudomonas syringae* pv. *syringae* van Hall on leaves of cowpea [*Vigna sinensis* (Torner) Savi] were reduced 93% by tartrate sprays. In the field, populations of *E. amylovora* were reduced by tartrate sprays and blossom blight on pear caused by *P. s.* pv. *syringae* was reduced by streptomycin or tartaric acid sprays. These results suggest pesticides that lower the pH of plant surfaces may be beneficial, particularly if the pH affects are not phytotoxic and acidity is maintained during periods of rainfall.

III. USE OF CHEMICALS TO REDUCE INOCULUM

Several application methods have been developed for treating plants to control diseases caused by phytopathogenic prokaryotes. Spray treatments are the most widely used, but seed treatment and injection treatments are also important. Generally, spray treatments are protective, being applied before infection occurs; seed and injection treatments are eradicative, being applied to reduce or eliminate pathogens located on and in plant tissues.

A. Seed Treatments

Infected seed are a significant source of primary infection for a number of bacterial incited diseases of vegetable and field crops. Use of disease-free seed is the best method of control, but the supply of such seed is not always adequate to meet the demand. Even when supplies are sufficient, there is a chance the seed has low but sometimes significant levels of infection. Therefore, there is interest in seed treatment methods for eliminating infected seed from seed lots with low levels of infection and as a precautionary measure for seeds considered to be disease-free.

Hot water treatments or treatments with mercurial compounds have been used to eradicate bacterial pathogens from seeds. Although hot water treatments are effective, they frequently reduce seed germination and seedling vigor. Treatment with compounds containing mercury have been banned by regulatory agencies in most countries and were often of doubtful value for controlling bacterial pathogens. There has been considerable interest in seed treatments with antibiotics to replace hot water and mercury treatment methods.

For seed treatments with antibiotics to be effective, they must be applied as a solution or slurry, not as a dry powder. For example, pelleting French bean (*Phaseolus vulgaris* L.) seed with streptomycin failed to control seed-borne *P. syringae* pv. *phaseolicola* (Burkholder) Young *et al.*, while soaking the seeds in a streptomycin sulfate solution was effective (Ralph, 1976). Streptomycin dust applied to pea (*Pisum sativum* L.) seeds failed to prevent primary infection of bacterial blight, caused by *P. syringae* pv. *pisi* (Sackett) Young *et al.* However, slurry treatments with streptomycin sulfate were effective and were less toxic than soaking the seed in streptomycin sulfate (Taylor and Dye, 1975). Slurries of streptomycin or kasugamycin were more effective and less phototoxic than soak or dust treatments to bean to control *P. s.* pv. *phaseolicola* (Taylor and Dudley, 1977). A soak in aureomycin, terramycin, or streptomycin eradicated *Xanthomonas campestris* pv. *campestris* (Pammel) Dowson from *Brassica* seed, but the treatments were phytotoxic. However, eradication of *X. c.* pv. *campestris* without damage to seeds was obtained when antibiotic soaks were followed by a 30-min soak in sodium hypochlorite (Humaydan *et al.*, 1980). This treatment was also compatible with a thiram soak for control of *Phoma lingam* (Tode ex Fr.) Desm.

Although seed treatments are limited primarily to situations where it is possible to eradicate bacteria borne within the seed, they can also be used to remove external contamination on seed free of internal bacteria. Currently, the Michigan Department of Agriculture tests about 1400 samples of dry edible bean seed annually for internal phytobacteria (Young, personal communication). Seed from lots without detectable internal infection can be sold as certified seed provided they are treated with streptomycin to kill any surface-borne bacterial pathogens.

B. Injection Treatments

Shortly after the initial report implicating mycoplasma-like organisms (MLO) as the probable causal agent for yellows diseases in plants, electron microscopic examinations and chemotherapy treatments were undertaken to provide additional evidence for an MLO etiology for a large number of plant diseases with unknown etiology. Recovery of trees with yellows type diseases was dramatic following transfusion of tetracycline compounds into the trunk. Because diseased trees were costly to remove and took years to replace, research efforts were expanded to develop injection treatments for use on a commercial basis. As a direct result of extensive research by several researchers, oxytetracycline–HCl was registered and is presently used for remission of symptoms of coconut lethal yellowing, pear decline, and X-disease.

Methods for injecting oxytetracycline into trees include infusion and pressure. Experimental applications to several tree species were made by gravity infusion of 1 to 4.7 liters per tree of the injection fluid (McCoy, 1972; Nyland and Moller, 1973; Rosenberger and Jones, 1977). To speed up injection, Sands and Walton (1975) suggested the use of small volumes (100 mg a.i. in 10 ml) of concentrated antibiotic solutions. This procedure caused unacceptable levels of trunk damage in peach trees (Allen and Davidson, 1978; Pearson and Sands, 1978; Rosenberger and Jones, 1977). However, infusion of pear trees with pipets was safe provided the concentration of the antibiotic solution was not too high (Lacy *et al.*, 1980). High pressure injection (14–18 kg/cm^2) was developed in California for the rapid injection of pear trees (Reil and Beutel, 1976). Although high pressure injections were effective for X-disease remission in peach, uptake of the solution was much slower than that reported for pear (Jones and Rosenberger, 1978).

On pear and peach, injection treatments were made in autumn to avoid detectable antibiotic residues in fruit. This timing was fortuitous because severe phytotoxicity to foliage noted with treatments made earlier in the season was not a problem (Rosenberger and Jones, 1977). However, injections made at or after leaf fall in late autumn were phytotoxic to foliage the next spring. Based on residue data from leaves, Rosenberger and Jones (1977) concluded that antibiotic injected in late autumn was stored at high levels in trees until spring. When injections are made very late in the growing season, little antibiotic enters the peach leaves before they fall to the ground. However, Lacy *et al.* (1980) detected tetracycline-like activity in pear leaves that abscised naturally. The trees were injected several weeks before leaf fall. Although late season injection may be desirable as a way of preventing antibiotic from entering orchard soils via fallen leaves, additional research is needed on procedures, such as lower rates of injection, to prevent phytotoxic effects the following spring.

Injection treatments also control other phytopathogenic prokaryotes in addition to mycoplasma. Copper sulfate injected into trunks of Jonathan apple trees 1–2 weeks before bud break reduced fire blight (Bushong *et al.*, 1964). Terramycin injected into trunks of peach trees under field and greenhouse conditions significantly reduced bacterial spot caused by *X. c.* pv. *pruni* (Dunegan *et al.*, 1953; Keil and Civerolo, 1979; Sands and Walton, 1975). Because trees injected with oxytetracycline when dormant have significant quantities of antibiotic in their leaves for a few weeks after growth starts, Keil and Civerolo (1979) suggested control takes place early in the season by preventing leaf infection. Injection treatments may also reduce overwintering of bacteria in twigs as suggested by Sands and Walton (1975). Injection of antibiotics for the control of bacterial canker of stone fruits, fire blight, and of other bacterial diseases of deciduous fruit crops should be attempted because it may indicate whether fall and/or early spring control measures are of value in the control of these important diseases.

C. Dormant Sprays to Perennial Crops

Growers of deciduous tree fruits often apply a late autumn or early season dormant spray application of copper compound to reduce the initial inoculum and to slow the rate of disease progress later in the season. For example, Bordeaux mixture or a fixed copper is applied at green tip on pear and apple to control fire blight, at early bud break on peach to control bacterial spot, and at leaf fall on cherries (*Prunus avium* L. and *P. cerasus* L.) to control bacterial canker. Although these recommendations persist, evidence is lacking that dormant sprays decrease the rate of disease progress compared to the rate without dormant sprays. Today, few growers apply them because modern orchard sprayers are not designed to apply copper compounds in dilute sprays. Moreover, copper compounds cause premature leaf fall unless an oil compound is added to reduce the problem (Allen and Dirks, 1979; Crosse and Bennett, 1957).

D. Spray Treatments during the Growing Season

Streptomycin, oxytetracycline, and copper compounds have been tested extensively as spray treatments for the control of bacterial incited diseases during the growing season. The results of these trials have been variable and are hard to interpret because the conditions of inoculum and climate under which the trials were conducted were not known. Despite considerable research on the factors affecting adsorption of antibiotics, these compounds have not given consistent control in practice, and many applications are required to achieve the control that is obtained. These bactericides would be quickly replaced if a compound became available that gave consistent control.

Tetracycline antibiotics were tested experimentally for the control of several yellows diseases (Chiykowski, 1972; Davis and Whitcomb, 1970). Disease symptoms were suppressed provided the plants were sprayed regularly, but symptoms reappear soon after treatments were discontinued. Only partial remission of X-disease symptoms was obtained in peach orchards sprayed regularly with oxytetracycline (Jones and Rosenberger, 1978). Antibiotics with good systemic properties are needed for the control of mycoplasma-like, rickettsia-like, and bacterial agents that are systemic in plants.

IV. DETERMINING THE NEED FOR AND TIMING OF CONTROL ACTION

Chemical control measures for bacterial diseases are usually applied on standard schedules, i.e., every 5–7 days, regardless of the status of the pathogen, vector populations, or the favorability or unfavorability of the weather for infection and disease development. Farmers are often disappointed in the performance of standard schedules. Infection either may not develop in unsprayed adjacent orchards, suggesting the program was unnecessary, or the program failed because of unusually favorable conditions for infection. Techniques for monitoring pathogen or vector populations, or for monitoring the weather conditions and using the data in forecasting systems, show promise for improving the effectiveness of chemical control treatments through better spray timing.

A. Monitoring Pathogen Populations

Selective media for isolating specific bacteria and differentiating them from other bacteria that might grow on the media have been developed for a number of bacterial pathogens. With these media, it becomes possible to monitor pathogen populations in the field and to relate population levels to needs for control. For example, a selective medium developed by Miller and Schroth (1972) was used in California's pear pest management program. Chemical control treatments were withheld until *E. amylovora* had colonized pear flowers in grower orchards (Moller *et al.*, 1981). This approach was effective because development of high epiphytic populations of the blight bacterium precede infection. Populations of *E. amylovora* develop slow enough to allow time for processing the samples and making control treatments. In the Northeast and Midwest, bacterial populations appear to develop quicker than in the West and sufficient time is not always available to provide growers with the results of monitoring before sprays should be applied (Beer and Opgenorth, 1976; Sutton and Jones, 1975). It may be possible using serological methods, such as immunofluorescence, to reduce the time needed to identify the bacteria.

B. Forecasting Based on Weather

For several fungal incited diseases, it is possible to monitor the weather in or near an orchard or field and forecast the need for and timing of control treatments. Forecasting systems for bacterial pathogens are limited, in part, because chemical control of bacterial incited diseases is much less developed than chemical control for fungal incited diseases. Also, current bactericides are protective rather than eradicative in control activity, and forecast systems are much more effective where the control chemical has good eradicative as well as protective properties.

Greatest progress has been made in the development of forecast systems for fire blight. Readers are referred to an article by Billing (1980) for a comparison of several systems currently in use. In the control of fire blight, spray treatments are aimed at reducing infection to blossoms during the bloom period. Infection in blossoms is sporadic, but control of blossom blight is essential to the success and cost effectiveness of a blight control program. Methods for timing streptomycin spray treatments based on environmental factors were initially developed in New York (Luepschen *et al.*, 1961; Mills, 1955) and later in Illinois (Powell, 1965), California (Thomson *et al.*, 1975), and England (Billing, 1979). In

California, daily mean temperatures are used to predict the appearance of epiphytic populations in blossoms and when to initiate bactericide treatments (Moller *et al.*, 1981; Thompson *et al.*, 1975). Development of similar forecast systems for other crops is needed to improve timing of control treatments.

C. Monitoring Insect Vector Species

The epidemiology of many diseases caused by phytopathogenic prokaryotes involves insect vectors. Mycoplasma- and rickettsial-like organisms are highly dependent on leafhopper or psyllid vectors. For a few bacterial pathogens, vectors play a significant and primary role in their epidemiology. Where vectors play a major role in disease spread, control strategies can be based on the status of the vector species. The potential for Stewart's wilt of corn, caused by *E. stewartii*, is related to survival of the corn flea beetle. Outbreaks of bacterial wilt were found by Stevens (1934) to follow mild winters favorable to survival of overwintering flea beetles, and a computer program was developed to forecast the severity of Stewart's wilt based on winter temperatures (Castor *et al.*, 1975).

New approaches to the detection of prokaryotes should make it possible to rapidly determine whether vectors are carrying specific disease agents. The enzyme linked immunosorbent assay (ELISA) procedure has already been developed to detect *Spiroplasma citri* Saglio *et al.* (Clark *et al.*, 1978; Saillard *et al.*, 1978), the corn stunt spiroplasma (Raju and Nyland, 1981), and the Pierce's disease bacterium (Nome *et al.*, 1980). Thus, with ELISA and other serological techniques, it should be possible to monitor species and time control measures based on the presence of the pathogen in the vector population.

V. THE FUTURE OF CHEMICAL CONTROL

A. Problems with Resistance

Development of resistance in the target organism and the potential for resistance in nontarget organisms are of concern where antibiotics are used for plant disease control. Resistance in the target organism results in the loss of control effectiveness while resistance in nontarget organisms is of potential significance in clinical situations. Resistance may result in losses to the grower and may greatly affect the profitability of a product to its manufacturer.

1. *Examples*

Resistance of phytopathogenic prokaryotes to streptomycin has resulted in poor control of bacterial spot of pepper (*Capsicum frutescens* L.) and tomato in Florida (Thayer and Stall, 1961) and of fire blight of pear in California, Washington, and Oregon (Coyier and Covey, 1975; Schroth *et al.*, 1979). Streptomycin-resistant *P. s.* pv. *syringae* were detected in apricot (*Prunus aremaniaca* L.) orchards in New Zealand sprayed with streptomycin, but control failures could not be attributed to epidemics of resistant strains (Young, 1977). Resistant *P. s.* pv. *syringae* were also selected on peach seedlings sprayed repeatedly with streptomycin and inoculated with a sensitive strain (Dye, 1958). However, the failure to control a leaf spot disease of cherry-laurel (*Prunus laurocerasus* L.) in a nursery was attributed to development of streptomycin resistance in *P. s.* pv. *syringae* (DeBoer, 1980). Streptomycin-resistant mutants of *P. s.* pv. *phaseolicola* were obtained *in vitro* but have not been detected in the field (Russell, 1975).

In *X. c.* pv. *vesicatoria* (Doidge) Dye, resistance contributed to erratic control of bacterial spot with streptomycin under field conditions. It appeared that resistant populations of the pathogen were selected out of mixed population after only 10 sprays (Stall and Thayer, 1962). In greenhouse tests, a field-collected resistant isolate was not controlled with sprays of 400 μg/ml streptomycin while a streptomycin-sensitive isolate was controlled (Thayer and Stall, 1961). Also, repeated streptomycin sprays in foliage nurseries resulted in the selection of streptomycin-resistant *X. c.* pv. *dieffenbachiae* (McCulloch and Pirone) Dye, the cause of bacterial leaf spot and tip burn of *Philodendron oxycardium* (Knauss, 1972).

2. *Mechanisms*

a. Streptomycin. Genetic resistance to streptomycin may arise in two ways. In the first, chromosomal mutations that impair the binding capacity of ribosomal proteins for the antibiotic (Ozaki *et al.*, 1969). In phytopathogens, this occurs spontaneously at frequencies of 10^{-9} to 10^{-8} resistant clones per colony-forming unit (CFU) (G. H. Lacy, personal communication). A second type of resistance is plasmid-borne. These plasmids may move conjugally from bacterium to bacterium at frequencies of 10^{-9} to 10^{-5} transconjugants/donor CFU. This type of resistance is mediated by periplasmic enzymes that adenylate or phosphorylate aminoglycosides such as streptomycin (Wallace *et al.*, 1979). Plasmid-borne streptomycin resistance has been transferred into *E. amylovora* in the laboratory (Bennett and Billing, 1975; Chatterjee and Starr, 1972), but was associated with attenuation or loss of virulence (Bennett and Billing, 1975).

Although the genetic basis for the natural streptomycin resistance occurring in *E. amylovora* causing fire blight on the West Coast of the United States has not been studied rigorously (Panopoulos *et al.*, 1978), *E. amylovora* strains with a high level of resistance were detected in California while in Washington and Oregon strains with intermediate and high levels of resistance were found. Generation times, virulence, and susceptibility to other antibiotics among resistant and sensitive strains were not significantly different (Moller *et al.*, 1981). Highly resistant strains persisted in orchards after streptomycin usage was discontinued, indicating a return to streptomycin after several years absence is unlikely to give effective control.

b. Tetracycline. Tetracycline and oxytetracycline resistance may develop among phytopathogenic bacteria by spontaneous chromosomal mutation (frequency = 10^{-9} to 10^{-8} resistant clones/CFU) (Lacy and Leary, 1975; Lacy and Sparks, 1979) or by conjugal transfer of plasmid-borne antibiotic resistance (frequency = 10^{-9} to 10^{-1} transconjugants/donor cell) (Reviewed in Lacy and Leary, 1979). The resistance mechanisms are probably similar for both genetic mechanisms; membrane permeability is altered to prevent intracellular accumulation of the antibiotic (Kaji and Ryoji, 1979). Virulence was not lost upon introduction of tetracycline resistance on conjugal plasmids (Lacy, 1979; Lacy and Leary, 1975).

3. *Frequency*

A major drawback to use of antibiotics is that pathogen resistance arises very quickly in contrast to the general biocide and alkylating agents mentioned previously. Since general biocides damage many bacterial systems simultaneously, resistance has relatively little chance to evolve. This is based on the observation that spontaneous single gene modifications to resistance usually occur at frequencies of 10^{-9} to 10^{-8} resistant clones per CFU. The chance that spontaneous resistance for several systems might arise simultaneously is factorial. For example, if we assume that simultaneous changes in 10 genes would give resistance to a general biocide, the chance that one cell would have spontaneous mutations for all 10 genes simultaneously is 10^{-90} to 10^{-80} or, practically, will not occur. Since only one gene change allows resistance to develop against antibiotics and a blighted pear shoot may easily contain 10^{9} to 10^{11} bacteria, one can understand how easily resistance to antibiotics may be selected.

For example, on the West Coast of the United States, streptomycin is practically useless for control of fireblight since resistance is so wide spread. On the East Coast, because of developmental differences in the disease, in cultural practices, and orchard sizes, less antibiotic is used. Streptomycin is still effective because the selection pressure for resistant strains is less intense (Moller *et al.*, 1981). One may predict, however, that streptomycin resistance will eventually appear in other areas either by spontaneous mutation or physical spread of antibiotic-resistant strains from the West Coast.

Tetracycline, theoretically, may suffer from the same drawback since *in vitro*, mutants of phytopathogens resistant to the antibiotics may be recovered readily. Therefore, one can also predict that resistance will eventually appear for this compound also. However, at this moment no resistance to tetracycline has been described among phytopathogenic prokaryotes. Additional antibiotic controls from bacterial pathogens must be developed and screened now so that if both streptomycin and tetracycline fail, new compounds will be available immediately to replace them.

Although resistance to streptomycin has developed, early studies indicate that the emergence of resistant strains in *E. amylovora* and *X. c.* pv. *vesicatoria* could be delayed by using a streptomycin and terramycin combination (English and Van Halsema, 1954). Unfortunately, such combinations are not used commercially. A combined treatment of streptomycin and terramycin is being developed for cabbage (*Brassica oleracea* var. *capitata* L.) seed since the combination is as effective as either singly and it is less likely that resistance will develop simultaneously to two antibiotics (Humaydan *et al.*, 1980).

B. Need for New Antibiotics

No new chemicals have been developed for the control of diseases caused by phytopathogenic prokaryotes since the introduction of streptomycin and tetracycline compounds, and almost no experimental compounds are available from chemical manufacturers for evaluation. As noted by Schroth and McCain (1981), potential sales for a highly effective new chemical cannot be estimated accurately based on current sales for available compounds. New chemicals for the control of phytopathogenic prokaryotes are also needed as tools for avoiding resistance problems. Development of strategies based on alternating or mixing compounds is very difficult to accomplish when only one or two chemical compounds are available.

VI. CONCLUSIONS

In the three decades since antibiotics were introduced, no new chemicals of significance have been developed for the control of bacterial diseases. However, there has been in the last decade a recognition that mycoplasma- and rickettsial-like organisms cause plant disease and that many of these diseases are amenable to chemical control. During this time, resistance problems with streptomycin have increased and some important bacterial pathogens have been detected in new areas. Thus, the need for highly effective chemical compounds to control phytopathogenic prokaryotes is greater than ever!

References

Allen, W. R., and Davidson, T. R. (1978). *Plant Dis. Rep.* **62,** 311–313.
Allen, W. R., and Dirks, V. A. (1979). *Can J. Plant Sci.* **59,** 487–489.
Beer, S. V., and Opgenorth, D. C. (1976). *Phytopathology* **66,** 317–322.
Bennett, R. A., and Billing, E. (1975). *J. Appl. Bacteriol.* **39,** 307–315.
Billing, E. (1979). *In* "Plant Pathogens" (D. W. Levelock, ed.), pp. 51–59. Academic Press, New York.
Billing, E. (1980). *Ann. Appl. Biol.* **95,** 365–377.
Bushong, J. W., Powell, D., and Shaw, P. D. (1964). *Phytopathology* **54,** 713–717.
Castor, L. L., Ayers, J. E., MacNab, A. A., and Krause, R. A. (1975). *Plant Dis. Rep.* **59,** 533–536.
Chatterjee, A. K., and M. P. Starr (1972). *J. Bacteriol.* **112,** 576–584.
Chiykowski, L. N. (1972). *Can. J. Plant Sci.* **52,** 29–33.
Coyier, D. L., and Covey, R. P. (1975). *Plant Dis. Rep.* **59,** 849–852.
Crosse, J. E., and Bennett, M. (1959). *Annu. Res. Rep. East Malling Res. Sta.* pp. 93–95.
Daines, R. H. (1980). *Plant Dis. Rep.* **44,** 826–827.
Davis, R. E., and Whitcomb, R. F. (1970). *Infect. Immun.* **2,** 201–208.
DeBoer, S. H. (1980). *Can. J. Plant Pathol.* **2,** 235–238.
Deep, I. W., and Young, R. A. (1975). *Phytopathology* **55,** 212–216.
Deep, I. W., McNeilan, R. A., and MacSwan, I. C. (1968). *Plant Dis. Rep.* **52,** 102–105.
Deiner, U. L., and Carlton, C. C. (1960). *Plant Dis. Rep.* **44,** 136–138.
Doi, Y., Teranaka, M., Yora, K., and Asuyama, H. (1969). *Ann. Phytopathol. Soc. Jpn.* **33,** 259–266.
Dunegan, J. C., Wilson, R. A., and Morris, W. T. (1953). *Plant Dis. Rep.* **37,** 604–605.
Dye, M. H. (1958). *N.Z. J. Agric. Res.* **1,** 44–50.
English, A. R., and VanHalsema, G. (1954). *Plant Dis. Rep.* **38,** 429–431.
Humaydan, H. S., Harman, G. E., Nedron, B. L., and DiNitto, L. V. (1980). *Phytopathology* **70,** 127–131.
Jones, A. L., and Rosenberger, D. A. (1978). *Proc. Symp. System. Chem. Treat. Tree Cult.* pp. 247–254.
Kaji, A., and Ryoji, M. (1979). *In* "Mechanism of Action of Antibacterial Agents" (F. E. Hahn, ed.), pp. 304–328. Springer-Verlag, Berlin and New York.
Keil, H. L., and Civerolo, E. L. (1979). *Plant Dis. Rep.* **63,** 1–5.
Knauss, J. F. (1972). *Plant Dis. Rep.* **56,** 394–397.

Lacy, G. H. (1978). *Phytopathology* **68,** 1323–1330.
Lacy, G. H., and Leary, J. V. (1975). *J. Gen. Microbiol.* **88,** 49–57.
Lacy, G. H., and Leary, J. V. (1979). *Annu. Rev. Phytopathol.* **17,** 181–202.
Lacy, G. H., and Sparks, R. B., Jr. (1979). *Phytopathology* **69,** 1293–1297.
Lacy, G. H., McIntyre, J. L., Walton, G. S., and Dodds, J. A. (1980). *Can. J. Plant Pathol.* **2,** 96–101.
Luepschen, N. S., Parker, K. G., and Mills, W. D. (1961). *Cornell Univ. Agric. Exp. Sta. Bull.* **963,** 1–19.
McCoy, R. E. (1972). *Plant Dis. Rep.* **56,** 1019–1021.
Miller, T. D., and Schroth, M. N. (1972). *Phytopathology* **62,** 1175–1182.
Mills, W. D. (1955). *Plant Dis. Rep.* **39,** 206–207.
Moller, W. J., Schroth, M. N., and Thomson, S. V. (1981). *Plant Dis.* **65,** 563–568.
Nome, S. F., Raju, B. C., Goheen, A. C., Nyland, G., and Docamp, D. (1980). *Phytopathology* **70,** 746–749.
Nyland, G., and Moller, W. J. (1973). *Plant Dis. Rep.* **57,** 634–637.
Ozaki, M., Mizushima, S., and Nomura, N. (1969). *Nature (London)* **222,** 333–339.
Panopoulos, N. J., Guimaraes, W. V., Hua, S. S., Sebersky-Lehman, C., Resnick, S., Lai, M., and Shaffer, S. (1978). *Microbiology* **1978,** 238–241.
Pearson, R. C., and Sands, D. C. (1978). *Plant Dis. Rep.* **62,** 753–757.
Powell, D. (1965). *Proc. Mich. State Hortic. Soc.* **94,** 1–7.
Powell, D. (1967). *Plant Dis. Rep.* **51,** 351–352.
Purcell, A. H. (1979). *J. Econ. Entomol.* **72,** 887–892.
Raju, B. C., and Nyland, G. (1981). *Curr. Microbiol.* **5,** 101–104.
Ralph, W. (1976). *Seed Sci. Technol.* **4,** 325–332.
Reil, W. O., and Beutel, J. A. (1976). *Calif. Agric.* **12,** 4–5.
Rosenberger, D. A., and Jones, A. L. (1977). *Phytopathology* **67,** 277–282.
Russell, P. E. (1975). *J. Appl. Bacteriol.* **39,** 175–180.
Saillard, C., Dunez, J., Garcia-Jurado, O., Nhami, A., and Bove, J. (1978). *C.R. Hebd. Seances Acad. Sci. Ser. D* **286,** 1245–1248.
Sands, D. C., and McIntyre, J. L. (1977a). *Plant Dis. Rep.* **61,** 311–312.
Sands, D. C., and McIntyre, J. L. (1977b). *Plant Dis. Rep.* **61,** 823–827.
Sands, D. C., and Walton, G. S. (1975). *Plant Dis. Rep.* **59,** 573–576.
Schroth, M. N., Thomson, S. V., and Moller, W. J. (1979). *Phytopathology* **69,** 565–568.
Schroth, M. N., and McCain, A. H. (1981). *In* "Handbook of Pest Management in Agriculture" (D. Pimentel, ed.), Vol III, pp. 49–58. CRC, Cleveland, Ohio.
Stall, R. E., and Thayer, P. L. (1962). *Plant Dis. Rep.* **46,** 389–392.
Stevens, N. E. (1934). *Plant Dis. Rep.* **18,** 141–149.
Sutton, T. B., and Jones, A. L. (1975). *Phytopathology* **65,** 1009–1012.
Taylor, J. D., and Dye, D. W. (1976). *N.Z. J. Agric. Res.* **19,** 91–95.
Taylor, J. D., and Dudley, C. L. (1977). *Ann. Appl. Biol.* **85,** 223–232.
Thayer, P. L., and Stall, R. E. (1961). *Phytopathology* **51,** 568–571.
Thomas, W. D., and Henderson, W. J. (1952). *Plant Dis. Rep.* **36,** 273–275.
Thomson, S. V., Schroth, M. N., Moller, W. J., and Reil, O. W. (1975). *Phytopathology* **65,** 353–358.
van der Zwet, T., and Keil, H. L. (1979). *U.S. Dep. Agric. Handbook* 510.
Wallace, B. J., Tai, P. C., and Davis, B. D. (1979). *In* "Mechanism of Action of Antibacterial Agents" (F. E. Nahn, ed.), pp. 272–303. Springer-Verlag, Berlin and New York.
Young, J. M. (1977). *N.Z. J. Agric. Res.* **20,** 249–252.

Part **V**

Cultivation and Preservation

The field of research concerning phytopathogenic prokaryotes is so wide that many important topics were not addressed specifically in this treatise. However, the chapters in this section are of vital importance to researchers in this field. T. A. Chen, J. M. Wells, and G. H. Liao (Chapter 20) discuss *in vitro* cultivation of nutritionally fastidious prokaryotes including spiroplasmas, plant mycoplasmalike organisms, and walled bacteria. J. P. Sleesman (Chapter 21) reviews preservation techniques that have been used with or may be applied to phytopathogenic prokaryotes.

Chapter **20**

Cultivation in Vitro: Spiroplasmas, Plant Mycoplasmas, and Other Fastidious, Walled Prokaryotes

T. A. CHEN, J. M. WELLS, *and* C. H. LIAO

I. INTRODUCTION

In recent years three distinguishable groups of prokaryotes, namely, spiroplasmas, mycoplasma-like organisms (MLOs), and rickettsia-like organisms [RLOs or bacteria-like organisms (BLOs)] have been associated with many plant diseases. These three groups of microorganisms

Phytopathogenic
Prokaryotes, Vol. 2

Copyright © 1982 by Academic Press, Inc.
All rights of reproduction in any form reserved.
ISBN 0-12-509002-1

share, in common, a number of properties. They are much smaller than Eubacteria and are difficult to isolate and grow *in vitro,* and thus are often referred to as "fastidious." In general, they are transmitted in nature from plant to plant through insect vectors, particularly by leafhoppers (Cicadellidae). Up to this point the study of these organisms has focused on their role in plant diseases although their association with the insect hosts might even be more significant in insect pathology. This area promises to be important in future studies for a better understanding of the ecology and evolution of these organisms. As plant pathogens, they are limited to the vascular tissues, i.e., either the phloem or xylem. For many years "yellows diseases" have been used to describe a group of plant diseases now known to be associated with phloem-limited prokaryotes. "Yellows" diseased plants are characterized by the symptoms of yellowing, stunting, virescence of floral petals, and the shortening of internodes. Plant diseases that are associated with xylem-limited prokaryotes generally exhibit symptoms including marginal necrosis or scorching of the leaves, decreased vigor, and dwarfing of shoot growth.

The discovery of mycoplasma as new plant pathogens in 1967 (Doi *et al.*, 1967; Ishiie *et al.*, 1967) and the subsequent isolation of spiroplasmas and other BLOs *in vitro* have yielded much information on these prokaryotes. To date, however, a major group of yellows agents, the MLOs, have not been cultured in artificial media. The difficulties encountered are largely due to our limited knowledge of the environment which these microbes inhabit. Without successful cultivation, studies to determine their etiology, taxonomic position, metabolism, and pathogenesis are impossible.

In this chapter we will review the information which is now available for the cultivation of these groups of prokaryotes associated with plant diseases and insects. We have also included information on spiroplasmas and mycoplasmas isolated from the plant surfaces. Most of these, if not all, are probably insect-associated. The nature of their relationship to insects has not been fully understood. But because of their ready cultivability a comparison of their nutritional requirements and those of the more fastidious ones will hopefully give us some insight on how to proceed in solving the problems of cultivation of other fastidious prokaryotes such as MLOs.

II. CULTIVATION OF SPIROPLASMAS

Spiroplasmas are easily identified by their helical morphology and contractile motility. Because the organism is bounded by a unit membrane and because of their minute size ($0.25 \times 2-15$ μm) they are usually seen only with dark-field or phase-contrast microscopy. At present, more than 40 spiroplasma isolates representing at least six serological groups (Davis *et al.*, 1979; Whitcomb, 1980) have been recovered from a variety of plants and arthropods. The spiroplasmas recovered from plants have been found to reside in the sieve-tube elements (Saglio and Whitcomb, 1979) and the nectar of the flowers (Davis, 1978a; Davis *et al.*, 1981). Spiroplasmas, if present in the insect body, are usually found in the hemolymph. Since spiroplasmas are transmitted by feeding leafhopper vectors, it is not surprising to find that the spiroplasmas also multiply in the salivary glands of the insect hosts. It was surprising, however, that the corn stunt spiroplasma was observed to reside intracellularly in the brain tissue of *Dalbulus elimatus* (Ball) and *D. maidis* (Delong and Wolcott) (Granados and Meehan, 1957).

Based on their natural habitats, the approaches to spiroplasma cultivation were determined by the use of media which not only consisted of ingredients for mycoplasma culture but also contained materials similar to the constituents of plant phloem sap or the insect hemolymph. The first acknowledged successful cultivation *in vitro* of spiroplasma was achieved for *Spiroplasma citri* Saglio *et al.* (Fudl-Allah *et al.* 1971, 1972; Saglio *et al.* 1971a,b).

In 1970, soon after the recognition of mycoplasma in plants infected by corn stunt, Chen and Granados (1970) isolated the disease agent from plant and maintained its infectivity for 43 days in an artificial medium (C-G medium). Although they were unable to subculture the corn stunt agent in the C-G medium it is now evident that, given proper isolation technique, incubation temperature, suitable microscopic observation, and the timing of subculturing passage, corn stunt spiroplasma can be cultured and repeatedly subcultured in the C-G medium (Chen, unpublished).

A. Media and Methods

1. Complex Media

In addition to the ingredients in the basic mycoplasma culture media (PPLO broth base, yeast extract, horse serum), many other enriched supplements have been added (Chen and Davis, 1979). These included DNA, tryptone, peptone, insect tissue culture medium (Schneider's *Drosophila* medium), animal cell culture medium (TC 199, CMRL-1066), and yeastolate. Carbohydrates, such as sucrose, glucose, fructose, and sorbitol, have been used in various complex media for the supply of energy sources and/or for regulating the osmolarity of the media. Since drastic pH changes occur in the medium during growth, a color indicator (phenol red) is routinely added to culture medium and the medium must be buffered to increase cell yield. It was demonstrated by Jones *et al.* (1977) that α-ketoglutaric acid and certain amino acids in the complex MIA medium could enhance the primary isolation of corn stunt spiroplasma from insect hemolymph.

Serum is probably the most important supplement of the culture medium. Although γ-globulin-free horse serum is generally used (15–20%) for mycoplasma cultivation, fetal bovine serum (FBS) has proved superior for most spiroplasmas (Chen, unpublished data). Batch sample testing for suitability for spiroplasma growth is particularly important prior to the purchase of horse sera. What factor(s) in the "unsuitable" sera fails to support spiroplasma growth, especially for the more fastidious strains, is not clear.

Purified agar (Ion agar, noble agar, etc.) has been used at 0.9–1.5% for solid culture media. However, regular agar–agar has been used with no apparent ill effects for spiroplasma growth.

2. *Simple Media*

After the successful cultivation of *S. citri* and corn stunt spiroplasma *in vitro,* Liao and Chen (1977) gradually removed ingredients from the medium and eventually formulated a simple medium (C-3G). They reported that *S. citri* and corn stunt spiroplasmas are able to grow in C-3G medium which contains only three ingredients: PPLO broth base, horse serum, and sucrose. This medium is easy to prepare and has been used to isolate and culture *S. citri,* corn stunt spiroplasma, honeybee spiroplasma, several flower spiroplasmas, and several spiroplasmas isolated from insects (Clark, 1978; Davis, 1978; Liao and Chen, 1977; McCoy *et al.*, 1979; Su *et al.*, 1978).

A recent slight modification of the C-3G medium has led to formulation of R_2 medium which contains PPLO broth (1.5%), fetal bovine serum or horse serum (15%), and sucrose (8–10%). R_2 has been used to make primary isolations and to grow all the cultivable spiroplasmas except the suckling mouse cataract agent (SMCA) which was originally isolated from rabbit ticks and shown to induce cataract in several rodents (Tully *et al.*, 1977). Although SMCA was isolated with and routinely maintained in the complex SP-4 medium (Tully *et al.*, 1977) it was found that this spiroplasma can also be cultured with a simple medium (R_8) which contains 2.1% PPLO broth base, 20% fetal bovine serum (or horse serum), and 0.5% glucose (Liao and Chen, unpublished data). It is, therefore, quite clear that a combination of three basic ingredients is sufficient to support the multiplication of any cultivable spiroplasma strains.

3. Chemically Defined Media

Recently, Chang and Chen (1981a,b, 1982) developed several chemically defined media to support the *in vitro* cultivation of spiroplasmas. The constituents of the media are complex and the preparation of the formulation is very tedious. They are useful, however, to investigate the nutritional requirements, metabolic pathways, and biosynthetic capabilities of spiroplasmas. Such results, when available, would lead us to a better understanding of why spiroplasmas such as the sex ratio organism (SRO) of *Drosophila* (Williamson and Poulson, 1979) and the fastidious spiroplasmas of *Oncometopia* (McCoy *et al.*, 1979) are still resistant to being cultured.

4. Isolation

Spiroplasmas can be isolated easily from young plant tissues showing early stages of disease symptoms (Chen and Davis, 1979). The young tissues usually contain spiroplasma at high concentration, are less likely to harbor other microbial flora, and the expressed sap appears to contain fewer factors inhibitory for the growth of primary isolates (Liao and Chen, 1980).

Plant pathogenic spiroplasmas are confined to the sieve-tube elements. Thus, surface sterilization of the plant host can be made without killing the spiroplasmas. $HgCl_2$ (0.1%) or sodium hypochloride (0.25–1.00%) is commonly used. After rinsing with sterile water, the tissues are placed in the culture medium. Commonly, many cuts are made crosswise along the vascular tissue to release the organisms from the phloem. This avoids pressing the tissue and producing unnecessarily great amounts of plant sap. To avoid growth inhibitors in plant sap, the primary culture may be subcultured immediately by making a 10-fold dilution in fresh medium. Evidence of spiroplasma growth is usually obtained in the diluted subcultures but not in the primary cultures. Another method involves centrifuging the primary cultures and resuspending the concentrated spiroplasmas from the sediment in fresh medium (Williamson and Whitcomb, 1975).

Isolation of spiroplasma from flower habitats is accomplished by simply rinsing the flower nectar with culture medium or submerging the flower in the medium for a length of time. The medium is then filtered through a 0.45-μm filter to remove other microbial contaminants.

Spiroplasmas are readily isolated from insect hosts. Using infected insect vectors as an alternate approach to isolate plant pathogenic spiroplasma avoids spiroplasmastatic inhibitors from plant sources (Liao and Chen, 1980). High concentrations of spiroplasmas are usually found in the insect hemolymph. Hemolymph can be collected using fine capillary glass tubing. Sometimes, hind legs pulled from the insect body and placed directly in the culture medium yield sufficient spiroplasmas for isolation. Finally, the whole insect body can be homogenized in the culture medium and filtered to eliminate other microorganisms.

In most cases, spiroplasmas are isolated and maintained in a broth medium. Several passages in broth are necessary to adapt the organism to the *in vitro* conditions. However, Kleopper (personal communication) has recently demonstrated that freshly isolated spiroplasmas from diseased plants can be inoculated directly on solid agar media.

5. *Growth in Culture*

The growth pattern of spiroplasmas in broth follows a sigmoid curve resembling those known for other microorganisms. The growth rate of spiroplasmas, however, varies greatly from one isolate to another and is also affected by medium composition, incubation temperature, pH, and osmotic pressure (Chen and Davis, 1979). Under the same conditions, for example, the doubling time for some flower spiroplasmas is 60–70 min whereas that of corn stunt spiroplasma is 7–8 hr (Chen, unpublished data).

Routine maintainence of established spiroplasma cultures is quite simple. Several precautions may be necessary during such maintainence. Spiroplasmas usually have a very short stationary phase in their growth since the medium becomes very acidic. When the pH in the medium drops to 5.4 or lower, which may be monitored by the phenol red indicator, the number of viable spiroplasmas in the culture decreases drastically (Liao and Chen, 1977). Liao and Chen (1977) reported that the incorporation of 0.06 *M* HEPES buffer in C-3G medium significantly increased the titer of corn stunt spiroplasma. In rapid-growing spiroplasmas, a delay of a few hours for subculturing may result in loss of the culture.

B. Nutrition

In the past, many workers have attempted to determine which substrates in the culture medium may be utilized by spiroplasmas (Chang and Chen, 1979, 1981c; Davis, 1979; Davis *et al.*, 1979; Freeman *et al.*, 1976; Igwegbe *et al.*, 1979; Jones *et al.*, 1977; Lee, 1977; Lee and Davis, 1978; Malloy and Chen, 1980; Mudd *et al.*, 1977; Saglio *et al.*, 1973; Townsend, 1976). Because the culture medium usually contains complex constituents like PPLO broth and serum, results of such studies were frequently different and sometimes conflicting. It is generally believed that PPLO broth and horse serum provide amino acids, fatty acids, nucleotides, and sterolic compounds (Razin, 1978). Thus, using a medium containing these two ingredients would at least allow one to investigate the substrate utilization of carbohydrates. Recently, however, results of such studies may be questioned when it was demonstrated that horse serum and PPLO serum fraction actually contain substances which could degrade di- or polysaccharides to their monomers (Malloy and Chen, 1982). It is clear that studies on the nutritional requirements of spiroplasmas will be limited until a chemically defined medium is made available.

In 1979, Chang and Chen (1979) showed that PPLO broth in C-3G medium can be replaced by two animal tissue culture media: Schneider's *Drosophila* medium and CMRL-1066. All the compounds in these media are defined except yeastolate, which was later substituted by asparagine, and horse serum, which has been replaced with fatty acids, lipids, and bovine serum albumin (Chang and Chen, 1981, 1982). Thus a completely chemically defined medium has been developed. Now carbohydrate, amino acid, nitrogenous base, lipid, fatty acid, and vitamin utilization may be determined in the growth of spiroplasmas.

C. Quantitation

1. *Direct Cell Counting*

In spite of their small size, viable spiroplasma are readily identified by their characteristic helical shape and the contractile motility. Using dark-field microscopy, direct observation has been applied to determine spiroplasma growth in liquid media (Liao and Chen, 1975, 1977) and in insect hemolymph (Whitcomb and Williamson, 1975). This method has the advantage of knowing immediately what has taken place in the culture. On the other hand, as culture age increases, spiroplasma become slender and elongated and gradually lose their helicity. Then it is difficult to determine whether such cells are still viable.

2. *Color-Changing Units (CCU)*

Jones *et al.* (1977) measured the viable cells in spiroplasma culture by the extent of acid production using a color indicator. For example, a broth culture with an unknown cell concentration may be serially 10-fold diluted in medium containing phenol red. After incubation, the highest dilution that shows a color change indicates spiroplasma multiplication and is considered as one color-changing unit (CCU). The cell titer of the undiluted culture is the reciprocal of dilution at the end point. Although this method is rapid, precision in enumeration is lost. The advantages and deficiencies of this method have recently been discussed by Whitcomb (1980).

3. *Colony-Forming Units (CFU)*

Spiroplasma in culture can produce colonies on solid agar media and may be used to enumerate viable spiroplasmas. In practice, however, some problems often arise. Many slow-growing isolates require 2–3 weeks to produce colonies, while the fast-growing ones often produce small satellite colonies or diffuse colonies at the peripheral areas of the primary colony. In addition, growth of the fastidious isolates tends to be more erratic on solid media than in the broth. The composition of the medium, amount of agar used, and dryness of the plate surface all can greatly affect the colony formation.

4. *Turbidity*

Measurement of turbidity as a function of spiroplasma growth has been used with limited success (Lee, 1977). The difficulty using turbidity of the culture medium as a parameter of spiroplasma growth may be attributed to several factors. Spiroplasmas, especially the slow-growing isolates, normally fail to form a high degree of turbidity in culture. As the culture ages, there is a tendency for spiroplasma to lengthen and to form twining clumps. Sometimes, precipitates may be observed in aged cultures when the pH of medium drops to 5.4 or under. However, Lee and Davis (personal communication) recently demonstrated that the log-phase growth of several spiroplasmas can be accurately measured by the absorbance at 660 nm when the cell population is in the range of 10^8–10^{10}/ml.

5. *Biochemical Measurements*

Direct measurement of the increase in cellular proteins or nucleic acids as a function of spiroplasma growth has not been fully explored. One problem encountered for determining changes in total protein or nucleic acid during growth is the limited yield in spiroplasma cultures. More sensitive methods that measure the amount of ^{32}P- or ^{14}C-labeled precursors incorporated into the cells have been proven to be useful to determine various stages of spiroplasma growth (Bové *et al.*, 1973; Bové and Saillard, 1979; Saglio *et al.*, 1973; Townsend *et al.*, 1977).

D. Cultivation in Nonnatural Hosts

1. *Cultivation in Nonvector Insects*

Several spiroplasmas which have been found to be borne by insects cannot be cultured by the techniques described above (McCoy *et al.*,

1978; Su *et al.*, 1978; Williamson and Whitcomb, 1974). Recent discoveries of spiroplasmas and other wall-less prokaryotes from flower surfaces (Davis, 1978b, 1981) and other insects (Chen, unpublished data; Whitcomb, personal communication) may eventually prove that most of spiroplasmas, if not all, are insect-borne. Since arthropods comprise the greatest number of species in the animal kingdom, one can safely predict that many more spiroplasma–insect associations will be discovered in the future. Why can some of them be easily cultivated *in vitro* while others not? One might suspect that some spiroplasmas are arthropod symbiotes and others are insect pathogens. In any case, the hemolymph of the insect hosts must provide the best conditions for spiroplasma growth. Surprisingly, it was found that even nonvector insects can also harbor spiroplasmas. Corn stunt spiroplasma adapted very well and grew to high titer when it was injected into the *Drosophila* hemolymph (Williamson and Whitcomb, 1974). Recently, McCoy *et al.* (1981) reported that hemolymph of the greater wax moth larvae (*Galleria mellonella* L.) can support the multiplication of several spiroplasmas of various origins. This *in vivo* culture technique may prove to be a useful alternative means to obtain large numbers of fastidious spiroplasmas or other wall-less prokaryotes.

2. *Cultivation in Organ and Cell Cultures*

Successful cultivation of SMCA in rabbit whole-lens organ culture was reported by Fabiyi *et al.* (1971). They found that infective titer of SMCA reached its peak in the lens organ culture fluids 5 days after inoculation. McBeath and Chen (1973) successfully established a monlayered cell culture of *Dalbulus elimatus,* the vector leafhopper of corn stunt disease. The culture medium, however, did not support the multiplication of corn stunt spiroplasma (unpublished data). A recent investigation made by Steiner and McGarrity (1980) indicated that a *Drosophila* cell culture supported the growth of several spiroplasmas of plant origin. Cytopathic effects of the *Drosophila* cell line was observed with some spiroplasma isolates (Steiner and McGarrity, 1980).

3. *Cultivation in Embryonated Hens Eggs*

The use of chicken embryonated eggs to propagate viruses, rickettsia, bacteria, and other prokaryotes has been a common practice in clinical and microbiological laboratories. Application of the same technique for culturing spiroplasma was first reported for SMCA which was maintained at high titer in allantoic and amniotic fluids of embryonated eggs and serially transferred for an indefinite number of passages (Clark, 1964; Picken *et al.*, 1968; Tully *et al.*, 1976). The chick embryos inoculated with SMCA died after 6–7 days incubation. Recently, Rose *et al.* (1979)

and Lin and Su (personal communication) have also used chick embryonated eggs to propagate *S. citri* and flower spiroplasma and demonstrated that the spiroplasmas exerted obvious pathogenicity to the inoculated embryos.

E. Preservation

Spiroplasmas are often maintained in the laboratory by continuous subculturing. This practice may become a nuisance when many strains of spiroplasma must be routinely maintained and contamination is often a problem. In addition, pathogenicity may be lost during *in vitro* passage (Whitcomb *et al.*, 1974). Fortunately, although spiroplasmas lack cell walls, they are quite hardy and may survive extreme conditions. Viable cells can be recovered from dried glass slides after 1 week (Whitcomb, unpublished data). Honeybee spiroplasmas can withstand the treatment of 0.05% phenol and 0.125% formaldehyde for 40 min (Stanek *et al.*, 1980). It was also demonstrated that several spiroplasmas survived after they were placed in the distilled water for 8 hr (Cotty *et al.*, 1978, 1980; Liao *et al.*, 1979). Several preservation methods are suggested here (also see Sleesman, this volume, Chapter 21).

1. *Freezing at −20 or −70°C*

Log-phase cultures of spiroplasma, both broth and agar, can be readily frozen and the cells can be preserved in the frozen state for months or years depending on the different isolates. No data are available on how long such frozen cultures remain viable. In general, the quicker a culture is frozen or thawed the higher is the chance for the cell to survive.

2. *Lyophilization*

In order to prevent loss of frozen cultures caused by power failure in the laboratory, spiroplasma cultures can be preserved by freeze-drying. Norman *et al.* (1970) have shown that the addition of sucrose at a final concentration of 12% before freeze-drying enhanced the recovery of lyophilized *Mycoplasma* sp. Since most spiroplasmas are cultured in media containing high concentration of sucrose (8–10%), cultures of log-phase growth can be used for freeze-drying directly. Lyophilized spiroplasma cells are expected to remain viable for several years.

3. *Drying on Paper Discs*

The method of drying microbial culture on paper discs was originally developed by Coe and Clark (1966) to preserve bacteria. This method has been used for *Mycoplasma pulmonis* (Sabin) Freundt (R-1) by Vogelzang (1975) who found that *M. pulmonis* cells remained viable on dried filter paper strips for at least 4 days. A similar method was adopted by Su and Chen (unpublished data) to preserve spiroplasmas. A drop (5 μl) of log-phase culture is deposited onto a sterile filter paper disc (3–4 mm diameter) which is air dried and then placed in a dessicator. Spiroplasmas can be recovered from the discs 6 weeks after storage at room temperature and 3–6 months after storage at -10°C. This method is most suitable for the transport of spiroplasma cultures by post.

III. CULTIVATION OF PLANT MYCOPLASMAS (MLOs)

Plant pathogenic mycoplasmas or mycoplasma-like organisms are wall-less prokaryotes. They are represented by the aster yellows (AY) agent. Plant diseases that are associated with the presence of these MLOs are called "yellows diseases." The plant to plant spread of yellows diseases in nature is accomplished by phloem-feeding insects, such as leafhoppers and psyllids. Like spiroplasmas, the MLOs also multiply within the insect hosts (Maramorosch, 1952). However, to this date, none of the MLOs associated with yellows diseases has been cultured.

Unlike spiroplasmas, morphologically the MLOs have never been observed to exist as a helical organism in plant hosts or in insect bodies by electron microscopy (Haggis and Sinha, 1978; Kloepper *et al.*, 1982). Recently, Lee and Davis (1981) developed a technique to isolate sieve tubes from the phloem tissue, thus allowing direct examination of the spiroplasmas or other agents in the vascular elements. So far, no filamentous helical organisms were seen in plants showing typical yellows symptoms (Lee, personal communication; Chen, unpublished data).

Besides the yellows disease agents, several MLOs have recently been isolated from plant surfaces and cultured *in vitro* (Davis *et al.*, 1977; McCoy, 1979; Su *et al.*, 1978; Whitcomb, personal communication). Apparently, these microorganisms share the same ecological niches as those for the flower spiroplasmas. Because of their suspected saprophytic nature almost no efforts have been made to study them. One cannot rule out, however, that these plant surface MLOs may comprise a large portion of the genus *Mycoplasma* and may also have a close relationship with arthropods.

Many attempts were made to isolate and cultivate the yellows agents but they have been met with failures. There were claims that mycoplasmas or spiroplasmas were obtained from several yellows-diseased plants (Charbonneau *et al.*, 1979; Giannotti, 1974; Giannotti and Giannotti, 1978; Giannotti *et al.*, 1979; Kondo *et al.*, 1977; Lowe and Raju, 1978; Maramorosch, 1979; Maramorosch and Kondo, 1978; Raju and Nyland, 1978; Raju *et al.*, 1979). According to these reports, the isolated mycoplasmas may be acholeplasmas or bovine mycoplasmas while the spiroplasmas are closely related or identical to *S. citri.* Proof of pathogenicity with some of the isolates was declared in some cases (Giannotti and Giannotti, 1979; Maramorosch, 1979). Unfortunately, those results could not be confirmed in other laboratories. Although spiroplasmas can be occasionally isolated from several yellows-diseased plants in California they failed to produce the typical yellows symptoms on the original host (Kloepper *et al.*, 1982).

Since the MLOs have resisted the axenic cultivation, alternative methods have been tried, with some success, to maintain the yellows agents in plant tissue cultures (Mitsuhashi and Maramorosch, 1964; Petru *et al.*, 1971; Jacoli, 1974; Maia and Beck, 1976; McCoy, 1978). Plant tissues grown in tissue culture media, whether initiated from healthy or diseased plants, must contain phloem tissues in which the MLO can be introduced and grow. Callus tissues with no vascular elements would not support the multiplication of yellows agents (McCoy, 1979).

Attempts have been made to culture the Western X-disease agent in the excised salivary glands of the vector leafhopper maintained in different culture media (Sugiura and Nasu, personal communication; Sugiura *et al.*, 1977, 1978). Although glandular cells were long considered dead, positive infectivity assay of the MLO was obtained from 2 weeks to several months after the salivary glands were dissected and kept *in vitro.* Their results also demonstrated that the Western X-disease agent could not multiply in the culture media for *S. citri* or for corn stunt spiroplasma but it could survive in the nonliving insect cells kept in the spiroplasma-growth media for a long period (Sugiura, personal communication). One wonders whether the glandular cells actually provided the MLO with certain nutrients which were not supplied in the various media? Or, on the other hand, whether the cell membranes of the insect act as a screen to prevent certain toxic or unfavorable materials in the medium to be in contact with the MLO. Sugiura *et al.* (1978) showed Western X-disease agents not only unable to utilize certain protein-rich ingredients such as PPLO broth, serum, and tryptone but also unable to tolerate their presence in the medium.

IV. CULTIVATION OF OTHER FASTIDIOUS, WALLED PROKARYOTES

An increasing number of plant pathogenic or plant-associated bacteria are being encountered which are fastidious, walled prokaryotes. They are distinct from mycoplasmas and spiroplasmas because of their smooth or ribbed cell walls. They are also persuasively different from other plant bacteria because of their inability to grow on common bacteriological media including potato–dextrose, nutrient, King's medium B, corn meal, dextrose–tryptose, malt extract, or tripticase agars. Similarly unsatisfactory are the complex and semisynthetic media containing components or extracts of coconut, blood, or brain tissues such as chocolate agar, brain–heart infusion, and Mueller–Hinton agar.

Biochemical studies of some of the fastidious bacteria reveal that their differences from other bacteria extend beyond their nutritional requirements. The cellular fatty acid profiles and DNA composition (percentage moles G + C) of the fastidious Gram-negative bacteria are significantly different from other known taxa (Wells *et al.*, 1982; Wells, unpublished data).

A. Organization by Habitat and Gram Reaction

The fastidious bacteria investigated to this date can be ordered into groups based on their habitat in the plant and their Gram reaction. Habitats are limited to xylem tissues or to phloem and parenchyma tissues. There are no confirmed reports of one type of fastidious bacterium naturally occupying both habitats. Xylem-limited bacteria are either Gram-positive or Gram-negative. The Gram-negative nature of the cell wall of some xylem inhabitants has been confirmed (Raju, 1982; Wells, 1981a) by the presence of a peptidoglycan or R layer in the periplasmic space, an ultrastructural feature characteristic of Gram-negative bacteria (Glankert and Thornley, 1969). The Gram reaction of the phloem-limited organisms has not yet been reported; however, based on *in planta* observations, they appear to fall into one of two morphological types depending on cell wall ultrastructure and on reproductive process—the Chlamydiae-like bacteria and the Rickettsia-like bacteria. The Chlamydiae-like organisms resemble the initial bodies of Chlamydiae (Gutter *et al.*, 1973), particularly the membrane-bound structures released upon budding (Tanami and Yamada, 1973). They also possess a smooth membranous wall (8 nm wide) separated from the cytoplasmic membrane (also 8 nm wide) by an electron transparent zone 5–15 nm wide (Moll and Martin, 1974). Binary fission has not been observed in this group. The Rickettsia-like organisms are generally characterized by a trilaminated double membrane cell wall composed of a conspicuously rippled outer membrane (8 nm wide), an electron transparent zone 10–15 nm wide in which a lightly stained R layer can generally be distinguished, and a cytoplasmic membrane 8 nm wide. In some members of this group there is evidence of binary fission.

1. Xylem Inhabitants

a. Fastidious Gram-Positive Bacteria. i. Ratoon stunting disease (RSD) bacterium. Filamentous rods (0.25–0.35 × 2–5 μm) present in sugarcane (*Saccharum officinarum* L.) affected with ratoon-stunting disease (RSD) have been isolated and cultured on artificial media (Davis *et al.*, 1980a; Liao and Chen, 1981). Morphological and biochemical tests indicated that the RSD bacterium is a coryneform bacterium of an undetermined species.

ii. Bermuda grass bacterium (BGB). Filamentous rods similar to the RSD bacterium were observed in Bermuda grass (*Cynodon dactylon* L.) by Chen *et al.* (1977) and cultured on artificial medium by Liao and Chen (1981). The similarity to the RSD bacterium was further strengthened by serological cross-reactions. The bermuda grass organism, however, does not cause RSD. RSD and BGB together have a host range that also includes sorghum (*Sorghum vulgare* Pers.), Sudan grass [*S. vulgare* var. *sudanense* (Piper) Hitch.], and maize (*Zea mays* L.).

b. Fastidious Gram-Negative Bacteria. i. Plum leaf scald bacterium. Rod-shaped bacteria (0.35 × 5 μm) shown by Raju *et al.* (1982) to cause plum leaf scald disease (PLS) were isolated from plum (*Prunus americana* Marsh) and cultured on a medium modified from that used to grow *Legionella pneumophila* Brenner *et al.* (Wells *et al.*, 1981b). Biochemical and serological properties of the PLS bacterium are shared by other members of this group (Wells *et al.*, unpublished data). Wild plum (*Prunus angustifolia* L.) and cherry (*P. avium* L.) are other hosts for this bacterium.

ii. Phony peach disease bacterium. Rod-shaped (0.35 × 2–5 μm) bacteria present in roots of peach (*Prunus persica* [L.] Batsch) trees affected with phony disease (PPD) were isolated and cultured on the same medium used for the PLS bacterium. Although the PPD and PLS bacteria share elements of a common etiology (Wells *et al.*, 1981a), the PPD bacterium can be distinguished biochemically by the presence of a distinct component in the cellular fatty acid profile (Wells *et al.*, 1982). This bacterium also infects nectarine [*Prunus persica* var. *nectarina* (Ait.) Maxim.] and has been found in cherry.

iii. Ragweed (RGW) bacterium. A rod (0.35 × 2–5 μm) morphologically like the PLS and PPD bacteria was isolated on BCYE medium by Timmer *et al.* (1981) from symptomless stems of ragweed (*Ambrosia artemisifolia* L.) adjacent to a citrus (*Citrus* spp.) orchard. The ragweed bacterium also resembles a rod observed in stems of Johnson grass [*Sorghum halepense* (L.) Pers.] collected near a peach orchard (Weaver *et al.*, 1980).

iv. Pierce's disease bacterium. The causal organism of Pierce's disease (PD) of grapevine (*Vitis* spp.) (Davis *et al.*, 1978) is a rod (0.25–5 × 1.1–2.3 μm) serologically related to the PLS and PPD bacteria (Raju *et al.*, 1982). The PD bacterium was isolated on JD-2 and JD-3 media but also grows on BCYE medium and its modifications (Raju *et al.*, 1982). Other hosts include almond (*Prunus amygdalus* Batsch) and alfalfa (*Medicago sativa* L.).

v. Elm leaf scorch bacterium. A rod (0.3–0.4 × 0.9–2.4 μm) associated with leaf scorch (ELS) of elm (*Ulmus america* L.) was cultured on S8 medium by Kostka *et al.* (1981). The ELS bacterium also grows on BCYE medium and is biochemically and serologically related to the PLS, PPD, PD, and RGW bacteria (Raju *et al.*, 1982; Wells *et al.*, 1982), and to morphologically similar bacteria in the xylem of oak (*Quercus alba* L.) and sycamore (*Platanus occidentalis* L.) (Hearon *et al.*, 1980).

vi. Periwinkle wilt bacterium. The bacterium causing Periwinkle wilt (PW) is a fastidious rod (0.25–0.4 × 2–5 μm) requiring BCYE or modifications for isolation and growth (McCoy *et al.*, 1978). As with the other members of this group, the PW bacterium shares similar morphological, biochemical, and serological characteristics with PLS, PPD, PD, and RGW bacteria (Wells and Raju, unpublished data).

vii. Clove wilt bacterium. A rod (0.2–0.3 × 1.5–3.0 μm) was isolated on JD-3 medium by P. Jones, Rothamstead Expt. Station England (personal communication) from stems of Sumatra clove [*Syzygium aromaticum* (L.) Merr. and Perry] affected by wilt (CW). The clove bacterium also grows on BCYE medium and is serologically related to the Pierce's disease bacterium.

viii. Johnson grass (JSG) bacterium. A rod (0.3–0.4 × 2–5 μm) serologically related to the PLS, PPD, and PD bacteria was found by Weaver *et al.* (1980) in stems of Johnson grass. This organism has not yet been reported as cultured on any artificial medium. Success may be impeded by low concentrations of the bacterium in Johnson grass stems rather than by any factor mitigating against its growth on media such as JD-3 or BCYE (Wells, unpublished data).

ix. Bentgrass wilt bacterium (BWB). Rod-shaped bacteria (0.5 × 1–1.5 μm) limited exclusively to xylem vessels were observed in Toronto creeping bentgrass (*Agrostis palustris* Huds. cv. 'Toronto') affected with bacterial wilt (BW) (Roberts *et al.*, 1981). Ultrastructural details, such as rippled cell wall, were similar to those of bacteria associated with PD, PPD, and PLS.

x. Almond leaf scorch bacterium. The organism causing almond leaf scorch (ALS) (Lowe *et al.*, 1976) has been shown to be the same as the PD bacterium (Davis *et al.*, 1980b; Raju *et al.*, 1980).

2. Phloem Inhabitants

a. Chlamydiae-like Organisms (Gram Reactions Not Yet Determined). i. Clover club leaf bacterium. Rod-shaped (0.2 × 2.0 μm), smooth walled bacteria, were observed in crimson clover (*Trifolium incarnatum* L.) showing symptoms of club leaf disease (Windsor and Black, 1973). Similar rods were also observed in phloem elements of periwinkle stems. Liu and Black (1974) noted that the bacteria were motile in solutions containing 30% glycerol and ceased to be motile upon the addition of 0.4% mercuric chloride.

ii. Citrus greening bacterium. Smooth walled rods (0.3 × 3.0 μm) were observed in phloem sieve tube elements of infected sweet orange [*Citrus sinensis* (L.) Osbeck] leaf midribs and in the hemolymph of the citrus psyllid vector (Moll and Martin, 1974). The bacteria had a double membranous wall. Binary fission was not observed, and reproduction appeared to be by a budding process.

iii. Potato leaflet stunt bacterium. Rod-shaped bacteria (0.2–0.3 × 1.0–2.4 μm) were found in phloem cells of potatoes (*Solanum tuberosum* L.) with leaflet stunt disease (Klein *et al.*, 1976). The thin and smooth membranous wall of the bacterium, as well as other ultrastructural details, resemble those of the clover club leaf organism.

b. Rickettsia-like Organisms. i. Infectious necrosis of grapevine bacterium. A rod-shaped bacterium (0.25–0.5 × 1.1–2.4 μm) with rippled cell walls was observed by Ulrychová *et al.* (1975) in association with infectious necrosis of grapevines. Although the bacterium was morphologically similar to the Pierce's disease bacterium (PD), it was considered distinct because of its habitat and because it could not be isolated or cultured on the medium used for the PD bacterium.

ii. Rugose leaf curl of clover bacterium. A rod-shaped bacterium (0.25 × 1–2 μm) was observed in phloem sieve tubes and phloem parenchyma of clover affected with rugose leaf curl disease (Behncken and Gowanlock, 1976). The bacterium was rickettsia-like possessing a darkly staining, trilaminar, rippled cell wall or outer membrane with a distinct R layer.

iii. Apple proliferation bacterium. A rickettsia-like rod (0.35 × 1–3 μm) was observed in phloem, tracheids, parenchyma, and occasionally in xylem of apple (*Malus sylvestris* Mill.) trees affected with proliferation disease (Petzold *et al.*, 1973). Morphology and ultrastructural details of the bacterium including a rippled cell wall bear resemblance to those of the Pierce's disease bacterium.

iv. Little leaf of Sida bacterium. A rickettsia-like rod inhabiting sieve tube elements of the phloem but not the xylem of *Sida cordifolia* L. affected with little-leaf disease was described by Hirumi and Maramorosch (1974) in a preliminary report.

B. Cultivation of Xylem Inhabitants

1. *Growth and Nutritional Requirements*

a. Semisynthetic Media. Certain generalizations may be made with regard to the growth requirements of the xylem-limited bacteria based on successful culture of some of these organisms on complex semisynthetic media. These generalizations apply with varying degrees of importance depending on the specific bacterium, strain, host source, culture conditions, or passage. Late-passage or media-adapted subcultures, for example, of some organisms are significantly less fastidious than primary colonies from original isolations (Wells *et al.*, 1981b).

Xylem inhabitants require a source of hydrolyzed peptones or of yeast extract. This is the chief undefined component of all semisynthetic formulations. Casein, soy meal or corn meal digests, acidicase, and beef infusions or extracts are the chief sources of peptones utilized. More fastidious organisms such as the PLS and PPD bacteria require yeast extract. The use of yeast extract with additional NaCl, however, was inhibitory (Wells, unpublished data), thus the working assumption is that the more fastidious bacteria require a medium free of sodium ions or of NaCl, or that the required ionic balance is disturbed with added sodium.

L-Cysteine or certain other amino acid supplements such as glutamine, glutamic acid, and serine are considered necessary for optimum growth of all the xylem-limited bacteria studied, except for the PD bacterium. The PD bacterium may meet any amino acid requirements from those present in peptone or yeast extract or the bacterium may be able to synthesize the required amino acids from the carbon skeletons provided by the organic acids included in the medium. IsoVitale X, a component of the media for the RSD bacterium, contains L-cysteine among 11 other ingredients.

The xylem-limited bacteria require an unusually large amount of available iron for growth. All formulations of media contain iron supplements of varying degrees of solubility. The most readily soluble form is ferric pyrophosphate (available from Centers of Disease Control, Atlanta, GA). Other sources of iron such as hemoglobin, hemin chloride, or ferric nitrate are satisfactory for all but the most fastidious strains. The PLS and PPD bacteria require ferric pyrophosphate specifically for primary isolation from host tissues, but will grow on media substituted with hemin-chloride once established as late-passage subcultures.

Successful isolation or culture of most of xylem-limited bacteria requires the incorporation of starch, bovine serum albumin, or acid-washed activated charcoal into the medium. Starch may be introduced as a component of Mueller–Hinton broth or agar or added in the soluble form. Charcoal is a necessary ingredient for primary isolation media for the highly fastidious bacteria (Wells *et al.*, 1981b) but may be replaced by albumin or starch in late passage subcultures. Although there is some evidence for starch hydrolysis during the growth of some fastidious Gram-negative bacteria (Feeley *et al.*, 1978), the primary function of this group of components is probably to absorb and sequester inhibitory factors in host tissues that contaminate the medium during primary isolation and in media components. The importance of inhibitors in host tissue extracts is recognized and is also controlled with charcoal additives for the isolation of *Legionella pneumophila*, a fastidious Gram-negative rod infectious to man (Feeley *et al.*, 1979). The charcoal requirement for this organism in growth in liquid medium, however, was reportedly overcome by the sterilization of media by filtration instead of autoclaving (Ristroph *et al.*, 1980). Inhibitors are also believed to be involved for the lack of success in the isolation of Gram-negative rods from cherry trees artificially inoculated with the bacteria by root grafts (Wells *et al.*, 1980).

The pH range for growth of the bacteria is relatively narrow and growth is inhibited by acidification. The pH of media successfully used for individual members of the group ranges from 6.6 in SC and S8 media (Davis *et al.*, 1980a) to 7.1 in the supplemented Mueller–Hinton broth (Liao and Chen, 1981) for the RSD bacterium. The range coincides with that independently determined for the PLS bacterium (Wells *et al.*, 1981b). Buffering is essential to sustain growth due to acidification of the media. Inorganic potassium phosphate buffer is generally used, however, an organic buffer 2-([2-amino-2-oxoethyl] amino)-ethanesulfonic acid (ACES) is necessary for the primary isolation of the PLS bacterium although the phosphate buffer is satisfactory once late-passage subcultures have been established (Raju *et al.*, 1982).

b. Chemically Defined Media. A thorough examination of the basic nutritional requirements of the fastidious Gram-negative bacteria from plants has not yet been reported. However, much can be gleaned from preliminary studies and from the investigations on the nutritional requirements of *Legionella* spp., a group of bacteria remarkedly similar to the Gram-negative rods from plants.

The PD bacterium and the ELS bacterium have basic growth requirements for as few as nine amino acids, including L-cysteine, a supplementary source of soluble iron, trace concentrations of minerals (available as contaminants in agar), and growth factors (Wells, unpublished data). Deletion of one amino acid or of the iron supplement will reduce growth by 75% or more in the first passage on defined medium, and will prevent growth in subsequent passages. There is also preliminary evidence that the growth factors are unnecessary. The other fastidious Gram-negative rods do not grow on an amino acid–iron medium and may thus require more than the nine amino acids or particular combinations and concentrations of amino acids. Research is now underway to illucidate these requirements.

The remarkable simplicity of the nutritional requirements of some of the Gram-negative rods from plants belie their designation as fastidious organisms. Their fastidiousness may therefore be attributable to their sensitivity to inhibitors in host extracts or to inhibitory concentrations of substances commonly found in standard bacteriological media such as carbohydrates, ions, and other undetermined factors. Their simple nutritional requirements suggest complex metabolic capabilities including that of synthesis of all growth factors.

The pattern of simple growth requirements repeats that of *Legionella pneumophila*. Pine *et al.* (1979) developed a chemically defined medium containing 20 amino acids, pyruvate, and α-ketoglutaric acid and carbon sources for *L. pneumophila*. Tesh and Miller (1981) refined the basic medium to one containing only L-arginine, L-isoleucine, L-leucine, L-methionine, L-serine, L-threonine, L-valine, and L-glutamic acid. This medium also supports the growth of the PD and ELS bacteria (Wells, unpublished data).

2. *Media Composition*

a. Semisynthetic Media. The media formulated for the various xylem-limited bacteria are presented in Table I. The semisynthetic media were originally prepared for the RSD bacterium, the PD, and the PLS bacteria and generally support maximal growth compared to more limited growth on chemically defined minimal media.

A semisynthetic medium for one type of organism may serve equally well or better for another. The ELS bacterium, for example, was isolated from the S8 medium originally prepared for the RSD bacterium (Kotska

Table I. Composition* of Semisynthetic Media for the Isolation and Growth of Fastidious, Xylem-Limited, Gram-Negative and Gram-Positive Rods

Bacterium	Medium designation	Peptone or yeast extract
1. RSD	SMH	Mueller–Hinton agar, 38 g[a]
2. RSD	SC	Cornmea agar, 17 g; Soytone, 8 g
3. RSD/ELS	S8	Soytone, 8 g
4. PD	JD-1	PPLO broth base, 10 g[d]
5. PD	JD-2	Casitone, 7 g; Soytone, 3 g
6. PD	JD-3	Casitone, 4 g; Soytone, 2 g
7. PLS/PPB	BCYE	Yeast extract, 10 g
8. PLS/RGW	BZYE	Yeast extract, 10 g
9. PPD/PW	PW	Phytone peptone, 4 g Trypticase peptone, 1 g

Carbon supplement	Iron source	Mineral supplements
1. Asparagine, 2 g; glutamic acid, 0.5 g; sodium citrate, 0.1 g	Hemoglobin, 10 mg[b]	$(NH_4)_2SO_4$, 0.5 g; KH_2PO_4, 1 g; K_2HPO_4, 2.5 g; $CaCl_2$, 0.5 g; $ZnSO_4$, 0.01 mg; $CuSO_4$, 0.01 mg
2. L-Cysteine, 0.1 g;[b] glucose, 0.5 g[b]	Hemin–chloride, 15 mg[b]	K_2HPO_4, 1g; KH_2PO_4, 1 g; $MgSO_4 \cdot 7H_2O$, 0.2 g
3. L-Cysteine, 0.1 g; glucose, 0.5 g	Hemin–chloride, 15 mg	K_2HPO_4, 0.5 g; KH_2PO_4, 1.5 g
4. (None)	Hemin–chloride, 0.04 g[d]	(None)
5. Trisodium citrate, 2 g; disodium succinate, 2 g	Hemin–chloride, 0.01 g,[d] $FeCl_3 \cdot 6H_2O$, 0.002 g	$MnSO_4$, 0.002 g; $(NH_4)_2SO_4$, 1 g; $MgSO_4 \cdot 7H_2O$, 1 g
6. Trisodium citrate, 2 g; disodium succinate, 0.01 g	Hemin–chloride, 0.01 g[d]	K_2HPO_4, 1.5 g; KH_2PO_4, 1 g; $MgSO_4 \cdot 7H_2O$, 1 g
7. L-Cysteine–HCl, 0.4 g[b]	Ferric pyrophosphate,[b] soluble, 0.25 g	(None)
8. L-Cysteine–HCl, 0.4 g[b]	Ferric pyrophosphate,[b] soluble, 0.25 g	K_2HPO_4, 1 g; KH_2PO_4, 1 g; $MgSO_4 \cdot 7H_2O$, 0.2 g
9. Glutamine, 0.4 g	Hemin–chloride, 10 mg[d]	K_2HPO_4, 1.2 g; $MgSO_4 \cdot 7H_2O$, 0.4 g; KH_2PO_4, 1 g

Table I (*Continued*)

Additional components	Agar	pH	Reference
1. Isovitalex, 10 g[b]	(Included in peptone source)	7.1[c]	Liao and Chen (1981)
2. (None)	(Included in peptone source)	6.6	Davis *et al.* (1980a)
3. (None)	(None)	6.6	Davis *et al.* (1980b); Kostka *et al.* (1981)
4. Bovine albumin, 0.5 g[b,d]	Bacto-agar, 15 g	6.5[c]	Davis *et al.* (1978)
5. BSA fraction V, 3 g	Bacto-agar, 15 g	6.8[c]	Davis *et al.* (1978)
6. BSA fraction V, 2 g	Bacto-agar, 15 g	7.0[c]	Davis *et al.* (1978)
7. ACES buffer, 10 g[f]; charcoal (Norit SG), 2 g	Bacto-agar, 17 g	6.7	Wells *et al.* (1981b)
8. Starch, soluble, 2 g	Bacto-agar, 17 g[g]	6.6	Raju *et al.* (1982)
9. BSA fraction V, 0.6 g, Phenol red, 0.002 g	Granulated agar, 12 g[g]	6.9	Davis *et al.* (1981)

* Per 1000 ml distilled water.
[a] Or Mueller–Hinton broth.
[b] Filter-sterilized and added after autoclaving of basal medium at 50°C.
[c] pH adjusted with 0.1 *N* KOH before autoclaving.
[d] Hydrated in 10 ml 0.5 *N* NaOH.
[e] Hydrolized in 100 ml H_2O.
[f] Hydrated at 50°C in 500 ml H_2O, then mixed with 40 ml 0.1 *N* KOH.
[g] May be omitted to prepare broth medium.

et al., 1981); and the medium for the PLS bacterium is used for bacteria associated with PPD (Wells *et al.*, 1981b), PD (Raju *et al.*, 1982), and RGW (Lee *et al.*, 1981). A thorough study of relative growth rates or suitability of the various media for all isolated bacteria of this group has not yet been reported.

b. Chemically Defined Media [Amino acid–STABA Medium (Wells, Unpublished)]. The PLS and RGW bacteria grow on a minimal amino acid medium (Tesh and Miller, 1981) supplemented with STABA, or stock preparation growth factors. Medium composition includes, per 1000 ml distilled water, ACES buffer (Sigma), 10 g; activated charcoal (Norit SG), 2 g; ferric pyrophosphate, 0.25 g; L-arginine, 0.9 g; L-cysteine Hcl · H_2O, 0.4 g; L-glutamic acid, 1.65 g; L-isoleucine, 0.55 g; L-leucine, 0.55 g; L-methionine, 0.3 g; L-serine, 0.65 g; L-threonine, 0.45 g; L-valine, 0.60 g; Bacto-agar, 17 g; and 10 ml STABA stock solution. The STABA stock solution contains, per 1000 ml distilled water, folic acid, 50 mg; biotin, 100 mg; choline chloride, 100 mg; calcium panathenate, 100 mg; thiamine–HCl, 100 mg; nicotinamiate, 200 mg; pyrodoxine–HCl, 200 mg; and *p*-aminobenzoic acid, 50 mg. The ACES buffer is first hydrated in 740 ml distilled H_2O at 50°C and then 40 ml 1 *N* KOH, the charcoal, and agar is added. The basal mixture is autoclaved and cooled to 50°C. After warming to 50°C, the amino acids (dissolved in 200 ml distilled water and sterilized through a 0.20-μm filter), 10 ml ferric pyrophosphate solution, and 10 ml STABA stock solution are then added to the basal mixture, and, finally, the pH is adjusted to 6.7 with 1 *N* KOH or HCl.

3. *Isolation Techniques*

Successful isolation of the fastidious, Gram-negative rods from plants requires a host source relatively rich in bacteria and asceptic laboratory technique. Wells *et al.* (1981a) reported that tissues containing about 25 to 34 rods per microscopic field at 400 × ($1.4–1.9 \times 10^7$ cells/cm^3) was minimum for repeatable isolations of the PLS bacterium. Peach and plum tissues with less than 5×10^6 cells/cm^3 were not good sources. Tissues should be stripped of bark, surface disinfested in sodium hypochlorite, and rinsed in sterile distilled water. There are four general isolation methods for establishment of uncontaminated primary colonies for most of the fastidious Gram-negative bacteria.

a. Blotting of Xylem Sap on Agar. Roots, stems, or twigs are cut into 2-cm sections, stripped of bark, surface disinfested (for 5 min in 1% sodium hypochlorite solution containing 3% ethyl alcohol), and rinsed in sterile water. The disinfestation procedure is repeated two to four times. Sections are then placed in a sterile Petri dish and the ends are shaved aseptically to expose fresh xylem tissue. Sections are then placed in a hand vice and gently crushed while expressed sap from exposed ends are blotted onto the agar medium. Each agar plate may be inoculated with as many impressions as desired, but four to six are recommended when highly contaminated sources such as root tissues are involved (Davis *et al.*, 1978; Wells *et al.*, 1981a).

b. Liquid Inoculum from Centrifuged Sap. Root, stem, petiole, or twig samples are cut into 2-cm sections, stripped of bark, surface disinfested (three to five times), transferred into a sterilized screw-capped centrifuge tube containing 5–10 ml of filter-sterilized phosphate-buffered saline (PBS, 0.1 *M*, pH 6.6), and centrifuged at 20,000 *g* for 10 min. After centrifugation, the tube is shaken well and each plate then inoculated with 0.5 to 1.0 ml of the saline (Davis *et al.*, 1978; Raju *et al.*, 1982).

c. Liquid Inoculum from Macerated Tissues. Tissues are sectioned, stripped of bark, surface disinfested (three to five times), transferred to a sterilized mortar and pestle in laminator flow-hood, 10 ml of filter-sterilized PBS is added, and the tissues ground. The supernatant is collected into sterilized screw-capped test tubes and serial two-fold dilutions (up to 1 : 4096) made in PBS or sterile distilled water. These dilutions are then used for inoculating plates (Raju *et al.*, 1982).

d. Isolations from Tissue Wedges. With some tissues containing relatively high concentrations of bacteria and a low incidence of extraneous or contaminating organisms, isolations have been made by incubating intact tissue sections or wedges in the medium. This method should not be used for root tissues. Stem, twig, or petiole sections stripped of bark, surface disinfested (three to five times), and placed in a sterile Petri dish are sliced into wedges. The wedges are then transferred to screw-capped test tubes containing the desired broth medium or imbedded directly into agar (Kostka *et al.*, 1981).

4. *Growth in Culture*

Successful culturing of primary colonies or of established stock cultures requires constant attention of the physical growth conditions and to the status of the colonies or cultures. On occasions intuitive judgments must be exercised in the modification of procedures or conditions to accommodate requirements of strains with slightly variant characteristics. General guidelines may be outlined, however, for the culture of the fastidious Gram-negative bacteria.

a. Growth Conditions. The fastidious Gram-negative bacteria from plants are aerobes and thus require an unmodified normal atmosphere for growth. The PLS bacterium is inhibited in atmospheres of 1% oxygen (O_2) but not by 5% (Wells *et al.*, 1981b). The enrichment of atmosphere with carbon dioxide (CO_2) is reported to stimulate the growth of *L. pneumophila* on a charcoal–yeast extract medium (Feeley *et al.*, 1978) but not of the PLS or PPD bacteria growing on BCYE medium. The bacteria require an incubation temperature close to 20–25°C for growth on artificial media. The PLS bacteria does not grow at 15 or at 35°C (Wells *et al.*, 1981b). There are reports of optimal growth at 28°C of strains of the PLS organism (G. W. Gorman, CDC, Bacteriology Div., Atlanta, personal communication).

b. Subculturing. Bacterial isolates must be streaked onto fresh media every 7–30 days depending on the particular strain and medium. Primary colonies in early passage (first to sixth) tend to grow in discrete, encapsulated microcolonies and must be individually transferred by needle microtechnique. Late passage cultures tend to grow as uniform mats ("lawns") or streaks on the agar and may be subcultured by loop transfers. The PD bacterium must be subcultured every 5–10 days when grown on JD-3 medium with the starch base. Culture viability is extended on JD-2 with BSA (M. Davis, personal communication). The PLS and most fastidious Gram-negative organisms retain viability on BCYE or BSZE agar and may be subcultured every 21–28 days. Periodically, subculture morphology should be examined microscopically at 25 × to note changes in gross characteristics or to detect changes that may indicate contamination.

c. Growth Patterns. Continuous growth of first-passage subcultures of the PLS bacterium was measured for 58 days on BCYE agar at 25°C. Growth curves tended to be sigmoid (Wells *et al.*, 1981b). Growth of late passage subcultures was more rapid, entering stationary phase after 7–10 days. Growth of the other fastidious bacteria is similarly patterned once stock cultures are established on their respective media.

5. *Quantitation*

The fastidious Gram-negative bacteria can be quantified by standard bacteriological techniques.

a. Cell Counts. Concentration of cellular suspension may be estimated by cell counting. The fastidious Gram-negative rods are best examined by a microscope with phase contrast optics, thus an ocular micrometer must be adapted for use with phase microscopy. Cell concentrations have been expressed in terms of "cells per microscopic field" where magnification and field of vision are specified (Wells *et al.*, 1981a). Such measurements can be quickly converted to cells per cubic centimeter by use of a micrometer or by calculations based on volume of suspension medium under the microscope coverslip and the fraction of that volume represented by the field of vision.

b. Turbidity (Optical Density). Cell suspensions harvested by centrifugation and resuspended or sampled directly from nonopaque culture medium can be measured in terms of light scattering at 660 nm. The tendency of some strains, however, to grow in tightly knit filamentous colonies or as filamentous forms limits the use of this method. Colonies and some filaments can be fragmented by partial grinding in a sintered glass hemogenizer to improve linearity.

c. Colony Counting. Bacterial isolates that tend to grow as discrete colonies on a particular medium or early passage subcultures of the PLS bacterium and others may be quantified by counting numbers and sizes of colonies. Wells *et al.* (1981b) plotted sigmoidal growth curves by this method, and Edelstein (1981) evaluated improved media for *Legionella pneumophila* in a similar manner.

C. Cultivation of Phloem Inhabitants

The isolation and culture of the phloem-limited Gram-negative bacteria on artificial media are developments that are anticipated, particularly with the recent progress in the cultivation of the xylem-limited organisms. It is unlikely that there are factors intrinsic to the bacteria that would prevent their eventual culture. The remarkable similarities in the morphology and ultrastructure of the rickettsia-like phloem organisms to the Gram-negative xylem-limited rods, and the vector-borne etiology of both groups are convincing evidence that further similarities will be found. The probability exists that the phloem-limited bacteria will have metabolic requirements somewhat different from those of the xylem-limited organisms due to the enriched nature of the phloem contents. The phloem inhabitants may have a greater tolerance if not a requirement for elaborated carbohydrates in particular. The cultivation of the phloem inhabitants will then provide the technology for metabolic and biochemical studies that will lead to a determination of their proper taxonomic classification.

V. CONCLUDING REMARKS

The study of spiroplasmas, mycoplasmas, and fastidious, walled prokaryotes from plants is still in an early stage of discovery. New forms or associations of these organisms with plants are steadily being reported in the scientific literature. The gratification of discovery, however, is quickly followed by the challenge of culturing the organism *in vitro*. A researcher may benefit from an awareness that this group of organisms may share certain basic requirements for growth *in vitro*, but in most cases must overcome special problems created by the fastidiousness of the particular form.

Cultivation *in vitro* is a necessary preliminary to any definitive study of the organism. Taxonomic associations or characterizations are particularly dependent or information on nutritional properties and biochemical profiles. The entire problem of classification is unresolved in the case of the fastidious, walled prokaryotes. Although much has been accomplished in the cultivation of spiroplasmas and the xylem-limited fastidious bacteria, the full definition of a minimal defined medium is necessary. The plant MLOs and the phloem-limited fastidious bacteria have yet to be successfully cultured *in vitro*.

Probably the most engaging question related to the culture of the fastidious prokaryotes is the nature of their fastidiousness. Progress with those forms that have been cultured has come in spite of the absence of this knowledge. Even with fastidious bacteria such as *L. pneumophila* in which there has been developed a minimal defined medium, we can only speculate as to why they are so difficult to grow in the laboratory. There is agreement, however, on the importance of inhibitors during isolation rather than on the lack of specific nutrients in artificial media. Indeed, basic nutritional requirements appear to be remarkably simple. Substances inhibitory to cultivation *in vitro* may be introduced as contaminants from host tissues outside of the specific habitat of the organism. Inhibitors may also originate from nonessential components or impurities in the culture medium. Fastidiousness, therefore, may simply be an expression of the highly specialized ecological niche occupied by these organisms in nature. As our understanding of the ecology of the fastidious prokaryotes increases, and as our knowledge develops of the basic nutritional requirements of the forms already cultured, researchers should be able to create laboratory environments conducive to the growth of the most fastidious of these organisms. Research efforts can then progress into the areas of biochemistry and metabolism.

References

Behncken, G. M., and Gowanlock, D. H. (1976). *Aust J. Biol. Sci.* **29,** 137–46.

Bové, J. M., and Saillard, C. (1979). *In* "The Mycoplasmas: Cell Biology of Spiroplasmas" (R. F. Whitcomb and J. G. Tully, eds.), Vol. 3, pp. 83–153. Academic Press, New York.

Bové, J. M., Saglio, P., Tully, J. G., Freundt, E. A., Lund, Z., Pillot, J., and Taylor-Robinson, D. (1973). *Ann. N.Y. Acad. Sci.* **225,** 462–470.

Chang, C. J. (1981). PhD dissertation, Rutgers University, New Brunswick, New Jersey.

Chang, C. J., and Chen, T. A. (1979a). *Int. Congr. Plant Protect, 9th* No. 647.

Chang, C. J., and Chen, T. A. (1979b). *Phytopathology* **69,** 1024.

Chang, C. J., and Chen, T. A. (1981a). *Phytopathology* **71,** 559.

Chang, C. J., and Chen, T. A. (1981b). *Phytopathology* **71,** 866.

Chang, C. J., and Chen, T. A. (1981c). *Phytopathology* **71,** 866.

Chang, C. J., and Chen, T. A. (1982). *Science* **215,** 1121–1122.

Charbonneau, D. L., Hawthorne, J. D., Ghiorse, W. C., and Vandemark, P. J. (1979). *Proc. ASM Annu. Meet., Los Angeles, May.*

Chen, T. A., and Davis, R. E. (1979). *In* "The Mycoplasmas: Cultivation of Spiroplasmas" (R. F. Whitcomb and J. G. Tully, eds.), Vol. 3, pp. 65–82. Academic Press, New York.

Chen, T. A., and Granados, R. R. (1970). *Science* **167,** 1633–36.

Chen, T. A., Su, H. J., Raju, B. C., and Huang, W. C. (1977). *Proc. Am. Phytopathol. Soc.* **4,** 231.

Clark, H. F. (1964). *J. Infect. Dis.* **114,** 476–487.

Clark, T. B. (1978). *Am. Bee J.* **118,** 18–19, 23.

Coe, A. W. K., and Clark, S. P. (1966). *Mon. Bull. Ministry Health* **25,** 97–100.

Cotty, P. J., Liao, C. H., and Chen, T. A. (1978). *Phytopathol. News* **12,** 234.

Cotty, P. J., Liao, C. H., and Chen, T. A. (1980). *Proc. Conf. Intl. Organ. Mycoplasmol., 3rd.*

Davis, M. J., Purcell, A. H., and Thompson, S. V. (1978). *Science* **199,** 75–77.

Davis, M. J., Gillaspie, A. G., Jr., Harris, R. W., and Lawson, R. N. (1980a). *Science* **210,** 1365–67.

Davis, M. J., Thomson, S. V., and Purcell, A. H. (1980b). *Phytopathology* **70,** 472–475.

Davis, M. J., French, W. J., and Schaad, N. W. (1981). *Curr. Microbiol.* **6,** 309–314.

Davis, R. E. (1978a). *Can. J. Microbiol.* **24,** 954–959.
Davis, R. E. (1978b). *Phytopathol. News* **12**(7), PO-7.
Davis, R. E. (1979). *Proc. ROC-US Coop. Sci. Semin. Mycoplasma Dis. Plants NSC Symp. Ser.* I, pp. 59–65.
Davis, R. E., Worley, J. F., and Basciano, L. K. (1977). *Proc. Am. Phytopathol. Soc.* **4,** 185–186.
Davis, R. E., Lee, I.-M., and Basciano, L. K. (1979). *Can. J. Microbiol.* **25,** 861–66.
Davis, R. E., Lee, I.-M., and Worley, J. F. (1981). *Int. J. Syst. Bacteriol.* **31,** 456–464.
Doi, Y., Teranaka, M., Yora, K., and Asuyama, H. (1967). *Ann. Phytopathol. Soc. Jpn.* **33,** 259–266.
Edelstein, P. H. (1981). *J. Clin. Microbiol.* **14,** 298–303.
Fabiyi, A., Elizan, T. S., and Pounds, J. E. (1971). *Proc. Soc. Exp. Biol. Med.* **136,** 88–91.
Feeley, J. C., Gorman, G. W., Weaver, R. E., Mackel, D. C., and Smith, H. W. (1978). *J. Clin. Microbiol.* **8,** 320–325.
Feeley, J. C., Gibson, R. J., Gorman, G. W., Langford, N. C., Rasheed, J. K., Mackel, D. C., and Blaine, W. B. (1979). *J. Clin. Microbiol.* **10,** 437–441.
Freeman, B. A., Sissenstein, R., McManus, T. T., Woodward, J. E., Lee, I.-M., and Mudd, J. B. (1976). *J. Bacteriol.* **125,** 946–54.
Fudl-Allah, A. E. A., Calavan, E. C., and Igwegbe, E. C. K. (1971). *Phytopathology* **61,** 1321.
Fudl-Allah, A. E. A., Calavan, E. C., and Igwegbe, E. C. K. (1972). *Phytopathology* **62,** 729–737.
Giannotti, J. (1974). *Colloq. Inst. Natl. Santé Rech. Med.* **33,** 99–106.
Giannotti, J., and Giannotti, D. (1978). *Ann. Phytopathol.* **10,** 489–92.
Giannotti, J., Vago, C., and Giannotti, D. (1979). *C. R. Acad. Sci. Ser. D* **288,** 85–87.
Glankert, A. M., and Thornley, M. J. (1969). *Microbiology* **23,** 159–198.
Granados, R. R., and Meehan, D. J. (1975). *J. Invertobr. Pathol.* **26,** 313–20.
Gutter, B., Asher, Y., Cohen, Y., and Becker, Y. (1973). *J. Bacteriol.* **115,** 691–702.
Haggis, G. H., and Sinha, R. C. (1978). *Phytopathology* **68,** 677–80.
Hearon, S. S., Sherald, J. L., and Kostka, S. J. (1980). *Can. J. Bot.* **58,** 1986–1993.
Hirumi, H., Himura, M., Maramorosch, K., Bird, J., and Woodbury, R. (1974). *Phytopathology* **64,** 581–82.
Igwegbe, E. C. K., Stevens, C., and Hollis, J. J., Jr. (1979). *Can. J. Microbiol.* **25,** 1125–1132.
Ishiie, T., Doi, Y., Yora, K., and Asuyama, H. (1967). *Ann. Phytopathol. Soc. Jpn.* **33,** 267–275.
Jacoli, G. G. (1974). *Can. J. Bot.* **52,** 2085–2088.
Jones, A. L., Whitcomb, R. F., Williamson, D. L., and Coan, M. E. (1977). *Phytopathology* **67,** 738–46.
Klein, M., Zimmerman-Gries, S., and Snek, B. (1976). *Phytopathology* **66,** 564–69.
Kloepper, J. W., Garrott, D. G., and Oldfield, G. N. (1982). *Phytopathology* **72,** 577–581.
Kondo, F., Maramorosch, K., McIntosh, A. H., and Varney, E. H. (1977). *Proc. Am. Phytopathol. Soc.* **4,** 190 (Abstr.).
Kostka, S. J., Sherald, J. L., Hearon, S. S., and Rissler, J. F. (1981). *Phytopathology* **71,** 768 (Abstr.).
Lee, I.-M. (1977). PhD thesis, University of California, Riverside.
Lee, I.-M., and Davis, R. E. (1978). *Phytopathol. News* **12,** 215.
Lee, I.-M., and Davis, R. E. (1981). *Annu. Meet. Am. Phytopathol. Soc.* **181.**
Lei, J. D., Su, H. J., and Chen, T. A. (1979). *Proc. ROC-US Coop. Sci. Semin. Mycoplasma Dis. Plants NSC Symp. Ser.* **I,** 89–98.
Liao, C. H., and Chen, T. A. (1975). *Proc. Am. Phytopathol. Soc.* **2,** 53.

Liao, C. H., and Chen, T. A. (1977). *Phytopathology* **67,** 802–807.
Liao, C. H., and Chen, T. A. (1980). *Can. J. Microbiol.* **26,** 807–811.
Liao, C. H., and Chen, T. A. (1981). *Phytopathology* **71,** 1303–1306.
Liao, C. H., Cotty, P. J., and Chen, T. A. (1979). *Proc. ROC-US Coop. Sci. Semin. Mycoplasma Dis. Plants.*
Liu, H. Y., and Black, L. M. (1974). *Colloq. Inst. Natl. Santé Rech. Med.* pp. 97–98.
Lowe, S. K., and Raju, B. C. (1978). *Phytopathol. News* **12,** 216.
Lowe, S. K., Nyland, G., and Mircetich, S. M. (1976). *Phytopathology* **66,** 147–151.
McBeath, J. H., and Chen, T. A. (1973). *Proc. Int. Congr. Plant Pathol., 2nd, Minneapolis.*
McCoy, R. E. (1978). *Proc. Int. Counc. Lethal Yellowing, 3rd, 1977, Univ. Fla. Agric. Res. Rep.* **78–2,** p. 20.
McCoy, R. E. (1979). *In* "The Mycoplasmas: Mycoplasmas and Yellows Diseases" (R. F. Whitcomb and J. G. Tully, eds.), Vol. 3, pp. 229–264. Academic Press, New York.
McCoy, R. E., Thomas, D. L., Tsai, J. H., and French, W. J. (1978a). *Plant Dis. Rep.* **62,** 1022–1026.
McCoy, R. E., Tsai, J. H., and Thomas, D. L. (1978b). *Phytopathol. News* **12,** 217.
McCoy, R. E., Williams, D. S., and Thomas, D. L. (1979). *Proc. ROC-US Coop. Sci. Semin. Mycoplasma Dis. Plants, NSC. Symp. Ser.* **I,** 75–81.
McCoy, R. E., Davis, M. J., and Dowell, R. V. (1981). *Phytopathology* **71,** 408–411.
Maia, E., and Beck, D. (1976). *Ann. Phytopathol.* **8,** 303–306.
Malloy, K. M., and Chen, T. A. (1980). *Phytopathology* **70,** 465 (Abstr.).
Malloy, K. M., and Chen, T. A. (1981). *Phytopathology* **71,** 892.
Maramorosch, K. (1952). *Nature (London)* **169,** 194–95.
Maramorosch, K. (1979). *Proc. Am. Soc. Microbiol.* **79,** 85.
Maramorosch, K., and Kondo, F. (1978). *Zentralbl. Bakteriol. Parasitenkd. Infektionskr. Hyg. Abt. 1 Orig. Reihe A* **241,** 196 (Abstr.).
Mitsuhaski, J., and Maramorosch, K. (1964). *Virology* **23,** 277–279.
Moll, J. N., and Martin, M. M. (1974). *Colloq. Inst. Natl. Santé Rech. Med.* pp. 97–98.
Mudd, J. B., Ittig, M., Roy, B., Latrille, J., and Bové, J. M. (1977). *J. Bacteriol.* **129,** 1250–56.
Norman, M. C., Franck, E. B., and Choate, R. V. (1970). *Appl. Microbiol.* **20,** 69–71.
Petru, E., Limberk, J., Ulrychová, M., and Break, J. (1971). *Biol. Plant.* **13,** 391–395.
Petzold, H., Marwitz, R., and Kunze, L. (1973). *Phytopathol. Z.* **78,** 170–81.
Pickens, E. G., Gerloff, R. K., and Burgdorfer, W. (1968). *J. Bacteriol.* **95,** 291–299.
Pine, L., George, J. R., Reeves, M. W., and Harrell, W. K. (1979). *J. Clin. Microbiol.* **9,** 615–626.
Raju, B. C., and Nyland, G. (1978). *Phytopathol. News* **12,** 216.
Raju, B. C., Purcell, A. H., and Nyland, G. (1979). *Proc. Meet. Int. Counc. Lethal Yellowing, 4th, Ft. Lauderdale* p. 12.
Raju, B. C., Nomé, S. F., Docampo, D. M., Goheen, A. C., Nyland, G., and Lowe, S. K. (1980). *Am. J. Enol. Vitic.* **31,** 144–148.
Raju, B. C., Wells, J. M., Nyland, G., Brylansky, R. H., and Lowe, S. K. (1982). *Phytopathology* **72** (in press).
Razin, S. (1978). *Microbiol. Rev.* **42,** 414–470.
Ristroph, J. D., Hedlund, K. W., and Allen, R. G. (1980). *J. Clin. Microbiol.* **11,** 19–21.
Roberts, D. L., Vargas, J. M., Jr., Detweiler, R., Baker, K. K., and Hooper, G. R. (1981). *Plant Dis.* **65,** 1014–1016.
Rodwell, A. W. (1974). *Inserm (Colloq. Inst. Natl. Santé Rech. Med.)* **33,** 79–86.
Rose, D. L., Tully, J. G., and Whitcomb, R. F. (1979). *Proc. Am. Soc. Microbiol.* **79,** 84.
Saglio, P., and Whitcomb, R. F. (1979). *In* "The Mycoplasmas: Diversity of All Lesser

Prokaryotes in Plant Vascular Tissue, Fungi, and Invertebrate Animals" (R. F. Whitcomb and J. G. Tully, eds.), Vol. 3, pp. 1–36. Academic Press, New York.

Saglio, P., Laflèche, D., Bonissol, C., and Bové, J. M. (1971a). *C. R. Hebd. Seances Acad. Sci. Ser. D* **272,** 1387–1390.

Saglio, P., Laflèche, D., Bonnisol, C., and Bové, J. M. (1971b). *Physiol. Veg.* **9,** 569–582.

Saglio, P. M., L'Hospital, M., Laflèche, D., Dupont, G., Bové, J. M., Tully, J. G., and Freundt, E. A. (1973). *Int. J. Syst. Bacteriol.* **23,** 191–204.

Stanek, G., Laber, G., and Hirschl, A. (1980). *Conf. IOM., 3rd Sept.*

Steindl, D. R. L. (1961). *In* "Sugarcane Disease of the World; Ratoon Stunting Disease" (J. P. Martin, E. W. Abbott, and C. G. Hughes, eds.), Vol. 1, pp. 433–459. Elsevier, Amsterdam.

Steiner, Th., Gamon, L., Levine, E., and McGarrity, G. (1980). *In Vitro* **16,** 216.

Su, H. J., Lei, J. D., and Chen, T. A. (1978). *Proc. Int. Congr. Plant Pathol., 3rd* p. 61.

Sugiura, M., Shiomi, R., Nasu, S., and Mizukami, T. (1977). *Trop. Agric. Res. Ser.* No. 10, 85–91.

Sugiura, M., Shiomi, T., and Nasu, S. (1978). *In* "Plant Diseases Due to Mycoplasma-like Organisms: Attempts at Axenic Culture of Some Mycoplasma-like Organisms," pp. 166–174. FFTC Book Series No. 13.

Tanami, Y., and Yamada, Y. (1973). *J. Bacteriol.* **114,** 408–412.

Tesh, M. J., and Miller, R. D. (1981). *J. Clin. Microbiol.* **13,** 865–869.

Timmer, L. W., Brlansky, R. H., Raju, B. C., and Lee, R. F. (1981). *Phytopathology* **71,** 909 (Abstr.).

Townsend, R. (1976). *J. Gen. Microbiol.* **94,** 417–420.

Townsend, R., Markham, P. G., Plaskitt, K. A., and Daniels, M. J. (1977). *J. Gen. Microbiol.* **100,** 15–21.

Tully, J. G., Whitcomb, R. F., Williamson, D. L., and Clark, H. F. (1976). *Nature* (*London*) **259,** 117–120.

Tully, J. G., Whitcomb, R. F., Clark, H. F., and Williamson, D. L. (1977). *Science* **195,** 892–94.

Ulrychová, M., Vanek, G., Jokes, M., Klobáska, Z., and Králik, O. (1975). *Phytopathol. Z.* **82,** 254–65.

Vignault, J. C., Bové, J. M., Saillard, C., Vogel, R., Farro, A., Venegas, L., Stemmer, W., Aoki, S., McCoy, R., Al-Beldri, A. S., Larue, M., Tuzcu, O., Ozsam, M., Nhami, A., Abassi, M., Bonfils, J., Moutous, G., Fos, A., Poutiers, F., and Viennot-Bourgin, B. (1980). *C. R. Acad. Sci. Paris Ser. D* **290,** 775–78.

Vogelzang, A. A. (1975). *Z. Versuchstierkd.* **17,** 240–246.

Weaver, D. J., Raju, B. C., Wells, J. M., and Lowe, S. K. (1980). *Plant Dis.* **64,** 485–487.

Wells, J. M., Weaver, D. J., and Raju, B. C. (1980). *Phytopathology* **70,** 817–820.

Wells, J. M., Raju, B. C., Thompson, J. M., and Lowe, S. K. (1981a). *Phytopathology* **71,** 1156–1161.

Wells, J. M., Raju, B. C., Nyland, G., and Lowe, S. K. (1981b). *Appl. Environ. Microbiol.* **42,** 357–363.

Wells, J. M., Raju, B. C., and Kostka, S. (1982). *Phytopathology* **72,** 267 (Abstr.).

Whitcomb, R. F. (1980). *Annu. Rev. Microbiol.* **34,** 677–709.

Whitcomb, R. F., and Williamson, D. L. (1975). *Ann. N.Y. Acad. Sci.* **266,** 260–75.

Whitcomb, R. F., Williamson, D. L., Rosen, J., and Coan, M. (1974). *Colloq. Inst. Natl. Santé Rech. Med.* **33,** 275–282.

Williamson, D. L., and Poulson, D. F. (1979). *In* "Mycoplasmas" (R. F. Whitcomb and J. G. Tully, eds.), Vol. 3, pp. 175–208. Academic Press, New York.

Williamson, D. L., and Whitcomb, R. F. (1974). *Colloq. Inst. Natl. Santé Rech. Med.* **33,** 283–290.

Williamson, D. L., and Whitcomb, R. F. (1975). *Science* **188,** 1018–20.

Williamson, D. L., Tully, J. G., and Whitcomb, R. F. (1979). *Int. J. Syst. Bacteriol.* **29,** 345–351.

Windsor, I. M., and Black, L. M. (1973). *Phytopathology* **63,** 1139–1148.

Chapter **21**

Preservation of Phytopathogenic Prokaryotes

JOHN P. SLEESMAN

I. INTRODUCTION

A. Problems

In vitro survival and preservation of prokaryotes have been intensively investigated by many workers, especially in medicine and food technology. Maintenance of surviving and unchanged microbes is a prerequisite for successful scientific investigation and for industrial ap-

Phytopathogenic Prokaryotes, Vol. 2

Copyright © 1982 by Academic Press, Inc.
All rights of reproduction in any form reserved.
ISBN 0-12-509002-1

plications. Type-culture collections are important as repositories of useful microbes. Clark and Loegering (1967), in their review of type-culture collections, pointed out that scientists have a responsibility to see that the particular organism used in their investigation be stored for possible future use and reference by others. Microbes developed by selection, mutation, and genetic manipulation may be inherently unstable (Breese and Sharp, 1980); this poses an additional problem for preservation.

Regrettably, many investigators have experienced the loss of important cultures during their careers. This is unfortunate from a scientific standpoint, since verification and other studies are then impossible. Some strains may be changed rather than lost. This might mean that important physical, biochemical, physiological, and/or pathogenic properties are not constant.

B. Objectives

First, I will examine the factors known to affect *in vitro* survival of prokaryotes. Because there has been little work on plant pathogens in this area, I will draw heavily on experiences with nonplant pathogenic bacteria for insights. Since any type of storage method used will inherently involve some selection factors, an understanding of these factors should aid in the design of preservation methods that maximize survival in an unchanged form. As more is learned about prokaryote survival, better and more efficient preservation methods will be discovered.

Methods for prokaryote maintenance and their relative effectiveness will be reviewed and discussed. Results of preservation of plant pathogenic bacteria will be examined in some detail, and experiences with nonplant pathogenic bacteria less, to help derive generalities. Although few wall-less plant pathogenic bacteria (mycoplasmas) have been cultured, mention is made of the various ways other members of this group have been preserved. Similarly, few plant pathogenic actinomycetes are recognized, but preservation of other actinomycetes is described.

A given method has advantages and disadvantages, depending on the needs of the individual investigator. Scientists working with plant pathogenic prokaryotes are faced with the problems of keeping and losing valuable strains. Since the working plant pathologist is often in a field situation with the minimum of instrumentation, he needs simple, reliable methods for prokaryote storage. In Section IV, I make suggestions based on my preference for various methods. Perhaps this discussion will inspire new ideas and stimulate further research.

II. FACTORS AFFECTING *in Vitro* SURVIVAL

A. General Considerations

Obviously, in agricultural systems, plant pathogenic prokaryotes are quite successful in season-to-season or natural survival. Our endeavors to enhance *in vitro* survival of phytopathogenic prokaryotes for preservation purposes could well be advanced by consideration of some of the principles involved in field survival.

Leben (1974, 1981) used the term hypobiosis to describe plant pathogens in a state of reduced metabolism. He suggested that plant pathogenic bacteria in nature survive environmental extremes in a hypobiotic state. Attainment of the hypobiotic condition is probably the result of natural aging and drying processes in diseased host tissue. He concluded that one important means of natural survival is presumably by hypobiotic cells in association with dry plant tissue. Perhaps cell survival is aided by protective chemicals produced in the host–pathogen interaction. In temperate regions, seasonal cold temperatures are undoubtedly important to survival since they reduce metabolic activity of tissue degrading saprophytes as well as pathogens. Structural characteristics of host tissue (e.g., woody stems) may also protect bacterial cells, aiding their survival. Pathogens on lesioned debris in the field are less likely to survive in soil than when they are on soil. Dry seed is an excellent vehicle for transfer of bacterial pathogens; epidemics of many annual crop plants begin this way.

Thus, in attempts to preserve prokaryotes, various workers have employed methods similar to natural survival. Two conditions favoring hypobiosis, desiccation and low temperature, are easily handled in the laboratory. In fact, they have long been recognized as the basis for the most successful preservation methods. Additionally, investigators have recognized the advantage of using suspending media that afford protection to stored cells. Conditions that induce hypobiosis *in vitro* as well as manipulations enhancing survival will be discussed in this section. Fundamental facts concerning hypobiosis presented here can and should be carefully considered as the different methods of preservation are discussed in the following section.

1. Temperature

a. General Effects. The relationship between low temperature and low metabolic activity is well established. The specific temperatures involved vary with the microbe, since temperature ranges for growth differ depending on the psychrophilic, mesophilic, and thermophilic nature of the organism. Whether microorganisms are stored on culture media, in host tissue, in water, by drying, or by freeze-drying, many workers combine these methods with low temperature storage. Low temperature is a relative term and I will adopt the following terminology: (1) refrigerator temperatures, ~5–10°C; (2) normal freezer temperatures, ~−20°C; (3) moderately low temperatures, ~−30 to −100°C, obtainable with special mechanical freezers; and (4) ultralow temperatures, the temperature of liquid nitrogen (−196°C). Not surprisingly, many organisms are stored successfully by freezing at moderately and ultralow temperatures.

The temperature comparisons in Table I for phytopathogenic bacteria indicate that, in nearly all cases, the best survival occurred at the lower temperatures; survival was favored by refrigerator versus room, freezer versus refrigerator, and ultralow versus freezer temperatures. A similar survival trend, which shows a positive correlation between an increase in temperature and death rate, has been reported for nonphytopathogenic prokaryotes (Table II). These studies show a survival advantage for moderately low versus freezer/refrigerator and ultralow versus moderately low temperatures. Several investigators have outlined temperatures that they felt would substantially favor storage. Wilson and Miles (1964) suggested that microbial cultures could be stored indefinitely below −70°C. Likewise, Calcott (1978) reported that bacteria exhibit a considerably reduced death rate below −80°C. Rates of chemical and physical changes in organisms are reduced to a minimum below −130°C (Martin, 1964) and all metabolic activity is suspended at −196°C (Wilson and Miles, 1964). Bridges (1966) stated that *Escherichia coli* (Migula) Castellani & Chambers could be maintained indefinitely at −196°C and that exponential growth of thawed cultures was restored within one normal generation time.

b. Mechanisms of Damage. Since prokaryote survival is favored by the use of moderately and ultralow temperatures, discussion of the possible mechanisms involved is in order. The problem with low temperature storage is successfully overcoming the concomitant stresses. Keeping in mind that remedies will be discussed at length later, let us examine the variables. The stresses encountered in low temperature storage include cold shock, freezing, thawing, ice crystal formation, and dehydration effects resulting from concentration of solutes (Calcott, 1978; MacLeod and Calcott, 1976).

These reviewers noted that cold shock, which can cause injury and death, occurred when sensitive organisms were chilled prior to actual freezing. Rapid cooling rates favored cold shock damage, whereas little

Table I. Effect of Temperature on Survival of Phytopathogenic Prokaryotes

Species	Storage temperature (°C) Most favorable	Less favorable	Preservation-method	References
Agrobacterium tumefaciens (Smith & Townsend) Conn	−20	5	Dried	Sleesman and Leben (1978)
	−172 to −196	−20	Frozen	Moore and Carlson (1975)
Corynebacterium michiganense (Smith) Jensen	5	20	Dried	Sleesman and Leben (1976a)
	−20	5 to 35	Soil	Basu (1970)
	−20	5	Dried	Sleesman and Leben (1978)
Corynebacterium nebraskense (Schuster *et al.*) emand Vidaver & Mandel	−20	5	Dried	Sleesman and Leben (1978)
Erwinia amylovora	1 to 16	20 to 40	Dried	Rosen (1938)
(Burrill) Winslow *et al.*	−172 to −196	−20	Frozen	Moore and Carlson (1975)
Erwinia carotovora (Jones) Bergey *et al.*	5	20	Dried	Sleesman and Leben (1976a)
	−20	5	Dried	Sleesman and Leben (1978)
	−172 to −196	−20	Frozen	Moore and Carlson (1975)
Erwinia stewartii (Smith) Dye	−20	5	Dried	Sleesman and Leben (1978)
Pseudomonas azadirachtae Desai *et al.*	5 to 10	19 to 39	Water	Srivastava and Patel (1968)
Pseudomonas cepacia (ex Burkholder) nom. rev. Palleroni & Holmes	5	20	Dried	Sleesman and Leben (1976a) (Antagonist AN 771)
Pseudomonas syringae pv. *glycinea* (Coerper) Young *et al.*	5	20	Dried	Sleesman and Leben (1976a)
	−20	5	Dried	Sleesman and Leben (1978)
Pseudomonas syringae pv. *lachrymans* (Smith & Bryan) Young *et al.*	−20	5	Dried	Sleesman and Leben (1978)
Pseudomonas syringae pv. *phaseolicola* (Burkh.) Young *et al.*	−20	5	Dried	Sleesman and Leben (1978)
	−172 to −196	−20	Frozen	Moore and Carlson (1975)
Pseudomonas solanacearum (Smith) Smith	−20	5	Dried	Sleesman and Leben (1978)
	Room	Refrigerator	Water	Berger (1970)

(*Continued*)

Table I. (*Continued*)

Species	Storage temperature (°C) Most favorable	Less favorable	Preser-vation-method	References
Pseudomonas syringae pv. *syringae* van Hall	−20	5	Dried	Sleesman and Leben (1978)
Xanthomonas campestris pv. *campestris* (Pammel) Dowson	−20	5	Dried	Sleesman and Leben (1978)
Xanthomonas campestris pv. *citri* (Hasse) Dye	10 to 13 (refrigerator)	12 to 39 (room)	Dried	Bagga (1967a,c)
Xanthomonas campestris pv. *malvacearum* (Erw. Smith) Dye	10 to 13	12 to 39	Dried	Bagga (1967a,c)
Xanthomonas campestris pv. *nigromaculans* f. sp. *zinniae* Hopkins & Dowson	−20	5	Dried	Sleesman and Leben (1978)
Xanthomonas campestris pv. *oryzae* (Uyeda & Ishiyama) Dye	1 to 16	20 to 40	Dried	Hsieh and Buddenhagen (1975)
Xanthomonas campestris pv. *phaseoli* (Erw. Smith) Dye	5	20	Dried	Sleesman and Leben (1976a)
	−20	5	Dried	Sleesman and Leben (1978)
	−25	5 and 20	Dried	Leach *et al.* (1957); Wilson *et al.* (1965)
Xanthomonas campestris pv. *pruni* (Smith) Dye	−172 to −196	−20	Frozen	Moore and Carlson (1975)
Xanthomonas rubrilineans (Lee *et al.*) Starr & Burkholder	10 to 13	12 to 39	Dried	Bagga (1967a,c)

injury occurred if chilling was slow. Cold shock increased cell permeability due to cytoplasmic membrane and cell wall damage. In studies with *E. coli*, Leder (1972) proposed that cold shock from rapid chilling may be related to crystallization of membrane lipids resulting in hydrophilic channels, permitting rapid efflux of permease-accumulated substrate; presumably, with a slow chilling rate, the membrane integrity is maintained by rearrangement of relatively mobile lipid chains.

The nature of damage due to freezing also has been linked to cell permeability changes (Calcott, 1978; MacLeod and Calcott, 1976). In studies with *E. coli*, Bretz and Hartsell (1959) found that frozen cells were osmosensitive upon thawing and postulated that this might be due to changes in the cell wall. In further work with *E. coli*, Rey and Speck

(1972) suggested freeze-thaw damage affects the outer lipopolysaccharide layer of the cell wall of Gram-negative bacteria, since frozen cells demonstrated increased sensitivity to surface-active agents and lysozyme. Evidence also exists that freezing–thawing can result in damage to the cytoplasmic membrane, as evidenced by leakage of materials from the cells (Calcott, 1978; MacLeod and Calcott, 1976).

The stresses of freezing and thawing are directly related to ice crystal formation and solute accumulation. Freezing constitutes the removal of pure water from an aqueous solution by formation of ice crystals (Meryman, 1956). From this simple definition, it is obvious that solute concentration of the unfrozen portion increases. Furthermore, with slow freezing and the resultant formation of intercellular ice, free water would be withdrawn from the cell, progressively increasing the concentration of cell constituents including electrolytes, proteins, and carbohydrates (Grieve and Povey, 1981; Meryman, 1956).

Table II. Effect of Temperature on Survival of Nonphytopathogenic Prokaryotes

Organism	Storage temperature (°C)		Preservation method	Reference
	Most favorable	Less favorable		
Actinomycetes, mycoplasmas	−20	4 to 37	Frozen	Ford (1962); Klienberger-Nobel (1962); Kuznetsov *et al.* (1972)
Bacteria	12	26 to 45	Water	Granai and Sjogren (1981)
	−20	−1 to −10	Frozen	Haines (1938); Mackey *et al.* (1980)
	−195	−1.5 to −78	Frozen	Weiser and Osterud (1945)
Bacteria, mycoplasmas	0 to 15	20 to 45	Dried	Annear (1970); Banno *et al.* (1978); Iijima and Sakane (1973); Koshi *et al.* (1977); McDade and Hall (1963a); Thorns (1979); Trollope (1975)
	4 to 10	21 to 43	Freeze-dried	Addey *et al.* (1970); Clement (1961); Marshall *et al.* (1974); Proom and Hemmons (1949)
Mycobacteria	−25 to −70	4	Freeze-dried	Lind (1967)
Treponemes, mycobacteria, mycoplasmas	−65 to −70	5 to −40	Frozen	Addey *et al.* (1970); Hollander and Nell (1954); Kelton (1964); Kim and Kubica (1972, 1973)

MacLeod and Calcott (1976) noted that the increase in solute concentration further reduced the freezing point of the remaining solution. This continues to occur as the temperature is lowered until the eutectic point is reached, below which the concentrated solution solidifies. The time period from initiation of freezing until this point is reached depends on the freezing rate (Mazur, 1966b). Thus, the rate of freezing also determines the duration of exposure to high solute concentrations. Haines (1938) hypothesized that damage due to freezing was a result of denaturation of macromolecules, possibly proteins, by high concentrations of salt.

Several persons noted that the most damaging temperature range for frozen storage of bacteria was −10 to −40°C because eutectic mixtures with water are formed (Ashwood-Smith, 1965; Bridges, 1966; LaPage *et al.*, 1970). In this range the deleterious effect of solute concentration overrides the more positive aspects of slowing metabolic activity (Meryman, 1956).

A second theory of freeze injury was put forth by Keith (1913) who felt that the lethal agent was ice crystal-caused membrane damage. Meryman (1956) associated rapid freezing with intracellular ice crystallization and mechanical damage. Mazur (1970) concluded that freezing exposed cells to loss of liquid water and increased concentrations of intra- and extracellular solutes, whether the cells equilibrate by dehydration (slow cooling) or by intracellular freezing (rapid cooling). Although very rapid freezing rates caused formation of small, unstable, nondamaging intracellular ice crystals, if cells are subjected to slow warming, these crystals grow by recrystallization, resulting in membrane damaging crystals (Mazur, 1966b). Thus, with rapidly cooled preparations, rapid warming is essential to minimize recrystallization; however, with slowly cooled cells, warming rate is less important. Mazur (1966b) felt that slow cooling rates preventing intracellular ice formation are less damaging. Optimum cooling rates will vary with the organism, but generally the optimum cooling rate for some bacteria ranges from 6 to 10°C/min (Calcott, 1978).

Mazur (1966a) proposed a two-factor hypothesis as a cause of cell death due to freezing and thawing. The first factor operates at slow freezing rates and is related to dehydration denaturation. The second operates at rapid freezing rates and is connected with the damaging effects of intracellular ice formation. Evidence to support this hypothesis was developed by Calcott and MacLeod (1974) in trials with *E. coli*. When frozen in water of saline, *E. coli* survival increased to a maximum at cooling rates of 6°C/min before decreasing to a minimum at 100°C/min. Survival increased to another peak with further increases in cooling rates to about 6000°C/min. At this ultrarapid cooling rate, rapid warming was essential to maintain the survival benefit of rapid cooling. Presumably with *E. coli,* cooling rates of less than 6°C/min would lengthen the time of detrimental exposure to concentrated solutes; rates of 100°C would involve formation of large, damaging intracellular ice crystals; and rates of 6000°C/min would result in formation of small, unstable but nondamaging ice crystals. Calcott *et al.* (1976) reported similar results with bacteria from five other genera.

In general, freezing and thawing deoxyribonucleic acid (DNA) does not result in genetic changes (Ashwood-Smith, 1965; Calcott, 1978). Working with *Salmonella gallinarium* (Klein) Bergey *et al.*, Sorrels *et al.* (1970) indicated that metabolically injured cells had increased nutrient requirements. Since properly handled injured cells repaired this damage, this change was not due to mutation. In one report, however, among 2135 *Enterobacter aerogenes* Hormaeche & Edward freeze-thaw survivors, 0.14% were auxotrophic mutants (Postgate and Hunter, 1963).

2. *Drying*

a. General Effects. Drying has been used extensively, either alone or, more commonly, in combination with lowered temperatures, as a means of preserving prokaryotic organisms. Successful utilization of desiccation for preservation depends on the species and the drying conditions. Certain plant pathogenic bacteria are extremely sensitive to drying (Jones, 1901; Kauffman, 1972; Kawamoto and Lorbeer, 1972; Nwigwe, 1973; Sleesman and Leben, 1976a). For efficient preservation of phytopathogenic prokaryotes, drying sensitivities must be taken into account. Other variables will be appraised here also, including responses to (1) different relative humidity (RH) and residual moisture levels, (2) drying with and without vacuum as related to drying rate and storage injury due to various gases, and (3) rehydration. Evidence for membrane and genetic damage as a result of desiccation will also be discussed.

Survival of most dried plant pathogenic bacteria was favored by storage at 0–34% RH; in one instance, *Xanthomonas campestris* pv. *phaseoli* (Smith) Dye survival was best at 51% RH (Table III). Survival was not promoted by the higher RHs and exposure of bacteria to 75% RH was lethal. A survival trend is apparent in relation to rate of drying. For quick dried bacteria, 71% of the most favorable RH entries in Table III were in the 0–5% range; with slow dried cells, only 29% of such entries were in the 0–9.5% range, whereas 71% were at 20–51% RH.

Reports on other dried bacteria confirm a general trend of decreasing

Table III. Effect of Desiccation on Survival of Phytopathogenic Bacteria

Species	Percentage relative humidity (RH)		Rate of drying[a]	Reference
	Most favorable	Less favorable		
Agrobacterium tumefaciens	0	34, 75	Quick	Leben and Sleesman (1981)
Corynebacterium michiganense pv. *michiganense*	34	0, 75	Slow	Sleesman and Leben (1976a)
Corynebacterium nebraskense	0, 34	75	Quick	Leben and Sleesman (1981)
Erwinia amylovora	0	Laboratory air	Slow	Rosen (1936)
	0, 9.5, 21	45	Slow	Rosen (1938)
Erwinia carotovora	34	0, 75	Slow	Sleesman and Leben (1976a)
Erwinia stewartii	0	34, 75	Quick	Leben and Sleesman (1981)
Pseudomonas cepacia	34	0, 75	Slow	Sleesman and Leben (1976a)
Pseudomonas syringae pv. *glycinea*	34	0, 75	Slow	Sleesman and Leben (1976a)
Pseudomonas syringae pv. *lachrymans*	34	0, 75	Quick	Leben and Sleesman (1981)
Pseudomonas syringae pv. *phaseolicola*	0	34, 75	Quick	Leben and Sleesman (1981)
Pseudomonas solanacearum	0	34, 75	Quick	Leben and Sleesman (1981)
Pseudomonas syringae pv. *syringae*	0, 34	75	Quick	Leben and Sleesman (1981)
Xanthomonas campestris pv. *campestris*	0, 34	75	Quick	Leben and Sleesman (1981)
Xanthomonas campestris pv. *citri*	0, 5	25, 50, 75	Quick	Bagga (1967a)
Xanthomonas campestris pv. *malvacearum*	0, 5	25, 50, 75	Quick	Bagga (1967a)
Xanthomonas campestris pv. *nigromaculans* f. sp. *zinnae*	0, 34	75	Quick	Leben and Sleesman (1981)
Xanthomonas campestris pv. *oryzae*	0, 20, 30	54, 68, 76, 100	Slow	Hsieh and Buddenhagen (1975)
Xanthomonas campestris pv. *phaseoli*	20	0, 51	Slow (5, 20°C)	Leach *et al.* (1957); Wilson *et al.* (1965)
	51	0, 20	Slow (−25°C)	Leach *et al.* (1957); Wilson *et al.* (1965)
	0, 20	51	Quick (5, −25°C)	Leach *et al.* (1957); Wilson *et al.* (1965)
	34	0, 75	Slow	Sleesman and Leben (1976a)
Xanthomonas rubrilineans	0, 5	25, 50, 75	Quick	Bagga (1967a)

[a] Quick dried, suspensions dried over calcium sulfate, calcium chloride, or silica gel prior to exposure to different RHs; slow dried, suspensions placed at different RHs and allowed to dry.

survival with increasing storage RH. Work with various species showed that survival was favored at 10–33% RH as compared to survival obtained at 53–85% RH (McDade and Hall, 1963a,b, 1964; Turner and Salmonsen, 1973). Monk and McCaffrey (1957) related different amounts of sorbed water to RH levels in which lyophilized bacteria were rewetted. Little effect on survival occurred with water contents below 15% and above 70%, but death rate increased in increasing water content to 33% and decreased thereafter up to 92%. In one test, the log death rate increased progressively through the RH values of 15, 29, 50, 70, and 94% (water content of 2.9, 4.8, 7.6, 15, and 19%, respectively) (Monk *et al.*, 1956). In the other test, survival was nearly equal at 15, 31, and 52% RH (5.2, 7.4, 11% water content, respectively), but became increasingly poorer at 75 and 94% RH (18 and 31% water content, respectively) (Monk and McCaffrey, 1957).

Residual moisture may be expressed in terms of water activity (a_w). In this work, optimum a_w for survival was determined by storing dried organisms in air or *in vacuo* over saturated salt solutions of known water activity. Presumably, the a_w value of the dried preparation came into equilibrium with the a_w value of the solutions (Asada *et al.*, 1980; Scott, 1958). Thus, a_w value can easily be related to percentage RH (e.g., 0.22 a_w corresponds to 22% RH). Survival of lyophilized bacteria after storage *in vacuo* was generally favored at 0.00–0.22a_w versus 0.33–0.53a_w. Optimum a_w for survival depended on the suspending medium and storage atmosphere (Scott, 1958). For example, cells suspended in water and stored in air survived best at 0.43a_w and worst at 0.00a_w. Studies on the interactions of various gases and a_w during storage indicated that the differences between gases are related to the level of residual water present; a residual water level of about 0.10a_w was recommended regardless of suspending medium or storage atmosphere (Marshall *et al.*, 1973).

Survival may be increased by storing prokaryotes at low residual moisture levels. With air-dried lactic acid streptococci milk cultures, preparations at 0.9 and 1.39% moisture survived storage better than those at 5.77% (Rogers, 1914). Strange and Cox (1976) recommended a residual moisture of 0.5–1.5% for optimum survival of freeze-dried bacteria. Likewise, LaPage *et al.* (1970) observed that complete dessication of cells resulted in total death of freeze-dried bacteria and that suspending media such as glucose enhance survival by retaining approximately 1% of the water content. Nei *et al.* (1965) also reported death of freeze-dried microbes in which nonfreezable water was removed during secondary drying after extensive desiccation. With *Streptomyces* species, it has been recommended that residual moisture of lyophilizates be maintained within a narrow range and at a low level for optimum survival (Kapetanovic and Pavletic, 1972).

Drying rate is important in prokaryote survival. Generally, rapid drying allows better survival (Martin, 1964). Quick-dried bacterial phytopathogens were less sensitive to a wider range of storage RHs and temperatures than slow dried cells (Leach *et al.*, 1957; Leben and Sleesman, 1981; Sleesman and Leben, 1976a; Wilson *et al.*, 1965). Survival of streptococci was greatly favored by rapid drying (Rogers, 1914). With L-drying (drying *in vacuo* from the liquid state without freezing), survival was less with larger volumes of cells and subsequent increased drying times (Fisher, 1950). Iijima and Sakane (1973) found that for *E. coli* to reach a 10% moisture level, L-drying required only 30 min compared to 3 hr for freeze-drying. These authors suggested that this rapid drying was less stressful than freeze-drying and might correlate with increased survival observed for bacteria sensitive to freeze-drying.

Storage atmosphere is another important variable. Martin (1964) recommended that dried microorganisms be preserved *in vacuo* in the cold. Various gases have been compared with air and *in vacuo* storage atmospheres. Several researchers reported better survival of dried bacteria *in vacuo* or in nitrogen as compared with storage in carbon dioxide, oxygen, air, argon, helium, neon, krypton, or xenon (Marshall *et al.*, 1973; Naylor and Smith, 1946; Proom and Hemmons, 1949; Rogers, 1914). The lethal effects of oxygen and air on dried bacteria have been shown (Morton and Pulaski, 1938; Stark and Herrington, 1931). An advantage of storing dried bacteria *in vacuo* is that absorption of moisture is prevented.

Another major stress encountered in drying of prokaryotes is rehydration. Anderson and Cox (1967) recommended the use of liquids of high osmotic pressure to rehydrate dried bacteria and lessen osmotic shock. Leach and Scott (1959) reported that slow rehydration of microorganisms by successive addition of small volumes of water lessened osmotic shock; survival was also enhanced by use of concentrated sugar or sugar alcohols as rehydrating solutions. Record *et al.* (1962) obtained much higher survival of freeze-dried bacteria by rehydrating in a solution of high osmotic pressure followed by slow dialysis to a more normal environment versus rehydration directly in water. In our survival studies with bacterial phytopathogens, we found that the dried bacteria were recovered in highest numbers by rehydrating in a 200 g/liter sucrose solution (Sleesman and Leben, 1976a).

b. Mechanisms of Damage. Probable sites of desiccation injury include membranes and genetic material. In their discussion of survival of microbes in aerosols, Anderson and Cox (1967) noted that the process of dehydration and hydration are likely to have a detrimental effect on proteins, structural elements, and nucleic acids. In collection of airborne bacteria, these workers suggested that rehydration, which results in an increase in osmotic pressure, may cause minor damage or may rupture membranes.

Three explanations for dehydration damage were proposed by Monk and McCaffrey (1957). First, physical damage to the structure of macromolecules or gross cellular organization may be involved. Second, depletion of sorbed water may result in denaturation of important cell substances. Third, partial metabolism may continue and either deplete the cell of the necessary substances or cause toxic compounds to accumulate. Partial metabolic activity has been detected at 33% water content (Monk *et al.*, 1957). They proposed that toxic hygroscopic substances may form which are in solution at 33% water content. At lower or higher water contents, these substances presumably would not be in solution in sufficient quantities to be toxic or their concentrations would be diluted.

It has been suggested that desiccation removes water from the protein structure resulting in collapse and some irreversible change (Webb, 1959). Certain compounds, when added to suspensions of bacteria prior to aerolization, protect cells during periods of desiccation (Webb, 1960a). This protective property may be due to the substance replacing water molecules in the protein structure through hydrogen bonding.

Desiccation damage may also be related to disruption of the cellular membranes (Webb, 1960b). In support of this hypothesis, the release of large amounts of UV light-absorbing materials and an increase in membrane permeability has been observed for lyophilized and rehydrated cells (Sinskey and Silverman, 1970; Wagman, 1960).

Nucleoprotein damage may contribute to death of bacteria from desiccation (Webb, 1961). Bacterial mutations as a result of desiccation have been reported (Ashwood-Smith, 1978; Servin-Massieu and Cruz-Camarillo, 1969; Tanaka, 1979; Webb, 1967). Likewise, physical damage to DNA including strand breakage has been observed (Asada *et al.*, 1980; Banno *et al.*, 1978). Mutations were induced by drying wild type *E. coli* to an a_w of 0.53 and below; mutation frequency increased as a_w decreased below 0.53 (Asada *et al.*, 1980). Ashwood-Smith (1978) indicated that with freeze-dried *E. coli*, maximum mutation rate may be between 3 and 4% residual moisture.

B. Manipulations to Enhance *in Vitro* Survival

1. *Growth Media*

The composition of growth media can have significant effects on bacteria, including survival and recovery from preservation stresses. Effects of growth medium have been noted with plant pathogenic bacteria. The number of *Pseudomonas solanacearum* (Smith) Smith variants detected after storage differed with the growth medium (Kelman, 1956). Extracellular polysaccharides in bacterial exudates have been reported to provide protection to bacteria from desiccation (Wilkinson, 1958; Wilson *et al.*, 1965). With *X. c.* pv. *phaseoli*, polysaccharide production was influenced by the carbon source; glucose, mannose, and sucrose proved best (Leach *et al.*, 1957). These investigators proposed that the increased resistance of *X. c.* pv. *phaseoli* in exudate to dessication was due to the retention of sufficient moisture by the hydrophilic polysaccharide.

Evidence indicates that the condition of bacteria prior to application of stresses can be influenced by the growth medium. Bacteria grown on a rich, complex medium or media allowing abundant growth were more tolerant to cold shock, freeze-drying, and exposure to an aqueous environment than those grown on simple, defined, or carbon-limited ones (LaPage *et al.*, 1970; Strange and Ness, 1963; Strange *et al.*, 1961). Such a survival advantage to cold shock may be related to an increased quantity of unsaturated fatty acid residues in the membrane lipid (Farrell and Rose, 1968). In the case of freezing and storage in liquid nitrogen, Smittle *et al.* (1974) observed increased survival of lactobacilli when sodium oleate supplemented the growth medium. Radioisotope data indicated that sodium oleate was incorporated solely into the lipid portion of the cells. They suggested that the protective characteristic associated with sodium oleate may be due to an effect on fatty acid composition in maintaining cell membrane integrity.

The fact that stresses employed in preservation techniques often cause sublethal or "reversible" injury to bacteria is well documented. Strange and Cox (1976) noted that reversibly injured microbes may fully recuperate if given an appropriate recovery environment. Both rich and minimal recovery media have been reported to favor bacterial recovery, depending on the organism and the stress involved. Various bacteria injured by freezing exhibited increased nutritional requirements; recovery was enhanced by use of rich recovery media (Arpai, 1962; Mossel *et al.*, 1980; Sorrells *et al.*, 1970; Yamasato *et al.*, 1973). In contrast, recovery of some freeze- or heat-injured bacteria was better in minimal media or one in which the nutrient concentrations had been diluted (Gomez *et al.*, 1973; Wilson and Davies, 1976; Yamasato *et al.*, 1978). Selective media may often be more toxic to injured than normal cells (Mossel *et al.*, 1980; Wilson and Davies, 1976).

Postgate (1976) discussed substrate accelerated death in which a particular substance, usually a carbon source or its metabolite, may be toxic under conditions where it was growth limiting in the medium from which the bacterial population was taken and present both in the starvation environment and the recovery medium. Therefore, a recovery medium enriched with this growth-limiting substance may be detrimental to accurate determination of cell viability.

2. *Culture Age*

Generally, bacterial cells from older cultures have been found to be more resistant to stress conditions than are cells from younger cultures. Some information is available on the effect of culture age on survival of plant pathogenic prokaryotes.

In studies with five plant pathogenic bacteria, survival to desiccation of cells from 1, 7, 14, 22, and 30 day cultures was compared; in general, superior survival was obtained with cells from 7 or 14 day cultures (Sleesman and Leben, 1976a). A similar trend was noted for *P. s.* pv. *glycinea* (Coerper) Young *et al.* cells from 7, 15, and 23–29 day lesions on soybean leaves. Survival was best with cells from the 15 day lesions. Similarly, *P. aeruginosa* (Schroeter) Migula cells from 7 day cultures survived desiccation best while cells from the exponential phase were most susceptible (Skaliy and Eagon, 1972).

The effects of culture age on survival of other prokaryotes have been observed for stresses including desiccation, L-drying, freeze-drying, cold shock, freezing, heat, aqueous environments, and chemicals. Many reports indicate that survival to these stresses are better endured by stationary phase cells rather than exponential phase cells (Calcott, 1978; Hurst *et al.*, 1974; Iijima and Sakane, 1973; Mackey *et al.*, 1980; Naylor and Smith, 1946; Sherman and Albus, 1923; Steinhaus and Birkeland, 1939; Strange and Cox, 1976). Conversely, with a mycoplasma strain, it has been found that survival after freeze-drying was better with cells from 24 versus 48 hr cultures (Addey *et al.*, 1970). The better survival of midstationary bacterial cells compared to logarithmic phase cells in an aqueous environment may be due to the fact that these older cells are better able to mobilize and use stored macromolecules (Granai and Sjogren, 1981).

3. *Cell Concentrations*

Another important variable affecting survival of prokaryotes is the cell concentration. In general, increased survival to stresses such as cold shock, freezing, freeze-drying, and aqueous environments is correlated with high cell populations.

Regarding cold shock, Strange and Dark (1962) observed that survival of *E. aerogenes* Hormaeche & Edwards at colony-forming units (CFU) greater than 10^9/ml was not significantly affected, but losses were much greater with lower cell concentrations. Use of dense populations in freezing and thawing favored survival of some bacterial species but not others (Major *et al.*, 1955). The cryoprotective effect of nonionic detergents was enhanced by high initial cell numbers, whereas cell density did not affect survival with the protectant glycerol (Calcott and Postgate, 1971). Calcott (1978) concluded that cell concentration does not affect immediate survival to freezing and thawing, but exerts its protective effect during frozen storage. LaPage *et al.* (1970) suggested that optimal survival with freeze-drying is favored by the use of dense cell suspensions; 10^{10} CFU/ml were recommended for *E. coli.* For successful preservation of mycobacteria by freeze-drying, cell concentrations of 10^5–10^7 CFU/ml were advised (Slosarek *et al.*, 1976).

In experiments with bacteria stored in aqueous suspension, Strange *et al.* (1961) suggested that survival was related to nutrients leaked from dead cells enabling survivors to grow and divide. Postgate (1976) proposed a threshold phenomenon; above a certain threshold cell concentration, either protective substances were exuded from dead cells or toxic compounds were rendered harmless by the population.

4. *Suspending Media*

As mentioned earlier, phytopathogenic bacteria often survive in nature in close association with some protective substance (exudate) and/or structure (host tissue). The principle of using a protective substance to enhance *in vitro* survival of prokaryotes is extensively documented in the literature. Various protective substances have been utilized to enhance survival to stresses including cold shock, freezing, drying, and freeze-drying.

a. Cold Shock Protectants. Cold shock injury to susceptible cells can be prevented by addition of substances such as magnesium, manganese, and calcium in the chilling fluid (Calcott, 1978). Additionally, susceptibility was decreased with increased osmolarity of the suspending medium (Leder, 1972).

b. Cryoprotectants. Cryoprotectants have been divided into two classes, those that penetrate cells and those that do not (Meryman, 1971). Glycerol and dimethyl sulfoxide (DMSO) are examples of penetrating types while nonpenetrating protectants include sucrose, Tween 80, and polyvinylpyrrolidone (MacLeod and Calcott, 1976).

Calcott (1978) further distinguished between substances that protected cells from freeze-thaw damage and those that protect against storage damage. Postgate and Hunter (1961) compared several compounds for protectant effect against these two types of stress. They found that glycerol, diethylene glycol, sucrose, and *i*-erythritol provided excellent protection (95–96% survival) against freeze-thaw damage; however, after storage at −20°C, only glycerol had maintained significant protective effect.

Little information is available on the effect of suspending media on survival of phytopathogenic prokaryotes for low temperature storage. Kennedy (1965), in trials with storage of *P. s.* pv. *glycinea* for 6–7 months at −15°C, found better survival with glucose as a suspending medium than water or glycerol. Moore and Carlson (1975) found that the best suspending medium for storage of *Agrobacterium tumefaciens* (Smith & Townsend) Conn and *Erwinia amylovora* (Burrill) Winslow *et al.*, at −20°C was skim milk when compared to distilled water, fresh yeast dextrose broth (YDP), fresh YDP + DMSO, or direct freezing in the culture medium (YDP). In the same publication, storage tests at −172 to −196°C with five genera of phytopathogenic bacteria showed that for most skim milk was superior but for others it was one of the worst medium. In even the worst medium, although bacterial numbers were often reduced greatly, sufficient cells survived for practical preservation.

Much more information is available on nonphytopathogenic prokaryotes relating to the beneficial effect of different suspending media. Glycerol and DMSO at concentrations of 10–15% were excellent cryoprotectants for many organisms (Bridges, 1966; Feltham *et al.*, 1978; Greiff and Meyers, 1961; Hollander and Nell, 1954; Sanfilippo and Lewin, 1970; Tanguay, 1959). Higher concentrations of both compounds were reported to be detrimental (Feltham *et al.*, 1978; Greiff and Meyers, 1961) and some bacteria have been found to be sensitive to these cryoprotectants (Hollander and Nell, 1954; Sanfilippo and Lewin, 1970). Glycerol was shown to be superior in cryoprotectant properties to water, gelatin, soluble vegetable oil, glucose, serum, and lactose (Boulanger and Portelance, 1975; Clement, 1961; Squires and Hartsell, 1955). Other compounds shown to be effective cryoprotectants include oxoid barley malt extract, sorghum malt extract, honey, sodium glutamate, sucrose, succinimide, and yeast extract (Johannsen, 1972; Yamasato *et al.*, 1973). Combinations of compounds such as dextran + sucrose + sodium glutamate and skim milk + L-malic acid, acetamide, succinimide, or apple juice have proved effective (Boulanger and Portelance, 1975; Gibson *et al.*, 1966).

Some information is available on the mechanism involved in cryoprotection of prokaryotes. Earlier we discussed the types and mechanisms of damage associated with freezing and thawing. Now we will discuss the basis for cryoprotectant effects.

Substances such as sugars and glycols have the characteristic in common of being strong hydrogen bonders and may limit the degree of dehydration in the cells by reducing the amount of water available to crystallize (Farrant, 1965; Meryman, 1956). Mazur (1970) proposed that most cryoprotectants protect cells from solute effects during freeze-thawing rather than against intracellular ice formation. Further, he stated that cryoprotectants may be capable of affording protection by acting at the cell surface and may not need to penetrate the cells to be protective. In support of this, Ray (1978) has reported that both penetrating and nonpenetrating cryoprotective compounds prevented damage to the lipopolysaccharide at the surface of *E. coli* cells and suggested that these two types of compounds may differ more in their mode of action than in their site of action. Nonpenetrating protectants protect cells from excessive osmotic gradients by allowing reversible influx and efflux of solute during the freeze-thaw process (Meryman, 1971). Calcott (1978), however, stated that nonpenetrating protectants act mainly with rapid freezing rates and suggested that they may minimize seeding of ice crystals across the cell membrane or may prevent extracellular ice formation.

c. Desiccation Protectants. Several authors have noted that protective media are of primary importance for successful use of drying or freeze-drying as maintenance methods (Annear, 1970; Fennel, 1960; Sourek, 1974). Two suspending media, 10% skim milk and 10% milk + 15% glycerol, have been compared for protective characteristics on 13 isolates of plant pathogenic bacteria to drying on silica gel (Leben and Sleesman, 1982; Sleesman and Leben, 1978). The milk–glycerol medium favored survival of several species after 18 and 60 months storage at 5 and −20°C, respectively.

Various substances have been reported to be protective against desiccation for some nonphytopathogenic prokaryotes. Stamp (1947) recommended nutrient gelatin plus ascorbic acid as a protectant for bacteria dried *in vacuo,* but Stephens (1957) found that casein, glucose, mucin, skim milk, and sucrose provided better protection. Scott (1958) reported survival of a dried bacterium was highest in sucrose, intermediate in glucose, and poorest in arabinose and water.

d. Freeze-Drying Protectants. Suspending media for freeze-drying should protect organisms during the various stages: freezing, dehydration, storage, and rehydration (Sourek, 1974). LaPage *et al.* (1970) noted that suspending media for use in freeze-drying in addition to being protective, should allow easy recovery; substances which form a cake on drying and thus protect against mechanical damage were recommended. The best protective media vary with the organism to be stored (Sourek, 1974).

Simple protective substances include glucose, sucrose, lactose, galactose, sodium glutamate, and sodium aspartate; more complex suspending media included serum, serum proteins, gelatin, skim milk, broth, dextran, starch, polyvinylpyrrolidone, and peptone (Fry, 1966; Martin, 1964). Combinations of the above mentioned substances also are useful. These include *mist desiccans* (serum + broth + glucose), peptone + starch + glutamate + gelatin, skim milk + glutamate, horse serum + mesoinositol, sucrose + glutamate + semicarbazide, and blood + lactose + gelatin (Abe, 1973; Marshall *et al.*, 1974; Martin, 1964; Redway and LaPage, 1974; Slosarek *et al.*, 1976; Sourek and Kulhanek, 1969).

With mycoplasmas, Addey *et al.* (1970) found that freeze-drying in liquid growth medium was successful; addition of bovine plasma albumin resulted in a slight advantage but additives such as milk and dextrose-dextran were detrimental. Lyophilization of an actinomycete was favored in horse serum as compared with nonfat milk or a mixture of gelatin and glucose (Kuznetsov *et al.*, 1977).

In a detailed study of 45 compounds chemically related to the protectant glutamic acid, effective protection was related to the presence of a hydrogen bond generating group and two acid groups (Morichi *et al.*, 1963). Several researchers have suggested that the protective action of substances such as sugars and amino acids to desiccation-type stress may be related to maintenance of sufficient residual moisture (Fry and Greaves, 1951; Obayashi and Cho, 1957).

III. PRESERVATION METHODS

The effectiveness of various preservation methods will be examined in this section. Frozen storage at freezer and moderately low temperatures are compared in the same subsection; results with ultralow temperatures are discussed separately. Preservation at refrigerator temperatures is cited only in conjunction with one of the other storage techniques.

A. Freezer and Moderately Low Temperatures

Frozen storage techniques require maintenance of constant low temperatures since alternate freezing and thawing is often harmful (Tuite, 1969). Frozen storage can be especially useful with organisms that are particularly sensitive to desiccation or freeze-drying methods. A major disadvantage of this method is reliance on mechanical refrigerators and continuous electric power.

Information has been reported on several plant pathogenic bacteria stored at household freezer and moderately low temperatures. *P. s.* pv. *glycinea* survivors were pathogenic after 6–7 months storage in 10% glucose at −15°C, but repeated freezing and thawing was harmful (Kennedy, 1965). Pathogenicity and antibiotic resistance of *X. c.* pv. *phaseoli* was not affected by storage at −20°C in nutrient broth plus 15% glycerol; however, the number of survivors decreased with increasing length of storage (Quadling, 1960). Survival of *A. tumefaciens, E. amylovora, P. s.* pv. *phaseolicola* (Burkholder) Young *et al.*, and *X. c.* pv. *pruni* (Smith) Dye decreased progressively over a 6-month period of storage at −20°C in culture growth medium (Moore and Carlson, 1975). Strains of 20 bacterial species including *A. tumefaciens* and *X. c.* pv. *translucens* (Jones *et al.*) Dye were reported to survive over 2 years after storage in 15% aqueous glycerol at −40°C (Clement, 1964). Thirteen phytopathogenic bacteria from five genera survived and were pathogenic after 18–30 months storage in 15% aqueous glycerol at −70°C (Sleesman and Leben, 1978).

Much the same type of data has been reported for other prokaryotes. Moderately low temperatures in the range of −65 to −78°C seem more efficacious than freezer or moderately low temperatures of −55°C and above. Acetic acid bacteria and some mycobacteria have been stored in a stable state for 4 to 4.5 years frozen at −20 to −28°C (Gruft *et al.*, 1968; Yamasato *et al.*, 1973). Fifty percent of mycobacteria survived 2 years storage at −20°C (Kim and Kubica, 1973). Preservation of flexibacteria and marine bacteria at −19 to −22°C has not been satisfactory (Floodgate and Hayes, 1961; Greig *et al.*, 1970; Sanfilippo and Lewin, 1970). Actinomycetes survived 4–5 years at −20°C (Kutzner, 1972; Kuznetsov *et al.*, 1972).

Survival of prokaryotes stored in the range of −40 to −55°C appears somewhat better. For example, 70% of over one-half of the strains of mycobacteria stored at −55°C survived the 6-year test period (Boulanger and Portelance, 1975).

Storage in the range of −65 to −78°C has proven even more effective for prokaryotes. Kelton (1964) found that 10% of the original number of mycoplasmas survived with no apparent changes after storage at −65°C for 12 months; most of this loss occurred during the first month. Fourteen avian and mammalian mycoplasmas were stored successfully for 3.5 years at −70°C (Addey *et al.*, 1970). The viability titer of only three strains was reduced 10-fold.

Kim and Kubica (1973) reported quantitative survival of 100% for mycobacteria stored at −70 C for 2 yr in tween-albumin broth. In a later investigation, they presented evidence that the key genetic and taxonomic features used for identification of mycobacteria were not affected by 2.5–5 yr storage at −70 C (Kubica *et al.*, 1977).

Glass beads have also been coated with bacteria and stored at −70 to −78°C. Multiple samples can be taken from the same tube, since retrieval can be accomplished before visible thawing occurs (Feltham *et al.*, 1978; Nagel and Kunz, 1972). Feltham *et al.* (1978) has used blocks of paraffin wax with vertical holes for storage of vials containing glass beads. The whole block of wax was removed from the freezer for subsampling and was found to keep cultures frozen for up to 1 hour. Thus, use of this technique would greatly save on storage space since fewer multiple tubes would be needed. A color-coding system is also possible with the use of colored beads which could be classified to distinguish between various groups as deemed necessary (Feltham *et al.*, 1978).

B. Ultralow Temperatures

Temperatures in the range of liquid nitrogen (−196°C) have been used successfully for long-term storage of prokaryotic organisms. Care must be exercised with the use of liquid nitrogen storage since an explosion hazard exists upon warming of imperfectly sealed ampoules (Meryman, 1963). Safety precautions in conjunction with liquid nitrogen storage have been outlined by Loegering *et al.* (1966).

Martin (1964) stated that storage at ultralow temperatures is valuable for organisms sensitive to other techniques such as lyophilization. Disadvantages in addition to safety have been mentioned. Samples frozen in liquid nitrogen do not lend themselves to shipping (LaPage *et al.*, 1970). Also, a large amount of storage space is required since multiple vials of each organism are needed (Bullen, 1975); therefore, he developed a sampling device which can repeatedly sample from tubes stored in liquid nitrogen. A sample can be taken in 3.5 min. In 4 min, the temperature of these frozen samples was found to rise to −40 to −50°C. It would appear that dangers in this technique would be the possible detrimental effect of fluctuating temperatures and chance of contamination.

Limited data are available in the literature on storage of phytopathogenic prokaryotes at ultralow temperatures. Moore and Carlson (1975) reported on the survival of 14 isolates of phytopathogenic bacteria from the genera *Agrobacterium, Corynebacterium, Erwinia, Pseudomonas,* and *Xanthomonas* after storage in various suspending media for 12 and 30 months at −172 to −196°C. All organisms survived and were pathogenic with survival loss minimal after initial freezing shock. They felt that liquid nitrogen preservation was more convenient and reliable than storage by lyophilization, water blanks, oil overlay, or frozen host tissue at −20°C.

Results on storage of other prokaryotes including bacteria, actinomycetes, and mycoplasmas at ultralow temperatures have been reported. Twenty-four week survival of lactic streptococci was excellent at −196°C (Gibson *et al.*, 1966). Survival of flexibacteria was the same whether stored at −196°C for 1 hr or 1 year; these workers suggested that flexibacteria could be preserved for many years at this temperature (Sanfilippo and Lewin, 1970). After storage of 16 *E. coli* strains at −196°C for over 2 years, no damage to plasmid DNA could be detected (Breese and Sharp, 1980). Following initial survival loss due to freezing, little storage loss occurred with most strains of seven genera and 69 to 111% of the cells survived 1–2 years.

Norman *et al.* (1970) maintained 74 strains of 26 species of mycoplasmas at −150 to −196°C for up to 9 years. Survival of selected strains ranged from 8 to >100% after freezing. Daily and Higgens (1973) described successful storage of bacteria and actinomycetes in the gas phase (−160°C) of liquid nitrogen. Advantages that they specified included use of cotton-plugged or capped tubes instead of sealed ampoules, larger volume capacity, easier storage and retrieval, no explosion hazard, and repeated sampling of tubes would save space.

C. Drying

1. *Beads/Stones*

Several materials have served as carriers for bacterial suspensions to be desiccated. The technique consists of coating beads with a suspension of the bacterium to be stored and drying in a tube containing self-indicating silica gel. Cotton or glass wool can be used to separate the carrier and the silica gel. The tube should be capped and sealed. The method is relatively simple and efficient. A major advantage is the saving on storage space since each container can be repeatedly sampled.

Norris (1963) preserved 3–5 day broth cultures of *Rhizobium* on porcelain beads at laboratory temperature. All 10 strains survived 100–132 weeks. At 80 weeks, all *Rhizobium* strains appeared unchanged culturally and in their *in planta* properties. He suggested that this method would be useful in isolated field stations with limited resources. Two publications on lactic acid bacteria report successful preservation from 6 months to 3 years when stored dry on porcelain berl saddles or granular pumice stone (Juven, 1979; Pilone, 1979). Streptomycete spores dried on unglazed porcelain beads survived 1.5 years (Kutzner, 1972).

2. *Silica Gel Particles*

Direct use of nonindicating anhydrous silica gel particles is even simpler than the previous method, since cotton or glass wool and beads or stones are eliminated. The technique has been used successfully with 7 day cultures of *A. tumefaciens, C. nebraskense* Schuster *et al., C. michiganenese* pv. *michiganense* (Smith) Jensen, *E. carotovora* (Jones) Bergey *et al., E. stewartii* (Smith) Dye, *P. s.* pv. *glycinea, P. s.* pv. *lachrymans* (Smith & Byron) Young *et al., P. s.* pv. *phaseolicola, P. solanacearum, P. s.* pv. *syringae, X. c.* pv. *campestris* (Pammel) Dowson, *X. c.* pv. *nigromaculans* f. sp. *zinniae sensu* Hopkins & Dowson, and *X. c.* pv. *phaseoli.* These pathogens survived 5 years of storage at −20°C with no apparent change in pathogenicity (Leben and Sleesman, 1982). It is recommended that storage temperatures be as low as possible, since an earlier report indicated storage at −20°C was much superior to that at 5°C (Sleesman and Leben, 1978). Protective suspending media, such as 10% milk + 15% glycerol, and precooling all materials to reduce lethal heat buildup when the suspension is absorbed by the silica gel particles are important to the success of this procedure.

This method has also been used successfully for other prokaryotes. Grivell and Jackson (1969) reported 13–111 week survival of 9 strains of bacteria on silica gel particles at 2–4°C. *E. coli* was successfully stored by this procedure for the 36-month test period (Brown, 1971). After 2.7 to 3.7 years at 4°C, 20 out of 33 bacteria survived storage on silica gel (Trollope, 1975). Thorns (1979) has reported survival for 26 strains of mycoplasmas stored at 4°C for 80 weeks on silica gel particles. Flexibacteria and streptomycetes, however, have not survived this procedure (Kutzner, 1972; Sanfilippo and Lewin, 1970).

3. *Agar Discs*

Bagga (1967c) has described a technique where culture agar discs of *Xanthomonas* and *Streptomyces* sp. were dried over calcium chloride for 24 hr and stored at 10–13°C in sealed containers; the xanthomonads survived the 12-month test period, but the actinomycetes died in only 9–10 months. Another report indicated that *X. c.* pv. *malvacearum* (Smith) Dye from 10 day cultures maintained pathogenicity and original characters after 12 months of storage by this technique (Bagga, 1967b). Four nonphytopathogenic bacteria from 7 day cultures have been successfully preserved for 4 years in agar discs dried in the refrigerator over silica gel (Seaby, 1977).

4. Other Carriers

Materials such as soil, sand, paper discs, cellulose fibers, and bacterial exudate (ooze) have been used as vehicles for storage of prokaryotes. A moist, sterile 3 : 1 : 1 soil, peat, perlite mixture was used to preserve 45 *C. michiganense* pv. *insidiosum* (McCulloch) Dye & Kemp strains for 1 year at 4 and 21°C without occurrence of variants or loss of pathogenicity (Carrol and Lukezic, 1971b). Only a small percentage of avirulent *C. m.* pv. *insidiosum* cultural variants was detected on selective medium with soil storage compared to maintenance in water or on growth medium (Carrol and Lukezic, 1971a). Survival of *X. c.* pv. *phaseoli* in *in vitro* produced exudate at −25°C (20 or 51% RH) was sufficient to allow preservation for at least 10 years (Wilson *et al.*, 1965). Hsieh and Buddenhagen (1975) suggested that a convenient method for long-term preservation of *X. c.* pv. *oryzae* (Ishiyama) Dye would be in ooze droplets at 0% RH and 1–10°C; they attained survival in a pathogenic state for more than 2 years.

Actinomycetes have historically been preserved in sterilized soil. Kutzner (1972) reported that most of 165 streptomycetes preserved by this procedure survived after 8 years. In storage of 1500 actinomycetes in soil at room temperature for up to 17 years, 50% survived (Pridham and Lyons, 1973). These workers abandoned preservation in soil because of contamination, mite problems, and lack of sufficient survival. Others have reported 92–96% survival of actinomycetes after 4 years in soil culture; characteristics lost during laboratory culture were restored with the use of soil (Kuznetsov *et al.*, 1974). Soil type may have affected the efficacy of this method.

5. Vacuum Drying

Drying *in vacuo* and L-drying (drying *in vacuo* from the liquid state without freezing) are effective means of prokaryote preservation. Survival is favored by the rapid rate of drying which occurs with this method. L-drying has been used for organisms sensitive to lyophilization (LaPage *et al.*, 1970; Martin, 1964).

Rhodes (1950) reported survival of 83% of 2724 bacterial strains tested at varying intervals up to 14 years when cultures were dried in horse serum *in vacuo* over P_2O_5. Soriano (1970) described Sordelli's method of drying *in vacuo* and reported almost 30 years survival of desiccated bacteria stored at room temperature. Substances such as sand or glass beads have been used as carriers. Streptococci dried *in vacuo* on sand survived 4 years when stored at 4–10°C (Koshi *et al.*, 1977). Segerstrom and Sabiston (1977) described a method whereby bacteria coated glass beads are cooled to near freezing and dried *in vacuo*. They reported up to 5 year survival.

Annear (1970) has described the apparatus and procedure for L-drying by which bacteria survived storage at 25 and 37°C for 4 years. To increase the surface area exposed, suspensions were placed on cotton wool or glass beads. Residual moisture measurements suggested that the cotton plug, which is inserted into tubes below the point of sealing in L-drying to prevent cross-contamination, aids survival during storage of sealed tubes by acting as a desiccant aiding maintenance of optimal moisture (Iijima and Sakane, 1973). A storage life of 10 years for L-dried *E. coli* was projected by these investigators.

D. Freeze-Drying

The mechanics of freeze-drying or lyophilization have been well reviewed by Tuite (1969). Others have also presented much information on this commonly used technique (Fry, 1966; LaPage *et al.*, 1970; Martin, 1964; Strange and Cox, 1976). Martin (1964) has noted the major advantages of lyophilization which include vacuum sealed containers eliminate contamination, most microbes survive for long periods, storage temperatures are not critical, the dried product can be easily shipped without special handling, and about 95% of all bacteria can be preserved by this method. Major disadvantages with this method include low quantitative survival and the fact that freeze-drying has been associated with induction of mutations (Tanaka *et al.*, 1979).

The principle of freeze-drying has been discussed by LaPage *et al.* (1970). The sample is first frozen forming a stable structure. This structure is maintained during drying which occurs by sublimation of water vapor from the ice surface. Because of the large surface area available, rehydration is rapid. Fry (1954) suggested that such a rigid structure of the drying product can prevent protein denaturation during desiccation. Important cellular proteins presumably would be prevented from coming into contact with high concentrations of other proteins or salt.

The suitability of lyophilization as a preservation technique varies with the organism. Kennedy (1965) reported a large decrease in the number of *P. s.* pv. *glycinea* survivors immediately after freeze-drying in water or lactose and a further decrease after 126 days at 27°C. Survival of this pathogen was increased by freeze-drying in leaf tissue, but still only 4% survival was recorded after 196 days at 7°C. Survival losses of 38–96% were recorded for lyophilized *E. coli* strains, although no loss of plasmid-borne antibiotic resistance was observed (Breese and Sharp, 1980). Only 50% of lyophilized mycobacteria cultures survived for 4 years (Gruft *et al.*, 1968). Antheunisse (1973) reported that after 6 years storage, 18 out of 30 lyophilized bacterial genera had 80–100% survival, 6 gave 50–70%, and 6 had 0–40%. Results with marine bacteria indicated that 91–100% of 45 strains survived in the freeze-dried state after 2–10 years (Floodgate and Hayes, 1961; Greig *et al.*, 1970).

Mycoplasmas can be preserved by freeze-drying, although sensitivity varies. One lyophilized mycoplasma isolate had 23.8% survival after 27 months storage at 4°C (Conrad, 1958). Norman *et al.* (1970) found that 15 mycoplasma strains varied in reaction to the freeze-drying process with survival values from 0.6 to 90%. Addey *et al.* (1970) reported all 10 isolates of lyophilized mycoplasmas stored at 4°C survived after 27–34 months, seven in undiminished numbers. Storage longevity of 3–4 years has been observed for 26 lyophilized mycoplasma strains stored at −26 to −65°C (Kelton, 1964).

Williams and Cross (1971) recommended freeze-drying as a suitable preservation method for almost all species of actinomycetes. Kutzner (1972) reported heavy growth from lyophilized streptomycetes after 1.5 years. Kuznetsov and Rodionova (1971) observed that many lyophilized actinomycetes survived for 12 years, but some species were sensitive. Morphological properties and antibiotic yields of lyophilized streptomycetes were found to remain stable after 4 years storage (Kapetanovic and Pavletic, 1972).

E. Sterile Distilled and Tap Water

This method of storage is exceedingly simple and requires little equipment or manpower. Because of its simplicity, large numbers of cultures can be preserved and repeated subsampling may be done from the same tube (DeVay and Schnathorst, 1963). The technique was described by Kelman and Person (1961) in which three to five loopfuls of the bacterium are suspended in water and stored. In this test they detected few avirulent variants of *P. solanacearum* after 18–24 months storage at 22°C.

Since then, many other workers have reported successful preservation of bacterial phytopathogens with this method. DeVay and Schnathorst (1963) recorded preservation of *C. m.* pv. *insidiosum, A. tumefaciens,* and *Pseudomonas* sp. in distilled water at 10°C. Pathogenic survivors of *P. azadirachtae* cells from 7 day and *X. c.* pv. *oryzae* from 3 day cultures were reported after 170–365 days storage in water at 5–10 and 19–39°C (Singh, 1971; Srivastava and Patel, 1968). Pathogenicity of *A. tumefaciens, C. m.* pv. *michiganense, P. aeruginosa, P. s.* pv. *lachrymans, P. sesami* Malcoff, *P. s.* pv. *syringae, X. marantae* Zagalto & Pereira, *X. passiflorae*

Pereira, and *X. c.* pv. *malvacearum* was constant after 30–40 months storage in distilled water or physiological solution at room temperature (DeVay and Schnathorst, 1963; Pereira *et al.*, 1970). Longer term pathogenic survival of 8 years and 7 months has been observed for *X. c.* pv. *vesicatoria* (Doidge) Dye (Doidge) Dowson from 72 hr slants maintained in sterile distilled tap water at 15°C (Person, 1969). No effect of distilled water storage for 10–20 months was noted on pigment or antibiotic production of 9 *X. albilineans* (Ashby) Dowson or 100 *P. s.* pv. *syringae* strains, respectively (DeVay and Schnathorst, 1963; Perez and Monllor, 1967).

Not all reports on use of water as a preservation method have been favorable. Preservation of 45 *C. m.* pv. *insidiosum* strains resulted in loss of 50% of the strains; survivors grew poorly, produced little pigment on growth medium, and cultural variants were detected (Carroll and Lukezic, 1971b). Since many avirulent colony types were detected on a selective medium, sterile water may not be a good storage medium for this bacterium (Carroll and Lukezic, 1971a).

Berger (1970) found that the number of *P. solanacearum* survivors falls off exponentially with age, but that eventually the viable fraction approaches a constant value. No support for his hypothesis that this bacterium survived in water through the oxidation of stored metabolizable material was found. Surviving cells evidently metabolized remains of cells and some low level multiplication may occur.

Granai and Sjogren (1981) postulated that the ability of bacteria to survive stress in an aqueous environment may be related to the ability to mobilize and use stored macromolecules. Endogenous glycogen has been related to the survival of *E. aerogenes* in water suspension; during storage, endogenous glycogen was degraded and oxidized (Strange *et al.*, 1961). Additionally, dead cells provided nutrients to survivors for growth and division.

F. Host Tissue

Many phytopathogenic bacteria have been successfully preserved in host tissue by drying or freezing. One obvious disadvantage of this procedure is that contaminants may impede recovery of the pathogen. Use of inoculated greenhouse plants, which usually are relatively free of other microbes, in conjunction with selective media are helpful aids with host tissue preservation. One *P. s.* pv. *glycinea* and five *P. s.* pv. *lachrymans* strains were maintained in a pathogenic state at 5°C in dried greenhouse inoculated host leaves for 5.5 to 12.5 years (Leben, unpublished). Chamberlain (1957) maintained *P. s.* pv. *glycinea* and *P. s.* pv.

tabaci (Wold & Foster) Young *et al.* in pathogenic form in dried greenhouse inoculated soybean [*Glycine max* (L.) Merr.] leaves for 3.5–7 years at 5–7°C. Plasmids were maintained in *X. c.* pv. *vesicatoria* when diseased greenhouse tomato (*Lycopersicon esculentum* Mill.) leaves were stored moist at 5°C, but plasmids were lost when this bacterium was maintained on an antibiotic-free medium (Lai *et al.*, 1977).

Preservation has also been successful utilizing naturally diseased host tissue *C. m.* pv. *insidiosum* and *X. c.* pv. *alfalfae* (Riker *et al.*) Dye survived and remained pathogenic in field collected alfalfa (*Medicago sativa* L.) stem, leaf, and shoot tissue stored at room temperature for 8–10 years (Claflin and Stuteville, 1973; Cormack, 1961). *X. c.* pv. *vesicatoria* has been reported to survive for 10 months at 10–38°C in diseased chilli (*Capsicum frutescens* var. *longum* Sendt.) leaves (Shekhawat and Chakravarti, 1978).

Freezing diseased host tissue also has been a successful preservation method. After 21 months, *C. m.* pv. *insidiosum* survived and was pathogenic at −20°C in diseased alfalfa tap roots (Kernkamp and Hemerick, 1952). Jones and Hartwig (1959) preserved *P. s.* pv. *tabaci* for 2 years and *X. c.* pv. *phaseoli* var. *sojense* (Hedges) Starr and Burkholder for 21 months in minced diseased leaves at −7 to −18°C without loss of virulence; however, virulence of *X. c.* pv. *phaseoli* var. *sojense* (Hedges) Starr & Burkholder was greatly reduced after 31 months storage.

Several workers have reported successful maintenance of *P. s.* pv. *glycinea* in frozen host tissue. Pathogenic survivors of *P. s.* pv. *glycinea* have been recovered after 31 months to 7 years storage in diseased soybean leaves at −10 to −18°C (Chamberlain, 1957; Frosheiser, 1956). Kennedy (1965) tested various suspending media in frozen storage of *P. s.* pv. *glycinea* in soybean leaves over a 6-month test period at −15°C. Quantitative data indicated that suspending in water gave 83% survival, much superior to suspending leaf tissue in glycerol, glucose, air, or ethyleneglycol. Survival in leaf tissue was superior to that obtained by suspending cells of the bacterium in the various suspending media. The protective effect of leaf tissue may be mechanical, nutritional, and/or related to exudates resulting from the host–pathogen interaction.

G. Serial Transfers

Although serial transfer has been commonly used as a preservation method, it seems less than desirable considering the earlier discussion of hypobiosis and past experience. The technique generally consists of storing organisms on growth medium at room temperature or refrigerator temperature (5°C) and transferring at periodic intervals. An advantage of this method is the ready availability of cultures for comparison and transfer; disadvantages include the substantial manpower and materials requirement, the possibility of mislabeling during the tedious task, dehydration, and the loss of cultures due to cultural variation, contamination, degeneration, and mutation (LaPage *et al.*, 1970; Tsuru, 1973). Serial transfer is rarely used for preservation of bacteria or organisms of industrial importance (Martin, 1964).

This technique may be inadequate for preservation of phytopathogenic bacteria. Examples of pathogens reported to have lost virulence when maintained by serial transfer include *C. m.* pv. *insidiosum, C. m.* pv. *sepodonicum* (Spieckermann & Kotthoff), Dye & Kemp, *P. s.* pv. *glycinea, P. s.* pv. *tabaci,* and *P. solanacearum* (Chamberlain, 1957; Frosheiser, 1956; Kelman and Jensen, 1951; Kernkamp and Hemerick, 1952; Sherf, 1943). Poor growth and cultural variants were recorded in *C. m.* pv. *insidiosum* cultures transferred every 14–21 days at 4 and 21°C (Carroll and Lukezic, 1971a,b; Fulkerson, 1960). Survival of *C. m.* pv. *sepodonicum* was uncertain after 30 day storage on agar medium (Sherf, 1943). Williams and Cross (1971) reported that serial transfer of actinomycetes resulted in changes in the organism. Nevertheless, use of a soft agar technique for storage of streptomycete spores has been reported successful after 3 years (Kutzner, 1972).

H. Oil Overlay

Storage life of prokaryotes on culture medium has been prolonged by overlaying with mineral oil, which serves to limit oxygen and thus slow metabolic activity. Fennell (1960) has listed some operating principles of the oil overlay procedure. Disadvantages of this method are bothersome handling of mineral oil, chance of contamination, and storage space required if several tubes of each organism are prepared (LaPage *et al.*, 1970).

Use of the oil overlay method has increased survival time of phytopathogens. Sherf (1943) reported that 10 day cultures of *C. m.* pv. *sepodonicum, P. s.* pv. *phaseolicola,* and *X. c.* pv. *phaseoli* survived under oil at room temperature for 10–18 months; however, all *C. m.* pv. *sepodonicum* cultures were dead at 21 months. No changes in pathogenicity or growth properties were noted with 24 hr *P. s.* pv. *phaseolicola* or 48 hr *P. solanacearum* cultures maintained under oil for 4 years (Jensen and Livingston, 1944; Kelman and Jensen, 1951).

Reports on other bacteria indicate some success with the procedure. After 3 years storage under oil, isolates of *Pseudomonas, Bacillus, Escherichia,* and luminous bacteria survived without any qualitative changes in morphological, cultural, or physiobiochemical properties (Nadirova and Zemlyakov, 1970; Vorobéva and Chumakova, 1973). Floodgate and Hayes (1961) reported 72% survival of 45 strains of marine bacteria stored under oil for 2 years. Antibiotic production by *Actinomyces roseolus* Preobrazhenskaya & Sveshnikova decreased with storage under oil for 2 years (Bushueva and Kuznetsov, 1974).

IV. DISCUSSION

Stopping or significantly lowering the metabolic activity of prokaryotes without causing excessive cellular damage is the foundation of superior preservation techniques. Preservation methods developed to date most commonly make use of adjustments in temperature and/or moisture to lower metabolism; less frequently, starvation (water storage) and oxygen limitation (oil overlay) have been utilized. It is probable that all preservation methods result in selection pressures from death or injury of sensitive cells. It is important, therefore, that the quantitative survival of the preserved prokaryote be as high as possible, ideally 100%. The methods, for which quantitative data are available, which have shown most consistently this capability are storage at moderate and ultralow temperatures. As a general trend, the lower the storage temperature, the higher the frequency rate of survival. Thus, temperatures from −70 to −196°C, which are below the eutectic temperature of most mixtures, appear to be very attractive as storage temperatures, whether used alone or in combination with desiccation. Methods based strictly on desiccation do not appear to provide such a high level of quantitative survival.

In addition to providing a high degree of prokaryote survival in an unchanged condition, the more useful preservation methods should provide a fairly long-term capability (5 years), be simple and inexpensive in procedure and equipment, provide for easy recovery, use a minimum of storage space, and offer optimum flexibility. For instance, preserved cultures should not be affected unduely by emergencies such as power outages. Also, shipment should be possible without elaborate preparation. All of the preservation methods we have reviewed appear to have limitations in at least one of these areas.

Rather than recommend one storage technique, it seems wise to use several methods to guard against loss of important cultures. To safeguard the cultures, important steps prior to preservation by any method are to ensure that the organism is pathogenic, in pure culture, and free of variant colony types. This requirement must be satisfied if pathogenic, pure cultures are to be recovered. From the plant pathologist's viewpoint, however, simple, quick, and inexpensive methods for storage are necessary. In this case, the method of choice, especially for field laboratory situations with little equipment, is storage dry on silica gel particles. I am impressed with the 5 year survival (in pathogenic form) that we have obtained with this method for storage of bacterial phytopathogens at ordinary household freezer temperatures. Although quantitative survival likely is not equivalent to frozen storage at moderate or ultralow temperatures, the technique is simple, reliable, allows repeated sampling from the same container, and is adaptable to other prokaryotes such as mycoplasmas. To increase survival of these bacteria to desiccation on silica gel, we suspended heavy suspensions of cells from 7 to 14 day cultures on sucrose nutrient agar in milk or milk + glycerol. Recovery was on the same rich medium. In a field situation I would choose preservation in host tissue, either dried or frozen, as a backup technique to silica gel; however, the disadvantage with this method is that the pathogen is not in pure culture.

When mechanical freezers or liquid nitrogen facilities are available, storage at -70 to $-196°C$ is recommended strongly. Unfortunately, in many cases the cost of these methods is prohibitive. Freeze-drying is a secondary choice, but equipment is expensive and the process time consuming. Methods such as serial transfer, oil overlay, and storage in water are not recommended for long-term storage, since in many instances metabolism is not sufficiently reduced to prevent death or changes of the stored culture.

In design of an ideal maintenance procedure, we shall review some of the facts about the two most useful tools for storage of prokaryotes; low temperature and desiccation. These two stresses have several similarities. Both procedures involve removal of free water from the cells, although dehydration of cells during freezing occurs at lower temperatures. Damage at slower rates of freezing may be due to solute buildup resulting in damage to cell walls and membranes. Most evidence indicates that little nucleic acid damage results from freezing. Desiccation also causes cell permeability changes, apparently related to cell membrane damage. Additionally, nucleic acids of desiccated cells are probably damaged. It is not clear whether this damage occurs during desiccation or during storage of desiccated cells. Dehydration and storage by freezing, however, apparently limit nucleic acid damage.

The time frame during which these various injuries occur needs further delineation. Does cell membrane or nucleic acid damage occur during the drying or freezing process, during long-term storage, or on recovery? It seems likely that cell damage may occur during any of these periods, depending on the particular sensitivity of each organism. Some facts are known. Survival to both stresses is affected by the condition of the microbe prior to treatment, treatment rate, protective compounds, storage conditions, stress removal rate, and the recovery environment. We have discussed general principles which help to alleviate some damage. Unfortunately, we do not know how many of these act. For example, what mechanism renders cells from older cultures less sensitive to stress? Is it due to induction of a hypobiotic condition in the cell triggered by starvation or accumulation of substances such as waste products in older cultures?

For desiccated cells, survival is usually best at a residual moisture level of about 1% for long-term storage. But what is the residual moisture condition of frozen cells? Does dehydration of frozen cells occur to the extent that only 1% residual moisture remains, or is the residual moisture level less critical with storage at lower temperatures?

Answers to these questions and development of more detailed information on cell damage during the various stages of preservation would aid greatly design of more efficient storage methods of prokaryotes. I propose that a hypothetical best preservation method might involve first desiccation and then long-term storage at low temperatures. To maximize survival to desiccation, the proposed method should involve use of high cell concentrations harvested at their greatest level of desiccation resistance, rapid desiccation, protective medium, controlled residual moisture, controlled storage atmosphere, appropriate protection during rehydration, and warming. Improvements over known methods appear possible in all these areas. Once survival to desiccation has been maximized, use of low temperatures (−70 to −196°C) support long-term survival.

An efficient storage technique should use a minimum of storage space. Drying bacteria on a carrier, possibly anhydrous silica gel particles, affords repeated sampling from the same container, thus saving on space. In addition to being simple, desiccation on silica gel appears to be relatively rapid. By dehydrating prior to frozen storage, fluctuating storage temperatures (power outages) would not expose cells to freezing and thawing effects. Shipment would be feasible since warming of dried bacteria would not be as harmful. Use of storage temperatures in the range of −70°C would likely be sufficient to maintain a high degree of long-term survival to properly desiccated cells.

In the use of silica gel, care must be used to control lethal heat buildup during absorption into the particles and the amount of suspension added per unit weight of silica gel must be closely monitored to assure appropriate levels of residual moisture. Container selection for long-term storage should be made with care since they should be sealed to prevent changes in residual moisture and/or storage atmosphere. Possibly, storage in the gas phase of liquid nitrogen would be suitable and also preclude necessity of sealing storage containers.

With the current emphasis on genetic engineering involving prokaryotes, development of proficient preservation methods is needed to preserve potentially unstable organisms and the large investments in time and money for their development. Storage of plasmids as pure DNA is also possible. Efficient preservation of industrially important engineered microbes which may produce important substances such as drugs, alcohol, amino acids, enzymes, pesticides, and other chemicals is imperative.

In agriculture, future research on conditions affecting survival of prokaryotes is needed and may prove useful in ways not related to their preservation. For instance, the lethal effect of 75% RH to plant pathogenic bacteria has been practically applied to reduce live *P. s.* pv. *lachrymans* cells in cucumber (*Cucumis sativus* L.) seed (Leben and Sleesman, 1981). Disease was prevented or its incidence reduced greatly in laboratory and field trials.

The future use of antagonistic prokaryotes for foliar disease control depends on their preservation. One limitation in the use of a bacterial antagonist to control *Bipolaris maydis* (Nisik.) Shoemaker on corn (*Zea mays* L.) was its sensitivity to desiccation (Sleesman and Leben, 1976b). Can manipulations be made to overcome this difficulty? Recently, plant growth-promoting rhizobacteria were formulated dry in xanthan gum plus talc and used successfully as potato seed piece treatments in the field (Kloepper and Schroth, 1981). Implications of prokaryote survival research for agriculture can be far reaching, from disease, insect, and weed control to use of prokaryotes as epiphytic nitrogen fixers and plant growth promoters.

Acknowledgments

Thanks are due the Agricultural Chemicals Division, MOBAY Chemical Corporation for their support of this work. Special appreciation is extended to Curt Leben for advice and counsel throughout the course of this project and for his critical review of the manuscript. I am also grateful to Lansing Williams and Phil Larsen for their helpful suggestions.

References

Abe, S. (1973). *Cryobiology* **10**, 468.

Addey, J. P., Taylor-Robinson, D., and Dimic, M. (1970). *J. Med. Microbiol.* **3**, 137–145.

Anderson, J. D., and Cox, C. S. (1967). *In* "Airborne Microbes" (P. H. Gregory and J. L. Monteith, eds.), pp. 203–226. Cambridge Univ. Press, London and New York.

Annear, D. I. (1970). *Cult. Collect. Microorgan. Proc. Int. Conf. 1968* pp. 273–279.
Antheunisse, J. (1973). *Antonie van Leeuwenhoek* **39,** 243–248.
Arpai, J. (1962). *Appl. Microbiol.* **10,** 297–301.
Asada, S., Takano, M., and Shibaski, I. (1980). *Appl. Environ. Microbiol.* **40,** 274–281.
Ashwood-Smith, M. J. (1965). *Cryobiology* **2,** 39–45.
Ashwood-Smith, M. J. (1978). *Cryobiology* **15,** 692.
Bagga, H. S. (1967a). *Plant Dis. Rep.* **51,** 1055–1058.
Bagga, H. S. (1967b). *Plant Dis. Rep.* **51,** 1058–1062.
Bagga, H. S. (1967c). *Plant Dis. Rep.* **51,** 747–750.
Banno, I., Sakane, T., and Iijima, T. (1978). *Cryobiology* **15,** 692–693.
Basu, P. K. (1970). *Phytopathology* **60,** 825–827.
Berger, L. R. (1970). *Cult. Collect. Microorgan. Proc. Int. Conf. 1968* pp. 265–267.
Boulanger, R. P., and Portelance, V. (1975). *Can. J. Microbiol.* **21,** 694–702.
Breese, M. D., and Sharp, R. J. (1980). *J. Appl. Bacteriol.* **48,** 63–68.
Bretz, H. W., and Hartsell, S. E. (1959). *Food Res.* **24,** 369–375.
Bridges, B. A. (1966). *Lab. Pract.* **15,** 418–422.
Brown, K. D. (1971). *J. Bacteriol.* **106,** 70–81.
Bullen, J. J. (1975). *J. Gen. Microbiol.* **89,** 205–207.
Bushueva, D. A., and Kuznetsov, V. D. (1974). *Antibiotiki* **19,** 1099–1100 (English Abstr.).
Calcott, P. H. (1978). "Freezing and Thawing Microbes." Meadowfield Press, Durham.
Calcott, P. H., and MacLeod, R. A. (1974). *Can. J. Microbiol.* **20,** 683–689.
Calcott, P. H., and Postgate, J. R. (1971). *Cryobiology* **7,** 238–242.
Calcott, P. H., Lee, S. K., and MacLeod, R. A. (1976). *Can. J. Microbiol.* **22,** 106–109.
Carroll, R. B., and Lukezic, F. L. (1971a). *Phytopathology* **61,** 1423–1425.
Carroll, R. B., and Lukezic, F. L. (1971b). *Phytopathology* **61,** 688–690.
Chamberlain, D. W. (1957). *Plant Dis. Rep.* **41,** 1039–1040.
Claflin, L. E., and Stuteville, D. L. (1973). *Plant Dis. Rep.* **57,** 52–53.
Clark, W. A., and Loegering, W. Q. (1967). *Annu. Rev. Phytopathol.* **5,** 319–342.
Clement, M. T. (1961). *Can. J. Microbiol.* **7,** 99–106.
Clement, M. T. (1964). *Can. J. Microbiol.* **10,** 613–615.
Conrad, R. D. (1958). *Avian Dis.* **2,** 132–138.
Cormack, M. W. (1961). *Phytopathology* **51,** 260–261.
Daily, W. A., and Higgens, C. E. (1973). *Cryobiology* **10,** 364–367.
DeVay, J. E., and Schnathorst, W. C. (1963). *Nature (London)* **199,** 755–777.
Duguid, J. R., and Wilkinson, J. F. (1953). *J. Gen. Microbiol.* **9,** 174–189.
Farrant, J. (1965). *Nature (London)* **205,** 1284–1287.
Farrell, J., and Rose, A. H. (1968). *J. Gen. Microbiol.* **50,** 429–439.
Feltham, R. K. A., Power, A. K., Pell, P. A., and Sneath, P. H. A. (1978). *J. Appl. Bacteriol.* **44,** 313–316.
Fennell, D. I. (1960). *Bot. Rev.* **26,** 79–141.
Fisher, J. P. (1950). *J. Gen. Microbiol.* **4,** 455.
Floodgate, G. D., and Hayes, P. R. (1961). *J. Appl. Bacteriol.* **24,** 87–93.
Ford, D. K. (1962). *J. Bacteriol.* **84,** 1028–1034.
Frosheiser, F. I. (1956). *Phytopathology* **46,** 526.
Fry, R. M. (1954). *In* "Biological Applications of Freezing and Drying" (R. J. C. Harris, ed.), pp. 215–252. Academic Press, New York.
Fry, R. M. (1966). *In* "Cryobiology" (H. T. Meryman, ed.), pp. 665–696. Academic Press, New York.
Fry, R. M., and Greaves, R. I. N. (1951). *J. Hyg.* **49,** 220–246.
Fulkerson, J. F. (1960). *Phytopathology* **50,** 377–380.
Gibson, C. A., Landerkin, G. B., and Morse, P. M. (1966). *Appl. Microbiol.* **14,** 665–669.

Gomez, R. F., Sinskey, A. J., Davies, R., and Labuza, T. P. (1973). *J. Gen. Microbiol.* **74**, 267–274.
Granai, C., and Sjogren, R. E. (1981). *Appl. Environ. Microbiol.* **41**, 190–195.
Greiff, D., and Meyers, M. (1961). *Nature (London)* **190**, 1202–1204.
Greig, M. A., Hendrie, M. S., Shewan, J. M. (1970). *J. Appl. Bacteriol.* **33**, 528–532.
Grieve, P. W., and Povey, M. J. W. (1981). *J. Sci. Food Agric.* **32**, 96–98.
Grivell, A. R., and Jackson, J. F. (1969). *J. Gen. Microbiol.* **58**, 423–425.
Gruft, H., Clark, M. E., and Osterhout, M. (1968). *Appl. Microbiol.* **16**, 355–357.
Haines, R. B. (1938). *Proc. R. Soc. London Ser. B* **124**, 451–472.
Hollander, D. H., and Nell, E. E. (1954). *Appl. Microbiol.* **2**, 164–170.
Hseih, S. P. Y., and Buddenhagen, I. W. (1975). *Phytopathology* **65**, 513–519.
Hurst, A., Hughes, A., and Collins-Thompson, D. L. (1974). *Can. J. Microbiol.* **20**, 765–768.
Iijima, T., and Sakane, T. (1973). *Cryobiology* **10**, 379–385.
Jensen, J. H., and Livingston, J. E. (1944). *Phytopathology* **34**, 471–480.
Johannsen, E. (1972). *J. Appl. Bacteriol.* **35**, 423–429.
Jones, J. P., and Hartwig, E. E. (1959). *Plant Dis. Rep.* **43**, 946.
Jones, L. R. (1901). *In* "Thirteenth Annual Report of Vermont Agricultural Experiment Station for 1900," pp. 299–332. Free Press Association, Burlington, Vermont.
Juven, B. J. (1979). *J. Appl. Bacteriol.* **47**, 379–381.
Kapetanovic, E., and Pavletic, Z. (1972). *Acta Bot. Croat.* **31**, 113–122 (English Summary).
Kauffman, P. H. (1972). M.S. thesis, Ohio State University.
Kawamoto, S. O., and Lorbeer, J. W. (1972). *Phytopathology* **62**, 1263–1265.
Keith, S. C. (1913). *Science* **37**, 877–879.
Kelman, A. (1956). *Phytopathology* **46**, 16–17.
Kelman, A., and Jensen, J. H. (1951). *Phytopathology* **41**, 185–186.
Kelman, A., and Person, L. H. (1961). *Phytopathology* **51**, 158–161.
Kelton, W. H. (1964). *J. Bacteriol.* **87**, 588–592.
Kennedy, B. W. (1965). *Phytopathology* **55**, 415–417.
Kernkamp, M. F., and Hemerick, G. (1952). *Phytopathology* **42**, 13.
Kim, T. H., and Kubica, G. P. (1972). *Appl. Microbiol.* **24**, 311–317.
Kim, T. H., and Kubica, G. P. (1973). *Appl. Microbiol.* **25**, 956–960.
Kleineberger-Nobel, E. (1962). "Pleuropneumonia-like organisms (PPLO) Mycoplasmataceae." Academic Press, New York.
Kloepper, J. W., and Schroth, M. N. (1981). *Phytopathology* **71**, 590–592.
Koshi, G., Rajeshwari, K., and Philipose, L. (1977). *Indian J. Med. Res.* **65**, 500–502.
Kubica, G. P., Gontijo-filho, P. P., and Kim, T. (1977). *J. Clin. Microbiol.* **6**, 149–153.
Kutzner, H. J. (1972). *Experientia* **28**, 1395–1396.
Kuznetsov, V. D., and Rodionova, E. G. (1971). *Antibiotica* **16**, 586–589 (English Abstr.).
Kuznetsov, V. D., Yangulova, N. V., and Rodionova, E. G. (1972). *Antibiotica* **17**, 790–793 (English Abstr.).
Kuznetsov, V. D., Rodionova, E. G., Yangulova, N. V., and Semenov, S. M. (1974). *Antibiotica* **19**, 1063–1069 (English Abstr.).
Kuznetsov, V. D., Filippopva, S. N., Murav'eva, S. A., and Fishman, V. M. (1977). *Microbiology* **46**, 265–270.
Lai, M., Shaffer, S., and Panopoulos, N. J. (1977). *Phytopathology* **67**, 1527–1530.
LaPage, S. P., Shelton, J. E., Mitchell, T. G., and Mackenzie, A. R. (1970). *In* "Methods in Microbiology" (J. R. Norris and D. W. Ribbons, eds.), Vol. 3A, pp. 135–228. Academic Press, New York.
Leach, J. G., Lilly, V. G., Wilson, H. A., and Purvis, M. R. (1957). *Phytopathology* **47**, 113–120.
Leach, R. H., and Scott, W. J. (1959). *J. Gen. Microbiol.* **21**, 295–307.

Leben, C. (1974). *Ohio Agric. Res. Dev. Cent., Wooster, Spec. Circ.* 100
Leben, C. (1981). *Plant Dis.* **65,** 633–637.
Leben, C., and Sleesman, J. P. (1981). *Plant Dis.* **65,** 876–878.
Leben, C., and Sleesman, J. P. (1982). *Plant Dis.* **66,** 327.
Leder, J. (1972). *J. Bacteriol.* **111,** 211–219.
Lind, A. (1967). *Scand, J. Respir. Dis.* **48,** 343–347.
Loegering, W. Q., Harmon, D. C., and Clark, W. A. (1966). *Plant Dis. Rep.* **50,** 502–506.
McDade, J. J., and Hall, L. B. (1963a). *Am. J. Hyg.* **77,** 98–108.
McDade, J. J., and Hall, L. B. (1963b). *Am. J. Hyg.* **78,** 330–337.
McDade, J. J., and Hall, L. B. (1964). *Am. J. Hyg.* **80,** 192–204.
Mackey, B. M., Derrick, C. M., and Thomas, J. A. (1980). *J. Appl. Bacteriol.* **48,** 315–324.
MacLeod, R. A., and Calcott, P. N. (1976). *Survival Veg. Microbes, Symp. Soc. Gen. Microbial* **26,** 81–109.
Major, C. P., McDougal, J. P., and Harrison, A. P., Jr. (1955). *J. Bacteriol.* **69,** 244–249.
Marshall, B. J., Coote, G. G., and Scott, W. J. (1973). *Appl. Microbiol.* **26,** 206–210.
Marshall, B. J., Coote, G. G., and Scott, W. J. (1974). *Appl. Microbiol.* **27,** 648–652.
Martin, S. M. (1964). *Annu. Rev. Microbiol.* **18,** 1–16.
Mazur, P. (1966a). *In* "Cryobiology" (H. T. Meryman, ed.), pp. 213–315. Academic Press, New York.
Mazur, P. (1966b). *Cryobiology* **4,** 181–192.
Mazur, P. (1970). *Science* **168,** 939–949.
Meryman, H. T. (1956). *Science* **124,** 515–521.
Meryman, H. T. (1963). *Fed. Proc., Fed. Am. Soc. Exp. Biol.* **22,** 81–89.
Meryman, H. T. (1971). *Cryobiology* **8,** 173–183.
Monk, G. W., and McCaffrey, P. A. (1957). *J. Bacteriol.* **73,** 85–88.
Monk, G. W., Elbert, M. L., Stevens, C. L., and McCaffrey, P. A. (1956). *J. Bacteriol.* **72,** 368–372.
Monk, G. W., McCaffrey, P. A., and Davis, M. S. (1957). *J. Bacteriol.* **73,** 661–665.
Moore, L. W., and Carlson, R. V. (1975). *Phytopathology* **65,** 246–250.
Morichi, T., Irie, R., and Yano, N. (1963). *J. Gen. Appl. Microbiol.* **9,** 149–161.
Morton, H. E., and Pulaski, E. J. (1938). *J. Bacteriol.* **35,** 163–183.
Mossel, D. A. A., Veldman, A., and Eelderink, I. (1980). *J. Appl. Bacteriol.* **49,** 405–419.
Nadirova, I. M., and Zemlyakov, V. L. (1970). *Microbiology* **39,** 973–976.
Nagel, J. G., and Kunz, L. J. (1972). *Appl. Microbiol.* **23,** 837–838.
Naylor, H. B., and Smith, P. A. (1946). *J. Bacteriol.* **52,** 565–573.
Nei, T., Araki, T., and Souza, H. (1965). *Cryobiology* **2,** 68–73.
Norman, M. C., Frack, E. B., and Choate, R. V. (1970). *Appl. Microbiol.* **20,** 69–71.
Norris, D. O. (1963). *Emp. J. Exp. Agric.* **31,** 255–258.
Nwigwe, C. (1973). *Plant Dis. Rep.* **57,** 227–230.
Obayashi, Y., and Cho, C. (1957). *Bull. W.H.O.* **17,** 255–274.
Pereira, A. L. G., Zagatto, A. G., and Figueiredo, M. B. (1970). *Biologico* **36,** 311–318.
Perez, J. E., and Monllor, A. C. (1967). *Plant Dis. Rep.* **51,** 739.
Person, L. H. (1969). *Plant Dis. Rep.* **53,** 927–929.
Pilone, G. J. (1979). *Am. J. Enol. Vitic.* **30,** 326.
Postgate, J. R. (1976). *Survival Veg. Microbes, Symp. Soc. Gen. Microbiol.* **26,** 1–18.
Postgate, J. R., and Hunter, J. R. (1961). *J. Gen. Microbiol.* **26,** 367–378.
Postgate, J. R., and Hunter, J. R. (1963). *J. Appl. Bacteriol.* **26,** 405–414.
Pridham, T. G., and Lyons, A. J. (1973). *Proc. Annu. Symp. East. Pa. Branch Am. Soc. Microbiol. 1971* p. 4.
Proom, H., and Hemmons, L. M. (1949). *J. Gen. Microbiol.* **3,** 7–18.

Quadling, C. (1960). *Can. J. Microbiol.* **6**, 475–477.
Ray, B. (1978). *Cryobiology* **15**, 691.
Record, B. R., Taylor, R., and Miller, D. S. (1962). *J. Gen. Microbiol.* **28**, 585–598.
Redway, K. F., and LaPage, S. P. (1974). *Cryobiology* **11**, 73–79.
Rey, B., and Speck, M. L. (1972). *Appl. Microbiol.* **24**, 585–590.
Rhodes, M. (1950). *J. Gen. Microbiol.* **4**, 450–456.
Rogers, L. A. (1914). *J. Infect. Dis.* **14**, 100–123.
Rosen, H. R. (1936). *Phytopathology* **26**, 439–449.
Rosen, H. R. (1938). *J. Agric. Res.* **56**, 239–258.
Sanfilippo, A., and Lewin, R. A. (1970). *Can. J. Microbiol.* **16**, 441–444.
Scott, W. J. (1958). *J. Gen. Microbiol.* **19**, 624–633.
Seaby, D. A. (1977). *Bull. Br. Mycol. Soc.* **11**, 55–56.
Segerstrom, N., and Sabiston, C. B., Jr. (1977). *J. Am. Med. Technol.* **39**, 22–23.
Servin-Massieu, M., and Cruz-Camarillo, R. (1969). *Appl. Microbiol.* **18**, 689–691.
Shekhawat, P. S., and Chakravarti, B. P. (1978). *Iran. J. Plant Pathol.* **14**, 11–19.
Sherf, A. F. (1943). *Phytopathology* **33**, 330–332.
Sherman, J. M., and Albus, W. R. (1923). *J. Bacteriol.* **8**, 127–139.
Singh, R. N. (1971). *Indian Phytopathol.* **24**, 153–154.
Sinskey, T. J., and Silverman, G. J. (1970). *J. Bacteriol.* **101**, 429–437.
Skaliy, P., and Eagon, R. G. (1972). *Appl. Microbiol.* **24**, 763–767.
Sleesman, J. P., and Leben, C. (1976a). *Phytopathology* **66**, 1334–1338.
Sleesman, J. P., and Leben, C. (1976b). *Phytopathology* **66**, 1214–1218.
Sleesman, J. P., and Leben, C. (1978). *Plant Dis. Rep.* **62**, 910–913.
Slosarek, M., Sourek, J., and Mikova, Z. (1976). *Cryobiology* **13**, 218–224.
Smittle, R. B., Gilliland, S. E., Speck, M. L., and Walter, W. M. (1974). *Appl. Microbiol.* **27**, 738–743.
Soriano, S. (1970). *Cult. Collect. Microorgan., Proc. Int. Conf. 1968* pp. 269–271.
Sorrells, K. M., Speck, M. L., and Warren, J. A. (1970). *Appl. Microbiol.* **19**, 39–43.
Sourek, J. (1974). *Int. J. Syst. Bacteriol.* **24**, 358–365.
Sourek, J., and Kulhanek, M. (1969). *Zentralbl. Backteriol. Parasitenkd. Infectionskr. Hyg. Abt. 2* **123**, 580–585.
Squires, R. W., and Hartsell, S. E. (1955). *Appl. Microbiol.* **3**, 40–45.
Srivastava, S. K., and Patel, P. N. (1968). *Indian Phytopathol.* **21**, 124–125.
Stamp, L. (1947). *J. Gen. Microbiol.* **1**, 251–265.
Stark, C. N., and Herrington, B. L. (1931). *J. Bacteriol.* **21**, 13–14.
Steinhaus, E. A., and Birkeland, J. M. (1939). *J. Bacteriol.* **38**, 249–261.
Stephens, J. M. (1957). *Can. J. Microbiol.* **3**, 995–1000.
Strange, R. E., and Cox, C. S. (1976). *Survival Veg. Microbes, Symp. Soc. Gen. Microbiol.* **26**, 111–154.
Strange, R. E., and Dark, F. A. (1962). *J. Gen. Microbiol.* **29**, 719–730.
Strange, R. E., and Ness, A. G. (1963). *Nature (London)* **197**, 819.
Strange, R. E., Dark, F. A., and Ness, A. G. (1961). *J. Gen. Microbiol.* **25**, 61–76.
Tanaka, Y., Yoh, M., Takeda, Y., and Miwatani, T. (1979). *Appl. Environ. Microbiol.* **37**, 369–372.
Tanguay, A. E. (1959). *Appl. Microbiol.* **7**, 84–88.
Thorns, C. J. (1979). *J. Appl. Bacteriol.* **47**, 183–186.
Trollope, D. R. (1975). *J. Appl. Bacteriol.* **38**, 115–120.
Tsuru, S. (1973). *Cryobiology* **10**, 471.
Tuite, J. (1969). "Plant Pathological Methods Fungi and Bacteria." Burgess, Minneapolis, Minnesota.
Turner, A. G., and Salmonsen, P. A. (1973). *J. Appl. Bacteriol.* **36**, 497–499.

Vorob'eva, T. I., and Chumakova, R. I. (1973). *Microbiology* **42,** 652–653.
Wagman, J. (1960). *J. Bacteriol.* **80,** 558–564.
Webb, S. J. (1959). *Can. J. Microbiol.* **5,** 649–669.
Webb, S. J. (1960a). *Can. J. Microbiol.* **6,** 71–87.
Webb, S. J. (1960b). *Can. J. Microbiol.* **6,** 89–105.
Webb, S. J. (1961). *Can. J. Microbiol.* **7,** 621–632.
Webb, S. J. (1967). *Nature (London)* **213,** 1137–1139.
Weiser, R. S., and Osterud, C. M. (1945). *J. Bacteriol.* **50,** 413–439.
Wilkinson, J. F. (1958). *Bacteriol. Rev.* **22,** 46–73.
Williams, S. T., and Cross, T. (1971). *In* "Methods in Microbiology" (C. Booth, ed.), Vol. 4, pp. 295–334. Academic Press, New York.
Wilson, G. S., and Miles, A. A. (1964). *In* "Principles of Bacteriology and Immunity" (W. Topley and G. Wilson, eds.), 5th Ed., Vol. I, pp. 127–172. Arnold, London.
Wilson, H. A., Lilly, V. G., and Leach, J. G. (1965). *Phytopathology* **55,** 1135–1138.
Wilson, J. M., and Davies, R. (1976). *J. Appl. Bacteriol.* **40,** 365–374.
Yamasato, K., Okuno, D., and Ohtomo, T. (1973). *Cryobiology* **10,** 453–463.
Yamasato, K., Okuno, D., and Ohtomo, T. (1978). *Cryobiology* **15,** 691–692.

Index

C

F

I

J

K

L

M

N

O

T